Promoting Healing and Resilience in People with Cancer: A Nursing Perspective

Mary Grossman

Promoting Healing and Resilience in People with Cancer: A Nursing Perspective

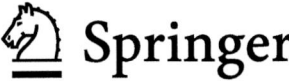

Mary Grossman, PhD (Retired)
Retired, Ingram School of Nursing
McGill University
Montreal, QC, Canada

ISBN 978-3-031-06100-4   ISBN 978-3-031-06101-1 (eBook)
https://doi.org/10.1007/978-3-031-06101-1

© The Editor(s) (if applicable) and The Author(s), under exclusive license to Springer Nature Switzerland AG 2022
This work is subject to copyright. All rights are solely and exclusively licensed by the Publisher, whether the whole or part of the material is concerned, specifically the rights of translation, reprinting, reuse of illustrations, recitation, broadcasting, reproduction on microfilms or in any other physical way, and transmission or information storage and retrieval, electronic adaptation, computer software, or by similar or dissimilar methodology now known or hereafter developed.
The use of general descriptive names, registered names, trademarks, service marks, etc. in this publication does not imply, even in the absence of a specific statement, that such names are exempt from the relevant protective laws and regulations and therefore free for general use.
The publisher, the authors, and the editors are safe to assume that the advice and information in this book are believed to be true and accurate at the date of publication. Neither the publisher nor the authors or the editors give a warranty, expressed or implied, with respect to the material contained herein or for any errors or omissions that may have been made. The publisher remains neutral with regard to jurisdictional claims in published maps and institutional affiliations.

This Springer imprint is published by the registered company Springer Nature Switzerland AG
The registered company address is: Gewerbestrasse 11, 6330 Cham, Switzerland

*To my family
and to all families who have traveled
cancer's pathways,
and to nurses and doctors who have paved
their way with compassion and competence*

Preface

Hope is a dimension of the soul...It is an orientation of the heart; it transcends the world that is immediately experienced, and it is anchored somewhere beyond the horizon.

Vaclav Havel

Nursing and medicine are the two pivotal healthcare professions with complementary and overlapping scientific knowledge and clinical skills which inform the care and treatment of patients with cancer across all its stages including the transition to survivorship. Shared professional goals include helping patients (with their loved ones) to tolerate their treatment to completion, live a healthy life disease free or live well with cancer, and or experience a peaceful end of life. As scientific evidence in cancer healthcare has mounted exponentially, it is almost axiomatic that both professions base their practice on this expanding repository of scientific knowledge, albeit filtered through the distinct perspectives of each profession, enabling both to complement one another in the shared goal of helping patients with cancer, and their loved ones.

Yet despite academic advances in the Nursing discipline since the latter half of the twentieth century, my professional observations over an academic career, are of a clinical practice too often bent toward the prevailing medical model of practice at the expense of exercising clinical expertise based on theoretical and empirical nursing knowledge of the *whole* person in the face of health-related adversity. It is my hope that in some very small way this book may encourage more nurses, particularly in the field of cancer care, to broaden the scope of their practice of the whole individual and loved one within a comprehensive scientific perspective.

The Gap Between Research Findings and Clinical Practice

Although the curriculum of university-prepared nurses consists of courses from the biological and psychosocial sciences, integrating this knowledge into a comprehensive understanding of the human experience of cancer, including the effects of diverse stressors on the whole person has proven challenging to actualize in clinical practice. Indeed, the process of incorporating the latest research findings into clinical interventions so that the people we care for receive timely clinical benefits based on the latest scientific evidence has been an uphill struggle throughout the healthcare field. Despite Nursing's purported legacy of caring for the *whole* person and *promoting healing* of both the mind and body, dating from Nightingale's papers [1], clinical practice in the majority of hospital centers has not fully embraced relevant research findings from related disciplines such as psycho-neuro-immunology nor developed a scientific body of stress-reducing and healing-inducing nursing interventions.

The panoply of *psychological stressors* that patients and caregivers are likely to experience along the clinical pathway to survivorship is an essential component of clinical care. Yet practice guided by scientific knowledge of the devastating effects of prolonged stress on neuroendocrinal and immune functions which adversely impact healing and resilient capabilities, and ultimately, the long-term health potential of cancer patients, appears to be lacking [2]. For instance, nursing tends to conceptualize *resilience* mainly from a generic psychological perspective (e.g., cognitive and behavioral coping efforts in response to psychological stress). Clinical interventions typically center around active listening and reframing that usually offer an important yet temporary clinical benefit. Because harmful stress-induced effects on the neural biology of the patient can threaten long-term survivability a multimodal, multitargeted nursing approach, is required.

The *point of transition from* a resilient (allostatic) to a toxic neurobiological response to stress is still unknown [3, 4]. However, evidence indicates that restored behavioral indicators of resilience in the aftermath of prolonged stress are not necessarily reflected by the underlying neurobiology [5]. This discrepancy can occur in individuals with a history of prolonged emotional distress in which the normal brain's architectural flexibility was compromised by previous chronic adversity. The brain's potential capacity for flexible neural remodeling in response to environmental stressors will determine how successfully the whole being may adapt in the future resulting in greater or poorer resilience. For this reason alone, it is a clinical imperative to leverage scientific knowledge of the spectrum of stress effects throughout the biology and behavior of the whole person, in order to mobilize relevant healing- and resilient-promoting interventions to alleviate their ill effects [6]. Knowledge of possible stress-related neurobiological impairments enables the nurse to identify meaningful biological and behavioral end points so that the effectiveness of tailored healing-inducing psychosocial interventions may be evaluated [3].

A case in point: A growing body of scientific evidence shows that clinical interventions which activate the dopaminergic reward circuitry strengthen resilience [3]. Positive memories through storytelling, cognitive expectations of a clinical benefit, promoting meaning and purpose in life, and strengthening supportive relationships have been empirically shown to trigger dopaminergic pathways that downregulate the stress response system (decreasing cortisol, catecholamines, and emotional distress). Despite the scientific evidence, these nursing interventions have *not been regularly brought to clinical prominence*, yet would provide a deep, *purposeful* therapeutic benefit to patients and their family caregivers. These healing promoting interventions are in keeping with nursing's domain of practice and should be mobilized to promote the resilience of patients and their caregivers across the continuum. Many are time efficient and easy to implement within the context of the nurse-patient relationship.

The Clinical Need for a Conceptual Model of Practice

Nursing's theoretical underpinnings were enriched by many conceptual models that flourished in the latter half of the twentieth century. Part of today's clinical challenge is to identify practice models with a patient-centered focus that promote the interrelated biological and behavioral health-related concepts that constitute the whole person with or without a chronic illness. A conceptual model is distinguished by a set of interrelated concepts, goals, desired clinical outcomes, and relevant interventions that delineate the scope, depth, and direction of the nurse's practice. Such a model may be used to evaluate the effectiveness of proposed psychosocial interventions by helping to interpret the significance of relevant clinical and research findings.

Stress, healing, coping, resilience, meaning, lifestyle behaviors, and health have been widely investigated as evidenced by a plethora of research findings. These results have led to the development of a few clinical interventions aimed at strengthening resilience, health, and overall well-being of patients and, to a lesser extent, their caregivers. This book offers a conceptual framework predicated on these indispensable human concepts which are embedded in the thoughts, beliefs, emotions, behavior and neurobiology of patients and their caregivers, so that scientifically justified nursing interventions may be purposefully developed and evaluated across the disease and recovery continuum, and results interpreted within a meaningful framework of practice. It is hoped that research findings may serve as stepping stones for further critical inquiry and evidentiary clinical practice shaped by the model of practice. This hope is made all the more probable when nurses experience their practice through a shared prism of goals, desired outcomes, and scientific evidence.

Without a coherent scientific context it is extremely challenging to establish meaningful goals and objectives of practice as well as to develop or implement relevant clinical interventions that complement rather than simply conform to medical goals and objectives. There continues to be a clinical disconnect between the biology and psychology of the person, when in fact both are integrally interrelated and taken together provide a deeper more comprehensive basis for understanding the dynamics of the whole person within the stressful context of living with cancer. A comprehensive nursing approach across the different phases of the cancer trajectory would be enhanced and made more purposeful by the use of a relevant conceptual model of practice that is grounded in a growing body of interrelated scientific findings.

Why This Book

The latest books on the nursing care of cancer patients and families tend to be organized around the latest medical research, principles of care, patient and family needs, procedures and/or techniques, and ethical considerations that are all important determinants of good nursing care. In contrast this book puts the whole person at the center of that care, meaningfully integrating the latest research findings within a conceptual model of nursing practice that delineates the extent and scope of humanistic practice within the clinical field of cancer. Because this book leaves the necessary component of the latest procedures and medical techniques to other excellent nursing's references, it may be argued that this book is ironically self-limiting. In deliberately doing so, its main message is that the core of the nurse's practice is the whole human being whose healing and resilient capabilities in the face of stress need to be amplified through a more comprehensive humanistic approach.

For that to occur we need to explicate adaptive processes of the whole person which dynamically interact with one another and are influenced by social, physical, and psychological environmental factors that either enhance or debilitate the health potential and long-term survivability of the patient [7]. In other words, the whole person (and the family) is the key clinical context of care, and the latest techniques, procedures, and related issues are valued as instruments that support but are not the defining focus of humanistic nursing care. This is only possible when a conceptual model of nursing is the predicate of practice.

A model's delineated scope of practice enables the further development and evaluation of theory and practice findings with clear relevance to the clinical care, quality of life, and survival of the whole patient. A *nursing* approach is derived from the clinical goals and concepts, and related findings delineated by the model. This practice-driven model facilitates the mobilization of relevant nursing interventions aimed at the patient's healing and resilient capabilities. In so doing, the nurse's clinical interventions also support the goals of medical treatment; and together are critical to the patient's ability to successfully adapt to cancer-related threats, tolerate the treatment to completion, live healthily in survivorship, or find acceptance and meaning at the end of life [8, 9].

What the Handbook Offers

For clinical researchers in the field of cancer, the conceptual model serves as a theoretical and empirical predicate for the development, evaluation, and interpretation of clinical interventions guided by the stated goals and objectives of the model. The model is meant to be a dynamic framework that both informs and is informed by research findings. It is hoped that research findings lead to modifications within the proposed relationships among the variables across the phases of the continuum. A growing repository of empirically demonstrated clinical interventions may eventually determine the optimal combination of conventional and complementary practices to consider for patients across varying phases of the disease and survivorship, and for their family caregiver. In other words, multimodal, multitargeted clinical strategies with shared and unique biological and behavioral endpoints may become the standard of nursing care, by effectively countering the corrosive effects of stress while also optimizing resilient capabilities of the person even in the absence of a cure.

As a clinical practice model it is hoped that the nursing goals, objectives, desired outcomes, delineated concepts, and proposed clinical approaches to patients and family caregivers may advance the practice of clinical nursing toward a more comprehensive understanding of the whole person with cancer and of loved ones. With a patient-centered humanistic focus anchored by *the quality of the nurse patient (family caregiver) relationships,* the nurse's technical, procedural, and medical expertise complements rather than defines the nurse's approach to patient and family care.

Because the Handbook delineates a contextual field of relevant theory and known findings based on its model of practice in cancer, it serves as an effective organizing framework for the nurse practitioner, nurse specialist, and student nurse. It can facilitate the purposeful acquisition of knowledge and skills that guide nursing approaches to the care of patients and the family caregiver. It also serves as a delineated context for seeking up-to-date research findings that continue to inform the goals and objectives of one's practice.

In summary, it is hoped that the nurses' *Model of stress, healing and resilience* based as it is on a practice model may serve as a scientific stepping stone toward providing informed, comprehensive nursing care to patients with cancer (and family caregivers) across all phases of the illness and recovery continuum. It is also hoped that in some small way, this book contributes in placing the patient with cancer (with his family caregiver) so that in optimal health in order to tolerate the treatment to completion, thrive in survivorship, live well with cancer, or experience a comforted, peaceful, and meaningful end of life. Although the subject of family is beyond the scope of this book, it is an important component of the patient experience.

How to Use the Handbook

The handbook is designed to describe the main concepts of the conceptual model of practice from theoretical and clinical perspectives. Each chapter highlights learning objectives and uses clinical and personal anecdotes, tables, and figures to illustrate the concepts under discussion. The Handbook is divided into five main parts, each part predicated on a specific theme with an introduction followed by corresponding chapters.

Part I is entitled The Stress, Healing and Resilience Nursing Model of the Whole Person Chapter 1 provides a review of the underlying theoretical tenets of the model, acknowledging the importance of preceding theory and concepts upon which this Model proudly stands. Chapter 2 defines and describes the key concepts of the whole person model. Topics include assumptions, the whole person, cancer-related stressors, health, processes of development, resilience and innate and self-induced healing; epigenetics, metabolism, sense of coherence, the biofield hypothesis, homeostasis, personal and social strengths (resources), lifestyle behaviors, the clinical environment, and Nursing goals and approaches.

Part II is entitled Resilience The Introduction orients the reader to the goals of Chaps. 3, 4 and 5. Chapter 3 defines different forms of psychological stress and its potential short term, resilient-promoting and or prolonged deleterious biological and behavioral effects on the whole person. Chapter 4 discusses *biological resilience* and the dynamic stress response system in relation to acute stressors of temporary duration in essentially healthy individuals. Topics include acute stressors of short duration, biological resilience (allostasis), brain and neural circuitry of resilience, and the biological stress response system (biological adjustments due to stress).

Chapter 5 focuses on *psychological resilience* in terms of the main emotion-regulating stress-coping system of resilience which characterizes the healthy person in the face of acute stress and daily demands. Topics include emotion-regulating stress-coping adaptation system of resilience, cancer-related threats (cognitive and emotional representations), health-related and post-traumatic growth outcomes, personal strengths (self-efficacy, optimism, hope), social strengths (support from family caregiver, family, and friends), relationship between support and coping, enabling versus cultivation hypothesis, coping and support over time, and clinical implications.

Part III is entitled Poor Resilience An introduction provides a brief overview of Part III. Chap. 6 addresses the concept of poor resilience by describing the deleterious effects of prolonged stress on the individual's biological and psychological resilience and health. Specific topics include characteristics of chronic stress, allostatic load, neural circuitry of the brain, HPA-axis, ANS and immune system, negative epigenetic changes, systemic inflammation, relationships between side effects, symptoms and underlying cytokines and other proinflammatory factors, metabolic and oxidative stress, and electromagnetic fields.

Chapter 7 on cancer addresses some of the key neural, endocrine, and immune dysregulating changes associated with cancer onset and its progression. Topics include major characteristics of chronic illness, cancer, cancer initiation, progression, invasion and metastases, tumor microenvironment and its key cancer-sustaining factors, and clinical implications.

Part IV is entitled Fostering Healing An introduction provides the overview of the chapters in Part IV. With the possible exception of Chap. 12 on the role of cognitive expectations in healing each chapter discusses a clinical intervention empirically known to promote healing and resilience based on theoretical underpinnings and or scientific evidence, mainly in individuals with cancer. Clinical strategies associated with enhancing positive cognitive expectations (Part IV Chap. 12) are based on experimental research with volunteers, as well as randomized controlled studies of patients with chronic illnesses. Nursing strategies to promote healing are discussed in chapters on (1) the quality of the nurse-patient relationship (Chap. 11) (2) enhancing adaptive coping efforts, self efficacy and self-management interventions (Chap. 9) (3) facilitating finding meaning or coming to terms with cancer (Chap. 10) (4) enhancing meaningful support (Chap. 11) (5) promoting the placebo or innate healing processes (Chap. 12) (6) fostering the relaxation response and mindful meditation (Chap. 13), and physical touch and biofield modalities (Chap. 14). Promoting healthy lifestyle behaviors has been incorporated as suggested nursing interventions across the continuum in Part V.

Part V is entitled Nursing Approaches Part V integrates the scientific knowledge and skills delineated by the conceptual model in Part, and elucidated by each subsequent chapter from Part II through Part IV. An introduction provides a brief description of the chapters devoted to the main phases of the cancer-related journey: the diagnostic (Chap. 15), treatment (Chap. 16), transition to survivorship (Chap. 17) and end of life (Chap. 18). Each chapter highlights the main issues faced by most patients and their family caregivers and suggests clinical interventions that have been shown to counter deleterious stress effects that can compromise the ability to complete medical treatment, threaten a cancer recurrence, the ability to live well with cancer, or experience a peaceful death. Chapter 19 considers the clinical feasibility, of incorporating the stress, healing, and resilient Nursing model into current clinical practice.

Although the book has been organized with the intention of first introducing the reader to the conceptual model, and then analyzing each main component in subsequent chapters from the perspective of relevant theory and research findings, the reader is encouraged to move in and out of sections and chapters in order to meet immediate learning needs. In an effort to minimize repeating content especially in Part V, I refer the reader to previous chapters that have covered certain content in depth.

What Distinguishes This Book from Others

This book reorients the clinical goals of nursing care toward a more patient-centered approach within which scientific knowledge is filtered through the prism of a practice model; and the latest medical treatments, techniques, procedures, and policies are relegated to an essential but *supporting role* of whole person care. This book was designed around key interrelated concepts and relevant nursing interventions, goals and desired outcomes of a practice model of the whole person, who happens to have cancer. As such, it serves as a relevant framework of the discipline's clinical, education, research and administrative arms of academic practice, and contributes to the

Nursing literature on cancer care of adults. Finally, I believe that my personal journey with cancer which converged with a lifelong academic and clinical career in Nursing ultimately provided the unwavering impetus to write this book, in the hope that it might facilitate, in some way, the quality of life of patients with cancer and their loved ones.

Reclaiming Nursing's Legacy

Over the last several decades, as hospital care has become more complex, Nursing has "given away parts of itself" to other professions: Patients who are not coping well tend to be transferred to psychology or to a massage therapist. Individuals with early stage cancers and basic questions about diet and exercise are readily sent for consultations to a dietician or exercise physiologist. There is nothing fundamentally wrong with that: Every individual has different needs, particularly patients with advanced disease. Yet the majority of individuals with cancer are healthy, and the information and strategies they seek fall within the health-promoting tenets of the nursing profession. Most individuals with cancer want to optimize their health during the treatment and afterward with the assistance of healthcare providers who know them best. People with cancer tend to first look to the nurse for this help, more than anyone else with the exception of their oncologist, because the nurse has seen them in vulnerable moments and understands the clinical implications and context within which the person with cancer now finds him- or herself. Moreover, it has been my clinical experience that most patients fear being pathologized or subjected to more fragmented care. "I may have cancer, but I am still healthy!" is a not unusual patient refrain.

Many nurses set aside meaningful time for patients and their informal caregivers, particularly at distressing moments. Although notable exceptions exist, mainstream nursing care has generally consisted of a limited repository of psychosocial interventions that include active listening, reframing patient perceptions, providing needed information, compassion, and comfort. These are all valuable interventions that may help to alleviate stress temporarily, but generally do not *sustain* relief. This Handbook strives to redress those parts of Nursing's legacy that may have been overlooked over the years, in part due to a paucity of research findings, but today are well documented and defensible components of nursing practice.

References

1. Skretkowicz V. Florence nightingale's notes on nursing and notes on nursing for the labouring classes. New York: Springer; 2010.
2. Wang M, Zhao J, Zhang L, Wei F, Lian Y, Wu Y, et al. Role of tumor microenvironment in tumorigenesis. J Cancer. 2017;8(5):761–73. PubMed PMID: 28382138. Pubmed Central PMCID: PMC5381164. Epub 2017/04/07. eng.

3. Fava GA, McEwen BS, Guidi J, Gostoli S, Offidani E, Sonino N. Clinical characterization of allostatic overload. Psychoneuroendocrinology. 2019;108:94–101. PubMed PMID: 31252304. Epub 2019/06/30. eng.
4. Seeman TE, Gruenewald TL, Cohen S, Williams DR, Matthews KA. Social relationships and their biological correlates: Coronary Artery Risk Development in Young Adults (CARDIA) study. Psychoneuroendocrinology. 2014;43:126–38. PubMed PMID: 24703178. Epub 2014/04/08. eng.
5. McEwen BS, Gray J, Nasca C. Recognizing resilience: learning from the effects of stress on the brain. Neurobiol Stress. 2015;1:1–11. PubMed PMID: 25506601. Pubmed Central PMCID: PMC4260341. Epub 2014/12/17. Eng.
6. Dutcher JM, Creswell JD. The role of brain reward pathways in stress resilience and health. Neurosci Biobehav Rev. 2018;95:559–67. PubMed PMID: 30477985. Epub 2018/11/28. eng.
7. Lutgendorf SK, Andersen BL. Biobehavioral approaches to cancer progression and survival: mechanisms and interventions. Am Psychol. 2015;70(2):186–97. PubMed PMID: 25730724. Pubmed Central PMCID: PMC4347942. Epub 2015/03/03. eng.
8. Antoni MH, Lutgendorf SK, Blomberg B, Carver CS, Lechner S, Diaz A, et al. Cognitive-behavioral stress management reverses anxiety-related leukocyte transcriptional dynamics. Biol Psychiatry. 2012;71(4):366–72. Pubmed Central PMCID: PMC3264698. Epub 2011/11/18. eng.
9. Andersen BL, Thornton LM, Shapiro CL, Farrar WB, Mundy BL, Yang HC, et al. Biobehavioral, immune, and health benefits following recurrence for psychological intervention participants. Clin Cancer Res. 2010;16(12):3270–8. PubMed PMID: 20530702. Pubmed Central PMCID: PMC2910547. Epub 2010/06/10. eng.

Montreal, QC, Canada　　　　　　　　　　　　　　　　　　　　Mary Grossman

Acknowledgments

Our becoming is a dynamic process of lifelong learning, replete with challenging experiences that stimulate our development. I have been blessed with extraordinary educators who were proactively engaged in their students' learning. Professor Margaret Hooton of the School of Nursing (SON) at McGill University (later known as the Ingram School of Nursing) was one such larger than life educator. Professor Hooton was a much beloved mentor, whose effortless ministrations enabled her students to "see" Nursing through her eyes: as an intellectually stimulating pursuit with a noble cause: enhancing the health and well-being of the whole person who needed our care. It was Marg who encouraged me to write my first article on professional practice as an undergraduate, and only reluctantly agreed to be a coauthor, such was her humility. Marg preferred to lead from behind, a phrase that Nelson Mandela made famous. In retrospect, I believe Marg's professional satisfaction emanated from seeing her students realize their professional potential to make a measurable difference in the nursing care of patients and families. It was also Marg who strongly encouraged me to take the first "nursing internship" program at McGill in the 1970s which included a 4-week rotation in Igloolik, Nunavut, where I had the opportunity to hone newly acquired scientific knowledge and clinical skills in a community nursing practice. There I learned a tremendous amount from the nurses who ran the station in the Innuit village; it was a clinical nursing experience that made my heart sing! I hope, somewhere in the firmament, Marg knows how much her students held her in high esteem.

I also have had the good fortune to work alongside wonderful colleagues and students with whom dialectical discussions, the pursuit of scientific knowledge and the practice of nursing to the full extent and scope of its profession, were worthy objectives, integral to our daily work. Specifically, I must thank with the deepest appreciation and gratitude a unique team of incredible advanced practice clinic nurses, Loretta Tyler, Rhonda Seidman, Patti O Connor, Terry Suss, Janet Kulczkyj, and Nancy Feeley, fellow comrades-in-arms with whom was developed the first ambulatory nursing pediatric practice for children and their families based on the acquisition of *scientific* knowledge and related clinical skills that were consistent with the goals, values, and substantive base of the nursing profession.

The mostly Master's-prepared nurses focused on development, health, support, distress, and coping of children with diverse health-related issues and their families, while their respective medical colleagues mainly treated illness. Nursing assistants were responsible for ancillary clinic-related services. At the very least, it was a cost-effective realignment of clinic services. But critically, it enabled nurses to practice to the full extent of their professional qualifications. The nurses not only cared for their patients and families in clinic but made visits on the unit when a child was hospitalized, and carried out family visits in the community, as needed. We held the first known regular journal club to deepen our scientific knowledge of key concepts relevant to our practice, and many of the nurses took an intense family intervention course in order to acquire additional clinical skills to work effectively with families. To my best knowledge it was the first clinic setting in Quebec in which nursing and medical colleagues promoted the comprehensive health and wellness of the children and families, through the complementary prism of their respective professions.

It could not have been implemented without the nurses' courageous commitment and demonstrated clinical competence. It could not have succeeded without the support of my medical colleague Nick Steinmetz who at the time was medical chief of ambulatory services. He quickly recognized what other healthcare providers were slower to grasp: that advanced practice nurses who practiced to the full extent of their profession benefited not only the patients and families, but enhanced the shared goals of their medical colleagues. Nick defended our professional goals and justified our complementary practice at critical moments, thereby supporting the shift from a medical to a collaborative nurse-physician model. And that made all the difference!

I also must thank Laurie Gottlieb, then Director of the School of Nursing at McGill, for the amazing opportunity I had to serve as the Co-director of Programs and Practice. I learned how a university curriculum and program are developed, the discipline-driven values and pedagogical thinking underlying decisions, and the imperative of disseminating the key principles of academic clinical practice throughout the community of hospitals and clinics. Thanks to Laurie who was the editor of the *CJNR*, a McGill peer-reviewed journal, I also had the added opportunity to serve as an Associate editor and got to experience, for the first time, the professional thrill of writing a few guest editorials. These experiences were indispensable to my personal growth as a person and a nurse, and for that I am deeply appreciative.

On faculty at McGill's School of Nursing I was immersed in activities related to academic programs, community nurse initiatives, government threats to the profession, the role of nurse practitioners, research projects, and the acquisition of clinical skills, in particular, working alongside Celeste Johnston, Helene Ezer, Laurie Gottlieb, Linda McHarg, Madeline Buck, Val Shannon, Franco Carnevale, Mimi O'Mansi, and Sara Frisch. I learned a tremendous amount about the diversity and scope of professional nursing practice and its national and international reach. I have no doubt that my experiences at the SON had an important effect on the way I think about health, illness and prevention, patients and families, and the need for universal academic Nursing practice.

During this phase of my career I was also a member of a clinical research team whose main goal was to improve the quality of nursing care for patients who had sustained a traumatic injury, and their families. In the 1990s this dedicated clinical team consisted of Virginia Lee, Jocelynne Van Neste Kenny, Linda McHarg, Maryse

Godin, and Jane Chambers-Evans. Together we sought to broaden conventional conceptualizations of nursing in caring for seriously injured patients. We focused on psychosocial concepts of emotional distress and cognitive processing (intrusive ideation), the meaning in life, support, coping, and health. We identified potential psychosocial interventions aimed at meaning making, enhancing support, cognitive restructuring, and dispelling distorted beliefs and generalizations. We reviewed the evidentiary data supporting complementary modalities such as reflexology and the use of imagery. It was an invaluable, stimulating period of theoretical and empirical exploration of these concepts in critically injured patients.

I also have to thank Gerry Batist, Medical Director of the Segal Cancer Centre at the Jewish General Hospital, and Lynne McVey, then Director of Nursing for the extraordinary opportunity to serve as Co-director of the Brojde Lung Cancer Centre. The greatest appreciation is given to Anna Brojde, who spearheaded the comprehensive approach to the care and treatment of patients and families at the Brojde Lung Cancer Centre. Anna's indefatigable determination to enhance the health-related care of the whole patient with cancer resulted in the first *integrative* center of its kind in Quebec, the eponymous clinic name now sadly commemorating the exceptional lives of both her husband Peter and Anna. Anna gave me the incredible opportunity to blend many nursing concepts and complementary therapies within the critical context of cancer care, which as a cancer survivor was close to my heart. The *integrative* multimodal, multitargeted approach aimed to improve the quality of life and well-being of patients with lung cancer (and their loved ones) in order to better tolerate treatment to its completion, optimize their health as survivors, live well with cancer as a chronic illness, and live in comfort and emotional equanimity at the end of life.

I learned so much about the potential therapeutic effects of acupuncture, massage, and physiotherapy especially from Thi Tran, Tracy Quinn, and Daniel Vales respectively who further informed my thinking about complementary therapies as part of multimodal, multitargeted psychosocial nursing and medical interventions to enhance the healing and resilient capabilities and reduce or eliminate disease in the whole person. It was an honor to collaborate on an integrative approach to care with Francine Manceau, an exceptional nurse who unfailingly went beyond the call of duty to optimize the well-being of her patients and loved ones. I was most grateful for the unwavering support of Tania Xenopoulos and Shelley Budd, the integrative team's administrative assistants par excellence. The ISON Master's student nurses who rotated through the Brojde Centre as part of their clinical stages, in particular, Tamar Amichai, Chloe Eustache, and Emily Jibb brought their dedication, stimulating questions, and creative thinking that energized the team and in so doing gave hope to our goals of practice. To all I am so thankful.

Working at the Brojde Centre presented the perfect synthesis of everything I was moving toward in Nursing. Cancer care of patients and family caregivers became the health-related context for my growing conceptualization of Nursing the whole person across the cancer trajectory, which eventually led me down the path toward writing this book.

As chapters started to take shape, four individuals in particular were instrumental in getting this book across the finish line. The first is Professor Heather Hart, Academic advisor in the Master's Program, Clinical Concentration, to whom this book owes its deepest gratitude and profound appreciation. Heather's invitations to give presentations to Master's students based on chapters in the book and or to supervise students' clinical work with families provided me with a fertile learning environment. I was able to share my thinking on a topic and engage in subsequent student discussions that invariably elucidated my thinking for the better. Heather was unfailingly supportive and encouraging, and a memorable nursing colleague who has been my great good fortune to know. Mark Ware and Adam Gavsie provided further opportunities to share my thinking with fourth-year medical students, which was also deeply appreciated.

The second person to whom I am indebted is Tom Hutchinson, Professor of Medicine and Professor of Oncology, and Director of the McGill Program in Whole Person Care. Tom's understated style and infectious sense of humor belie a brilliant mind and a profoundly generous colleague. In his typically witty and light-hearted way, Tom would ask me from time to time when I thought I might be finished! Always a good question, and even more, that he would be "delighted" to read it, and having done that, Tom facilitated the book's transfer to Springer Nature. Tom has been a wonderful colleague and friend to whom much is owed in gratitude.

This brings me to Springer-Nature and my wonderfully supportive Executive Editor, Nathalie Lhorset-Poulain, and her equally capable team which includes Manisha Rao and Cecile Schuetze-Gaukel. Nathalie and her team have a magical way of carrying the author effortlessly through each step along the way to publication. But just as importantly, Nathalie's incisive suggestions always made the manuscript better. She and her team have been a pleasure to work with, and I am eternally grateful for their assistance. Fourth, I must give lots of thanks to April Colosimo, librarian at the McGill University Library of Health and Biological Sciences. April was unfailingly helpful in sorting out glitches on end notes and retrieving critical research articles in an amazingly timely manner. April made the review of the literature a seamless exercise that immeasurably facilitated the writing of this book.

All endeavors truly take a village—My close friends Lisa Travis, Jill Martis, June Hutchinson, Barra McNeill, and Louise Carpenter unfailingly humored me by listening, supporting, cajoling, and encouraging my progress. They never tired of me sharing the latest research findings or discussing the finer points of different concepts in the model.

Last, but first and foremost, my family. My family was my greatest champion, taking an active interest in whatever I was writing about at the time. My brother Peter deeply entrenched in world markets, yet was unfailingly enthusiastic and often humorously prodded me onward. My daughter, Caroline, and her husband, Norm, started mindful meditation practices following a particularly passionate discussion. My son Matthew and his wife Sarah's frequent refrain was "How's the book going" their voices carrying across continents. And early in my writings, my sister-in-law, Sarah, a yoga enthusiast, demonstrated basic positions as a hoped for incentive for me to adopt this fine modality which shared many of the meditative characteristics of other mindfulness activities. Later as I rounded the bend toward the finish line, I could always count on Jan for a cooked meal almost every night! In big and little ways I was constantly reminded of the incredible energy-producing effects of support!

Above all, I must thank my remarkable and compassionate parents. Had they lived, they would have been the only individuals to predict that I would write a book one day in my professional field. As doctors, they devoted their lives to the common good, valued hard work, human decency, and a life of integrity. These were the principles they lived by and instilled in their children. Our weekly "parliamentary" debates around a Sunday family breakfast were emblematic of their credo. As children we were always called upon to share our ideas and later to justify our thinking. Above all we learned to stand up for what we believed in, and then to do something about it.

Contents

Part I The Stress, Healing, and Resilience Nursing Model of Whole Person Care

1 Theoretical Underpinnings 3
   1.1 Theoretical Underpinnings 3
   References 5

2 The Stress, Healing, and Resilience Nursing Model of Whole Person Care 7
   2.1 Introduction 7
   2.2 Objectives 8
   2.3 Core Values and Assumptions of Practice 8
   2.4 Goals of the Practice Model 9
   2.5 The Whole Person and the Environment 9
   2.6 Psychological Stress 10
   2.7 Health as an Essential Property of the Whole Being 12
        Health-Related Outcomes 12
        Key Internal Processes of Health 12
   2.8 Personal Strengths and Social Resources (Supportive Relationships) ... 16
        Social Resources (Supportive Relationships) 16
   2.9 Healthy Lifestyle Behaviors 17
   2.10 Epigenetics 17
   2.11 Homeostasis 17
   2.12 Energy and Metabolic Processes 18
   2.13 Sense of Coherence 19
   2.14 Nursing Approaches 20
        Quality of the Nurse–Patient Relationship 21
        Timing of Interventions 22
        Format 22
   References 23

Part II Resilience

3 Psychological Stress 31
    3.1   Introduction 31
    3.2   Definitions 32
           Properties of Psychological Stress 33
           Benefits or Harmful Effects 33
    3.3   Acute Stressor Effects 34
    3.4   Prolonged Psychological Stress 35
           Early Childhood Adversity (ECA) 36
    3.5   Need for Measurable Terminology for "Stress" 38
    3.6   Cumulative Measures of Stress 39
    3.7   Nursing Implications 41
    References 42

4 Biological Processes of Resilience 47
    4.1   Introduction 47
    4.2   Objectives 48
    4.3   Definitions 48
           Resilience 48
           Stressors 50
    4.4   Key Neural Structures and Mediators 51
           Brain Plasticity 52
           The Stress-Related Systems and Mediators 53
           Negative Glucocorticoid Feedback System 54
    4.5   The Biphasic Process of Biological Resilience 55
           The First Phase: The Process of Stress-Induced Neural
           and Physiological Adjustments 55
           The Second Phase, Healing, and Restoration 56
    4.6   Other Processes That Influence Biological Resilience 57
           Age 57
           Sex Differences 58
           Epigenetics 58
           Circadian Rhythm 59
           Energy 59
    4.7   Nursing Implications 60
    References 62

5 Psychosocial Processes of Resilience 65
    5.1   Introduction 65
    5.2   Objectives 66
    5.3   Definition: Psychological Resilience 67
    5.4   Theoretical Tenets and Model of Psychological Resilience:
          The Emotion-Regulating Stress-Coping Adaptation System of
          Psychological Resilience 67

		Antecedent Factors	67
		Cognitive and Emotional Schemas or Representations	68
		Cognitive and Behavioral Coping Strategies	68
		Personal Resources, Social Resources, and Risk Factors	69
		Health-Related Outcomes	72
	5.5	Research Findings among the Key Variables of the Stress Adaptation Coping System of Resilience	73
		A Meta-Analyses Based on the CSM	73
		The Stress-Coping Adaptive Process of Resilience	74
	5.6	Nursing Implications	83
	References		85

Part III Poor Resilience

6	**Poor Resilience**		95
	6.1	Introduction	95
	6.2	Objectives	95
	6.3	Definitions	96
		Poor Resilience	96
		Allostatic Load (AL)	96
		Allostatic Overload	98
	6.4	The Four Conditions of Chronic Stress	99
	6.5	Pervasive Neurobiological Maladaptive Disruptions	100
		Brain, Neural Circuitry, and Threat to Brain's Plasticity	100
	6.6	Impaired HPA Axis, ANS, and Immune Functioning	103
		Impaired Negative Feedback Inhibition System and Damaged Glucocorticoid (GR) Receptors	103
		Impaired PNS Healing Processes	104
		Dysregulated Immune System	104
	6.7	Other Dysregulated Mediators	104
	6.8	The Impaired Dopaminergic Reward System	106
	6.9	Dysregulated Circadian Rhythm	106
	6.10	Chronically Stress-Induced Epigenetic Changes	106
	6.11	Systemic Inflammation	107
	6.12	Metabolic Oxidative Stress	108
	6.13	Weakened Bioelectromagnetic Field	109
	6.14	Behavioral Indicators of Poor Resilience	109
	6.15	Nursing Implications	110
	References		112

7	**Cancer**		119
	7.1	Introduction	119
	7.2	Objectives	119
	7.3	Chronic Illness	120
	7.4	Cancer	120
		Definition	120

	7.5	Factors Conducive to the Development of Cancer.	121
		The Microbiome	122
	7.6	The Development of Cancer	123
		Cancer Stem Cells (CSCs).	124
		The Role of ROS in Tumorigenesis and Cancer Progression	125
		The Tumor Microenvironment (TME).	127
	7.7	Progression, Invasion, and Metastases.	129
		Chemoresistance	130
		Epithelial-to-Mesenchymal Transition (EMT) in Tumor Progression and Recurrence	130
		Metastases	131
	7.8	Nursing Implications	132
	References.	133	

Part IV Fostering Healing and Resilience

8	**The Quality of the Nurse–Patient Relationship**	139	
	8.1	Introduction	139
	8.2	Objectives.	140
	8.3	Why Patients Need a Quality Relationship with the Nurse	140
	8.4	Definition.	141
	8.5	The Quality of the Nurse–Patient Relationship	142
		Clinical Research.	143
	8.6	Relational Characteristics of the Nurse–Patient Relationship	143
		Being Present.	144
		Communication	145
		Compassion	148
		A Sense of Connectedness with Patients and Family Caregivers . .	149
		Evidence-Based Practice (EBP)	154
	References.	156	

9	**Promoting Emotion-Regulating Coping Resilience**	163	
	9.1	Introduction	163
	9.2	Objectives.	164
	9.3	Definitions: The Emotion/Self-Regulating Coping System of Psychological Resilience	164
	9.4	Randomized Controlled Intervention Studies (RCTs): Enhancing Coping Efforts	166
		Cognitive–Behavioral Strategies (CBS)	166
		Self-Management Interventions (SMI)	166
	9.5	Suggested Nursing Approaches	168
		Nursing Assessment.	168
		Nursing Interventions: Promoting Emotion-Regulating Coping Efforts	172
		The Nurse's Essential "Resilient-Promoting Toolbox"	173

	9.6	Final Thoughts	185
		Appendix: Psychosocial Interventions—Cognitive–Behavioral Therapy/Cognitive–Behavioral Stress Management Interventions/Self-Efficacy	186
		References	193
10	**Fostering Meaning Making**		**201**
	10.1	Introduction	201
	10.2	Objectives	201
	10.3	Definitions	202
	10.4	Emotional and Existential Distress	203
		Emotional Distress	203
		Existential Distress	203
	10.5	Conceptual Underpinnings	204
		Global Meaning-Orienting System	204
		Situational Meaning	205
		Search for Meaning: Adjusted Global and Situational Meanings	205
		Found Meaning or Meaning Made	208
		Moderators and Mediators of Meaning	210
	10.6	Meaning-Making Clinical Interventions	213
		The Life Review	214
		Meaning-Made Interventions	215
	10.7	Nursing Approaches	215
		Nursing Assessment	215
		Nursing Interventions: Global Assumptions, Situational Meanings, and Meaning Making	216
		Meaning-Making Strategies	217
		Facilitating Deliberate Rumination	220
		A Word About Causal Attributions	221
		A Matter of Personal Choice	222
	10.8	Final Thoughts	223
		Appendix: Psychosocial Interventions—Meaning-Related Studies	224
		References	231
11	**Strengthening Supportive Relationships**		**239**
	11.1	Introduction	239
	11.2	Objectives	239
	11.3	Definitions	240
		Family Support	241
		Partner and Spousal Support	241
	11.4	Models of Support and Clinical Findings	242
		Stress-Buffering Model	242
		Main Effects Model	243
		Mediating Effects	244

	11.5	Support and Personal Resources	245
		Support and Attachment	245
		Support and Self-Efficacy	246
		Support and Optimism	246
		Support and Resilience	247
		Support and Coping Behaviors	248
		Not All Support Is Supportive	248
		When Patients Lack Support	249
		Support and Neurobiological Effects	249
	11.6	The Importance of a Patient- Family Caregiver Dyad as the Focus of a Supportive Intervention	251
	11.7	Controlled Trials: Supportive Expressive Intervention Studies	252
		SEGT and Survivability	253
	11.8	Nursing Approaches	254
		Nursing Assessment of Patients and Family Caregivers	254
		Nursing Interventions	258
	11.9	Final Thoughts	262
		Appendix: Psychosocial Support-Related Interventions	263
		References	278
12	**Psychological Healing and Leveraging the Placebo Effect**		**287**
	12.1	Introduction	287
	12.2	Objectives	288
	12.3	Definitions	288
	12.4	How Cognitive Expectations Are Formed	289
		Positive and Negative Expectations: Side Effects	289
		Cognitive Expectations: Drug Conditioning	292
	12.5	Unconscious Conditioning Associated with Treatment-Induced Immunosuppression	294
	12.6	Mechanisms of Action: Psychosocial-Neurobiological Systems of Healing	295
		Learning and Conditioning	295
		The Brain's Reward System	296
		Neuroimaging and the Stress Response System and Immune Responses	297
		MOA and Nocebo Pathways	297
	12.7	Nursing Approaches	299
		The Quality of the Nurse-Patient Relationship	300
		Verbal Suggestions and Open/Closed Treatments	302
		Open/Hidden Clinical Condition	304
		Promoting Cognitive Expectations: RCTs	306
		Strategies to Minimize the Nocebo Effect	306
		Managing Informed Consent	307
		Modulating Unconscious Conditioning	308
	12.8	Final Comments	309
		References	310

13 Mindfulness-Based Practice and Eliciting the Relaxation Response... 317
- 13.1 Introduction ... 317
- 13.2 Objectives... 317
- 13.3 Definitions ... 318
- 13.4 Mindful Meditation ... 319
  - Benson's Relaxation Response (RR) Technique ... 320
  - Mindfulness-Based Cancer Recovery (MBCR)... 320
- 13.5 Mechanism of Action... 321
- 13.6 Research Findings ... 321
  - Mindful Techniques on Neural Structural Regions ... 321
  - Physiological Outcomes... 323
  - Immune Functions ... 323
  - Molecular Changes... 324
  - Psychological and Behavioral Outcomes... 325
  - Cognitive Functions ... 326
- 13.7 MM as a Self-Care Skill for Nurses... 328
- 13.8 Nursing Implications ... 329
- 13.9 Final Thoughts... 331
- Appendix: MBSR. Psychosocial and Behavioral Interventions—Mindful Meditation (MM), Relaxation Response Technique (RR), Mindfulness-Based Stress Reduction Intervention (MBSR), and Mindfulness-Based Cancer Recovery (MBCR) ... 332
- References... 345

14 Physical Touch and Healing Touch ... 351
- 14.1 Introduction ... 351
- 14.2 Objectives... 351
- 14.3 Physical Touch... 352
  - Definitions ... 352
- 14.4 Contextual Factors ... 354
- 14.5 Attachment and Embodiment Theories ... 355
- 14.6 Buffering and Main Effects ... 356
- 14.7 Neurobiological Processes of Physical Touch ... 356
- 14.8 Experimental Research ... 357
  - Touch and Healthy Volunteers ... 357
- 14.9 Clinical Research Findings ... 360
  - Physical Touch Within the Context of the Nurse-Patient Relationship ... 360
  - Facilitating Affectionate Touch Within a Close Patient-Family Caregiver Relationship... 364
- 14.10 Nursing Implications ... 365
  - Nursing Take-aways... 366
- 14.11 Final Comments... 368
- 14.12 Therapeutic Touch (TT), Healing Touch, and Reiki ... 368
  - Definitions ... 369
- 14.13 Conceptual Underpinnings... 371

	14.14	Research Findings 372
		Symptom Relief 372
		Quality of Life (QOL) 374
		Healthcare Providers and Reiki 375
		Experimental Animal Research 377
	14.15	Clinical Research Caveats 377
	14.16	Final Thoughts 378

Appendix: Mind-Body (MBSR). Psychosocial
Interventions—Multimodal Interventions—Mind-body
(MBSR), Energy, and Other CTs 379
References 392

Part V Nursing Approaches

15 The Diagnostic Phase 405
15.1 Introduction 405
15.2 Objectives 405
15.3 Definitions: The Diagnostic Prehabilitation Phase 406
15.4 Emotional Distress 407
        Factors Underlying Patient and Caregiver Distress 408
15.5 Physical Functioning, Fitness, and Activity 408
15.6 Neurophysiological Dysregulation 409
15.7 Clinical Research Findings: Prehabilitation Interventions 409
        Presurgery 410
15.8 Nursing Implications 413
        Nursing Assessment 414
        Establishing a Nurse-Patient/Caregiver Relationship 417
        Provide Relevant Information 418
        Cognitive Beliefs and Expectations 419
        Enhancing Cognitive-Behavioral and Meaning-Making Coping
        Strategies 422
        Self-Management Interventions 427
        Strengthening Supportive Relationships 427
        Healthy Lifestyle Behaviors with a Focus on Physical
        Fitness, Physical Activity, Healthy Diet, and Nutrition 428
15.9 Managing Consent 433
References 433

16 Treatment Phase 441
16.1 Introduction 441
16.2 Objectives 441
16.3 Definition 442
16.4 Clinical Issues 442
        Lifestyle Health-Related Risks 443

	16.5	Treatment: Chemotherapy and Radiation-Related Therapy and Surgery 444

- 16.5 Treatment: Chemotherapy and Radiation-Related Therapy and Surgery 444
  - Perisurgical Phase Review 445
  - Symptoms and Side Effects 446
  - Body Image Impairments................................... 448
- 16.6 Psychosocial Interventions and Related Research.............. 449
  - Perceived Support 449
  - Cognitive-Behavioral Interventions (CB) 450
  - MBSR/MBCTs... 451
  - Self-Management Interventions (SMI) 452
  - Progressive Relaxation and Imagery 452
  - Massage, Foot Reflexology 453
  - Exercise, Weight, and Nutrition........................... 454
  - Therapeutic Healing..................................... 457
- 16.7 Family Caregivers 457
  - Cognitive-Behavioral Strategies CBT 458
  - Mindfulness-Based Interventions (MB)..................... 458
  - Nursing Approaches..................................... 459
  - The Nurse–Patient Relationship........................... 460
  - Promoting Self-Management (Problem-Solving) Capabilities ... 461
  - Cognitive-Behavioral Coping Approaches................... 462
  - Enhancing the Quality of Supportive Relationships 463
  - Managing Positive/Negative Expectations of Treatment 464
  - Promoting Immune Functioning 465
  - Supporting Diet, Relevant Nutrition, and Physical Activity 467
  - Facilitating Wound Healing in the Perioperative Period 470
  - Symptom/Side Effects 471
  - Family Caregivers 474
- References... 475

17 The Transition to Survivorship 491
- 17.1 Introduction 491
- 17.2 Objectives.. 491
- 17.3 Definition.. 492
- 17.4 Common Patient Concerns 493
  - Feelings of Medical Abandonment 493
  - An Altered Self-Identity.................................. 494
  - Fear of a Cancer Recurrence (FCR)........................ 494
  - Changes in Family Support 495
  - Enduring Symptoms and Side Effects of Treatment or Cancer .. 495
  - Lifestyle Behaviors 498

	17.5	Clinical Research: Psychosocial Interventions 499
		Cognitive-Behavioral (CB) Strategies 499
		Mind–Body Stress Reduction (MBSR) and Mindfulness-Based Cancer Recovery (MBCR) 500
		Massage and Foot Reflexology 502
		Self-Management Interventions (SMI) 502
		Health-Related Education 503
		Health-Promoting Lifestyle Interventions 504
	17.6	Proposed Nursing Approaches........................... 507
		Maintain a Sense of Connectedness between Nurse and Individual and Family 507
		Promote Self-Management Capabilities 508
		Fear of a Cancer Recurrence 508
		The Quality and Quantity of Informal Support 509
		Managing Symptoms and Side Effects of Treatment and the Cancer 510
		Finding Meaning in the New Normal Life 512
		Promoting a Healthy Lifestyle.......................... 513
	References... 518
18	**Supportive Care and End of Life**............................. 531
	18.1	Introduction 531
	18.2	Objectives... 532
	18.3	Definition 532
	18.4	Cessation of Treatment 533
	18.5	Transition to Supportive Care Services 533
		Nature of Transition and Lack of Information............... 533
		Timing 534
	18.6	Patient Concerns, Distress, and Symptom Burden 535
		Emotional Distress and Existential Suffering 535
		Symptom Burden 536
	18.7	Family Caregiver Concerns 536
	18.8	Clinical Benefits of Early Integrated Oncology-Supportive Care Services 537
	18.9	RCTs: Psychosocial Interventions........................ 539
		Patient-Focused Studies................................ 539
		Focus on Patient and Caregiver Dyads..................... 541
		Focus on the Family Caregiver........................... 542
	18.10	Nursing Approaches................................... 544
		Quality of the Nurse–Patient/Family Relationship 545
		Cognitive-Behavioral Emotion-Regulating Coping Strategies ... 545
		More Cognitive Strategies 547
		Strengthening Supportive Relationships 551

		Symptom Management	553
		Health Education	558
		Self-Management Interventions	559
	18.11	Unique Needs of Caregivers	560
		Bereavement.	561
	References.		562

19 Is It Feasible. 575
	19.1	Introduction	575
	19.2	Nursing Objectives.	577
	19.3	Definitions	577
	19.4	Barriers to Evidence-Based Nursing Practice	577
		Peer-Reviewed Research Versus Clinical Nursing Journals.	578
		A Paucity of Patient-Centered Conceptual Practice Models	578
		Definitions of Evidence-Based Practice.	579
		Work-Related Stress.	580
		The Quality of the Nurse–Patient Relationship	581
		A Lack of Scientific Knowledge and Psychosocial Skills Among Clinical Nurses.	582
	19.5	Toward Academic Practice.	583
		The Nursing Leadership.	584
		Implementing the Model	585
		Team Values	586
		Critical Analytic Research Skills	586
		Clinical Skills.	587
		Staffing, Schedules, and Assignments	591
		A University-Affiliated Clinical Learning Environment	592
		Nurturing the Nurse's Wholeness	593
	References.		595

Closing Remarks. 601

Clinical Approaches: Appendices 605

Part I

The Stress, Healing, and Resilience Nursing Model of Whole Person Care

Introduction

What we say, how we say it, and what we do convey our core beliefs about illness, health, and wellness, and in so doing, may trigger or suppress innate processes of healing in those we care for. Part I introduces the stress, resilience, and healing nursing model of whole person care. Chapter 1 provides the historical theoretical underpinnings of the model. Chapter 2 presents the key conceptual tenets of the model of whole person care, the nursing goals, desired outcomes, and proposed psychosocial interventions empirically known to enhance healing and resilience in patients with cancer and their family caregivers.

Theoretical Underpinnings 1

1.1 Theoretical Underpinnings

My earliest memories about cancer and healing come from a true story my father once told me. He was an ENT surgeon working at an academic hospital in the early 1950s when a curious event concerning one of his patients occurred. A priest had made an appointment to see my father because of a chronic problem with hoarseness that had befuddled previous doctors. My father located a tumor of the larynx. As per the protocol of the newly established hospital tumor board, my father presented the diagnostic evidence, and the board members fully concurred with his diagnosis.

A cancer diagnosis was dire in those days, so the evening before the surgery, my father dropped by the priest's hospital room with the nurse in charge. The priest was praying, but stopped on seeing his surgeon and the nurse. My father, who was not particularly religious, but respectful of the priest's devotion to his faith, asked if they could all pray together, which they did in the priest's room. They were three individuals from different faiths praying to their own higher being encompassing the priest with their presence, caring, and support. The next morning, my father and the medical residents started the operation. But they soon discovered to their amazement that the tumor had disappeared. It was inexplicable.

When I have shared this story with nursing students, it has been met, unsurprisingly, with the highest degree of skepticism. A couple of students have had the courage to say what I am certain many others were thinking: that it could be explained away by poor diagnostic tools in those days or medical incompetence! Still, it was equally difficult to dismiss, out of hand, the diagnostic capabilities of a group of surgeons working at an eminent university hospital in Montreal, all members of the tumor board, who had arrived at the same conclusion. It was a mystery.

Years later, doing research for this book, I came across a scientific review of the placebo effect in oncology, now recognized as an innate healing effect, triggered by strongly held cognitive expectations of a positive clinical outcome. Based on WHO criteria, the review reported that the cancer tumors were significantly reduced in about 2.4% or 10 out of 375 patients from 10 trials [1]. From a scientific perspective, it was an unimpressive result to be normally discounted out of hand.

Yet the finding left open the possibility for the medically inexplicable. Although humans throughout history have been known to heal physical and psychic wounds, it is only recently that medical scientists have come to realize that strongly held human beliefs can trigger innate processes of healing via various physiological pathways. These include the reward system and a downregulated stress response system that enable the reemergence of healing processes which can also enhance cell-mediated immunity, a critical anticancer defense (e.g., [2–4]).

Healing and health in the whole person have been much revered core concepts of the nursing discipline, since Florence Nightingale's Notes on Nursing, which was published over 100 years ago [5]. Nightingale's scientific observations suggested that distressed patients possessed an innate ability to heal or restore wholeness, when certain environmental conditions, such as uninterrupted sleep, a clean, restful or quiet environment, and a caring and thoughtful approach were met. These observations led her to hypothesize that the mind influences physical well-being, and conversely, physical health has a significant impact on the mind [5]. Both involve reparative processes within the interactive context of the patient's environment. These mind–body connections laid down the first essential ideas about what constituted the whole person (an integrated mind-body) in relation to stress, health, and healing within the discipline of nursing.

Since then, nurse scientists have argued that human beings are more than the sum of their parts, in staunch contrast to a healthcare system mostly shaped by a reductionist perspective in which the clinical focus remains the illness and treatment. Their thinking was influenced by Selye's theory of stress [6], Lazarus' and Folkman's work on stress and coping [7, 8], von Bertalanffy's general systems theory [9], and Roger's conceptualization of the human being as an "irreducible whole, fueled by homeodynamic energy interrelating with the environment" [10]. Von Bertalanffy [9] argued that systems are distinguished by nonlinear interactions among their constituent parts, which was a prescient idea that has since been supported by research findings that highlight the human's nonlinear process of biological adjustments in response to environmental stressors [11]. In other words, the whole person both influences and is influenced by the environment.

McGill University's School of Nursing under the leadership of Moyra Allen developed the key concepts of the McGill Model of Nursing. In contrast to prevailing thinking in the 1960s that health and illness were at opposite ends of the same continuum, the McGill model envisioned health as co-existing with illness [12]. Influenced by the work of Spiegel [13] and Bronfenbrenner [14], health was described in terms of multidimensional developmental processes that grow toward greater complexity and self-actualization while maintaining coherence over the life span [15].

Around the same time, research in the field of environmental stress and psychoneuroendocrine and immune sciences provided scientific legitimacy to nursing's foundational beliefs about the mind–body relationship, healing, and resilience (in terms of both biological and psychological processes of adaptation in relation to the environment (e.g., [16, 17]). McEwen and colleagues built upon earlier landmark research on stress by introducing concepts of allostasis (healthy resilience) to exemplify the adaptive changes that occur in response to stress, and allostatic load (maladaptive changes) to reflect the measurable burden caused by chronic stress on the whole person [11, 17]. They have advanced knowledge of the whole person through their work on the main biological regulator of stress and the dynamic nonlinear networks of biological mediators that trigger widespread temporary or prolonged changes to neural structures, pathways, and functions throughout the whole being. These stress-induced changes suppress neurobiological processes (e.g., the parasympathetic nervous system) associated with regeneration, reparation, and restoration (healing) of myriad biological functions including cell-mediated immunity, which is vital for promoting long-term health particularly in patients with cancer [18–20]. Knowledge of these stress-induced neurobiological impairments negatively affecting healing and resilient processes has added immeasurably to the clinical context within which resilient- and healing-promoting clinical interventions may be developed and evaluated.

These scientific advances underscore Nursing's need for an integrated formulation of the whole person based on stress, healing, resilience, and related concepts delineated by a conceptual model so that nursing interventions may target relevant unique and overlapping endpoints that promote or protect the individual's resilience and health. This is a clinical imperative in caring for patients with cancer and their family caregiver who must confront diverse stressors along the continuum.

References

1. Chvetzoff G, Tannock IF. Placebo effects in oncology. J Natl Cancer Inst. 2003;95(1):19–29. https://doi.org/10.1093/jnci/95.1.19; PubMed PMID: 12509397. Epub 2003/01/02. eng.
2. Benson H, Stark M. Timeless healing: the power and biology of belief. New York: Simon & Schuster; 1997.
3. Dutcher JM, Creswell JD. The role of brain reward pathways in stress resilience and health. Neurosci Biobehav Rev. 2018;95:559–67. https://doi.org/10.1016/j.neubiorev.2018.10.014; PubMed PMID: 30477985. Epub 2018/11/28. eng.
4. Colloca L, Barsky AJ. Placebo and nocebo effects. N Engl J Med. 2020;382(6):554–61. https://doi.org/10.1056/NEJMra1907805; PubMed PMID: 32023375. Epub 2020/02/06. eng.
5. Skretkowicz V. Florence Nightingale's notes on nursing and notes on nursing for the labouring classes. New York: Springer Publishing Co; 2010.
6. Selye H. Stress without distress. New York: Springer; 1976.
7. Lazarus R. Psychological stress and the coping process. New York, NY: McGraw Hill International Books Co.; 1966.
8. Lazarus RS, Folkman S. Stress, appraisal and coping. New York: Springer; 1984.
9. Bertalanffy L. General system theory: foundations, development, applications. New York: G. Braziller; 1973.
10. Malinski VM. In: Rich JBBAKL, editor. Models and theories focused on human existence. Sudbury, MA: Jones & Bartlett Learning; 2011.
11. McEwen BS. Physiology and neurobiology of stress and adaptation: central role of the brain. Physiol Rev. 2007;87(3):873–904; PubMed PMID: 17615391. Epub 2007/07/07. eng.

12. Gottlieb L, Rowat K. The McGill model of nursing: a practice derived model. Adv Nurs Sci. 1987;9(4):51–61.
13. Spiegel D. The developing mind. New York: The Guilford Press; 1997.
14. Bronfenbrenner U. The ecology of human development: experiments by nature and design. Cambridge, MA: Harvard University Press; 1981.
15. Gottlieb L, Gottlieb B. The development/health framework within the McGill model of nursing: 'Laws of nature' guiding whole person care. Adv Nurs Sci. 2007;30(1):E43–57.
16. McEwen B. Central effects of stress hormones in health and disease: understanding the protective and damaging effects of stress and stress mediators. Eur J Pharmacol. 2008;583:174–85.
17. McEwen BS, Stellar E. Stress and the individual. Mechanisms leading to disease. Arch Intern Med. 1993;153(18):2093–101; PubMed PMID: 8379800. Epub 1993/09/27. eng.
18. Lutgendorf SK, Sood AK, Antoni MH. Host factors and cancer progression: biobehavioral signaling pathways and interventions. J Clin Oncol Off J Am Soc Clin Oncol. 2010;28(26):4094–9; PubMed PMID: 20644093. Pubmed Central PMCID: PMC2940426. Epub 2010/07/21. eng.
19. Wang M, Zhao J, Zhang L, Wei F, Lian Y, Wu Y, et al. Role of tumor microenvironment in tumorigenesis. J Cancer. 2017;8(5):761–73; PubMed PMID: 28382138. Pubmed Central PMCID: PMC5381164. Epub 2017/04/07. eng.
20. Lutgendorf SK, Andersen BL. Biobehavioral approaches to cancer progression and survival: mechanisms and interventions. Am Psychol. 2015;70(2):186–97; PubMed PMID: 25730724. Pubmed Central PMCID: PMC4347942. Epub 2015/03/03. eng.

The Stress, Healing, and Resilience Nursing Model of Whole Person Care

2

Volumes are now written and spoken upon the effect of the mind upon the body. Much of it is true, But I wish a little more was thought of the effect of the body on the mind ... The sick suffer from painful thoughts as well as bodily pain and illness—F Nightingale [1].

Our task must be to free ourselves by widening our circle of compassion to embrace all living creatures and the whole of nature and its beauty—Albert Einstein.

2.1 Introduction

The stress, healing and resilience model of the whole person posits that health captured at a point in time is influenced by the effect(s) of environmental stresses on dynamic processes of healing and resilience (adaptation). Successful biological and behavioral adjustments in response to environmental stresses across the lifespan depend on the quality, intensity, duration, recurrence and frequency of stressful exposures as well as by the presence of personal and social resources. Stressful experiences causing widespread impairments that adversely affect neural flexibility result in poor resilient capabilities that ultimately compromise health. The model offers a delineated scientific context to assess patients with cancer and their loved ones for the purpose of determining relevant psychosocial nursing interventions that may strengthen healing and resilient capabilities as they confront various stressors along the illness and recovery continuum. Although not the purpose of this book, this conceptual nursing model is appropriate for individuals with other chronic illness and to promote the health of healthy populations.

2.2 Objectives

At the end of this chapter, you will be able to

1. Explain what is meant by the *whole* human being.
2. Describe the concept of health in relation to its multilayered dimensions, attributes, and processes.
3. Identify key health-related outcomes of resilience.
4. Describe the relationships among psychological stress, healing, and resilience.

2.3 Core Values and Assumptions of Practice

The healing and resilience nursing model of whole person care is predicated on a number of assumptions.

First, the quality of the nurse–patient (and caregiver) relationship provides an important therapeutic context.

Second, nursing is centered on the whole person within a 'family' context. The primary focus of care is promoting psycho-social, neurobiological, behavioral and spiritual processes conducive to optimizing healing, resilience and health, in part by effectively managing the potential effects of environmental stress on the person. *Accordingly, procedures and techniques are regarded as important albeit ancillary nursing functions.*

Third, nursing is guided by professional values of compassion, continuity of care, knowing the patient and family, presence, the relief of suffering, and a nurse–patient–caregiver relationship based on mutual respect, trust, and understanding within which healing may be optimized [2–5].

Fourth, from a systems perspective, the model recognizes the bidirectional interrelationships among the environment, individual, family, and nursing. In the special context of cancer, the patient, informal caregiver (family), and nurse influence and are influenced by one another. Humans tend to seek proximity to loved ones in stressful times and become distressed when separated: When a cancer-related threat is present it impacts the patient and family (the informal caregiver) with reciprocating effects [4, 6]. Thus, the unit of nursing care is the patient and partner or family caregiver as emotions, thoughts, and feelings tend to be mutually shared and experienced within this relationship [7]. This unit of care recognizes bidirectional influences within the broader context of family. For the purpose of this handbook, however, "family" is represented mainly by the person's family caregiver (or significant other).

Fifth, the individual is conceptualized as a complex and dynamic, *integrated whole* throughout all the organizational levels of being from the molecular to the spiritual in which the totality of the person is greater than the sum of all parts and from which spiritual and creative expressions cannot be compartmentalized [8]. From *tenets of complexity theory*, the model recognizes that the human organism's health depends on its ability to maintain biological stability, homeostasis,

2.5 The Whole Person and the Environment

and internal coherence while dynamically adapting to environmental stresses as it continues to develop biological and behavioral complexity throughout the lifespan [9–11]. Biological and behavioral *variability* is an integral adaptive property of overall resilience.

Sixth, health and illness coexist in the whole person. People with acute, chronic, and even life-threatening illnesses can be healthy, even as they live with a life-threatening, progressive illness [12].

Seven, innate biological processes and functions of healing are integral to the process of adaptation or resilience, governed by the reemergence of the parasympathetic nervous system (PNS), vagal nerve, and cholinergic activity throughout the human organism in the aftermath of psychological stress (e.g., [13]). Other healing processes may be triggered by conscious expectations or beliefs in a clinical benefit or by finding meaning in a stressful situation [14–16], as well as by acquiring effective emotion-regulating coping strategies [17, 18]. Another form of healing may be healing touch, therapeutic touch, or Reiki based on the intentional mobilization of energy to remove blockages and restore energy balance throughout the whole person, thereby facilitating processes of healing (e.g., [19]). Social and physical factors within the clinical environment can consciously or unconsciously promote or suppress the individual's healing capabilities [20].

Eight, biological stability of the human organism is associated with energy conservation, healing, resilience, and health at basal levels of physiology [13].

Nine, an electromagnetic biofield of the person intercommunicates with the energy fields of the external environment which may account, in part, for the human ability to sense other human's thoughts, feelings, and sensations [21, 22]. Biofield therapies such as Reiki or healing touch also may interact with the human's energy field (chi or qi) so that changes in the energy field may result in healing-inducing changes in the physiology and mood of the person ([23] p. 1229).

2.4 Goals of the Practice Model

The first goal is to provide the theoretical and empirical basis for a more comprehensive and substantive clinical approach to the care of the whole person with cancer within the context of his family caregiver. A second goal is to facilitate the development and evaluation of nursing interventions aimed at reducing emotional stress and enhancing resilient and healing capabilities in order to promote the patient's health across the cancer and survival trajectory, and especially, at identified periods of vulnerability: diagnosis, treatment, transition to survivorship, and end of life.

2.5 The Whole Person and the Environment (See Part II, Chap. 3; Part IV Chaps. 8 and 11)

The person: According to Von Bertalanffy's general system theory (1969) and his conceptualization of the human being, the whole person is an "irreducible whole, fueled by homeodynamic energy and interacting with the environment." The whole person is a complex, dynamic, and integrated biological and behavioral entity of systems, subsystems, pathways, signaling molecules, metabolic processes, and functions across multiple interrelated levels ranging from the genome to the individual's macroorgans. All is interconnected and maintained via a dynamic, ubiquitous, and nonlinear, mostly bidirectional network of mediating enzymes, hormones, cytokines, transcription factors, and other neurotransmitters [24, 25]. This network is modulated by the neuroendocrinal and immune-based stress response system responsible for maintaining homeostasis and internal coherence, as well as the development, defense, healing, and resilience of the whole being. The whole person is also greater than the sum of its parts. For instance, the person's thoughts, ideas, and spiritual sensations exceed the delineated parameters of the corporeal being [8, 11, 12]. *Environment:* The whole person is influenced by interactions between the genome and the environment. The whole person influences and is influenced by the internal and external environment. The physical environment such as the quality of air, housing, other buildings, transportation vehicles, land, and/or water can impact the health of the individual. Similarly, physical and social factors in the clinical environment can also cause conscious and unconscious neurophysiological responses that can either promote or interfere with the patient's therapeutic goals of treatment [20]. Factors such as social and economic stressors, daily demands and hassles, acute stressors, life-threatening accidents, or a chronic illness mediated by the brain impact the whole being. Similarly, internal environmental factors such as viruses, nonsymbiotic bacteria, or cancer can adversely impact the whole person, whereas internal interrelated healing, resilient, immune, and metabolic processes strive to maintain homeostasis and a coherent whole as developmental processes drive the actualization of the whole being.

2.6 Psychological Stress (See Part II Chaps. 3, 4 and 5)

In this book, psychological stress and psychosocial stress are used interchangeably. Psychological stress is "the human response" to internal and external environmental threats causing neurobiological, biochemical, epigenetic, cognitive, and behavioral changes that have the potential to disrupt homeostasis, resilience, healing, and development (Fig. 2.1) [10, 26]. For instance, chronic stress can damage neural structures, pathways, and even DNA, causing mutations that result in the onset of a chronic illness such as cancer [26–28]. Stress is typically described in terms of its acuity, chronicity, intensity, frequency, duration, and controllability. Psychological stress varies over the lifespan, including across the different stages of the cancer and survival continuum. The extent to which it has a negative effect on the individual depends on the type of stressor(s), and the individual's meaning of the stressor self-efficacy beliefs, coping capabilities, personal strengths or resources, perceived support, and healthy lifestyle behaviors which facilitate the individual's overall dynamic capacity for resilience. In such contexts, perceived stress of normally short duration can be the impetus for personal growth.

2.6 Psychological Stress

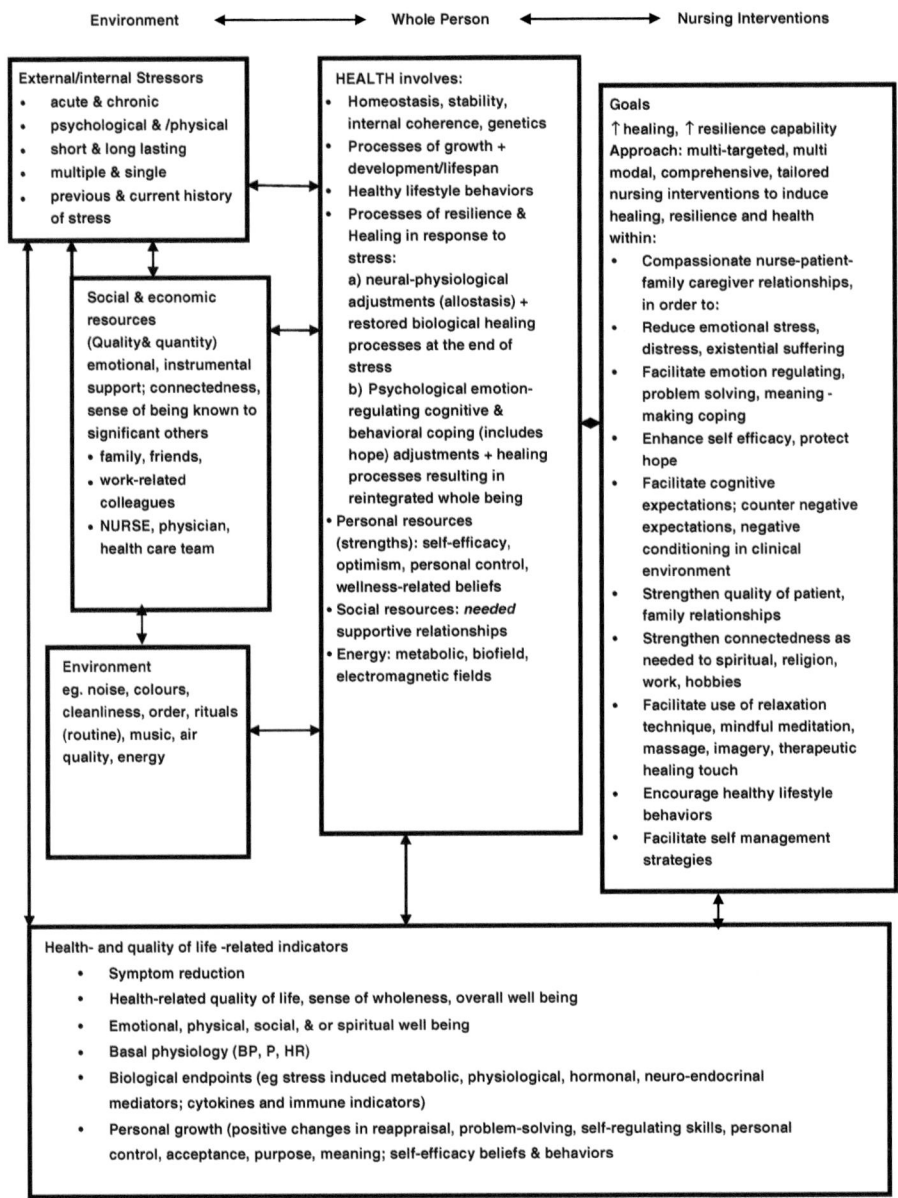

Fig. 2.1 Key components of the stress, healing and resilience nursing model of the whole person

2.7 Health as an Essential Property of the Whole Being

An essential property of the whole person is health, captured at a moment in time. Health is described as "a *state* of optimal physical, mental, social and spiritual well-being, and perceived wholeness" (adapted from WHO https//www.who.int/about/who-we-are/constitution. Accessed May 23, 2019). Health is a function of the individual's dynamic ability to maintain relative social, physical, biological, behavioral, and emotional stability, internal coherence, energy, and *homeostasis* in the face of adversity, including a life-threatening illness, such as cancer [29].

Health-Related Outcomes

Health refers to the optimal neurobiological, psychosocial, cognitive, physical and metabolic systems, processes, and functions of an individual taken at one moment in time. Indicators of health typically involve measures of quality of life, overall well-being, wholeness, personal growth, and symptomatology. For instance, well-being is the overall cumulative effect of the individual's neurobiological and behavioral processes of healing and adaptation, and personal and social resources, including beliefs about the world and the self's place in it [30]. Psychological well-being is the realization of a positive attitude, a purposeful life, the self-actualization of personal goals, capabilities, and growth over the lifespan [30].

Stress induced neurobiological impairments tend to be associated with symptoms of disease; Early clinical knowledge of neurophysiological changes may be leveraged to mount tailored clinical interventions to optimize resilience and health. [31]. Interrelationships among symptoms, cytokines, and immune functions within the patient's clinical context may highlight altered neurobiological pathways to be targeted by healing-promoting or resilient-enhancing psychosocial interventions [32, 33]. Postoperative patients with cancer are known to be fatigued and immunosuppressed during the six-week recovery phase before the start of adjuvant chemotherapy. In the absence of chemotherapy, the suppressed NK cell state enables roving cancer cells to travel unimpeded, thereby predicting a future cancer recurrence [33, 34]. Equipped with this biological and behavioral scientific knowledge, the nurse might develop a nursing intervention aimed at strengthening the individual's innate NK cell activity and cell-mediated immune functions, including the critical functions of the cytotoxic natural killer cells (i.e., CD 8+ T cells) in the immediate postoperative period in order to protect and or enhance the individual's future health (e.g., [35]) (Review Parts IV and V, Chap. 16).

Key Internal Processes of Health

Significantly, health depends on timely and orderly integrated and dynamic processes of: development, adaptation (resilience), healing, and metabolism, which affect all dimensions, systems, subsystems, functions, and behaviors, including homeostatic operations, coherent biorhythms, and an intact human biofield, as the whole individual dynamically intersects with the environment [36]. For instance, health depends on the dynamic nonlinear compensatory variations (adjustments) in the interrelationships among biological constituents in response to various stressors of variable duration and intensity, as well as by the ability of the human organism to maintain synchrony among cellular and system biorhythms throughout the person so that energy is conserved in order to fuel other needed biological and developmental processes [10, 29].

Processes of Development
Development is a genetically programmed orderly process starting in utero that progressively grows toward greater biological and behavioral differentiation, complexity, and function stimulated by its mediating interactions with the social–cultural environment as it is propelled toward greater maturity and self-actualization [9, 11, 37]. Developmental processes from the molecular to the spiritual shape the process of becoming and of self-actualization of the whole being. This is driven by epigenetic changes that are induced by interactions at the gene–environmental interface, and all these dynamic processes and interactions are fueled by metabolic processes.

Developmental resilience is the essential process of developing or learning more adaptive or resilient-promoting capabilities in response to an expanding environment of challenging stressors in order to successfully and flexibly confront similar stressors in the future. Processes of development and resilience may be viewed as interdependent in that individuals learn to overcome various developmental challenges (such as learning to ride a bike) while acquiring adaptive coping strategies and personal and social capabilities to successfully manage emotions and use more effective coping behaviors in the future. These adaptive capabilities also appear to protect future developmental processes from the potentially corrosive effects of environmental stresses. Both interrelated processes have overlapping yet distinct functions (stress stability and protection versus progressive maturation) that are mediated by continuous gene–environment interactions which induce corresponding epigenetic instructions [38, 39].

Processes of Resilience (See Part II)
Another essential process of health is biological and behavioral resilience, due to its adaptive and protective functions in the face of manageable, short-term adversity across the lifespan [40, 41]. Resilient processes are triggered by *manageable,* adverse events, environmental demands, acute stressors, and threats of short duration. Resilience is the "ability of the human organism to successfully adapt to environmental challenges in order to maintain stability and homeostasis" [41]. At the biological level, the stress response system consisting of the hypothalamus–pituitary–adrenal axis (HPA axis), autonomic nervous system (ANS), and immune systems and their nonlinear network of interacting mediators are involved. At the psychological level, adaptive emotion-regulating stress-coping systems are implicated [17, 42]. And both are integrally involved in promoting resilience and by extension and health.

The process of resilience depends on these critical, interrelated processes of adaptation:

1. Temporary biological, cognitive, emotional, and behavioral adjustments made in response to stress [38].
2. Reemergence of biological and behavioral healing processes at the end of stress that restore neurophysiological adjustments to near-normal structures and parametric values while embedding adaptive physical and psychosocial changes within corresponding neural circuitry that guide the individual's growing flexibility and adaptive responses to future stressors [38, 41]. In the aftermath of acute short-term stress-induced conditions, the whole person can achieve a higher integrated level of adaptive functioning and capability (for instance, learned strategies or evidence of personal growth) [10, 13, 43].
3. Biological and behavioral flexibility is reflected by structural plasticity of neural and neuroendocrine processes as well as cognitive and behavioral flexibility in critical thinking capabilities, decision making, or problem solving [38, 44]. Adaptive plasticity refers to the ability of the neural structures of the brain to continuously remodel itself so that the individual may continue to adapt to stress exposures over the lifetime [38, 39].

The continuous accumulation of adaptive neural–biological and coping responses to stress is embedded in neural circuits that guide adaptive cognitive and behavioral responses to similar stressors in the future, providing protection against future deleterious stress effects on the biology and behavior of the person [10]. Personal and social resources such as a sense of self-efficacy, finding meaning and purpose, supportive interrelationships, and cognitive expectations of clinical benefits all help to buffer resilience from the potentially deleterious effects of the stressor and in so doing support the individual's acquisition of resilient-promoting capabilities (e.g., [42, 45]).

In summary, resilience is triggered by exposure to stress and is driven mainly by the integrated biological stress response system and emotion-regulating, stress-coping adaptive processes of resilience (which are discussed in greater detail in Part II Chaps. 4 and 5). Both work in tandem to protect the human organism from the deleterious effects of stress on homeostasis and health.

Processes of Innate and Self-Induced Healing (Review Part IV)

Healing may occur anytime in the aftermath of various psychosocial (and physical) stressors and is an integral part of the adaptive processes of biological and behavioral resilience.

Innate Biological Healing Processes after Stress Innate biological healing processes are an integral part of the restorative functions of resilience and are triggered by the downregulation of the stress response system. *Biological healing processes* involve the reactivation of the parasympathetic nervous system (PNS) and its vagal nerve and acetylcholine) in a time-ordered fashion [13, 46]. The reemergence of these restorative, healing pathways in the aftermath of the stress event enables *the* *near* restoration of stress-induced adjustments to neural–endocrine and immune structures, functions, and pathways. This includes the restoration to normal parametric values of compensatory adjustments made by stress mediators and other biological constituents in response to stress [38].

Physical Wound Healing (See Part V Chap. 16) As nurses, we have all cared for individuals recovering from physical wounds, for instance, associated with surgery. Scientific evidence indicates that physical wound healing is negatively affected by psychosocial stress, as reflected by a longer healing duration, suggesting that this innate process of healing is inhibited by psychosocial stress [47, 48]. A patient with a hostile spousal relationship may experience unremitting distress that may potentially slow wound healing. This has important clinical implications for postoperative individuals with cancer whose wounds must heal before starting adjuvant chemotherapy and/or radiation therapy. A prolonged healing rate can also predispose the patient's future health to life-threatening clinical implications of untreated circulating residual cancer cells after surgery.

Self-Induced Healing Healing may occur as a function of *the self-induced* adoption of effective emotion-regulating coping processes of resilience which downregulate the biological stress response system, in order to improve feelings of anxiety, fear, and/or depression (e.g., [42, 49, 50]). Self-induced healing is an integral part of the stress-coping system of resilience, of which meaning making also plays a central healing-inducing role [14]. Self-induced healing also may occur when an individual connects with the spiritual or something greater than the self or engages in known stress-reducing activities, such as Benson's relaxation response technique, mindful meditation, yoga, or prayer. Healing is also enhanced by a sense of *connectedness* to significant others [51–54]. Other ways to stimulate healing is by adopting a healthy lifestyle [55].

Cognitive Expectations Promote Healing Processes (Review Part IV Chap. 12) Healing may be elicited via conscious beneficial expectations of a treatment especially for symptoms of nausea, pain, depressed mood, and motor functions [56, 57]. It used to be referred to as the placebo effect which was controlled for in clinical trials of pharmaceutical agents. In recent years, the potential for facilitating healing processes associated with a person's cognitive expectation of wellness or a clinical benefit has been scientifically recognized to strengthen overall resilience, reduce stress, and improve treatment efficacy (e.g., [45]) (see Part IV Chap. 12). The classic example is the adult who makes an appointment to see the doctor because of a terrible cold. But on arrival at the doctor's office, the patient feels much better. The expectation of clinical benefit on arrival to the doctor is based on previously learned positive health-related experiences. But research findings also suggest that a patient's positive expectations for a clinical benefit not only may improve pain and anxiety, for instance, but even some immune cell functions [58, 59].

Conversely, self-fulfilling negative clinical expectations known as the nocebo effects can suppress the restorative functions of healing processes and interfere with the therapeutic benefit of some medications. Both positive and negative expectations within the context of clinical conditions are now better understood and have important clinical implications for nurses caring for patients (see Part IV Chap. 12).

2.8 Personal Strengths and Social Resources (Supportive Relationships) (See Part IV, Chaps. 8–11)

Health is a function of the individual's personal strengths which may directly or indirectly mediate the relationship between environmental stressors and resilience and health. Personal *strengths* **or** *resources* influence the use of adaptive coping efforts (i.e., psychological resilience) and protect the individual from the toxic effects of stress [60, 61]. Personal strengths include resilience, a sense of optimism, a sense of personal control, self-efficacy, and possibly hope [62–64]. Resilience is also a strength as well as an adaptive process. Personal resources may change as a function of the environmental or clinical context (Chaps. 5 and 9).

Social Resources (Supportive Relationships) (Review Part IV Chaps. 8 and 11)

Strengths also refer to the social resources and, in particular, supportive relationships and support behaviors individuals perceive and receive across the lifespan as individuals *learn to successfully* adapt to various stressors. The individual influences and is influenced by his or her social surroundings. The social environment includes work-related colleagues, neighbors, community, friends, family, partners, spouses, and loved ones and the quality and quantity of supportive (social, emotional, instrumental) relationships. However, the quality of the individual's relationships with loved ones or "informal supports" is particularly important for patients with cancer and their informal caregivers. Supportive relationships influence the person's use of coping strategies in the face of adversity. Informal support has been shown to predict a longer survivorship among patients with breast cancer [51, 52, 65].

The nurse and other healthcare providers are an integral part of the individual's clinical environment through the quality of their relationships with the patient and caregiver (and significant family) within the clinic or hospital setting and/or the patient's home (e.g., [53, 66, 67]). The nurse is an important source of support to the patient and family especially within a connected nurse–patient (and caregiver) relationship. A nurse's support can promote resilience and health in part by reducing emotional distress, downregulating the biological stress response system but also by providing relevant knowledge and skills to cope effectively (e.g., [53, 68, 69]). What a nurse says and does, for instance, regarding a medical treatment or the cancer can influence the patient's conscious expectations of a clinical benefit based on findings from related studies [20, 70–72].

2.9 Healthy Lifestyle Behaviors

Healthy lifestyle behaviors facilitate the growth and development of the individual across biological, social, emotional, psychological, physical, and metabolic processes independent of stress. It also strengthens physical fitness and facilitates the restoration or healing of stress-induced neurophysiological and molecular pathways. Critical components include a good night's sleep, daily physical activity, healthy dietary pattern of eating and nutrition, a significant reduction in the consumption of alcohol, and maintenance of a normal weight and waist circumference [55]. A healthy lifestyle also involves healthy ways to cook foods in order to preserve their beneficial nutrients and minimize carcinogenic-producing molecules.

The original manuscript of this book included a chapter on healthy lifestyle behaviors which turned out to be a huge chapter, deserving a nursing book in its own right! Promoting healthy lifestyle behaviors is part of nursing's legacy that sadly appears to have fallen by the wayside, but is vital to the overall health of the whole person that we care for. Consequently, each chapter of Part V includes the latest research findings and nursing suggestions related to recommended lifestyle behaviors at each phase of the continuum.

2.10 Epigenetics

Resilience is seamlessly regulated by epigenetic mechanisms, described as continuous interactions at the environmental–gene nexus which influence reversible "bioactive molecular events" situated above the genome (i.e., in promoter regions) [38]. For instance, environmental factors such as glucocorticoids, cytokines, and chemokines and other neuromodulators are in continuous interaction with the genome, which involves changes to histones, cytosine methylation, chromatin remodeling, and RNA-based mechanisms. These changes modify gene expression without altering the DNA sequence in response to environmental stresses (such as good stress, tolerable stress, allostatic load, and toxic allostatic overload). The selected genes that are expressed subsequently modify the activities and functions of the human organism based on their biological instructions. Both nurturing and stressful environments and lifestyle behaviors cause epigenetic changes with consequential but generally reversible implications for healing and resilience [38, 73]. Significantly, knowledge of the *reversibility* of epigenetic processes should encourage the nurse to promote adaptive coping efforts and healthy changes in lifestyle behaviors in patients and caregivers [38, 41].

2.11 Homeostasis

Homeostasis is a property of cells, tissues, organs, and interrelated mediators functioning within a network of biochemical intercommunications and homeostatic modulating functions. The human organism's ability to maintain homeostasis lies in its ability to dynamically adapt to environmental demands while ensuring relative stability, equilibrium, and integrity (cohesiveness and coherence) as the human organism moves toward developmental actualization [13, 74]. This continuous adaptive process based on nonlinear changes in the patterns of interrelationships among biological mediators depends on energy [13, 74]. Homeostasis generally requires low energy consumption, but requires greater metabolic energy to sustain homeostasis during stressful situations [13].

Although biological resilience and homeostasis complement one another and share interrelated physiological functions that are essential for health, homeostasis in principle refers to specific, regulatory physiological adjustments that are essential for maintaining life (such as regulating body temperature, blood pressure, and glucose and calcium levels). Homeostatic adjustments may be stimulated by changes, for instance, in body position or activity level, or need for energy to sustain cellular functions involving "redox" homeostasis (i.e., maintaining a nucleophilic tone) (e.g., [27]).

Conversely, allostasis or resilience tends to refer to more widespread adaptive adjustments in response to environmental stressors across neuroendocrine, cardiovascular, and immune systems in order to maintain homeostasis and the stability of the human organism.

2.12 Energy and Metabolic Processes

The health of the whole person is described as a *dynamic*, integrative entity in which growth and developmental complexity, resilient and healing processes and functions, biorhythms, and homeostasis, for example, *are driven by energy and metabolic processes of the person*. Energy is produced biochemically, metabolically, electrically, and electromagnetically [13, 21, 74, 75]. For instance, energy is observed in electric charges within the brain captured by EEG, the heartbeat recorded by an ECG, the coherent maintenance of various circadian rhythms throughout the human, as well as in myriad biochemical processes that underlie development, resilience, healing, and homeostasis. Transformation of energy from one form to another occurs at all levels of the human organism and is known as *transduction*. Each time a stress mediator or emotion-carrying neuropeptide (ligand) binds to their specific cell receptor it "transduces" neurochemical information into another form that can be used by the cell. Energy is required to transport and process biological information and induce biomodulating adaptive changes among biological interrelationships while maintaining the stability, cohesiveness, and optimal functioning of the person [13, 74, 76, 77].

Metabolic Processes Living cells depend on metabolic processes to obtain and utilize energy from the chemical bonds in food, specifically from carbohydrates (especially glucose) and lipids (monoacylglycerols and long-chain fatty acids) as well as to utilize protein (small peptides and amino acids) for cellular building and reparation. Sugar and fat molecules for instance are broken down to produce energy in the form of ATP, and NADH, an electron donor molecule implicated in myriad anabolic reactions [78]. Metabolic processes are essential for homeostasis, growth and development, healing, resilience, and reproduction.

Although an in-depth description of metabolic processes, circadian rhythms, and electromagnetic fields is beyond the scope of this book, energy is included in the model in growing recognition that there are many forms of energy in the human organism including subtle energy fields and electromagnetic fields which influence biological functions throughout the human body (e.g., [75, 79]) (Part IV Chap. 14). Today, the use of mechanical energy via ultrasound devices is used to promote healing [80]. And some energy-driven therapies, though controversial, such as acupuncture and therapeutic touch appear to contribute to some forms of dynamic healing as well [19, 81, 82].

When environmental demands are short term, the healthy human organism is easily able to replenish its energy stores. When stress is long term, these energy stores can become depleted, compromising the body's ability to execute normal resilient adaptations throughout the biology of the person and to maintain homeostasis.

2.13 Sense of Coherence (See Fig. 2.1)

A personal sense of coherence is a well-described psychological phenomenon of the person and refers to a general orientation or feeling of overall confidence that internal and external environmental stimuli are predictable and explainable and that personal and social resources are available to manage these stimuli successfully [83]. For example, Antonovsky's sense of coherence refers to an overall sense of meaning, comprehensibility and manageability of a situation. A recent study reported that a high sense of coherence in breast cancer survivors was predictive of survival [84].

Coherence may also be understood biologically. In a review of research on the variation and amplitude of autonomous biological rhythms (such as the heart rate, respirations, blood pressure, EEGs), Thayer and Sternberg (2006) deduced that a state of coherence, an indicator of resilience and health, was reflected by optimal variation in biological rhythms throughout the person. Bernardi's earlier research (2001) on biological rhythms noted that the slightest perceived stress disturbed this harmonious variation, whereas prayer appeared to amplify the variation across different rhythms such that they fell into "synchrony or resonance." These variations in amplitude may be seen as a measure of the extent to which the body is using energy efficiently to fuel the myriad functions of the body.

Every cell in the body vibrates with energy exchanges including the electrically charged particles associated with biological interactions [85, 86]. When dynamic biological systems and natural oscillators, such as heart rate, *function in harmony*, optimal well-being exists [86, 87]. Accordingly, one way to gather information about the resilience of the human organism is by recording the amplitude and variations in the body's biological rhythms associated with the heart rate, respiration, and brain waves (e.g., [88]). Thayer and Sternberg's review (2006) showed that coherent, regular, and variable rhythms with greater amplitude were associated with lower systemic inflammation, lower blood sugar levels, and more effective immune functioning compared to controls. Systemic inflammation can be a marker of advanced cancer.

Coherent variability in the body's biorhythms has also been related to autonomic nervous system balance (SNS/PNS) at basal physiology and signifies conservation of energy and optimal resilience [89, 90]. In contrast, biorhythms distinguished by *irregular variations with short or reduced amplitudes* have been associated with chronic negative emotions. The Framingham Heart Study among others has shown that reduced heart rate variability (HRV) is associated with increased risk for mortality [16, 91]. HRV refers to the generally equivalent length of time between heart beats characterized by greater consistent amplitudes (e.g., [88]).

2.14 Nursing Approaches (See Parts IV and V)

Nursing aims to put the patient and family caregiver in his or her optimal overall biological and behavioral condition of resilience and health in order to enable successful management of cancer-related stresses throughout the diagnostic, treatment, transition to survivorship and end-of-life phases. Each phase may have overlapping and unique goals, but in principle, the main overall nursing goals of practice are to:

1. Develop a meaningful nurse–patient and caregiver relationship within which patient and caregiver goals may be optimally realized (separately and together).
2. Reduce the emotional distress of patients and caregivers.
3. Provide symptomatic relief.
4. Strengthen the patients' (and caregiver's) biological and behavioral resilience across the disease, treatment, recovery, and supportive care continuum in order to: (a) enhance quality of life and well-being; (b) support the goals of treatment; (c) enhance the patient's ability to tolerate and complete treatment; and (d) lengthen the patient's survival, ability to live well with cancer, and/or experience a sense of well-being at the end of life.
5. Provide emotional and physical comfort and solace.

Specific nursing goals regarding the caregiver: Given the health-related interdependence between patients and caregivers, and converging evidence that caregiver health declines as cancer progresses, nurses must act to ensure that the caregivers' unmet needs are also addressed from diagnosis. Beyond establishing a meaningful nurse–patient and caregiver relationship, these needs may include:

1. Education about the disease and treatment.
2. Information about caregiving skill preparedness (e.g., self-management).
3. Strategies to manage patient symptoms and how to work effectively with the nurse.
4. Strategies to reduce caregiver's psychological distress and caregiver burden at various phases, but especially during the terminal phase.
5. Strategies to enhance caregiver quality of life by addressing pertinent self-care and lifestyle behaviors (e.g., [55, 92]).
6. Providing the caregiver with emotional support, active listening, and access to relevant resources.

The suggested psychosocial nursing approaches described in Part IV of the book were selected due to their safety for patients (do no harm) and growing scientific consensus of their therapeutic benefit based on cumulative evidence from meta-analyses, systematic reviews, clinical trials as well as qualitative studies, and prospective and cross-sectional studies.

Quality of the Nurse–Patient Relationship (Part IV Chaps. 8 and 19)

It is within the context of a meaningful nurse–patient and caregiver relationship that healing moments may be optimized and resilience enhanced [16, 53, 56]. Psychosocial nursing approaches are predicated on a compassionate, collaborative approach with the patient and caregiver distinguished by a shared sense of purpose, mutual respect, effective communication, and sense of connectedness (Part IV, Chap. 11). These relationships are further strengthened through the nurse's demonstrated competence (skills) in the use of appropriate conventional and complementary nursing strategies, including communication techniques [67, 93].

Table 2.1 summarizes the clinical objectives to consider in promoting healing and resilience tailored to the needs of each individual. The successful realization of each objective depends on the quality of the nurse's relationship with the patient (and family caregiver), the nurse's scientific knowledge of stress, healing, and resilience, and effective psychosocial skills. It depends on *the nurse knowing* the patient and caregiver in terms of developmental age, spiritual and supportive connections, beliefs, values, and assumptions about the world and the individual's place in it,

Table 2.1 General nursing objectives

• Decrease the biological and psychological stress response
• Effectively manage patient symptoms
• Promote emotion-regulating stress-coping adaptive cognitive and behavioral capabilities
• Enhance self-regulation behaviors
• Cultivate self-efficacy beliefs, and skills such as problem solving (self-management skills); other strategies tailored to the cancer experience; and use of relevant resources
• Help patient cultivate new meanings, purposes, and hopes anchored in clinical reality
• Protect patient hope
• Encourage healthy resilient-promoting lifestyle behaviors (physical activity, nutrition and diet, and weight)
• Optimize patient's positive beliefs about wellness and placebo-inducing healing capabilities
• Identify potential physical and social environmental stimuli that may impede the individual's innate healing capabilities (nocebo effects)
• Use of the relaxation response, mindful meditation, yoga, therapeutic use of touch, and reiki
• Share relevant disease and treatment-related information
• Promote family support, sense of connectedness, and use of strategies to seek and obtain needed support
• Support greater self and spiritual awareness
• Encourage, as appropriate, advance care planning

their current and past life experiences which have a bearing on resilient capabilities, and their fears, anxieties, coping efforts, and resources. Knowing the patient combined with scientific knowledge of cognitive expectations may be leveraged by the nurse to strengthen treatment efficacy and promote symptom management (e.g., [20]).

The nature of the nurse–patient/caregiver relationship will be shaped by the nurse's own sense of wholeness, past experiences, compassion, sensitivity, resilience, scientific knowledge, clinical expertise, communication skills, decision-making skills as well as by feeling supported by the nursing leadership and team, and by collaborative working relationships with the oncology team (e.g., [53, 94]).

Timing of Interventions

Scientific data suggest that the patient and caregiver benefit from nursing interventions that are implemented *early in the illness and treatment* trajectory so that fears, concerns, and potential obstacles to optimizing their health goals including how to manage their stress may be properly addressed. Cancer patients who received *early* clinical interventions to promote resilience were shown to adhere better to their treatment and demonstrate longer survival rates [51, 65, 95, 96]. Moreover, patients with the highest levels of perceived informal support in baseline measures of resilient-promoting interventions also had the highest rates of survival. This finding suggests that support should be assessed during the diagnostic phase, and as indicated, an intervention to strengthen the patient's supportive relationships, would be carried out [52].

What may be most clinically beneficial to the patient and caregiver is to offer an integrated, multimodal resilient-promoting psychosocial intervention that starts in the diagnostic phase and continues regularly throughout each phase of the continuum, providing the patient and caregiver with relevant information and skills and emotional support to effectively manage the diverse challenges they must face. Each phase offers an opportunity for the nurse to anticipate, reinforce, or introduce stressor-specific knowledge and skills to reduce emotional distress and strengthen healing and resilient adaptive processes.

Format

Clinical approaches may be offered one-on-one or in group workshops. The psychosocial nursing strategies in this book are summarized in Part IV and provide evidenced-based suggestions that will hopefully serve as a clinical incentive for developing further defensible clinical interventions. These clinical interventions may contribute to comprehensive multitargeted, multimodal nursing approaches that target both unique and overlapping endpoints to promote the whole individual's healing and resilient capabilities at each phase of the illness trajectory. In essence, the book consists of a foundational repository of psychosocial interventions based on the latest scientific evidence that may be evaluated across clinical contexts, altered, improved, and supplanted by future clinical interventions based on well-designed randomized controlled studies.

References

1. Skretkowicz V. Florence Nightingale's notes on nursing and notes on nursing for the labouring classes. New York: Springer Publishing Co; 2010.
2. Nightingale F. Notes on nursing: what it is, and what it is not. New York: Dover Publications, Inc; 1969.
3. Sinclair S, Beamer K, Hack TF, McClement S, Raffin Bouchal S, Chochinov HM, et al. Sympathy, empathy, and compassion: a grounded theory study of palliative care patients' understandings, experiences, and preferences. Palliat Med. 2017;31(5):437–47; PubMed PMID: 27535319. Pubmed Central PMCID: PMC5405806. Epub 2016/08/19. eng.
4. von Bertalanffy L. General system theory: foundations, development, applications. New York: Braziller; 1968.
5. Brito Pons G, Librada Flores S. Compassion in palliative care: a review. Curr Opin Support Palliat Care. 2018;12(4):472–9.
6. Kershaw T, Ellis KR, Yoon H, Schafenacker A, Katapodi M, Northouse L. The interdependence of advanced cancer patients' and their family caregivers' mental health, physical health, and self-efficacy over time. Anna Behav Med. 2015;49(6):901–11; PubMed PMID: 26489843. Pubmed Central PMCID: PMC4825326. Epub 2015/10/23. eng.
7. Johansen S, Cvancarova M, Ruland C. The effect of cancer patients' and their family caregivers' physical and emotional symptoms on caregiver burden. Cancer Nurs. 2018;41(2):91–9; PubMed PMID: 28426539. Epub 2017/04/21. eng.
8. Erickson HL. Modeling and role-modeling: a view from the client's world. Cedar Park, TX: Unicorns Unlimited; 2006.
9. Gottlieb L, Gottlieb B. The development/health framework within the McGill model of nursing: 'Laws of nature' guiding whole person care. Adv Nurs Sci. 2007;30(1):E43–57.
10. McEwen BS. Physiology and neurobiology of stress and adaptation: central role of the brain. Physiol Rev. 2007;87(3):873–904; PubMed PMID: 17615391. Epub 2007/07/07. eng.
11. Bronfenbrenner U. The ecology of human development: experiments by nature and design. Cambridge, MA: Harvard University Press; 1981.
12. Gottlieb L, Rowat K. The McGill model of nursing: a practice derived model. Adv Nurs Sci. 1987;9(4):51–61.
13. Thayer JF, Sternberg E. Beyond heart rate variability: vagal regulation of allostatic systems. Ann N Y Acad Sci. 2006;1088:361–72; PubMed PMID: 17192580.
14. Park CL. Making sense of the meaning literature: an integrative review of meaning making and its effects on adjustment to stressful life events. Psychol Bull. 2010;136(2):257–301; PubMed PMID: 20192563. Epub 2010/03/03. eng.
15. Kaptchuk TJ, Friedlander E, Kelley JM, Sanchez MN, Kokkotou E, Singer JP, et al. Placebos without deception: a randomized controlled trial in irritable bowel syndrome. PLoS One. 2010;5(12):e15591; PubMed PMID: 21203519. Pubmed Central PMCID: PMC3008733. Epub 2011/01/05.
16. Benson H, Stark M. Timeless healing : the power and biology of belief. New York: Simon & Schuster; 1997.
17. Folkman S, Lazarus RS, Dunkel-Schetter C, DeLongis A, Gruen RJ. Dynamics of a stressful encounter: cognitive appraisal, coping, and encounter outcomes. J Pers Soc Psychol. 1986;50(5):992–1003; PubMed PMID: 3712234. Epub 1986/05/01. eng.
18. Folkman S. Positive psychological states and coping with severe stress. Soc Sci Med. 1997;45(8):1207–21; PubMed PMID: 9381234. Epub 1997/09/25. eng.
19. Reeve K, Black PA, Huang J. Examining the impact of a healing touch intervention to reduce posttraumatic stress disorder symptoms in combat veterans. Psychol Trauma. 2020;12(8):897–903; PubMed PMID: 33346680. Epub 2020/12/22. eng.

20. Colloca L, Barsky AJ. Placebo and nocebo effects. N Engl J Med. 2020;382(6):554–61; PubMed PMID: 32023375. Epub 2020/02/06. eng.
21. Jaross W. Hypothesis on interactions of macromolecules based on molecular vibration patterns in cells and tissues. Front Biosci (Landmark Ed). 2018;23:940–6; PubMed PMID: 28930582. Epub 2017/09/21. eng.
22. Rubik B. Energy medicine and the unifying concept of information. Altern Ther Health Med. 1995;1(1):34–9; PubMed PMID: 9419791.
23. Jain S, Mills PJ. Biofield therapies: helpful or full of hype? A best evidence synthesis. Int J Behav Med. 2010;17(1):1–16; PubMed PMID: 19856109. Pubmed Central PMCID: PMC2816237. Epub 2009/10/27. eng.
24. McEwen B. Central effects of stress hormones in health and disease: understanding the protective and damaging effects of stress and stress mediators. Eur J Pharmacol. 2008;583:174–85.
25. McEwen BS. Protective and damaging effects of stress mediators: central role of the brain. Dialogues Clin Neurosci. 2006;8(4):367–81; PubMed PMID: 17290796. Pubmed Central PMCID: PMC3181832. Epub 2007/02/13. eng.
26. Juruena MF. Early-life stress and HPA axis trigger recurrent adulthood depression. Epilepsy Behav. 2014;38:148–59; PubMed PMID: 24269030. Epub 2013/11/26. Eng.
27. Kirtonia A, Sethi G, Garg M. The multifaceted role of reactive oxygen species in tumorigenesis. Cell Mol Life Sci. 2020;77(22):4459–83; PubMed PMID: 32358622. Epub 2020/05/03. eng.
28. Sillar JR, Germon ZP, DeIuliis GN, Dun MD. The role of reactive oxygen species in acute myeloid leukaemia. Int J Mol Sci. 2019;20(23):6003; PubMed PMID: 31795243. Pubmed Central PMCID: PMC6929020. Epub 2019/12/05. eng.
29. McEwen BS. Stress, adaptation, and disease. Allostasis and allostatic load. Ann N Y Acad Sci. 1998;840:33–44; PubMed PMID: 9629234. Epub 1998/06/18. eng.
30. Ryff CD. Psychological well-being revisited: advances in the science and practice of eudaimonia. Psychother Psychosom. 2014;83(1):10–28; PubMed PMID: 24281296. Pubmed Central PMCID: PMC4241300. Epub 2013/11/28. eng.
31. Dantzer R, O'Connor JC, Freund GG, Johnson RW, Kelley KW. From inflammation to sickness and depression: when the immune system subjugates the brain. Nat Rev Neurosci. 2008;9(1):46–56; PubMed PMID: 18073775. Pubmed Central PMCID: PMC2919277. Epub 2007/12/13. eng.
32. Wang H, Unternaehrer JJ. Epithelial-mesenchymal transition and cancer stem cells: at the crossroads of differentiation and dedifferentiation. Dev Dyn. 2019;248(1):10–20; PubMed PMID: 30303578. Epub 2018/10/12. eng.
33. Yang J, Antin P, Berx G, Blanpain C, Brabletz T, Bronner M, et al. Guidelines and definitions for research on epithelial-mesenchymal transition. Nat Rev Mol Cell Biol. 2020;21(6):341–52; PubMed PMID: 32300252. Pubmed Central PMCID: PMC7250738. Epub 2020/04/18. eng.
34. Angka L, Khan ST, Kilgour MK, Xu R, Kennedy MA, Auer RC. Dysfunctional natural killer cells in the aftermath of cancer surgery. Int J Mol Sci. 2017;18(8):1787; PubMed PMID: 28817109. Pubmed Central PMCID: PMC5578175. Epub 2017/08/18. eng.
35. Cohen L, Parker PA, Vence L, Savary C, Kentor D, Pettaway C, et al. Presurgical stress management improves postoperative immune function in men with prostate cancer undergoing radical prostatectomy. Psychosom Med. 2011;73(3):218–25; PubMed PMID: 21257977. Epub 2011/01/25. eng.
36. Fava GA, McEwen BS, Guidi J, Gostoli S, Offidani E, Sonino N. Clinical characterization of allostatic overload. Psychoneuroendocrinology. 2019;108:94–101; PubMed PMID: 31252304. Epub 2019/06/30. eng.
37. Spiegel D. The developing mind. New York: The Guilford Press; 1997.
38. McEwen BS, Gray J, Nasca C. Recognizing resilience: learning from the effects of stress on the brain. Neurobiol Stress. 2015;1:1–11; PubMed PMID: 25506601. Pubmed Central PMCID: PMC4260341. Epub 2014/12/17. Eng.
39. McEwen BS, Nasca C, Gray JD. Stress effects on neuronal structure: hippocampus, amygdala, and prefrontal cortex. Neuropsychopharmacology. 2016;41(1):3–23; PubMed PMID: 26076834. Pubmed Central PMCID: PMC4677120. Epub 2015/06/17. eng.

40. Karatsoreos IN, McEwen BS. Annual research review: the neurobiology and physiology of resilience and adaptation across the life course. J Child Psychol Psychiatry. 2013;54(4):337–47; PubMed PMID: 23517425. Epub 2013/03/23. eng.
41. McEwen BS. In pursuit of resilience: stress, epigenetics, and brain plasticity. Ann N Y Acad Sci. 2016;1373(1):56–64; PubMed PMID: 26919273. Epub 2016/02/27. eng.
42. Leventhal H, Phillips LA, Burns E. The common-sense model of self-regulation (CSM): a dynamic framework for understanding illness self-management. J Behav Med. 2016;39(6):935–46; PubMed PMID: 27515801. Epub 2016/08/16. eng.
43. Mount BM, Boston PH, Cohen SR. Healing connections: on moving from suffering to a sense of well-being. J Pain Symptom Manag. 2007;33(4):372–88; PubMed PMID: 17397699. Epub 2007/04/03. eng.
44. McEwen BS, Morrison JH. The brain on stress: vulnerability and plasticity of the prefrontal cortex over the life course. Neuron. 2013;79(1):16–29; PubMed PMID: 23849196. Pubmed Central PMCID: PMC3753223. Epub 2013/07/16. eng.
45. Dutcher JM, Creswell JD. The role of brain reward pathways in stress resilience and health. Neurosci Biobehav Rev. 2018;95:559–67; PubMed PMID: 30477985. Epub 2018/11/28. eng.
46. Sapolsky RM. Stress and plasticity in the limbic system. Neurochem Res. 2003;28(11):1735–42; PubMed PMID: 14584827. Epub 2003/10/31. eng.
47. House SL. Psychological distress and its impact on wound healing: an integrative review. J Wound Ostomy Continence Nurs. 2015;42(1):38–41. PubMed PMID: 25549307. Epub 2014/12/31. eng.
48. Kiecolt-Glaser JK, Loving TJ, Stowell JR, Malarkey WB, Lemeshow S, Dickinson SL, et al. Hostile marital interactions, proinflammatory cytokine production, and wound healing. Arch Gen Psychiatry. 2005;62(12):1377–84; PubMed PMID: 16330726. Epub 2005/12/07. eng.
49. Carlson LE, Tamagawa R, Stephen J, Drysdale E, Zhong L, Speca M. Randomized-controlled trial of mindfulness-based cancer recovery versus supportive expressive group therapy among distressed breast cancer survivors (MINDSET): long-term follow-up results. Psycho-Oncology. 2016;25(7):750–9; PubMed PMID: 27193737. Epub 2016/05/20. eng.
50. van Vulpen JK, Peeters PH, Velthuis MJ, van der Wall E, May AM. Effects of physical exercise during adjuvant breast cancer treatment on physical and psychosocial dimensions of cancer-related fatigue: a meta-analysis. Maturitas. 2016;85:104–11; PubMed PMID: 26857888. Epub 2016/02/10. eng.
51. Andersen BL, Thornton LM, Shapiro CL, Farrar WB, Mundy BL, Yang HC, et al. Biobehavioral, immune, and health benefits following recurrence for psychological intervention participants. Clin Cancer Res. 2010;16(12):3270–8; PubMed PMID: 20530702. Pubmed Central PMCID: PMC2910547. Epub 2010/06/10. eng.
52. Lutgendorf S, De Geest K, Bender D, Ahmed A, Goodheart M, Dahmoush L, Zimmerman M, et al. Social influences on clinical outcomes of patients with ovarian cancer. J Clin Oncol. 2012;30(23):2885–90.
53. Thorne SE, Kuo M, Armstrong EA, McPherson G, Harris SR, Hislop TG. 'Being known': patients' perspectives of the dynamics of human connection in cancer care. Psycho-Oncology. 2000;14(10):887–98; discussion 99-900. PubMed PMID: 16200520. Epub 2005/10/04. eng.
54. Buber M. I thou. New York, New York: Simon & Schuster; 1970.
55. World Cancer Research Fund AIfcr. Diet, nutrition, physical activity and cancer: a global perspective. Summary of 3rd expert report. Continuous update project expert report. dietandcancerreport.org; 2018.
56. Benson H, Friedman R. Harnessing the power of the placebo effect and renaming it "remembered wellness". Annu Rev Med. 1996;47:193–9; PubMed PMID: 8712773.
57. Petrie KJ, Rief W. Psychobiological mechanisms of placebo and nocebo effects: pathways to improve treatments and reduce side effects. Annu Rev Psychol. 2019;70:599–625; PubMed PMID: 30110575. Epub 2018/08/16. eng.

58. Ben-Shaanan TL, Azulay-Debby H, Dubovik T, Starosvetsky E, Korin B, Schiller M, et al. Activation of the reward system boosts innate and adaptive immunity. Nat Med. 2016;22(8):940–4; PubMed PMID: 27376577. Epub 2016/07/05. eng.
59. Ben-Shaanan TL, Schiller M, Azulay-Debby H, Korin B, Boshnak N, Koren T, et al. Modulation of anti-tumor immunity by the brain's reward system. Nat Commun. 2018;9(1):2723; PubMed PMID: 30006573. Pubmed Central PMCID: PMC6045610. Epub 2018/07/15. eng.
60. Hagger MS, Koch S, Chatzisarantis NLD, Orbell S. The common sense model of self-regulation: meta-analysis and test of a process model. Psychol Bull. 2017;143(11):1117–54; PubMed PMID: 28805401. Epub 2017/08/15. eng.
61. Seiler A, Jenewein J. Resilience in cancer patients. Front Psych. 2019;10:208; PubMed PMID: 31024362. Pubmed Central PMCID: PMC6460045. Epub 2019/04/27. eng.
62. Chirico A, Lucidi F, Merluzzi T, Alivernini F, Laurentiis M, Botti G, et al. A meta-analytic review of the relationship of cancer coping self-efficacy with distress and quality of life. Oncotarget. 2017;8(22):36800–11; PubMed PMID: 28404938. Pubmed Central PMCID: PMC5482699. Epub 2017/04/14. eng.
63. Trevino KM, Prigerson HG, Epstein RM, Duberstein PR. Reply to Hope, optimism, and the importance of caregivers in end-of-life care. Cancer. 2019;125(23):4330–1; PubMed PMID: 31381145. Epub 2019/08/06. eng.
64. Henselmans I, Fleer J, de Vries J, Baas PC, Sanderman R, Ranchor AV. The adaptive effect of personal control when facing breast cancer: cognitive and behavioural mediators. Psychol Health. 2010;25(9):1023–40; PubMed PMID: 20204948. Epub 2010/03/06. eng.
65. Andersen BL, Yang HC, Farrar WB, Golden-Kreutz DM, Emery CF, Thornton LM, et al. Psychologic intervention improves survival for breast cancer patients: a randomized clinical trial. Cancer. 2008;113(12):3450–8; PubMed PMID: 19016270. Pubmed Central PMCID: PMC2661422. Epub 2008/11/19. eng.
66. Hartley S, Raphael J, Lovell K, Berry K. Effective nurse-patient relationships in mental health care: a systematic review of interventions to improve the therapeutic alliance. Int J Nurs Stud. 2020;102:103490; PubMed PMID: 31862531. Pubmed Central PMCID: PMC7026691. Epub 2019/12/22. eng.
67. Thorne S, Hislop TG, Kim-Sing C, Oglov V, Oliffe JL, Stajduhar KI. Changing communication needs and preferences across the cancer care trajectory: insights from the patient perspective. Support Care Cancer. 2014;22(4):1009–15; PubMed PMID: 24287506. Epub 2013/11/30. eng.
68. Hostinar CE. Recent developments in the study of social relationships, stress responses, and physical health. Curr Opin Psychol. 2015;5:90–5; PubMed PMID: 26366429. Pubmed Central PMCID: PMC4562328. Epub 2015/09/15. Eng.
69. Wiechula R, Conroy T, Kitson AL, Marshall RJ, Whitaker N, Rasmussen P. Umbrella review of the evidence: what factors influence the caring relationship between a nurse and patient? J Adv Nurs. 2016;72(4):723–34; PubMed PMID: 26692520. Epub 2015/12/23. eng.
70. National Comprehensive Cancer Network. Distress management. Clinical practice guidelines. J Natl Compr Canc Netw. 2003;1(3):344–74; PubMed PMID: 19761069. Epub 2003/07/01. eng.
71. Colloca L, Finniss D. Nocebo effects, patient-clinician communication, and therapeutic outcomes. JAMA. 2012;307(6):567–8; PubMed PMID: 22318275. Pubmed Central PMCID: PMC6909539. Epub 2012/02/10. eng.
72. Colloca L, Lopiano L, Lanotte M, Benedetti F. Overt versus covert treatment for pain, anxiety, and Parkinson's disease. Lancet Neurol. 2004;3(11):679–84; PubMed PMID: 15488461. Epub 2004/10/19. eng.
73. McEwen BS, Eiland L, Hunter RG, Miller MM. Stress and anxiety: structural plasticity and epigenetic regulation as a consequence of stress. Neuropharmacology. 2012;62(1):3–12; PubMed PMID: 21807003. Pubmed Central PMCID: PMC3196296. Epub 2011/08/03. eng.
74. McEwen BS, Wingfield JC. What is in a name? Integrating homeostasis, allostasis and stress. Horm Behav. 2010;57(2):105–11; PubMed PMID: 19786032. Pubmed Central PMCID: PMC2815096. Epub 2009/09/30. eng.
75. Kučera O, Cifra M. Radiofrequency and microwave interactions between biomolecular systems. J Biol Phys. 2016;42(1):1–8; PubMed PMID: 26174548. Pubmed Central PMCID: PMC4713408. Epub 2015/07/16. eng.

76. Accardi MV, Daniels BA, Brown PM, Fritschy JM, Tyagarajan SK, Bowie D. Mitochondrial reactive oxygen species regulate the strength of inhibitory GABA-mediated synaptic transmission. Nat Commun. 2014;5:3168; PubMed PMID: 24430741. Epub 2014/01/17. eng.
77. Vijgen GH, Bouvy ND, Leenen L, Rijkers K, Cornips E, Majoie M, et al. Vagus nerve stimulation increases energy expenditure: relation to brown adipose tissue activity. PLoS One. 2013;8(10):e77221; PubMed PMID: 24194874. Pubmed Central PMCID: PMC3806746. Epub 2013/11/07. eng.
78. Alberts B, Johnson A, Lewis J. Molecular biology. 4th ed. New York: Garland Science; 2002.
79. Skarja M, Jerman I, Ruzic R, Leskovar RT, Jejcic L. Electric field absorption and emission as an indicator of active electromagnetic nature of organisms--preliminary report. Electromagn Biol Med. 2009;28(1):85–95; PubMed PMID: 19337899. Epub 2009/04/02. eng.
80. Shimizu T, Fujita N, Tsuji-Tamura K, Kitagawa Y, Fujisawa T, Tamura M, et al. Osteocytes as main responders to low-intensity pulsed ultrasound treatment during fracture healing. Sci Rep. 2021;11(1):10298; PubMed PMID: 33986415. Pubmed Central PMCID: PMC8119462. Epub 2021/05/15. eng.
81. Lutgendorf SK, Mullen-Houser E, Russell D, Degeest K, Jacobson G, Hart L, et al. Preservation of immune function in cervical cancer patients during chemoradiation using a novel integrative approach. Brain Behav Immun. 2010;24(8):1231–40; PubMed PMID: 20600809. Pubmed Central PMCID: PMC3010350. Epub 2010/07/06. eng.
82. Miller KR, Patel JN, Symanowski JT, Edelen CA, Walsh D. Acupuncture for cancer pain and symptom management in a palliative medicine clinic. Am J Hosp Palliat Care. 2019;36(4):326–32; PubMed PMID: 30286611. Epub 2018/10/06. eng.
83. Antonovsky H, Sagy S. The development of a sense of coherence and its impact on responses to stress situations. J Soc Psychol. 1986;126(2):213–25; PubMed PMID: 3724090. Epub 1986/04/01. eng.
84. Lindblad C, Langius-Eklöf A, Petersson LM, Sackey H, Bottai M, Sandelin K. Sense of coherence is a predictor of survival: a prospective study in women treated for breast cancer. Psycho-Oncology. 2018;27(6):1615–21; PubMed PMID: 29528529. Epub 2018/03/13. eng.
85. Lednyiczky G, Zhalko-Tytarenko O, Topping S, Buzasi T. Human endogenous electromagnetic field fluctuation in relation to an organism's reaction to the EMF of body constituent substances. http//wwwenergetic-medicinenet/research/HumanEMfieldfluctuation.pdf. Accessed 18 Oct 2011. 1998.
86. Rubik B. The biofield hypothesis: its biophysical basis and role in medicine. J Altern Complement Med. 2002;8(6):703–17; PubMed PMID: 12614524.
87. Pert CB, Dreher HE, Ruff MR. The psychosomatic network: foundations of mind-body medicine. Altern Ther Health Med. 1998;4(4):30–41; PubMed PMID: 9656499.
88. Diaz-Rodriguez L, Arroyo-Morales M, Fernandez-de-las-Penas C, Garcia-Lafuente F, Garcia-Royo C, Tomas-Rojas I. Immediate effects of reiki on heart rate variability, cortisol levels, and body temperature in health care professionals with burnout. Biol Res Nurs. 2011;13(4):376–82; PubMed PMID: 21821642. Epub 2011/08/09. eng.
89. Bhasin MK, Dusek JA, Chang BH, Joseph MG, Denninger JW, Fricchione GL, et al. Relaxation response induces temporal transcriptome changes in energy metabolism, insulin secretion and inflammatory pathways. PLoS One. 2013;8(5):e62817; PubMed PMID: 23650531. Pubmed Central PMCID: PMC3641112. Epub 2013/05/08. eng.
90. Dusek JA, Benson H. Mind-body medicine: a model of the comparative clinical impact of the acute stress and relaxation responses. Minn Med. 2009;92(5):47–50; PubMed PMID: 19552264. Pubmed Central PMCID: PMC2724877. Epub 2009/06/26. eng.
91. Tsuji H, Venditti FJ Jr, Manders ES, et al. Reduced heart rate variability and mortality risk in an elderly cohort: the Framingham heart study. Circulation. 1994;90(2):878–83.
92. Sun V, Grant M, Koczywas M, Freeman B, Zachariah F, Fujinami R, et al. Effectiveness of an interdisciplinary palliative care intervention for family caregivers in lung cancer. Cancer. 2015;121(20):3737–45; PubMed PMID: 26150131. Pubmed Central PMCID: PMC4592403. Epub 2015/07/08. eng.
93. Wittenberg E, Reb A, Kanter E. Communicating with patients and families around difficult topics in cancer care using the COMFORT communication curriculum. Semin Oncol Nurs.

2018;34(3):264–73; PubMed PMID: 30100368. Pubmed Central PMCID: PMC6156926. Epub 2018/08/14. eng.
94. Banerjee SC, Manna R, Coyle N, Shen MJ, Pehrson C, Zaider T, et al. Oncology nurses' communication challenges with patients and families: a qualitative study. Nurse Educ Pract. 2016;16(1):193–201; PubMed PMID: 26278636. Pubmed Central PMCID: PMC4961044. Epub 2015/08/19. eng.
95. Bakitas MA, Tosteson TD, Li Z, Lyons KD, Hull JG, Li Z, et al. Early versus delayed initiation of concurrent palliative oncology care: patient outcomes in the ENABLE III randomized controlled trial. J Clin Oncol. 2015;33(13):1438–45; PubMed PMID: 25800768. Pubmed Central PMCID: PMC4404422 online at www.jco.org. Author contributions are found at the end of this article. Epub 2015/03/25. eng.
96. Dionne-Odom JN, Azuero A, Lyons KD, Hull JG, Tosteson T, Li Z, et al. Benefits of early versus delayed palliative care to informal family caregivers of patients with advanced cancer: outcomes from the ENABLE III randomized controlled trial. J Clin Oncol. 2015;33(13):1446–52; Epub 2015/03/25. eng.
97. Servan-Schreiber D. Anticancer: a new way of life. New York: Viking; 2008.
98. Bernardi L, Sleight P, Bandinelli G, Cencetti S, Fattorini L, Wdowczyc-Szulc J, et al. Effect of rosary prayer and yoga mantras on autonomic cardiovascular rhythms: comparative study. BMJ. 2001;323(7327):1446–9; PubMed PMID: 11751348. Pubmed Central PMCID: 61046.

Part II

Resilience

Introduction

Part II examines resilience or human adaptation to environmental challenges from both biological and psychological perspectives in Chaps. 3, 4, and 5, respectively [1]. Resilience develops over the lifespan prompted by the need to adapt to environmental stressors. The growing person learns to successfully adjust to age-appropriate challenges in his or her increasingly complex environment through the growing acquisition of emotion-regulating, cognitive, emotional, and behavioral coping responses with guidance from supportive relationships. In the person's ongoing interactions with the environment, he or she develops an expanding repertoire of behavioral skills and cognitive flexibility that also enable better management of similar stressors in the future. Chapter 3 discusses the diverse forms of psychological stress and its cumulative effects on the whole person. Chapter 4 presents a review of biological processes of resilience; Chapter 5 reviews psychosocial processes of resilience. Although the biology and behavior of resilience are interrelated and integrated within the human organism, Part II presents each resilient process separately due to the amount of scientific information to cover. It is hoped that in this way clinical awareness of key biological and psychological clinical targets and processes associated with resilience will be heightened [2].

References

1. McEwen BS. Physiology and neurobiology of stress and adaptation: central role of the brain. Physiol Rev. 2007;87(3):873–904; PubMed PMID: 17615391. Epub 2007/07/07. eng.
2. McEwen BS. Biomarkers for assessing population and individual health and disease related to stress and adaptation. Metabolism. 2015;64(3 Suppl 1):S2–S10; PubMed PMID: 25496803. Epub 2014/12/17. eng.

Psychological Stress

3.1 Introduction

Human resilience occurs across the lifespan in response to environmental stressors and daily experiences. In the past, "perceived stress" was often dismissed as part of the daily reality of a busy life. If you stopped to acknowledge feelings of stress, you were apt to be met with phrases such as "you'll get over it" or "we all get stressed from time to time, you just have to deal with it." Meanwhile, the corrosive effects of repeatedly experienced acute and/or chronic stress on the neurophysiology of the person proceeded unabated at subclinical levels, disrupting critical signaling pathways so that the individual was made more vulnerable over time to the onset of various chronic illnesses such as cancer (e.g., [1]).

Today, the scientific evidence testifies to the potentially debilitating effects of unregulated stress to the whole individual. Key factors include whether the stress exposure is experienced over a short or prolonged period and is perceived to be manageable or unmanageable. How stress is managed across the lifespan not only influences later quality of life, but also is empirically known to influence adherence to treatment and even long-term survivability in patients with cancer (e.g., [2, 3]).

This chapter describes different forms of environmental stress; some serve to trigger the development and maintenance of resilience; others that are perceived as a profound threat to personal survival or well-being may be more difficult to overcome, contributing to widespread neurophysiological disruptions and even damage to cells and DNA that predispose the individual to chronic illness such as cancer.

Objectives
At the end of the chapter, you will be able to:
- Describe characteristics of acute and chronic forms of psychological stress.
- Learn about the relationships among stress, development, and resilience in early childhood and adulthood.
- Describe stress in terms of allostasis, allostatic load, and allostatic overload.

Clinical Anecdote 3.1
In those days, the biological dangers of living with stress every day was given short shrift for a career woman in her 30's. The ability to juggle half a dozen responsibilities was a 'can do' source of personal pride for the 60's generation. At the height of this madness, I had two young children under 10, was working part time and studying for a PHD in Nursing. In retrospect, I should have known better, but in those days no one really understood stress; it was a moniker for all the nonspecific symptoms that we really did not pay much attention to like headaches or fatigue. Certainly the biological link to illness did not figure prominently in one's daily life. In the 1980's women were expected to multi task without complaint. Being a workaholic was a kind of badge of pride. It never occurred to any of us that the stress of trying to juggle many hats in order to achieve personal goals could also be altering neural structures and physiological pathways even as we thought that we were coping well.

3.2 Definitions

According to Lazarus and Folkman (1984) [4], perceived stress occurs when environmental demands exceed one's ability to cope. A more comprehensive definition is that psychological stress is the "human response" to internal and external environmental stressors that result in myriad disruptions across interacting socioemotional, cognitive, and behavioral dimensions anchored by neurostructural, physiological, and molecular pathways and functions of the whole person [1]. Psychological stress also refers to human responses to social or physical threats that cause biochemical, epigenetic, cognitive, and behavioral changes which have the potential to disrupt homeostasis, resilience, and healing [5, 6]. Psychological stress ultimately has to do with how the individual perceives stressors and the meanings they attribute to them which launch consequential effects throughout the whole being.

Sources of stress occur within the individual's extrinsic and intrinsic environment: Extrinsic sources include social, physical, financial, work-related stressors, and/or medically related treatment. Intrinsic sources include viruses, bacteria, oxidative stress, debilitating, or life-threatening chronic illnesses such as cancer.

Emotional Distress An estimated 20–52% of patients with cancer experience some level of distress which is associated with underlying neurobiological adjustments as a response to a stressful event or situation (e.g., [7]). Distress typically refers to an "unpleasant experience of a psychological (i.e., cognitive, behavioral, emotional) social, spiritual and/or physical nature that interferes with the ability to cope effectively with a threat such as cancer, its physical symptoms and its treatment" ([8] p. 6). Distress can range from "typical common feelings of vulnerability, sadness, fear, depression, anxiety, panic social isolation, to emotional distress and existential and/or spiritual crisis" ([8] p. 6). Emotional distress within the context of cancer care tends to be triggered by the cancer diagnosis or recurrence, and cancer-related treatments including major surgeries, chemotherapy and radiation therapy. A history of early childhood adversity predicts greater emotional reactivity to stressors, such as depression in individuals who experience a cancer diagnosis in adulthood [9, 10].

Existential Distress (Review Part IV Chap. 10) This form of distress refers to a demoralized state characterized by symptoms of hopelessness, and a lack of purpose, or meaning in life [11]. Existential distress may be observed at any phase of the continuum, with one half to one-third of cancer survivors having reported experiencing such distress [12]. It is especially evident in individuals facing progressive disease and a shortened life which profoundly challenge global assumptions and beliefs about the world and the self [13–15]. These individuals may be identified by their sense of hopelessness, meaninglessness, lack of purpose, and a desire for a hastened death.

Properties of Psychological Stress

Psychological stress varies in its intensity, frequency, duration, predictability, and meaning significance to the individual within the context of his/her perceived ability to cope effectively. It may be described in terms of the individual's cognitive perceptions of the stressor and emotional reactions to it, such as a cancer- or treatment-related perceived threat. The individual's subsequent behavioral response will depend in part on whether the stressor is perceived to be manageable or uncontrollable [16, 17]. Individuals with cancer are also exposed to the physiological stress effects of the tumor and the treatment causing the release of inflammatory cytokines associated with various symptoms that may also influence the individual's experience of psychological stress [1, 18].

Benefits or Harmful Effects (Review Parts II and III)

Stressors may have beneficial or deleterious effects that impact resilience and health across the lifespan (Fig. 3.1). Stressors such as learning to ride a bike or studying for an exam generally facilitate the acquisition of cognitive and behavioral coping skills and cultivate experiential knowledge that is the predicate of cognitive flexibility and greater resilience, often to a higher level of adaptive integration. Conversely

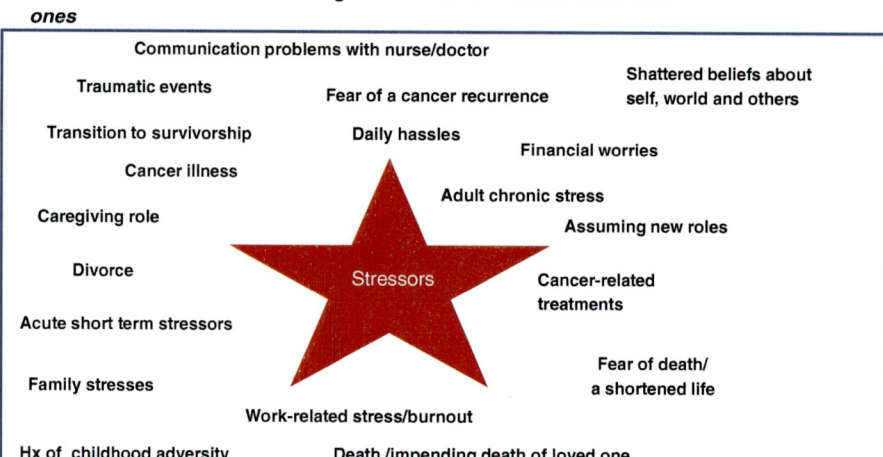

Fig. 3.1 Sources of stress/distress (e.g., [8, 9, 12, 19, 20])

stressors which exceed the individual's perceived ability to cope can cause disruptive and potentially damaging biological and psychological effects throughout the whole person. If stress is prolonged and untreated, it leads to serious pathophysiological impairments that promote the development of chronic illnesses, cancer, and even a shortened life [21, 22].

Stress has also been shown to have a biphasic effect with differential beneficial and harmful effects on the human organism as a function of the duration and intensity of the stress. As we will discuss below and in Chaps. 4 and 5, an acute stressor initially activates the biological stress system (HPA axis, ANS) including an immune response via released glucocorticoids and noradrenaline in order to respond effectively to the perceived challenge which has an overall adaptive and resilient-promoting effect, short term [23]. Conversely, chronic exposure to the same stressor over several weeks may lead to immune suppression.

3.3 Acute Stressor Effects (Review Part II Chaps. 4 and 5)

Acute stressors refer to short-lived, stressful situations causing a rise in negative emotional reactions such as increased tension, anxiety, fearfulness, and/or distress. In the main, an acute stress response of limited duration promotes resilience and survival through neural–endocrine, autonomic, immune, metabolic, and cardiovascular adjustments that are restored or healed in the aftermath of the stress and result in adaptive neural circuitry [24]. An acute stressor event may also refer to the demands and hassles characterized by minor, stress-induced but manageable situations [6].

Examples of an acute stressor event include getting children dressed and to school before going to work, ensuring supper is on the table and helping with homework, going to a job interview, an exam, or failing an important exam. But the impact again is usually limited in duration and is generally manageable. Over time, a healthy stress response becomes accustomed to similar demands, and with an effective coping and supportive system, the activated biological stress response tends to diminish [6].

Conversely, a singular often unpredictable, even life-threatening acute event such as a cancer diagnosis may cause prolonged anxiety distinguished by posttraumatic stress-related symptoms of uncontrollable intrusive ideation and behavioral avoidance that if unaddressed may lead to progressive neurobiological impairments throughout the whole person [25]. Stress-induced sleeplessness even for a few nights can cause circadian disruptions that are associated with increased appetite, increased evening cortisol levels, increased release of inflammatory cytokines, increased sympathetic activity with a corresponding decrease in the parasympathetic nervous system associated with neurophysiological healing and restorative processes [26].

Acute stress effects go beyond behavioral manifestations of anxiety and emotional distress or depressive symptoms to underlying usually reversal neurobiological changes in the aftermath of stress in healthy brains. Challenges of short duration that are effectively managed and result in the acquisition of cognitive and behavioral skills associated with a belief in one's ability to manage similar stressors in the future are sometimes referred to as "good" stress (Part II Chaps. 4 and 5).

3.4 Prolonged Psychological Stress (Review Part III, Chaps. 6 and 7)

Chronic psychological stress causes widespread neurobiological, emotional, social, and behavioral disruptions throughout the human organism. Over time, the chronic stress of a hostile work environment or marriage or even ineffectively managed daily demands and hassles over a lifetime cause changes to the neural architecture of the brain such as the hippocampus, prefrontal cortex (PFC), and amygdala, and also alters physiological and molecular pathways, functions, and behavior [6, 27]. Even when repeated demands become habituated over time, epigenetic changes may persist for instance in the dentate gyrus of the hippocampus with long-term possible consequences for how effectively individuals may manage future stresses [6, 18, 28]. The dentate gyrus plays an important role in memory formation and learning.

Unregulated chronic stress can be associated with a damaged negative glucocorticoid feedback system that normally regulates the on/off switch for the stress response system (i.e., HPA and SAM axes) [29]. The toxic effects of ongoing circulating glucocorticoids and other mediators result in structural remodeling of neurons in the hippocampus with dendritic culling, synaptic alterations, and suppression of neurogenesis in the dentate gyrus. It may also lead to a decrease in neural flexibility, a critical factor in maintaining biological and consequently behavioral resilience.

Similarly, the PFC undergoes stress-induced changes to neural structures such as dendritic culling and a decrease in apical dendritic spine density in the medial PFC pyramidal neurons. These changes are associated with difficulties in cognitive capability, decision making, learning, and memory. Conversely, stress mediated by glucocorticoid levels causes dendritic hypertrophy and an increase in spine density in the basolateral amygdala, causing increased anxiety and other mood alterations [29].

Elevated circulating glucocorticoids can lead to glucose intolerance and insulin insensitivity, obesity, and altered metabolism of the extracellular matrix [30]. Other serious consequences include the suppression of cell-mediated immune functions, critical for cancer cell surveillance and eradication [31, 32]. The impaired stress response system continues to promote a systemic inflammatory environment conducive to the eventual manifestation of diverse chronic illnesses, including tumorigenesis, cancer progression, and metastases in genetically predisposed individuals [21, 32].

Chronic psychological stress ultimately threatens homeostasis by suppressing restorative healing processes and by over taxing metabolic processes essential for adaptive resilience, internal coherence, development, and health [29, 33, 34]. Unmanaged, acute, and chronic forms of stress produce widespread biochemical, epigenetic, neurophysiological, cognitive, and behavioral impairments threatening the health and survivability of the individual [29]. These neurobiological changes may proceed unknowingly by both the distressed individual fighting cancer and his or her healthcare provider treating him, potentially further compromising the ability to tolerate treatment to completion or even prolong survivorship.

Early Childhood Adversity (ECA)

How the individual copes with current stressors depends in part on previously developed resilience and life experiences. Positive experiences in early childhood play a critical role in developing a healthy brain architecture with the capacity for flexibly adapting to future challenges throughout life mediated by corresponding gene expression and epigenetic changes [18]. Conversely early childhood adversity tends to limit the brain's capacity for flexible adaptation in the face of future stressors. As will be discussed in chapters on resilience the brain is the main organ of stress and adaptation which directs the biological and behavioral responses to environmental challenges. The most vulnerable stages of development are the prenatal, infancy, childhood, and adolescence, although every phase of the lifespan exposed to chronic stress and related stress mediators causes deleterious impairments to the neurobiology of the individual with potential long-lasting consequential effects [18, 35, 36].

Studies of early chronic adversity experienced during the sensitive prenatal phase, infancy, early childhood, and adolescence have been shown to exert profound and long-lasting effects on the growing individual's development and adaptive capabilities in adulthood [35, 36]. These individuals may have endured maternal or caregiver deprivation, neglect, constant conflict, aggression, hostility, physical and/or emotional abuse, and/or extreme poverty (low SES) and tend to be at most risk for developing adult depression, cognitive difficulties, and emotional reactivity as well as chronic illnesses, such as cancer or diabetes. The higher risk of chronic illness in these adults may be caused by low-grade systemic inflammation and immune dysfunction (e.g., [9, 37, 38]). A cross-sectional study of 92 patients with metastatic lung cancer showed that early childhood maltreatment appeared to be significantly and positively associated with physical problems, depression, distress, and increased C-reactive protein (CRP) in adult patients [10]. Multivariate analyses strongly suggested that this sustained adversity ($\beta = 0.37, p = 0.001$) and elevated CRP ($\beta = 0.30, p = 0.004$) independently accounted for depression in these adult patients. Early childhood adversity was also found to explain a significant proportion of physical symptoms ($\beta = 0.35, p = 0.004$).

Early childhood adversity appears to have long-lasting deleterious effects on an individual's emotional reactivity to stress and resilient capabilities in adulthood, strongly suggesting that these adults once diagnosed with cancer may be particularly vulnerable in the face of significant health-related and existential challenges. Although healing processes reemerge when chronic stress ends, biological differences persist, compared to humans with a nurturing, nondistressed upbringing [18, 29]. The findings point toward the importance of assessing for early childhood adversity in patients newly diagnosed with cancer. It also underscores the need for RCTS that evaluate the effectiveness of psychosocial interventions tailored to patients with cancer and a history of early childhood adversity in order to optimize their healing and resilient processes.

Animal Research can illuminate what happens at a biological and molecular level under conditions of early chronic stress that may help to explain the potentially devastating consequences observed in adulthood. Rat models indicate that the expression of numerous genes in the aftermath of stress appears to differ from the pattern of gene expression associated with prechronic stress and also compared to never chronically stressed controls [18, 29]. The brain's morphology or structural plasticity which is altered in response to chronic and acute stress may heal almost to its prestressed size and structure given optimal conditions, but nonetheless still demonstrates evidence of nonhealing. Dendrites, for instance, in the prefrontal cortex appear pruned compared to their normal dendritic display, while dendrites in the amygdala are fuller and more dense compared to controls suggesting greater negative emotional reactions in response to subsequent stressors (e.g., [6]).

These neural changes, observed in animal studies, may inform the emotional behaviors of some individuals who appear to overreact emotionally at the cancer diagnosis, are not easily consoled, and persist in showing signs of emotional distress and even depressive symptoms when other cancer patients have already accepted their clinical reality and are coping well.

Summary

Emotional distress and existential distress are two forms of psychological stress that are typically experienced by patients with cancer, with progressively consequential neurobiological sequelae as psychological stress progresses from a relatively temporary state to a prolonged unregulated state in the absence of coping and supportive resources [1, 8]. The extent to which stressors impact the individual's emotional or existential distress is influenced by the stage of development, sex, environmental context, early childhood adversity, the meaning attributed to the stressor, its perceived manageability, the type and stage of the cancer, coping efforts, as well as one's use of personal and social resources, and healthy lifestyle behaviors. For instance, prolonged stress may be reflected and exacerbated by not eating healthily, neglecting to exercise, lack of sleep, and being overweight. Finally, two additional biological systems contribute to the widespread life-threatening effects of chronic stress: pro-inflammatory epigenetic changes, and the metabolic burden caused by maintaining homeostasis in the presence of widespread impairments, including the overproduction of extremely toxic reactive oxygen species (ROS) (Review Part III Chaps. 6 and 7).

3.5 Need for Measurable Terminology for "Stress"

Because descriptions of human stress tend to be ambiguous, a scientific initiative was undertaken to develop cumulative measures based on interrelated indicators of relevant physiological systems and behaviors in order to optimize clinical knowledge of the impact of the stress experience on the whole person (e.g., [1, 39, 40]). As a consequence, psychological stress has been operationalized in terms of allostasis, allostatic load, and allostatic overload (Table 3.1) [41, 42]. These terms describe the extent to which changes in interactive physiological (and behavioral) systems have been impacted by stress. The intent is to create a cumulative index based on biopsychosocial and behavioral indicators that would contribute to clinical understanding of the individual's potential stress-related risks to resilience and health based on their biological and behavioral profile (e.g., [43]). A few clinical tools based on either biological markers of stress and/or combined with psychosocial, cognitive, and behavioral markers of stress continue to be developed in order to identify individuals with the stress-related burden of allostatic load and, in particular, allostatic overload [1, 39].

Table 3.1 Measurable terms used to describe various forms of stress effects in relation to resilience (Review Part II Chaps. 4 and 5; Part III Chaps. 6 and 7)

Scientific terms to describe stress effects on mind and body	Definition
Allostasis	Neurobiological, social, physical, and behavioral adjustments triggered by manageable, short-term stressors that are restored (healed) to their normal parametric range when stress ends. Includes good and tolerable forms of stress effects [39]
Allostatic load (AL)	AL refers to the cumulative chronic effects of daily stresses and moderate-to-major stressful experiences associated with neural–biological impairments and inadequate psychosocial, cognitive, and lifestyle behaviors which may be reflective of psychosocial stresses that exceed or severely strain the ability to cope [1] may also be described as toxic stress defined as "strong, frequent stressors and/or prolonged activation of the stress response system in the absence or paucity of personal and social resources" ([1] p. 95)
Allostatic overload (OL)	OL is the result of chronic toxic stress that *exceeds the individual's coping capabilities*, causing progressive systemic neurophysiological and metabolic impairments and psychosocial, cognitive, and behavioral disturbances which lead to disease [1]

3.6 Cumulative Measures of Stress (Table 3.2)

A clinical stress profile *should* include psychosocial and behavioral stress effects such as emotional reactions (anxiety, depression, emotional distress, existential suffering), cognitive and behavioral coping responses, personal resources (e.g., optimism, self-esteem), supportive relationships, lifestyle behaviors (i.e., physical activity, diet, and weight) as well as empirically known stress-related neurobiological and immune mediators that together serve as biosocial and behavioral markers of interrelated systems of resilience (Table 3.2) [1, 39, 55]. Altogether the

Table 3.2 Key biological and behavioral indicators to consider in assessing allostatic load, allostatic overload [1, 6, 13, 44, 45]

History of stressful experiences [1, 29, 33, 42, 46]
– Recent, past, early life adversity
– Threat, emotional distress, existential distress, anxiety, depressed mood, fear
Sources of stress: Identify
– Short acute stressors or prolonged and chronic (e.g., family, career, financial, cancer, treatment, partner/spouse)
Adaptive versus maladaptive coping and support behaviors [13, 47–51] (See Chaps. 5, 9–11)
– Evidence of coping strategies (positive reappraisal, use of emotion-focused, problem-focused, meaning-focused coping and behavioral coping strategies, success reaching out and maintaining meaningful informal and formal supportive relationships
– Maladaptive behaviors such as blaming, escape/avoidance
– Sees illness as a challenge versus a source of distress
Personal resources/strengths and supportive relationships (self-efficacy, optimism,) (see Chaps. 9–11)
Poor versus *healthy lifestyle behaviors* [52]
– Diet, physical activity/exercise, sleep, weight, use of alcohol and drugs, smoking
Stress mediators [1, 53, 54]
– Levels of urinary NOR, cortisol
– Serum measure of DHEA-S inflammatory cytokines (IL-6, IL-2, NK cells, cytotoxic T cells)
– C-reactive protein (↑ed. response to inflammation)
Other physiological biomarkers [1]
– Resting systolic and diastolic blood pressure, body mass index, waist–hip ratio, high-density lipoprotein (HDL) and low-density lipoprotein (LDL) cholesterol triglycerides, fasting glucose
Symptoms/side effects [1, 8]
– Emotional distress, anxiety, fear, sadness, depressive mood, existential distress, pain (e.g., lack of meaning, purpose), difficulty concentrating and or making health-related decisions, fatigue, difficulty sleeping, suppressed cell-mediated immunity, loss of appetite, loss of weight, difficulty breathing
Distress thermometer ≥ 4 severe distress; < minimal to small–moderate distress [8]
Health-related outcomes (see Chaps. 6, 7, and 9–11)
– Increased vulnerability to chronic illness according to genetic predisposition: cancer progression, cancer recurrence
– QOL, psychological well-being, PTG
Clinical implications
Identifying stress-inducing vulnerability during the cancer continuum: at diagnosis, presurgery and postsurgery, pre and during other medical treatments, transition to survivorship, and end of life

multidimensional cumulative measure, in principle, would capture stress-induced changes in the pattern of parametric values implicated in an individual's resilient adaptation to stress, providing clinical insights into healing processes and health status.

A cumulative measure of stress might point toward allostatic load signaling a clinical (and nursing) urgency to identify potential sources of biological and psychosocial stress, and intervene accordingly ([1] p. 95). For instance, glucocorticoids (cortisol) measured at different times of the day might show a lack of variation in parametric values that would normally vary in association with normal circadian rhythm. Circulating glucocorticoids are also part of the network of mutually regulating mediators involved in the biological stress response system. Among its functions is to signal the downregulation of the stress regulating HPA axis via negative feedback loops to the pituitary (ACTH) and the hypothalamus (CRH) when stress ends. Stress-related mediators are either restored to normal function in the aftermath of stress or contribute to systemic inflammation due in part to glucocorticoid dysregulation. The use of psychosocial criteria alone provides only a partial clinical profile of the cumulative effects of stress on the whole person [1, 8, 56]. A combination of biological and behavioral indicators allows for the identification of distinct patterns of interrelationships among the variables as a function of the impact of stress on the whole person. If a cumulative measure is reflective of allostatic load, this may signal the potential for cancer progression, or a cancer recurrence.

Eventually, a cumulative measure may be used to identify dysregulated endpoints that can serve as the intentional targets of multimodal medical and nursing interventions to enhance resilience and health-related outcomes (Review Part III Chaps. 6 and 7). Patient findings based on a cumulative index may enable researchers and clinicians to prognosticate across the various patterns of endpoints and/or discern critical biological tipping points, for instance, between allostatic load and allostatic overload, the latter of which could signal the likely onset of a cancer recurrence. The research data strongly underscore the importance of doing clinical assessments of psychological distress and their underlying causes in all patients with cancer, and their caregivers at regular intervals across the disease and treatment spectrum, starting at diagnosis [8, 57, 58].

NCCN Guidelines on distress management recommends the use of the distress thermometer (DT), a 10-point screening tool for identifying the level of distress and its underlying causes (that is sources of patient distress) through its follow-up "Problem List" of clinical concerns based on a yes/no format ([8] p. 8). All "yes" responses signal the clinical need to investigate further, and to subsequently intervene immediately, starting at the diagnostic phase. The DT is a validated tool that has been used numerous times in patients with various cancers. A meta-analysis of 42 studies and 14,000 patients revealed a pooled sensitivity of 81% and a pooled specificity of 72% at a diagnostic cut off of "4" [59]. However, findings from a Dutch study suggested using a cutoff of "7" to reduce the number of false-positive results [60]. As a well-known, widely used diagnostic measure of emotional distress, the DT items are similar to the diagnostic, psychosocial "clinimetric" criteria used to identify individuals with allostatic overload [1].

Cancer and Allostatic Load/Overload Because most individuals with cancer experience psychological stress throughout the stages of the disease and treatment, the use of a cumulative index of allostatic load (AL) could be more helpful than a single measure, such as C-reactive protein (C-RP) or IL-6, to evaluate the magnitude of stress effects or its burden throughout the whole individual [61]. A systematic review ($n = 12$) of allostatic load in cancer and a "mini" meta-analysis found significant correlations between AL and (a) cancer-related stress, (b) a positive cancer history, (c) posttraumatic growth, (d) resilience, and v) cancer-specific mortality and cancer pathology [61]. The meta-analysis ($n = 4$) of patients with cancer showed that a 1-unit augmentation in AL was related to a 9% increase in cancer-related mortality. The results lacked clarity regarding causal direction between cancer and AL and could not reliably identify the set of optimal variables that should be included in a cumulative index to assess AL (or chronic stress). Nonetheless, a cumulative index based on selected immune (e.g., inflammatory cytokines), cardiovascular (e.g., heart rate variability—HRV) and metabolic as well as neuroendocrinal indicators should be added to lifestyle behaviors in further research using actual patient data (see Table 3.2).

3.7 Nursing Implications

The disruptive effects of stress throughout the whole being particularly when long standing pose an important potential risk to health, to treatment completion and even to survivorship of patients with cancer and their caregivers. The impact of a stress exposure depends on: the types of stressors (psychological or physical, unpredictable, or predictable, manageable or not), the duration, frequency and intensity of the stressor(s), past and present history of adversity, gender, genetic makeup, epigenetic alterations, coping strategies, other personal resources, perceived supportive relationships, and the developmental stage of the stress exposure(s). Cancer is both a reflection of cumulative stress and a source of current physiological stress.

Given the prevalence of episodic distress among individuals with cancer, the important takeaways from this chapter are as follows:

1. Do a distress screening as part of regular clinical assessments on all individuals diagnosed with cancer throughout the continuum and especially around points of clinical vulnerability such as at diagnosis, before and after a cancer-related surgery, the beginning of chemotherapy, a cancer recurrence and transition to palliative care or survivorship.
2. Individuals scoring below "4" on the DT suggesting minimal or manageable stress-related levels nonetheless should be offered nursing interventions that would protect, buffer, and/or strengthen their resilient capabilities along the continuum. These folks may benefit from suggested strategies to manage various stressors over the course of treatment and recovery (To be discussed in Parts IV and V).
3. Incorporate into clinical assessments biological as well as behavioral indicators of stress (markers or endpoints). These assessments may eventually help to estimate the

impact of stress throughout the whole person. Use indicators that reflect interrelated systems of resilience known to be critically impacted by stress, for instance, immune functioning the glucocorticoid negative feedback system. These indicators also may be used to evaluate whether targeted nursing interventions have the intended neurophysiological as well as psychosocial effect. In the absence of a standardized index, consider generating your own index of lifestyle behaviors, physiological measures, and biological mediators associated with resilient capabilities based on meta-analyses and reviews of key endpoints in cancer care (Table 3.2) [61].
4. As prolonged chronic stress (allostatic load) leads to pervasive and destructive neurobiological effects exacerbated by dysfunctional lifestyle behaviors, poor coping skills, and inadequate support from important relationships, interventions to improve their behavioral resilient capabilities must be considered and evaluated with both behavioral and biological indicators of resilience (Review Clinical approaches in Part IV).
5. Deleterious effects of early life chronic stress appear to be long-lasting, as evidenced by the manifestation of chronic illnesses and cognitive and psychological difficulties in managing stress as adults [9, 10, 38]. These individuals deserve our particular attention and, especially, the opportunity to benefit regularly from the quality of the nurse–patient relationship as well as other therapeutic approaches described in Part IV.

On a final note, the seamless and reversible interactions between environmental stresses and gene expression continue throughout each developmental stage as individuals are affected by diverse life experiences. Current thinking is that these epigenetic changes provide *opportunities for nurses to "redirect"* unhealthy behavioral tendencies toward more adaptive interactions with the environment, via a number of nursing interventions to be discussed throughout this book [18]. According to developmental resilience studies, nursing interventions may promote compensatory pathways toward better resilient capabilities even when chronic stress effects, such as heightened emotional reactivity in individuals with a history of early childhood adversity, appear to be long-lasting. Notwithstanding, the first clinical imperative is to assess and offer clinical interventions that reduce the patient's psychological stress in order to protect his/her overall ability to fight cancer, optimally tolerate the medical treatments, live well during survival, and/or optimize his quality of life during the end-of-life phase.

References

1. Fava GA, McEwen BS, Guidi J, Gostoli S, Offidani E, Sonino N. Clinical characterization of allostatic overload. Psychoneuroendocrinology. 2019;108:94–101; PubMed PMID: 31252304. Epub 2019/06/30. eng.
2. Bakitas M, Lyons KD, Hegel MT, Balan S, Brokaw FC, Seville J, et al. Effects of a palliative care intervention on clinical outcomes in patients with advanced cancer: the project ENABLE II randomized controlled trial. JAMA. 2009;302(7):741–9; PubMed PMID: 19690306. Pubmed Central PMCID: PMC3657724. Epub 2009/08/20. eng.

3. Temel JS, Greer JA, Muzikansky A, Gallagher ER, Admane S, Jackson VA, et al. Early palliative care for patients with metastatic non-small-cell lung cancer. N Engl J Med. 2010;363(8):733–42; PubMed PMID: 20818875. Epub 2010/09/08. eng.
4. Lazarus RS, Folkman S. Stress, appraisal and coping. New York: Springer; 1984.
5. Juruena MF, Agustini B, Cleare AJ, Young AH. A translational approach to clinical practice via stress-responsive glucocorticoid receptor signaling. Stem Cell Investig. 2017;4:13; PubMed PMID: 28275643. Pubmed Central PMCID: PMC5334557. Epub 2017/03/10. eng.
6. McEwen BS. Physiology and neurobiology of stress and adaptation: central role of the brain. Physiol Rev. 2007;87(3):873–904; PubMed PMID: 17615391. Epub 2007/07/07. eng.
7. Mehnert A, Hartung TJ, Friedrich M, Vehling S, Brähler E, Härter M, et al. One in two cancer patients is significantly distressed: prevalence and indicators of distress. Psychooncology. 2018;27(1):75–82; PubMed PMID: 28568377. Epub 2017/06/02. eng.
8. Riba MB, Donovan KA, Andersen B, Braun I, Breitbart WS, Brewer BW, et al. Distress management, version 3.2019, NCCN clinical practice guidelines in oncology. J Natl Compr Canc Netw. 2019;17(10):1229–49; PubMed PMID: 31590149. Pubmed Central PMCID: PMC6907687. Epub 2019/10/08. eng.
9. Miller GE, Chen E, Parker KJ. Psychological stress in childhood and susceptibility to the chronic diseases of aging: moving toward a model of behavioral and biological mechanisms. Psychol Bull. 2011;137(6):959–97; PubMed PMID: 21787044. Pubmed Central PMCID: PMC3202072. Epub 2011/07/27. eng.
10. McFarland DC, Nelson C, Miller AH. Early childhood adversity in adult patients with metastatic lung cancer: cross-sectional analysis of symptom burden and inflammation. Brain Behav Immun. 2020;90:167–73; PubMed PMID: 32791210. Pubmed Central PMCID: PMC7544656. Epub 2020/08/14. eng.
11. Kissane DW, Clarke DM, Street AF. Demoralization syndrome--a relevant psychiatric diagnosis for palliative care. J Palliat Care. 2001;17(1):12–21; PubMed PMID: 11324179. Epub 2001/04/28. eng.
12. Vehling S, Philipp R. Existential distress and meaning-focused interventions in cancer survivorship. Curr Opin Support Palliat Care. 2018;12(1):46–51; PubMed PMID: 29251694. Epub 2017/12/19. eng.
13. Park CL. Making sense of the meaning literature: an integrative review of meaning making and its effects on adjustment to stressful life events. Psychol Bull. 2010;136(2):257–301; PubMed PMID: 20192563. Epub 2010/03/03. eng.
14. Park CL, Edmondson D, Fenster JR, Blank TO. Meaning making and psychological adjustment following cancer: the mediating roles of growth, life meaning, and restored just-world beliefs. J Consult Clin Psychol. 2008;76(5):863–75; PubMed PMID: 18837603. Epub 2008/10/08. eng.
15. Robinson S, Kissane DW, Brooker J, Burney S. A systematic review of the demoralization syndrome in individuals with progressive disease and cancer: a decade of research. J Pain Symptom Manag. 2015;49(3):595–610; PubMed PMID: 25131888. Epub 2014/08/19. eng.
16. Hagger MS, Koch S, Chatzisarantis NLD, Orbell S. The common sense model of self-regulation: meta-analysis and test of a process model. Psychol Bull. 2017;143(11):1117–54; PubMed PMID: 28805401. Epub 2017/08/15. eng.
17. Leventhal H, Phillips LA, Burns E. The common-sense model of self-regulation (CSM): a dynamic framework for understanding illness self-management. J Behav Med. 2016;39(6):935–46; PubMed PMID: 27515801. Epub 2016/08/16. eng.
18. McEwen BS, Gray J, Nasca C. Recognizing resilience: learning from the effects of stress on the brain. Neurobiol Stress. 2015;1:1–11; PubMed PMID: 25506601. Pubmed Central PMCID: PMC4260341. Epub 2014/12/17. Eng.
19. Park CL, Cho D, Blank TO, Wortmann JH. Cognitive and emotional aspects of fear of recurrence: predictors and relations with adjustment in young to middle-aged cancer survivors. Psychooncology. 2013;22(7):1630–8; PubMed PMID: 23060271. Epub 2012/10/13. eng.
20. Wilson J, Kirshbaum M. Effects of patient death on nursing staff: a literature review. Br J Nurs. 2011;20(9):559–63; PubMed PMID: 21647017. Epub 2011/06/08. eng.

21. Kirtonia A, Sethi G, Garg M. The multifaceted role of reactive oxygen species in tumorigenesis. Cell Mol Life Sci. 2020;77(22):4459–83; PubMed PMID: 32358622. Epub 2020/05/03. eng.
22. McEwen BS, Eiland L, Hunter RG, Miller MM. Stress and anxiety: structural plasticity and epigenetic regulation as a consequence of stress. Neuropharmacology. 2012;62(1): 3–12; PubMed PMID: 21807003. Pubmed Central PMCID: PMC3196296. Epub 2011/08/03. eng.
23. Holzel BK, Carmody J, Evans KC, Hoge EA, Dusek JA, Morgan L, et al. Stress reduction correlates with structural changes in the amygdala. Soc Cogn Affect Neurosci. 2010;5(1): 11–7; PubMed PMID: 19776221. Pubmed Central PMCID: PMC2840837. Epub 2009/09/25. eng.
24. McEwen B. Central effects of stress hormones in health and disease: understanding the protective and damaging effects of stress and stress mediators. Eur J Pharmacol. 2008;583: 174–85.
25. Chan CMH, Ng CG, Taib NA, Wee LH, Krupat E, Meyer F. Course and predictors of post-traumatic stress disorder in a cohort of psychologically distressed patients with cancer: a 4-year follow-up study. Cancer. 2018;124(2):406–16; PubMed PMID: 29152719. Epub 2017/11/21. eng.
26. McEwen BS, Karatsoreos IN. Sleep deprivation and circadian disruption: stress, allostasis, and allostatic load. Sleep Med Clin. 2015;10(1):1–10; PubMed PMID: 26055668. Epub 2015/06/10. eng.
27. McEwen BS. Sleep deprivation as a neurobiologic and physiologic stressor: Allostasis and allostatic load. Metab Clin Exp. 2006;55(10 Suppl 2):S20–3; PubMed PMID: 16979422. Epub 2006/09/19. eng.
28. Hunter RG, Murakami G, Dewell S, Seligsohn M, Baker ME, Datson NA, et al. Acute stress and hippocampal histone H3 lysine 9 trimethylation, a retrotransposon silencing response. Proc Natl Acad Sci U S A. 2012;109(43):17657–62; PubMed PMID: 23043114. Pubmed Central PMCID: PMC3491472. Epub 2012/10/09. eng.
29. McEwen BS. Neurobiological and systemic effects of chronic stress. Chronic stress (Thousand Oaks). 2017;1:2470547017692328; PubMed PMID: 28856337. Pubmed Central PMCID: PMC5573220. Epub 2017/09/01. eng.
30. Cain DW, Cidlowski JA. Immune regulation by glucocorticoids. Nat Rev Immunol. 2017;17(4):233–47; PubMed PMID: 28192415. Epub 2017/02/14. eng.
31. Shimba A, Ikuta K. Control of immunity by glucocorticoids in health and disease. Semin Immunopathol. 2020;42(6):669–80; PubMed PMID: 33219395. Epub 2020/11/22. eng.
32. Wang M, Zhao J, Zhang L, Wei F, Lian Y, Wu Y, et al. Role of tumor microenvironment in tumorigenesis. J Cancer. 2017;8(5):761–73; PubMed PMID: 28382138. Pubmed Central PMCID: PMC5381164. Epub 2017/04/07. eng.
33. McEwen BS. Protective and damaging effects of stress mediators: central role of the brain. Dialogues Clin Neurosci. 2006;8(4):367–81; PubMed PMID: 17290796. Pubmed Central PMCID: PMC3181832. Epub 2007/02/13. eng.
34. McEwen BS, Nasca C, Gray JD. Stress effects on neuronal structure: hippocampus, amygdala, and prefrontal cortex. Neuropsychopharmacology. 2016;41(1):3–23; PubMed PMID: 26076834. Pubmed Central PMCID: PMC4677120. Epub 2015/06/17. eng.
35. Pervanidou P, Chrousos GP. Metabolic consequences of stress during childhood and adolescence. Metab Clin Exp. 2012;61(5):611–9; PubMed PMID: 22146091. Epub 2011/12/08. eng.
36. Pervanidou P, Chrousos GP. Early-life stress: from neuroendocrine mechanisms to stress-related disorders. Horm Res Paediatr. 2018;89(5):372–9; PubMed PMID: 29886495. Epub 2018/06/11. eng.
37. Fagundes CP, Glaser R, Kiecolt-Glaser JK. Stressful early life experiences and immune dysregulation across the lifespan. Brain Behav Immun. 2013;27(1):8–12; PubMed PMID: 22771426. Pubmed Central PMCID: PMC3518756. Epub 2012/07/10. eng.
38. Danese A, McEwen BS. Adverse childhood experiences, allostasis, allostatic load, and age-related disease. Physiol Behav. 2012;106(1):29–39; PubMed PMID: 21888923. Epub 2011/09/06. eng.

References

39. McEwen BS. Biomarkers for assessing population and individual health and disease related to stress and adaptation. Metab Clin Exp. 2015;64(3 Suppl 1):S2–S10; PubMed PMID: 25496803. Epub 2014/12/17. eng.
40. Seeman TE, McEwen BS, Rowe JW, Singer BH. Allostatic load as a marker of cumulative biological risk: MacArthur studies of successful aging. Proc Natl Acad Sci U S A. 2001;98(8):4770–5; PubMed PMID: 11287659. Pubmed Central PMCID: PMC31909. Epub 2001/04/05. eng.
41. McEwen BS. Stress, adaptation, and disease. Allostasis and allostatic load. Ann N Y Acad Sci. 1998;840:33–44; PubMed PMID: 9629234. Epub 1998/06/18. eng.
42. McEwen BS. Allostasis and allostatic load: implications for neuropsychopharmacology. Neuropsychopharmacology. 2000;22(2):108–24; PubMed PMID: 10649824. Epub 2000/01/29. eng.
43. Walker FR, Pfingst K, Carnevali L, Sgoifo A, Nalivaiko E. In the search for integrative biomarker of resilience to psychological stress. Neurosci Biobehav Rev. 2017;74(Pt B):310–20; PubMed PMID: 27179452. Epub 2016/05/18. eng.
44. Dunkel-Schetter C, Feinstein LG, Taylor SE, Falke RL. Patterns of coping with cancer. Health Psychol. 1992;11(2):79–87; PubMed PMID: 1582383. Epub 1992/01/01. eng.
45. World Cancer Research Fund AIfcr. Diet, nutrition, physical activity and cancer: a global perspective. Continuous update project expert report. dietandcancerreport.org: wcrf; 2018.
46. McEwen B, Stellar E. Stress and the individual. Mechanisms leading to disease. Arch Intern Med. 1993;153(18):2093–101; PubMed PMID: 8379800. Epub 1993/09/27. eng.
47. Folkman S, Lazarus RS, Dunkel-Schetter C, DeLongis A, Gruen RJ. Dynamics of a stressful encounter: cognitive appraisal, coping, and encounter outcomes. J Pers Soc Psychol. 1986;50(5):992–1003; PubMed PMID: 3712234. Epub 1986/05/01. eng.
48. House JS, Kahn RL. Measures and concepts of social support. New York: Academic Press; 1985.
49. House JS, Landis KR, Umberson D. Social relationships and health. Science. 1988;241(4865):540–5; PubMed PMID: 3399889. Epub 1988/07/29. eng.
50. House J. Work, stress and social support. Reading, MA: Addison-Wesley; 1981.
51. Folkman S, Lazarus RS, Gruen RJ, DeLongis A. Appraisal, coping, health status, and psychological symptoms. J Pers Soc Psychol. 1986;50(3):571–9; PubMed PMID: 3701593. Epub 1986/03/01. eng.
52. World Cancer Research Fund AIfcr. Diet, nutrition, physical activity and cancer: a global perspective. Summary of 3rd expert report. Continuous update project expert report. dietandcancerreport.org; 2018.
53. Seeman TE, Gruenewald TL, Cohen S, Williams DR, Matthews KA. Social relationships and their biological correlates: coronary artery risk development in Young adults (CARDIA) study. Psychoneuroendocrinology. 2014;43:126–38; PubMed PMID: 24703178. Epub 2014/04/08. eng.
54. Seeman TE MB, Rowe JW, Singer BH. Allostatic load as a marker of cumulative biological risk. Proc Natl Acad Sci U S A. 2001;98:4770–5.
55. Latino-Martel P, Cottet V, Druesne-Pecollo N, Pierre FH, Touillaud M, Touvier M, et al. Alcoholic beverages, obesity, physical activity and other nutritional factors, and cancer risk: a review of the evidence. Crit Rev Oncol Hematol. 2016;99:308–23; PubMed PMID: 26811140. Epub 2016/01/27. Eng.
56. Ruini C, Vescovelli F, Albieri E. Post-traumatic growth in breast cancer survivors: new insights into its relationships with well-being and distress. J Clin Psychol Med Settings. 2013;20(3):383–91; PubMed PMID: 23229823. Epub 2012/12/12. eng.
57. Ferrell BR, Twaddle ML, Melnick A, Meier DE. National Consensus Project Clinical Practice Guidelines for quality palliative care guidelines, 4th edition. J Palliat Med. 2018;21(12):1684–9; PubMed PMID: 30179523. Epub 2018/09/05. eng.
58. Ferrell BR, Temel JS, Temin S, Alesi ER, Balboni TA, Basch EM, et al. Integration of palliative care into standard oncology care: American Society of Clinical Oncology clinical practice. J Clin Oncol. 2016;34:1–19.

59. Ma X, Zhang J, Zhong W, Shu C, Wang F, Wen J, et al. The diagnostic role of a short screening tool--the distress thermometer: a meta-analysis. Support Care Cancer. 2014;22(7):1741–55; PubMed PMID: 24510195. Epub 2014/02/11. eng.
60. Ploos van Amstel FK, Tol J, Sessink KH, van der Graaf WTA, Prins JB, Ottevanger PB. A specific distress cutoff score shortly after breast cancer diagnosis. Cancer Nurs. 2017;40(3):E35–40; PubMed PMID: 27135753. Epub 2016/05/03. eng.
61. Mathew A, Doorenbos AZ, Li H, Jang MK, Park CG, Bronas UG. Allostatic load in cancer: a systematic review and mini meta-analysis. Biol Res Nurs. 2021;23(3):341–61; PubMed PMID: 33138637. Epub 2020/11/04. eng.

Biological Processes of Resilience

4

> *… it is the brain's plasticity that gives hope for therapies that utilize brain-body interactions [1, p. 1]*

4.1 Introduction

How well an individual adapts to various environmental challenges depends on a healthy brain structure, its capacity for neural plasticity, and the timely activation and shutdown of interacting mediators from relevant neural, autonomic, immune, metabolic, and cardiovascular systems and functions [2]. Newly diagnosed individuals with cancer tend to experience greater vulnerability to diverse stressors along the disease and recovery continuum due to a number of factors, including the potentially life-threatening nature of the cancer, unfamiliar clinical contexts in which they find themselves, their age, and even sex [2, 3].

Clinical knowledge of the *dynamic role of the healthy brain, key neural circuits, processes, and mediators of* resilience can inform the nurse's clinical assessments and the use of purposeful and tailored clinical interventions to protect and promote resilience, particularly at empirically known points of clinical vulnerability. The aim of this chapter is to provide knowledge about allostatic resilience so that practitioners are motivated to protect and/or strengthen the resilience of the patient throughout each phase of the cancer trajectory.

4.2 Objectives

At the end of this chapter, you will be able to:

1. Describe the neurobiological adjustments made in response to manageable sources of stress and the role of stress mediators
2. Describe epigenetics and its relationship to resilience
3. Explain the biphasic role of cortisol
4. Describe the processes of biological healing that are integral to biological resilience
5. Define allostasis and its relationship to biological resilience

Clinical Anecdote 4.1
T was a vibrant and sporty individual in her early 30's whose life was happily humming along. She tried to stay healthy by eating lots of vegetables, fruits and grains, less red meat, more fish. She ran every day after work in order to 'decompress' before starting her evening, caring with her husband for their two children. So it came as a shock when an annual medical exam revealed she had stage 1 breast cancer. She could not imagine why she had fallen ill. Her childhood had been equally happy. The only sadness in their family history were grandparents who had to live through the last months of the war in Holland, when the city of Amsterdam was starving. But T's resilient capabilities enabled her to successfully overcome the shock of early stage cancer and to make a full recovery.

4.3 Definitions

Resilience

Resilience refers to the dynamic ability of the human organism to ***adapt*** to stressful albeit manageable events of relatively short duration in order to maintain relative homeostasis and internal coherence across neurobiological structures, systems, pathways, and functions (as well as psychological, socioemotional, and physical functions). Biological processes of resilience are triggered by a stressor, maintained for an appropriate (temporary) duration and then shut off at the end of stress [4]. In healthy brains, adaptive responses to an acute stressor promote resilience and survival [2].

Allostasis
Allostasis refers to the biological (and behavioral) processes of resilience involved in responding to an environmental challenge of short duration with mediators from autonomic, metabolic, neuroendocrinol, and immune systems that interact with one another within a dynamic compensatory nonlinear network that promotes adaptation so long as these mediators are turned on and off promptly as a function of the duration of the stressor [3, p. 2].

Resilience or allostasis protects the human organism from the potential toxic effects of stress and through its adaptive capabilities also develops flexibility to

4.3 Definitions

Table 4.1 Scientific terms used to measure/describe various stress effects (Review Chap. 3)

Scientific terms to describe stress effects on mind and body	Definition
Allostasis	Neurobiological, social, physical, and behavioral adjustments triggered by manageable and short-term stressors that are restored (healed) to their normal structures and parametric range when stress ends. Includes good and tolerable forms of stress effects (e.g., [4])
Allostatic load (AL)	Conversely, AL refers to the cumulative chronic effects of daily stresses and moderate-to-major stressful experiences associated with neural–biological impairments and the consequences of maladaptive psychosocial, cognitive, and lifestyle behaviors which exceed or severely strain the ability to cope [5]. May also be described as **toxic stress** defined as "strong, frequent stressors and/or prolonged activation of the stress response system in the absence of personal and social resources" and possibly impaired brain structure with limited flexibility to respond adaptively [5, p. 95]

successfully adapt to future challenges (Table 4.1) [6, 7]. Essential properties of biological resilience include neuroplasticity (section "Brain Plasticity") and dynamic changes in parametric values among relevant mediators of nonlinear interrelationships (section "The Stress-Related Systems and Mediators (Review Also Part III Chap. 6)") in response to stress that can be restored to normal and/or near-normal neural structures and parametric values after stress [3]. Another property is the ability of the stress response system to habituate its adaptive responses to familiar demands over time, thereby both conserving metabolic energy and reducing the magnitude or intensity of these acute stress effects on the biology of the person, underscoring a biological as well as behavioral learning function [4]. An important property of resilience is thought to be the development of biological and behavioral flexibility which underlies successful adaptations to future challenges.

Flexibility

Flexibility refers to the ability of the healthy brain's neural structures to dynamically *remodel or positively adapt* to environmental challenges throughout life within the context of previous experiences and personality characteristics. The development of a healthy brain architecture is largely due to positive life experiences especially in early childhood which promote flexible neural circuitry mediated by gene expression and epigenetic processes that determine biological and subsequently behavioral resilience, including cognitive flexibility [3, p. 2]. These dynamic stress-activated processes include changes in stress-related mediators. Whereas these structural changes and levels of circulating mediators are restored to their previous near-normal architecture and range of parametric values, underlying epigenetic changes may persist as a function of environmental stimuli and may play a role in regulating the brain's plasticity or flexibility across the lifespan.

From a clinical perspective, neural structural flexibility may be reflected by the ability to learn from past experiences, adapting what has worked from different experiences guided by adaptive neural circuitry that is continuously modulated by gene expression and epigenetic modulation [3].

Stressors (Review Part II Chap. 3)

As previously discussed, adaptation to stress is influenced by myriad factors, which include the duration, frequency and intensity of the stressor(s). Resilient-promoting stressors tend to be of short duration and generally experienced as low-to-moderate in intensity [8]. Manageable stresses meet goals of strengthening and developing psychological and biological resilience [9]. Major life events might include a diagnosis of cancer, a divorce, loss of a loved one, or difficulty finding a job. Other stressors include daily demands and hassles of work, spouse, children, other family members, and friends. These daily challenges may be attenuated through learning effective coping strategies and by having supportive relationships. The stressful experience may be low impact yet prolonged in its repeated nature and sometimes even appear to be beyond our control, as reflected, perhaps by expectations at work or an ill child at home. But in the main, the individual believes he is successfully managing the stresses that come his way. McEwen [3] has noted however, that these tolerable, long-term stress effects have cumulative deleterious effects on our underlying neurobiology that eventually manifest in frequent illnesses such as the common cold or flu, but also chronic illnesses, and a hastened aging process.

The clinical difficulty is to ascertain the cutoff between the ability of the whole being to sustain tolerable biological adjustments with elevated circulating stress mediators (e.g., cortisol, norepinephrine) and the point of conversion from protective and buffering effects into toxic effects. The point of transition between tolerable and toxic stress (allostatic load; Review Chap. 6) is not easily discernible at a biological level [3, 9].

Good Stress and Resilience
"Good stresses refers to developmentally challenging learning experiences that increase function and performance" [10, p. 576]. Good stress leads to the acquisition of cognitive, behavioral, and social skills associated with growth and developmental milestones, often supported by a nurturing figure.

Early childhood is replete with examples of good stress, for instance, the doting father who encourages a toddler who wants to climb up the slide rather than use the ladder, or a parent who encourages an unwilling toddler to share his toys. Later, examples of good stress may be observed with a teacher who tutors a student in mathematical problems, a nursing student who does his/her first intravenous insertion with the quiet support of the clinical professor, and a college student training for the 100-m dash. Good stress enables the development of cognitive, physical, social, and other self-efficacy skills, resulting in a higher integrated level of resilience [11, 12].

Tolerable Stress and Resilience
Tolerable biological stress refers to potentially impaired biological resilient processes in which the magnitude and/or scale of the stress-induced neurophysiological alterations are ultimately attenuated by the individual's personal and social resources and short-lived duration of the stress exposure [5] (Review Part II Chap. 5). Daily demands and challenges interspersed by moderate to severe major events may ultimately be manageable due to the presence of resources and effective coping efforts that enable successful adaptation with minimal allostatic load (Fig. 4.1) [3].

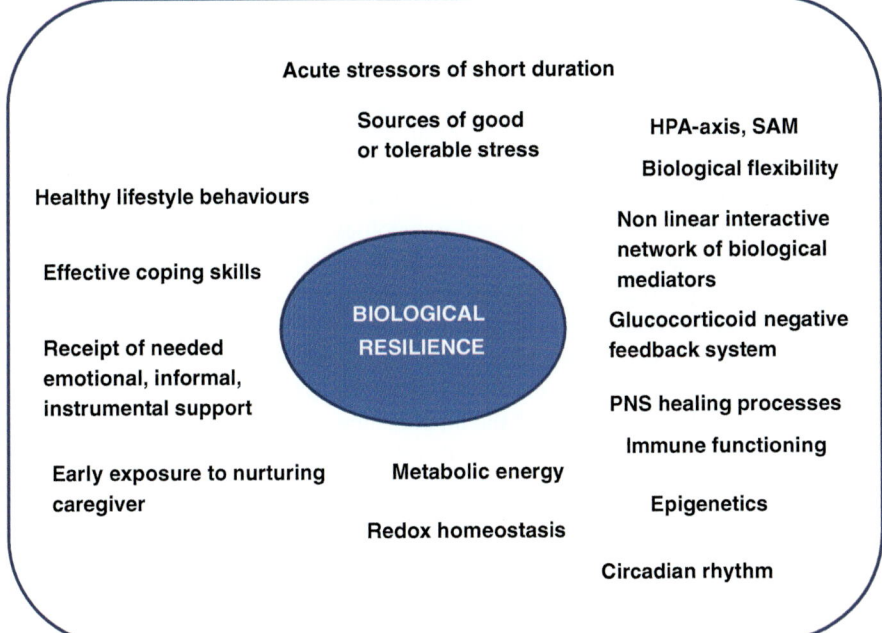

Fig. 4.1 Determinants of biological resilience

4.4 Key Neural Structures and Mediators

The brain is the central organizing top-down regulator of resilience and adaptation to daily life demands, challenges, and perceived stressors. A healthy brain continuously receives and interprets environmental stressors that subsequently drive the neurophysiological adjustments across neuroendocrinol, autonomic, immune, metabolic, kidney, and cardiovascular systems and behaviors as a function of underlying epigenetic changes regulating gene expression [6]. Neurophysiological mediators in different brain regions also modulate cognitive function, emotion regulation, and self-regulation [13].

The prefrontal cortex (PFC), hippocampus, and amygdala constitute a dynamic and interactive neural circuitry which processes, coordinates, and adjusts biological and behavioral responses to external and internal threats to homeostasis and health [12]. Whereas the PFC is the central organ of cognition and executive function, the hippocampus is the center for learning and memory formation, and the amygdala and striatum are the regions of emotionality and learning (e.g., [14]). The hippocampus and amygdala are limbic brain structures that process experiences by interacting with brain areas such as the hypothalamus and brainstem as well as the higher-order prefrontal cortex [12].

Brain Plasticity

An essential property of resilience is the brain's dynamic neuroplasticity, modulated by epigenetic changes and gene expression triggered by internal and external environmental demands. The brain as the central organ of stress and adaptation determines which stimuli are a threat to the human organism and how to respond. Its stress-induced dynamic remodeling of neural circuitry coordinates the flexible adjustments made throughout its neural physiology, functions, and behaviors [3, p. 2]. Stress-induced brain plasticity involves remodelling neural structures, synapses, and neural pathways and adjusting its neural functions in response to environmental demands. When stress ends, the brain's neural remodeling is restored to its prior or near prior neural structures while also embedding new or altered neural circuitry that supports the brain's plasticity in adapting to future stressful experiences.

For instance the gyrus dentate of the hippocampus adapts to short term stress by suppressing neurogenesis. The brain can also shift neural pathways from a damaged area of the brain to an undamaged area (functional plasticity) over the lifespan. Several brain regions are likely involved, but most research has concentrated on the prefrontal cortex (PFC), hippocampus, amygdala, and nucleus accumbens, and, increasingly, the periaqueductal gray region of the brain [15, p. 11].

Neural Remodeling Neural remodeling typically occurs at neuronal synapses as evidenced by alterations to the number and length of dendrites (branching/debranching), spine density, and size and number of excrescences associated with a nerve cell. Neural remodeling also involves neural cell replacement and changes in neurogenesis in the dentate gyrus of the hippocampus, which plays an important role in memory and learning [16, 17]. Other potential neuronal–structural changes may be reflected by a stress-induced smaller brain volume as a function of the duration, intensity, and frequency of stress.

Brain Volume Whereas the prefrontal cortex (PFC) and hippocampus show a stress-induced *reduction* in volume size due to neuronal culling at the synapses, and corresponding suppression of neurogenesis in the CA3 dentate gyrus of the hippocampus, the volume size of the stress-activated amygdala *increases* as neuronal interconnections are made more complex (e.g., [4, 18]). These changes lead to temporary disruptions in the PFC, hippocampus, and amygdala neural circuitry reducing the normal control of the PFC over the amygdala, with the more stress-activated amygdala subsequently inhibiting normal hippocampal and PFC functions.

Stress-induced dendritic growth in the amygdala's neurons has been attributed to unconditioned and uncontrollable expressions of fear and anxiety, and to heightened emotional reactivity due also to the fact that the PFCs overriding functions on the amygdala's functions are reduced during the stressor event (see McEwen [4] excellent review). In contrast, the stress effects in the PFC and the CA3 dentate gyrus of the hippocampus are manifested by dendritic pruning which contribute to difficulties in critical thinking, decision making, difficulty with working memory, and memory formation [19].

Function Findings from mice studies suggest that in the healing aftermath of stress, when behaviors have generally returned to normal, gene expression does not reflect its prestress patterns of expression and epigenetic changes still persist in the brain [3, 16, 17]. Although the clinical implications are unclear, it may be that these changes reflect modified neural circuits that provide adaptive flexibility in responding to future stressors akin to the ongoing processes of biological and behavioral development that are thought to alter aspects of neural circuits in order to continue to shape the brain's subsequent interactions with the environment via epigenetic changes.

The Stress-Related Systems and Mediators (Review Also Part III Chap. 6)

The hypothalamic–pituitary–adrenal axis (HPA axis), sympathetic nervous system (SNS), sympathetic adrenal medullary (SAM) axis, and immune systems are interrelated through a dynamic nonlinear network of mutually regulating biological mediators that make needed adjustments within their respective range of parametric values, in response to a stress exposure [20]. The network is said to be nonlinear in that a change in one mediator results in compensatory adjustments in the other interrelated mediators of systems and subsystems according to each mediator's respective range of parametric values. This *biological network* directs the functions and various physiological activities of the human organism in order to maintain homeostasis and internal coherence [18, 21].

Stress-related mediators typically include glucocorticoids, corticotropin-releasing hormone (CRH), adrenocorticotropic hormone (ACTH), dehydroepiandrosterone (DHEA), (cortisol), mineralocorticoids, catecholamines such as noradrenaline (NOR), serotonin (5-HT), dopamine, as well as insulin, glucagon, brain-derived neurotrophic factor (BDNF), and neuropeptide-Y (NPY) (e.g., [12, 17]). They include excitatory neurotransmitters such as glutamate, inhibitor transmitters such as GABA, neurotrophic factors, and intercellular signaling molecules such as the neural cell adhesion molecule (NCAM) and endocannabinoids. Stress-induced mediators also consist of cytokines, growth factors, and pro-inflammatory transcription factors (e.g., NFkB) and other mediating factors affected by stress within a nonlinear bidirectional network of regulating effects (e.g., [20]). For instance, pro- and anti-inflammatory cytokines regulate one another, but are also modulated by glucocorticoids and catecholamines [4, 20, 22]. In the initial adjustment phase of acute psychological stress, catecholamines stimulate pro-inflammatory cytokine production, while glucocorticoids are known to inhibit or restrain production.

Biphasic Stress Response: Protection Versus Damage Stress mediators such as glucocorticoids and NOR are biphasic and can either protect or damage the human organism depending on the phase, and the duration, frequency, and intensity of the stress experience [13]. For instance, the elevated circulation of cortisol and NOR initially serves a protective function that facilitates resilient adaptation. But when these same mediators, especially glucocorticoids, remain stress-elevated beyond a critical time frame, they inflict widespread damages to neural cells, pathways, and functions, which if not reversed compromise biological resilience, health outcomes, and even survival (see Part III, Chaps. 6 and 7) (e.g., [19, 23]).

Mediators such as brain-derived neurotrophic factor (BDNF) exert differential effects depending *on where* it is released in the body. During stress BDNF is suppressed in the dentate gyrus (DG) of the hippocampus so that neurogenesis is also inhibited, thereby negatively affecting learning capabilities. Conversely BDNF levels are increased in the nucleus accumbens which is associated with depressive-like effects [16]. These stress-induced temporary adjustments highlight why, for instance, a patient facing a stressful operation or poor prognosis may experience a depressed mood and demonstrate difficulties processing information being conveyed by the doctor or nurse. In the moment, the individual may struggle to process the clinical consequences of a stressor event, but with appropriate support, this is generally temporary and part of the process of adaptation.

Negative Glucocorticoid Feedback System

Glucocorticoids are involved in a number of physiological processes that have important implications for the resilience, health, or illness of an individual. Glucocorticoids exert regulating roles in immune functioning, metabolic processes, and learning (via hippocampus) [24, 25]. A healthy glucocorticoid-driven negative feedback inhibition system is also critical for turning off the stress response mechanism in an efficient manner when the source of stress is over [26].

The glucocorticoids activate their biological activities by binding with two types of cell membrane receptors: The low-affinity glucocorticoid receptors (GRs) tend to be expressed throughout most regions of the brain. The high-affinity mineralocorticoid receptors (MRs) are concentrated mainly in the limbic regions (hippocampus, central amygdala, and lateral septum) [25, 27]. A glucocorticoid MR/GR balance in their mediated activities is thought to be protective against stress-related diseases.

Exposure to a stressor induces two phases in the stress response system. First, an *immediate* autonomic nervous system (ANS)-driven response followed by *a delayed* HPA axis activated response mediated by the release of glucocorticoids [27]. *In the initial response* to an acute stressor, the activated adrenal cortex releases glucocorticoids that rapidly access the brain, where the MRs have a high binding affinity with the naturally occurring endogenous glucocorticoids, which rapidly occupy the MRs until receptor saturation occurs. Being high-affinity receptors for glucocorticoids, these sites are almost constantly occupied at low levels of HPA activity suggesting that the MRs tend to mediate glucocorticoid effects mainly under conditions of basal HPA activity.

Notwithstanding, the rapid action glucocorticoid (ligand)–MR receptor linkage is also thought to precipitate *the cognitive appraisal and behavioral responsiveness to the stressor* [25–27]. During mild stress, it seems that MR saturation also is responsible for the negative feedback of the HPA axis which subsequently downregulates cortisol production to basal levels of functioning [25, 27]. Conversely, the GR's low-affinity binding sites for glucocorticoids account for their relatively *lower occu*pancy at basal HPA conditions [25].

In the "delayed" phase of an acute stressor event, glucocorticoid circulating levels continue to rise, forcing glucocorticoid (ligand) binding with the GR receptors (which normally have a low affinity for endogenous glucocorticoids). *GR activation/saturation* is responsible for downregulating the stress response mechanism by switching off glucocorticoid production via the "negative feedback control" of the HPA axis when stress ends. For instance, 1 h or so after the initiation of stress, the gene-mediated activities of the GR in the hippocampus lead to downregulation of adrenergic actions, with increased inhibitory effects of serotonin resulting in adaptive processes that involve consolidating memory.

4.5 The Biphasic Process of Biological Resilience

The centrally integrated neurobiological system of adaptation (resilience) consists of the brain, hypothalamic–pituitary–adrenal axis (HPA axis), autonomic nervous system (ANS), sympatho-adrenal medullary pathway (SAM), immune system, and the critical nonlinear network of biological mediators that are mobilized throughout the human organism in response to stress. The process of resilience encompasses two interrelated dynamic processes: *The first phase* sees neurobiological *adjustment*s made in response to stress (section "Age"). *The second phase*, initiated by the end of the stressful experience and the downregulation of the biological stress response system (review the negative glucocorticoid feedback), enables the reemergence of relative PNS dominance over SNS activities (section "Sex Differences" (Review McEwen [3, 4])). The healing processes of the PNS and vagal nerve and its cholinergic activities (via acetylcholine) govern the *near restoration and/or healing* of the stress-altered neural structures and the disrupted nonlinear interrelationships among mediators, restoring levels within normal parametric values [28].

The First Phase: The Process of Stress-Induced Neural and Physiological Adjustments

A stress-induced HPA axis, sympatho-adrenal medullary axis (SAM), autonomic nervous system (ANS), immune system, and metabolic system are mobilized to respond to an acute stressor exposure driven by underlying epigenetic changes [4, 15]. In particular, the central neural circuit of the PFC, hippocampus, and amygdala undergo temporary changes to its neural architecture, physiological and molecular pathways, gene expression, and functions in response to a stress exposure.

The hypothalamus releases corticotrophin-releasing hormone (CRH) which activates the whole stress response system: The SNS overrides and essentially suppresses the healing and anti-inflammatory functions of the parasympathetic nervous system (PNS) which normally modulates SNS activity at basal levels of resilience [4]. The activated SNS also suppresses the normally controlling functions of the PFC over the amygdala as well as anticancer cell functioning of the immune system. Suppressed functioning of the mPFC has been associated with temporary problems in executive functions such as problem solving and decision making during short-term experiences of acute stress. In contrast, the functions of the amygdala (responsible for emotional responses) become unregulated and uncontrollable driving the continuation of the biological stress response system [20].

The Second Phase, Healing, and Restoration

In the aftermath of stress, the PNS and vagal nerve activity reemerge in relative dominance over SNS activities. Restoration of the PNS, vagus nerve, and cholinergic activity enable innate healing or restoration of the stress-induced dynamic adjustments made to neural structures to normal or near-normal parameters [4, 28]. This restorative process of resilience driven by underlying epigenetic changes and gene expression is thought to produce adaptive neural circuits which guide biological and behavioral adaptation to future stressors [3]. Although the process is not clear, these adaptive changes may contribute to the individual's biological, cognitive, and behavioral flexibility in order to adapt more easily to future stressors, not previously exposed to in the past. Research findings suggest that after stress ends, residual stress-induced alterations may persist; for instance, a neuron's dendritic branches may look slightly different compared to its prestress state, although at a behavioral level, no such difference may be apparent [3].

McEwen [13, p. 58] refers to the healing of neural architecture as "a form of neuroplastic adaptation" which may be facilitated by the reemergence of resilient-promoting or healing mediators such as BDNF which occurs in the dentate gyrus of the hippocampus although BDNF in the nucleus accumbens is downregulated. The healing phase also involves embedding adaptive neural circuits which include myriad cellular and molecular pathways that likely result in more flexible resilient capabilities in the future.

The vagal nerve and its neurotransmitter, acetylcholine, also enable the restoration of stress-induced alterations in the values of nonlinear interrelationships among mediators, to normal parametric ranges [3, 29]. Cholinergic activity downregulates inflammatory factors, restoring the relative balance of inflammatory to anti-inflammatory cytokines [30]. Thus, PNS healing processes restore the normal pattern of basal physiological values among biological mediators as well as the brain's neural architecture to near-normal prior structures and functions, thereby also reducing metabolic energy requirements [28, 31].

The quality of the healing or restoration determines whether the stress-induced adjustments result in (1) adaptive resilience, (2) poor resilience (maladaptation), or even (3) a higher level of adaptation as experienced by individuals who have learned something meaningful through adverse experiences (as in managing the consequences of cancer and its treatments) or "good stress" (as in the stress-inducing process toward academic achievement).

The process of biological resilience is facilitated by the presence of personal and social resources which buffer the human organism from the potentially strained effects of tolerable stress [3, 13].

4.6 Other Processes That Influence Biological Resilience

Other processes that influence biological resilience include normal functioning of circadian rhythms and epigenetic processes. Factors also influencing resilience include SES, developmental history, and early life experiences (e.g., [3, 32]). Personal resources, coping responses, supportive relationships, and lifestyle behaviors are also important modulating processes, to be discussed in Part II, Chap. 5.

Age

Young adults with healthy brains and exposed to repeated stress are generally thought to restore stress-induced neurobiological adjustments to normal structures and parametric values, based on rodent models (e.g., [33, 34]). However, adults exposed to the same repeated stresses such as the normal demands of life over the lifespan are thought not to make the same adaptations to prestress levels due in part to the "wear and tear" of daily stresses over time, which may also correspond with the aging process, again based on rodent studies [35]. Bloss and colleagues [35] showed that younger rodents appeared to make an almost complete recovery of neural remodeling in the aftermath of chronic stress, while adult rodents appeared to have lost significantly more of their neural remodeling adaptability. The findings suggest that adults with cancer and a history of allostatic stress may be more vulnerable at a biological level in the process of adapting to the new challenges of cancer and its treatment over the trajectory.

In summary, resilience is the ability to adapt to environmental challenges and contributes to future resilience through a dynamic process of flexible neuro structural and physiological alterations which also provide internal stability in the face of changing environmental demands. A number of internal and external factors influence the human organism's capacity to successfully adapt to stress, such as the stressful experience of cancer, treatment, and recovery, underscoring the clinical need to assess the potential impact of these illness and recovery phases on the resilience and health of each patient.

Sex Differences (Review McEwen [3, 4])

Sex is genetically assigned and is also mediated by the actions of sex hormones at genomic receptors (ie DNA) and nongenomic receptors (such as on cell membranes and or in the cell cytosol) [15]. Rodent studies showed that females and males displayed different dendritic patterns in the hippocampus in the aftermath of chronic restraint stress (CRS) [3, p. 5]. Whereas females did not show any changes to their CA3 dendrites, males did. Furthermore, the males also were observed to have hippocampal-associated memory impairment, which females did not. Conversely, whereas female rats showed greater dendritic growth in projections into the amygdala in the aftermath of CRS, males showed dendritic remodeling of the mPRC, which the females did not. Just these few findings raise the issue of potential clinical implications in caring for male and female patients with cancer. It suggests that women may be more predisposed to emotional reactivity in the face of a stressor, whereas men tend to go into executive thinking mode! Further studies with humans are needed as most studies have been based on male populations (e.g., [4]).

Epigenetics

Epigenetics is a central reversible biological system in the development and maintenance of human resilience. It refers to bioactive "events" occurring above the genome (i.e., the individual's complete set of genetic instructions) which regulate gene expression across the lifespan without changing the DNA sequence [36, 37]. This involves continuous interactions between environmental factors, such as hormones, cytokines, chemokines and neuromodulators, and the genome resulting in gene expression which directs the physiological functions and behaviors of the individual. These environmental factors induce a genomic response, for instance, via histone modifications (i.e., the proteins in the chromatin of chromosomes), DNA methylation of cytosine residues on DNA, and other environment–genome interactions that involve various modifications to the expression of mRNA molecules [38]. For instance, DNA cytosine methylation is an example of an epigenetic change that prevents certain genes from being expressed, thereby altering subsequent biology and behaviors [3, p. 5]. Another epigenetic activity that alters gene expression may include changes to histone proteins by methylation/demethylation and acetylation/deacetylation which remodel chromatin structures so that, for instance, other proteins may either be prevented from being "read" or enabled to be read [3, 38].

Epigenetics is triggered by a number of factors including lifestyle and external/internal environmental factors such as pollution, age, disease state, and a nurturing upbringing. For instance, early exposure to a nurturing environment predisposes an individual to unique epigenetic patterns of turning on/off genes associated with stress responses conducive to health-promoting development of resilience throughout life. Environmentally driven epigenetic regulation influences which genes will respond/not respond to novel stimuli and challenges, which will subsequently determine the nature of overall development, including the lifelong development of resilience.

Epigenetics plays an essential role in either strengthening or undermining biological resilience depending on *the nature of the environmental challenge*. For instance, epigenetics contributes to biological resilience when a stressor is of short duration, deemed manageable due to appropriate use of coping behaviors and support, backed by a resilient-promoting nurturing history and healthy neural–endocrine structures, processes, and functions [3, 36]. The seamless epigenetic changes driving resilience for better or worse across the developmental lifespan is indicative of the human capacity for adaptation or maladaptation. Even individuals with severe early life stress may benefit from resilient-promoting interventions given the property of neural plasticity (e.g., [39]). These interventions may not restore the individual to normal, prestress levels of resilience, but may promote changes in neural circuitry that may provide different strategies for improving adaptive capabilities.

Circadian Rhythm

The master circadian pacemaker for the brain and the body is the suprachiasmatic nucleus (SCN), located in the anterior hypothalamus. The SCN is responsible for synchronizing all the biological "clocks" that reside in every cell of the body. Emanating from the SCN are modulating neural–endocrine and molecular signaling pathways that travel throughout the human organism, regulating the systems involved in maintaining resilience or allostasis and homeostasis [40]. Circadian rhythm refers to the natural physical, mental, and behavioral cyclical changes that respond to darkness and light within a 24-h period.

The physiological systems and signaling factors that regulate allostasis, such as cortisol and melatonin, are also implicated in the circadian rhythms associated with the sleep–wake cycle [32, 41]. The SCN modulates the timing between sleep and wakefulness and synchronizes the "biological" clocks in every cell of the body. Disruptions in circadian rhythms, for instance, due to lack of sleep, even short-term appear to promote allostatic load and reduce metabolic, neural–endocrine, and behavioral resilience [32, 41]. A shortened night sleep can reduce parasympathetic tone (i.e., enable the acceleration of sinus node activity), increase the flow of inflammatory cytokines and evening cortisol levels, increase appetite at night (via increased ghrelin with reduced leptin levels), and alter cognitive acuity. These changes and other neuroendocrine disruptions if prolonged over time increase the risk of allostatic load and destabilize resilience, but can be overturned with a good night's sleep.

Energy

At basal physiological levels, energy is conserved and directed at promoting normal metabolic functions throughout the human organism, such as growth and development, healing processes, and immune defenses that search the human organism for circulating cancer cells, viruses, and other pathogens (e.g., [42]). These functions are temporarily suppressed during acute (and chronic) stress as energy levels are increased and redirected toward responding to the threat, *thereby temporarily increasing the individual's vulnerability* to further illness or disease progression during that short interval caused by the acute stressor event.

Reactive Oxygen Species Mitochondrial respiration consists of a sequence of metabolic reactions and processes that need oxygen in order to convert energy stored in food (macronutrients) into adenosine triphosphate, the main energy provider to the cell. The by-product of this essential metabolic process is reactive oxygen species (ROS). ROS are highly reactive radicals or oxidants. ROS refers to reactant oxygen-carrying molecules that consist of radicals (such as the superoxide $O2^-$), which is the product of an electron reduction, leaving a charged ionic species or hydroxyl (HO) as well as nonradical species such as H_2O_2 (hydrogen peroxide) which is both an oxidizing and reducing agent [43]. ROS also is generated by human exposure to external environmental toxicities as well as by various metabolic processes in the mitochondria and endoplasmic reticulum (ER), cytokines (e.g., tumor necrosis factor-alpha or TNF-α), and pathogenic viruses and bacteria.

Redox Homeostasis Redox homeostasis is the balance between the rate of production of ROS oxidants and their removal from the body [44]. At low basal levels of energy as part of redox homeostasis, ROS serves as essential signaling oxidants which interact with signaling molecules along cellular pathways that regulate normal cellular functions such as cell growth, differentiation, inflammation, immune functioning, the stress response, survival, and aging (e.g., [43]). Redox homeostasis ensures that cellular biological systems conduct these normal functions and processes. Redox refers to the process in which one molecule is oxidized (i.e., loses electrons) such as the highly reactive ROS, and another molecule is reduced (i.e., gains electrons); oxidation and reduction are complementary processes that help to promote redox homeostasis [44]. In a resilient individual with personal resources and supports, antioxidant defense systems of the mitochondria play an important role in controlling the main ROS signaling species, H_2O_2, which under prolonged stressful conditions becomes unregulated, causing considerable widespread damage to cell structures, tissues, and DNA [45]. (Discussed in Chap. 6).

4.7   Nursing Implications

This chapter highlights the critical role of biological resilience to the ongoing health of individuals but especially to those individuals who have cancer but are essentially healthy, and whose resilience and energy levels must be protected and strengthened. The health of the brain and specifically its ability for neural structural remodeling in response to environmental demands, modulated by epigenetic changes and gene expression, is critical for enabling flexible neurophysiological stress-related responses, functions, and behaviors of the individual to further promote adaptation to environmental demands in the future.

4.7 Nursing Implications

Although the majority of patients with cancer possess resilient capabilities across developmental, psychological, behavioral, and biological domains, living with cancer is fraught with various disease- and treatment-related stressors so that each stress exposure in principle can emotionally and biologically wear on the patient's neuronal plasticity (flexibility) and adaptive capabilities. This biological knowledge in itself provides an informed context for acting to ensure that the individual's adaptive capabilities are protected, especially during this stressful episode in their life. Parts IV and V discuss these clinical approaches.

Knowledge that the activated biological stress response system is also modulated by allostatic nonlinear interrelationships among interrelated stress mediators that are deeply implicated in the widespread stress response of the whole person (i.e., neural–endocrine, immune, metabolic, and cardiovascular systems) provides a number of biomarkers that may be considered to more closely assess the overall resilience of patients at different phases of the continuum. These mediators also serve as endpoints to evaluate clinical interventions aimed at downregulating stress and/or strengthening the individual's overall adaptive capabilities.

This chapter has also described the impact of acute stress of short duration on the temporary suppression of the parasympathetic system and cholinergic healing related pathways. It is also worth noting that conventional treatments for cancer, such as chemotherapy, medical radiation therapy, and surgery are also known stressors that have been shown to temporarily suppress immune cell functions associated with hunting down and eliminating rogue cancer cells and other pathogens, even in resilient individuals. This scientific evidence highlights the imperative of implementing psychosocial interventions that down regulate stress and induce healing processes throughout the person, thereby restoring or improving their biological (and behavioral) resilience (e.g., [42]).

Widespread neural–endocrinal changes are thought to be temporary and restored to normal parametric values in the aftermath of short-term stress exposure. However, some evidence, albeit from rodent studies, found that neural remodeling, physiological alterations, and gene expression denotative of resilient capabilities were restored to near but not completely prestress neurophysiology although anxiety levels improved [33, 46, 47]. Perhaps, these almost completely restored structural parameters signify adaptive plastic flexibility that enables the human organism to respond successfully to future stresses. But it may also be indicative of stress-induced mild changes that over the lifespan become cumulative, eventually posing a potential risk to an individual's adaptive capabilities. For instance, whereas young adult rats appear to return to normal neural structures and physiology in the aftermath of acute short-term stress, older middle-aged adults show a loss of resilience [17, 47]. Although not directly transferable to human behavior, these findings at a minimum highlight the clinical importance of assessing over the continuum the ability of adult patients with cancer and their loved ones to maintain their resilient capabilities.

As we shall discuss in greater depth throughout Parts IV and V, a clinical imperative would be to strengthen patient and family caregiver resilience through specific psychosocial interventions that can reduce the ill effects of stress and strengthen resilience in the face of biological vulnerability, starting from the diagnostic phase through the treatment phase, and continuing into survivorship and supportive care.

References

1. McEwen BS. Neurobiological and systemic effects of chronic stress. Chronic Stress (Thousand Oaks, Calif). 2017. PubMed PMID: 28856337. Pubmed Central PMCID: PMC5573220. Epub 2017/09/01. eng.
2. McEwen B. Central effects of stress hormones in health and disease: understanding the protective and damaging effects of stress and stress mediators. Eur J Pharmacol. 2008;583:174–85.
3. McEwen BS, Gray J, Nasca C. Recognizing resilience: learning from the effects of stress on the brain. Neurobiol Stress. 2015;1:1–11. PubMed PMID: 25506601. Pubmed Central PMCID: PMC4260341. Epub 2014/12/17. Eng.
4. McEwen BS. Physiology and neurobiology of stress and adaptation: central role of the brain. Physiol Rev. 2007;87(3):873–904. PubMed PMID: 17615391. Epub 2007/07/07. eng.
5. Fava GA, McEwen BS, Guidi J, Gostoli S, Offidani E, Sonino N. Clinical characterization of allostatic overload. Psychoneuroendocrinology. 2019;108:94–101. PubMed PMID: 31252304. Epub 2019/06/30. eng.
6. McEwen BS, Nasca C, Gray JD. Stress effects on neuronal structure: hippocampus, amygdala, and prefrontal cortex. Neuropsychopharmacology. 2016;41(1):3–23. PubMed PMID: 26076834. Pubmed Central PMCID: PMC4677120. Epub 2015/06/17. eng.
7. Muehsam D, Lutgendorf S, Mills PJ, Rickhi B, Chevalier G, Bat N, et al. The embodied mind: a review on functional genomic and neurological correlates of mind-body therapies. Neurosci Biobehav Rev. 2017;73:165–81. PubMed PMID: 28017838. Epub 2016/12/27. eng.
8. Aschbacher K, O'Donovan A, Wolkowitz OM, Dhabhar FS, Su Y, Epel E. Good stress, bad stress and oxidative stress: insights from anticipatory cortisol reactivity. Psychoneuroendocrinology. 2013;38(9):1698–708. PubMed PMID: 23490070. Epub 2013/03/16. eng.
9. Dekker J, Braamse A, Schuurhuizen C, Beekman ATF, van Linde M, Sprangers MAG, et al. Distress in patients with cancer - on the need to distinguish between adaptive and maladaptive emotional responses. Acta Oncol. 2017;56(7):1026–9. PubMed PMID: 28145789. Epub 2017/02/02. eng.
10. Karatsoreos IN, Bhagat S, Bloss EB, Morrison JH, McEwen BS. Disruption of circadian clocks has ramifications for metabolism, brain, and behavior. Proc Natl Acad Sci U S A. 2011;108(4):1657–62. PubMed PMID: 21220317. Pubmed Central PMCID: PMC3029753. Epub 2011/01/12. eng.
11. Kalisch R, Muller MB, Tuscher O. A conceptual framework for the neurobiological study of resilience. Behav Brain Sci. 2015;38:e92. PubMed PMID: 25158686. Epub 2014/08/28. eng.
12. McEwen BS, Gianaros PJ. Stress- and allostasis-induced brain plasticity. Annu Rev Med. 2011;62:431–45. PubMed PMID: 20707675. Epub 2010/08/17. eng.
13. McEwen BS. In pursuit of resilience: stress, epigenetics, and brain plasticity. Ann N Y Acad Sci. 2016;1373(1):56–64. PubMed PMID: 26919273. Epub 2016/02/27. eng.
14. Fareri DS, Tottenham N. Effects of early life stress on amygdala and striatal development. Dev Cogn Neurosci. 2016;19:233–47. PubMed PMID: 27174149. Pubmed Central PMCID: PMC4912892. Epub 2016/05/14. eng.
15. McEwen BS, Morrison JH. The brain on stress: vulnerability and plasticity of the prefrontal cortex over the life course. Neuron. 2013;79(1):16–29. PubMed PMID: 23849196. Pubmed Central PMCID: PMC3753223. Epub 2013/07/16. eng.
16. Gray JD, Milner TA, McEwen BS. Dynamic plasticity: the role of glucocorticoids, brain-derived neurotrophic factor and other trophic factors. Neuroscience. 2013;239:214–27. PubMed PMID: 22922121. Pubmed Central PMCID: PMC3743657. Epub 2012/08/28. eng.
17. Gray JD, Rubin TG, Hunter RG, McEwen BS. Hippocampal gene expression changes underlying stress sensitization and recovery. Mol Psychiatry. 2014;19(11):1171–8. PubMed PMID: 24342991. Epub 2013/12/18. Eng.
18. Karatsoreos IN, McEwen BS. Annual research review: the neurobiology and physiology of resilience and adaptation across the life course. J Child Psychol Psychiatry. 2013;54(4):337–47. PubMed PMID: 23517425. Epub 2013/03/23. eng.

19. McEwen BS. The ever-changing brain: cellular and molecular mechanisms for the effects of stressful experiences. Dev Neurobiol. 2012;72(6):878–90. PubMed PMID: 21898852. Pubmed Central PMCID: PMC3248634. Epub 2011/09/08. eng.
20. McEwen BS. Protective and damaging effects of stress mediators: central role of the brain. Dialogues Clin Neurosci. 2006;8(4):367–81. PubMed PMID: 17290796. Pubmed Central PMCID: PMC3181832. Epub 2007/02/13. eng.
21. MacPhee D, Lunkenheimer E, Riggs N. Resilience as regulation of developmental and family processes. Fam Relat. 2015;64(1):153–75. PubMed PMID: 26568647. Pubmed Central PMCID: PMC4642729. Epub 2015/11/17. eng.
22. McEwen BS. Stress, adaptation, and disease. Allostasis and allostatic load. Ann N Y Acad Sci. 1998;840:33–44. PubMed PMID: 9629234. Epub 1998/06/18. eng.
23. Eiland L, McEwen BS. Early life stress followed by subsequent adult chronic stress potentiates anxiety and blunts hippocampal structural remodeling. Hippocampus. 2012;22(1):82–91. PubMed PMID: 20848608. Epub 2010/09/18. eng.
24. Cain DW, Cidlowski JA. Immune regulation by glucocorticoids. Nat Rev Immunol. 2017;17(4):233–47. PubMed PMID: 28192415. Epub 2017/02/14. eng.
25. Mifsud KR, Reul J. Mineralocorticoid and glucocorticoid receptor-mediated control of genomic responses to stress in the brain. Stress. 2018;21(5):389–402. PubMed PMID: 29614900. Epub 2018/04/05. eng.
26. Raison CL, Miller AH. When not enough is too much: the role of insufficient glucocorticoid signaling in the pathophysiology of stress-related disorders. Am J Psychiatry. 2003;160(9):1554–65. PubMed PMID: 12944327. Epub 2003/08/29. eng.
27. Juruena MF, Agustini B, Cleare AJ, Young AH. A translational approach to clinical practice via stress-responsive glucocorticoid receptor signaling. Stem Cell Investig. 2017;4:13. PubMed PMID: 28275643. Pubmed Central PMCID: PMC5334557. Epub 2017/03/10. eng.
28. Thayer JF, Sternberg E. Beyond heart rate variability: vagal regulation of allostatic systems. Ann N Y Acad Sci. 2006;1088:361–72. PubMed PMID: 17192580. Epub 2006/12/29. eng.
29. Grote V, Levnajić Z, Puff H, Ohland T, Goswami N, Fruhwirth M, Moser M. Dynamics of vagal activity due to surgery and subsequent rehabilitation. Front Neurosci. 2019;13:1116.
30. Pavlov VA, Tracey KJ. The vagus nerve and the inflammatory reflex--linking immunity and metabolism. Nat Rev Endocrinol. 2012;8(12):743–54. PubMed PMID: 23169440. Pubmed Central PMCID: PMC4082307. Epub 2012/11/22. eng.
31. Thayer JF, Sternberg EM. Neural aspects of immunomodulation: focus on the vagus nerve. Brain Behav Immun. 2010;24(8):1223–8. PubMed PMID: 20674737. Pubmed Central PMCID: PMC2949498. Epub 2010/08/03. eng.
32. McEwen BS, Karatsoreos IN. Sleep deprivation and circadian disruption: stress, allostasis, and allostatic load. Sleep Med Clin. 2015;10(1):1–10. PubMed PMID: 26055668. Epub 2015/06/10. eng.
33. Radley JJ, Rocher AB, Janssen WG, Hof PR, McEwen BS, Morrison JH. Reversibility of apical dendritic retraction in the rat medial prefrontal cortex following repeated stress. Exp Neurol. 2005;196(1):199–203. PubMed PMID: 16095592. Epub 2005/08/13. eng.
34. Radley JJ, Sisti HM, Hao J, Rocher AB, McCall T, Hof PR, et al. Chronic behavioral stress induces apical dendritic reorganization in pyramidal neurons of the medial prefrontal cortex. Neuroscience. 2004;125(1):1–6. PubMed PMID: 15051139. Epub 2004/03/31. eng.
35. Bloss EB, Janssen WG, McEwen BS, Morrison JH. Interactive effects of stress and aging on structural plasticity in the prefrontal cortex. J Neurosci Off J Soc Neurosci. 2010;30(19):6726–31. PubMed PMID: 20463234. Pubmed Central PMCID: PMC2888496. Epub 2010/05/14. eng.
36. Schuebel K, Gitik M, Domschke K, Goldman D. Making sense of epigenetics. Int J Neuropsychopharmacol. 2016;19(11):1–10.
37. Mehler MF. Epigenetic principles and mechanisms underlying nervous system functions in health and disease. Prog Neurobiol. 2008;86(4):305–41. PubMed PMID: 18940229. Pubmed Central PMCID: PMC2636693. Epub 2008/10/23. eng.

38. Gibney ER, Nolan CM. Epigenetics and gene expression. Heredity. 2010;105(1):4–13. PubMed PMID: 20461105. Epub 2010/05/13. eng.
39. Iacona J, Johnson S. Neurobiology of trauma and mindfulness for children. J Trauma Nurs. 2018;25(3):187–91. PubMed PMID: 29742631. Epub 2018/05/10. eng.
40. Rosenwasser AM, Turek FW. Neurobiology of circadian rhythm regulation. Sleep Med Clin. 2015;10(4):403–12. PubMed PMID: 26568118. Epub 2015/11/17. eng.
41. McEwen BS. Sleep deprivation as a neurobiologic and physiologic stressor: allostasis and allostatic load. Metab Clin Exp. 2006;55(10 Suppl 2):S20–3. PubMed PMID: 16979422.
42. Wang M, Zhao J, Zhang L, Wei F, Lian Y, Wu Y, et al. Role of tumor microenvironment in tumorigenesis. J Cancer. 2017;8(5):761–73. PubMed PMID: 28382138. Pubmed Central PMCID: PMC5381164. Epub 2017/04/07. eng.
43. Kirtonia A, Sethi G, Garg M. The multifaceted role of reactive oxygen species in tumorigenesis. Cell Mol Life Sci. 2020;77(22):4459–83. PubMed PMID: 32358622. Epub 2020/05/03. eng.
44. Panieri E, Santoro MM. ROS homeostasis and metabolism: a dangerous liaison in cancer cells. Cell Death Dis. 2016;7(6):e2253. PubMed PMID: 27277675. Pubmed Central PMCID: PMC5143371. Epub 2016/06/10. eng.
45. del Pilar Sosa Idelchik M, Begley U, Begley T, Melendez J. Mitochondrial ROS control of cancer. Semin Cancer Biol. 2017;47:57–66.
46. Radley JJ, Anderson RM, Hamilton BA, Alcock JA, Romig-Martin SA. Chronic stress-induced alterations of dendritic spine subtypes predict functional decrements in an hypothalamo-pituitary-adrenal-inhibitory prefrontal circuit. J Neurosci Off J Soc Neurosci. 2013;33(36):14379–91. PubMed PMID: 24005291. Pubmed Central PMCID: PMC3761048. Epub 2013/09/06. eng.
47. Goldwater DS, Pavlides C, Hunter RG, Bloss EB, Hof PR, McEwen BS, et al. Structural and functional alterations to rat medial prefrontal cortex following chronic restraint stress and recovery. Neuroscience. 2009;164(2):798–808. PubMed PMID: 19723561. Pubmed Central PMCID: PMC2762025. Epub 2009/09/03. eng.

Psychosocial Processes of Resilience 5

> *It is not the strongest species that survive, nor the most intelligent, but the ones most responsive to change*
>
> Charles Darwin

5.1 Introduction

Psychosocial resilience refers to the emotion-regulating, cognitive–behavioral system of adaptation which is seamlessly related to the neuro plasticity and processes of biological resilience. As discussed in Chap. 4, the brain's architecture directs in a top down manner, mediated by continuous epigenetic changes and gene expression how the whole person's neurobiology and subsequent psychosocial behavior will successfully or unsuccessfully adapt to environmental experiences throughout the lifespan (A healthy brain and its dynamic stress-responsive neural architecture is developed through positive life experiences which promote the biological flexibility needed for the successful adaptation of the whole person [1]. This biological flexibility shapes subsequent behavior such as cognitive flexibility which is needed to promote adaptive psychosocial processes of resilience. In other words, stress-induced remodeling of neural structures driven by positive experiences, epigenetic changes and gene expression modulates the nonlinear compensatory pattern of physiological adjustments made among the biological mediators that interact with one another and also regulate resilient-promoting behaviors, including health-related behavioral choices [1]. Changes in the brain's architecture are continuously shaped by the individual's social and physical environment as well as cumulative life experiences that propel the individual toward either psychosocial and physical resilience or greater illness-related vulnerability.

The majority of patients with cancer and their family caregivers successfully adapt cognitively and behaviorally to the various cancer- and treatment-related stressors along the continuum, with only periodic manifestations of short-term psychological distress [2]. Because psychosocial resilience is also shaped by the individual's history of stressful experiences, quality of supportive relationships, SES, early childhood adversity, personal resources, and coping strategies used in the past, some individuals with cancer and their family caregivers may find that the challenges they must face during the cancer experience exceed their ability to cope effectively. Stressed behaviors may be manifested by sleepless nights, lack of exercise, poor eating habits, too much alcohol, and anxiety. As the brain changes in response to acute as well as chronic stress, it may at different points along the cancer trajectory conceivably respond with less neural structural and functional flexibility. Among essentially resilient individuals, their fundamental biological and psychosocial adaptive capabilities may be restored and strengthened via targeted psychosocial interventions that can improve psychosocial and biological flexibility [3, p. 57]. Learning how to effectively manage anxiety or distress in the face of adversity using both cognitive and behavioral emotion-regulating strategies within a supportive context promotes neural remodeling and relevant neural circuitry, enabling more flexible management of stressors in the future [1]. Learning to regulate one's emotions and by extension, modulate stress-induced inflammatory pathways and constituents, may interfere or counter inflammatory processes that drive cancer growth and proliferation [4].

Because resilience has been recognized as a critical neurobiological and psychosocial adaptive process of human health, there is a clinical imperative to understand its complex and interrelated factors and systems in order to identify relevant targets or endpoints for psychosocial interventions that can strengthen the individual's resilience, especially in those experiencing distress during the diagnosis, treatment, survivorship, and end-of-life phases of the continuum [5–7]. This chapter focuses on the adaptive, emotion-regulating, stress-coping processes of psychological resilience.

5.2 Objectives

At the end of this chapter, you will be able to:

1. Describe the adaptive process of psychological resilience and healing
2. Explain the relationship between resilience and health
3. Identify direct, buffering, and mediating effects in the psychological stress-coping adaptation system of resilience

Clinical Anecdote 5.1
In retrospect my initial response to the cancer diagnosis was a personal revelation I could never have imagined. I immediately defaulted to a problem-solving response. This helped me to calm down and focus on all that could be done to achieve a more hopeful result. I also shared this news with family and a couple of very close friends

who would regularly accompany me on daily walks, in the service of normalizing daily life that helped to attenuate feelings of anxiety. We discussed everything except my illness. This was extremely therapeutic, and kept me guardedly optimistic while focused on the here and now. We talked about books, children, politics, and shows we had seen. But when one dear friend, out of concern for my health, inquired about my clinical results and whether I was experiencing various symptoms, it triggered renewed anxiety. And ever so delicately, I tried to explain that it was better not to discuss my illness unless I raised it. These small cognitive and behavioral adjustments to a devastating diagnosis enabled me to manage my emotional reactions while providing a perceived sense of normalcy and control over my life.

5.3 Definition: Psychological Resilience

Resilience refers to psychological and biological interrelated processes of adjustment in response to various stressors resulting in adaptation in the aftermath of the stressful experience [1]. Psychological resilience refers to the dynamic, emotion-regulating, cognitive, and behavioral adaptive processes and coping strategies that are activated by adverse events in order to protect the individual's physical, mental, cognitive, and social health [1, 2]. Each successful cognitive and behavioral coping adaptation increases the individual's flexibility to respond more successfully to stressors in the future due to continued changes in the brain's structure and neural circuitry that enable greater cumulative flexibility in confronting stressful experiences in the future [1].

5.4 Theoretical Tenets and Model of Psychological Resilience: The Emotion-Regulating Stress-Coping Adaptation System of Psychological Resilience

Psychological resilience is based on a dynamic emotion-regulating stress-coping system of adaptation [6–8]. The *proposed* model is derived from theoretical tenets of the (1) stress and coping models of Folkman and Lazarus [6] and Folkman and Greer [9], (2) the common sense model of self-regulation, of Leventhal [8], and (3) the meaning-making model of Park et al. [7].

Antecedent Factors

The individual's mental schema of the self in combination with an illness-related schema identifies and interprets physical and somatic deviations from normal such as unusual symptoms that are interpreted by previous knowledge, experience, or illness-related discussions. These antecedent factors generate cognitive and emotional schemas or representations of the illness- and treatment-related threats that influence initial appraisals and coping responses [8].

Cognitive and Emotional Schemas or Representations

Cancer- or treatment-related cognitive schema or representations inform the individual's initial appraisal which is predicated on five sets of beliefs about the threat or stressor event [8]: (1) the source of the perceived threat (for instance, cancer) and perception of associated symptoms; (2) expected timeline of the threat: ie. duration, onset, and end; (3) Consequences: experienced or anticipated physical, cognitive, and social disruptions; (4) causes for the threat; and (5) the controllability of threat. Cognitive representations also inform the individual's emotional reactions such as anxiety, fear, distress, or composure. Both cognitive and emotional representations of the threat influence the subsequent pattern of coping responses and by extension resilient capability and health-related outcomes.

Cognitive and Behavioral Coping Strategies

Cognitive and emotional representations of the threat trigger cognitive and behavioral coping efforts that are *directly* aimed at (1) managing the threat, for instance, via problem-solving efforts and (2) downregulating the distressing emotional reactions, for instance, via use of distraction and meaning-making or relaxation response techniques [6, 10–13]. Coping efforts mediate the relationship between the deleterious effects of a perceived threat and health-related outcomes.

The key to psychological **resilience** is the effective mobilization of resilient-promoting emotion-regulating cognitive and behavioral coping strategies in response to stressors associated with the cancer diagnosis, treatment, survivorship, and supportive care phases. Patients and family caregivers must make necessary cognitive and behavioral coping adjustments in response to these and other stressors in order to maintain or improve their overall emotional and functional well-being [8, 14].

Coping efforts are typically described in terms of problem-focused, emotion-focused, and meaning-making coping efforts [6, 12, 13, 15]. Problem-focused adjustments refer to the strategies used to successfully manage the stressor, for instance, when a patient is unexpectedly short of breath and takes action by going to emergency. Emotion-focused coping refers to the strategies used to reduce the emotional distress associated with the stressor. An example is the use of distraction or focusing on one's breath on the way to the hospital. Meaning-making coping efforts reappraise the stressor experience in a way that enables the person to make sense of the cancer diagnosis or find meaning in adversity in order to maintain psychological well-being, acceptance, or personal growth [7, 10]. Meaning making is implicated at all levels of a stress exposure. Both appraisal and reappraisal induce interpretations of the stressor, the emotional reaction, and potential consequences. An individual may be described as being either directly engaged in managing a stressor (as in cognitive reappraisal or problem solving) or disengaged (as in use of avoidance and denial).

Patients and families generally use a range of coping strategies according to their appraisals of the threat and their personal and social resources. Five clusters of coping strategies were identified in a study of 603 patients with cancer: (1) seeking or using support, (2) focusing on the positive, (3) distancing, (4) cognitive escape/avoidance, and (5) behavioral escape/avoidance. Both problem-focused and emotion-focused strategies were identified with in each cluster [16]. Notwithstanding, as part of the meaning-making literature, the use of spiritual/religious coping is increasingly recognized as an important strategy for maintaining well-being in individuals with cancer [17].

Coping efforts typically include cognitive reappraisal, reframing, avoidance, emotion venting, generic problem solving, specific problem solving, seeking support, use of hope, acceptance, a sense of spiritual/religious connectedness, and meaning making. For instance, positive reappraisal (a cognitive coping strategy) may reinterpret the cancer (consequences, time frame, controllability) in a more positive light that is less threatening to the self which also serves to reduce the emotional distress and enhance well-being.

Hope

An important cognitive coping strategy is hope, although it has sometimes been taken as a personal resource. A meta-analysis of optimism and hope revealed that the two concepts were distinct despite some conceptual similarities [18]. Whereas optimism appears to be rooted in generalized global assumptions and beliefs, hope refers to a "reciprocally-derived sense of agency (or goal-directed determination) and pathways (planning ways to achieve goals)" [19, p. 571]. Hope is about having workable paths to realistic, desired goals (pathway thinking) and the motivation to use those paths (agency thinking) to achieve those goals that may be realized even in the terminal phase of life [20]. Hope influences appraisals of the stressor (its meaning and potential implications) [21]. Hope triggers behaviors that take advantage of opportunities to achieve desired goals. Contrary to being optimistic, hope can motivate an individual to action.

Hope has been related to quality of life, support, and spiritual and existential well-being in patients on treatment or palliative care [22, 23]. In contrast, a sense of hopelessness has been associated with increased symptom burden, psychological distress, and depression [24]. Patients have also been shown to lose hope but find it again *when they are able to modify their perceptions and see possibilities* [25]. Hope is not tethered to a cure or to some absolute goal in the future. It is capable of being reoriented to goals in the present as a function of the state of illness [26, 27]. Given the ability of hope to keep emotional distress at bay, it is important for patients to remain hopeful; one clinical strategy is to supportively help the patient or caregiver to reframe their hopes within a realistic clinical context that may change as the disease progresses. Other factors that contribute to coping capabilities include cultural beliefs and values as well as the patient's age and personal goals [14, 28].

Personal Resources, Social Resources, and Risk Factors

The adaptive process of psychological resilience (via the use of coping efforts) is influenced by interacting and modifiable personal and social resources (Fig. 5.1) (e.g., [17, 29, 33–35]). These resources serve as protective and/or enabling factors

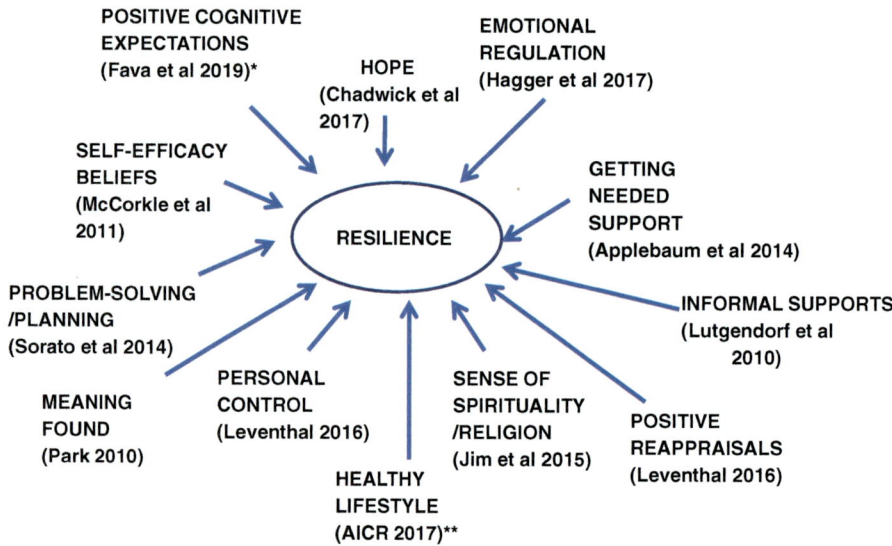

Fig. 5.1 Factors that promote resilience [7, 8, 14, 17, 21, 28–32]

that can positively influence resilience and health outcomes or serve as risk factors to be discussed below.

Personal Resources (PR)

Personal resources refer to modifiable personal strengths that enable an individual to realize goals that promote health-related outcomes [36]. PRs include self-efficacy beliefs, sense of coherence, optimism, cognitive flexibility, self-esteem, purpose in life, and/or a sense of spirituality (e.g., [37–40]). PRs play a critical role in modulating the stress-coping adaptation system of resilience, by positively influencing an individual's appraisals and reappraisals of the stressful event, and subsequent choice of coping efforts at each stressful phase of the cancer trajectory. Perhaps, for this reason, these personal attributes are also regarded as personal strengths.

Perceived strengths, however, tend to be context-driven; they benefit an individual in stressful situations that are perceived as manageable, but may be ineffective when stress is prolonged, uncontrollable, and beyond the individual's beliefs in his or her ability to cope effectively. Among personal strengths, there are three that regularly influence the adaptive resilience of patients with cancer and their family caregiver.

1. *General Self-Efficacy Beliefs:* An essential personal strength that influences the stress-coping adaptation response is belief in one's own competence to act effectively in highly stressful situations. General self-efficacy has been defined as beliefs in one's ability to mobilize the cognitive, behavioral, and social resources needed to act capably in a given situation [34, 41]. Individuals who believe in their ability to find solutions to manage the implications of their disease (problem-

solving coping behaviors) and to successfully obtain the help they need are more likely to mobilize effective coping strategies, achieve their goals of reducing toxic stress effects, and enhance their health potential [30, 42]. Generalized self-efficacy has its likely beginnings in the developmental relationships of growing infants and children with nurturing parents who help to interpret the expanding environment and help develop the appropriate coping skills to effectively adjust to perceived stressors.
2. *Sense of Optimism:* Sense of optimism or dispositional optimism refers to the belief or global assumption that life generally holds more favorable than unfavorable outcomes and that desired outcomes are usually attainable [39, 43]. Sense of optimism as a consequence is thought to be accompanied by a positive affect even when life circumstance becomes challenging. Optimism is thought to be an important component of self-regulation theory [44].
3. *Resilience:* In principle, an individual's psychological resilience may be regarded as a modifiable personal resource that refers to an overall perceived ability to successfully adapt to stress [2]. Significant positive relationships between a measure of resilience as a personal resource and health-related outcomes, specifically, global quality of life, posttraumatic growth (PTG), vitality, and well-being, *suggest that the individual's perceived resilience is a key determinant of health and posttraumatic growth* (e.g., [45]).

A number of cumulative indexes offer a summary measure of overall resilience assessed at a moment in time, recognizing that it may change as a function of environmental demands (e.g., [46, 47]). These indexes, however, offer added benefit by including psychosocial behavioral as well as biological biomarkers of resilience that may highlight areas of clinical vulnerability which could benefit from targeted clinical interventions [1, 31].

Social Resources
Social resources include family, friends, and healthcare providers who encourage and facilitate the patient's and caregiver's coping-related efforts in order to achieve optimal resilience, well-being, and health. Social support refers to the giving and receiving of caring, reassuring, material, compassionate, and loving behaviors within an emotionally connected and meaningful relationship that provides a sense of security, validation, belonging, and self-esteem. Support also refers to being part of a social network and to the availability and receipt of instrumental and informational as well as emotional support [48]. Informal support in particular has been found to be effective in promoting relevant cognitive and behavioral coping efforts (Fig. 5.1) [49, 50].

Risk Factors
Personal and social resources may also behave as risk factors, such as the lack of perceived support, an impaired coherent self, or a pessimistic worldview [51]. Personal and social risk factors negatively influence coping pathways (e.g., [28, 50, 52]). An individual who lacks the personal and/or social resources (such as a

resilient family) to effectively confront cancer-related challenges is likely to experience poor coping capabilities and neural endocrine and other biological disruptions increasing a biological threat to resilience and even survival (e.g., [31, 53]). From a nursing perspective, these findings albeit based mostly on cross-sectional with some longitudinal data nevertheless suggest the importance of assessing the potential effects of personal and social resources strengths/risk factors on stress-coping adaptive capabilities during the cancer experience.

Health-Related Outcomes

Psychological resilience has been assessed in terms of four main indicators of health: First is health-related quality of life (HRQOL) and overall well-being [54]. Health-related quality of life is defined in various ways but typically refers to how well a patient is functioning in his or her physical, cognitive, emotional, and social domains of life. Studies have identified thresholds of clinical importance for four quality of life scales from the EORTC QLQ-C30: physical functioning, emotional functioning, pain, and fatigue. The quality of life scales may be used to measure the current status of patients with cancer [55, 56].

Second is emotional distress, existential suffering, and symptoms and side effects that include *cancer-related biomarkers and pathophysiological indicators of disease* [14, 31, 53].

Third is psychological well-being (PWB) which refers to a sense of positive psychological functioning based on the perception of purposefully and meaningfully growing toward self-actualization, realizing life goals, coping with life challenges and finding acceptance in new clinical realities [57, 58].

Fourth is posttraumatic growth (PTG) which refers to positive changes in cognitive and behavioral responses to a traumatic event, such as cancer [59, 60]. PTG may emerge from cognitive efforts to find positive meaning in a stressful experience. The traumatic event stimulates the individual to cognitively reflect upon and analyze what has happened, its impact on the self, the impact of the self in relation to others and the larger world, from which new meanings may lead to a sense of personal growth and psychological healing [2] (Review Part IV, Chap. 10). Although related, a measure of psychological well-being provides an overall sense of well-being of the whole person, whereas a measure of personal growth is about demonstrated and identifiable sources of positive change.

Examples include meaningful changes in life philosophy that influence values and priorities; the development of more meaningful personal relationships; a new appreciation of life; new spiritual insights, a sense of connectedness to something greater than the self; an enhanced sense of personal strengths (e.g., self-efficacy) and/or personal meanings derived from the cancer experience (e.g., [7, 15, 59, 61]). PTG may also be illustrated by new health-promoting lifestyle behaviors that have been integrated into daily life. PTG ultimately signifies that something about the self has been learned at a deeply personal, meaningful level. It is thought that the experience of posttraumatic growth helps to restore resilience at a higher level of integrated functioning (e.g., [49, 62]).

PTG and Psychological Well-Being (PWB) The relationship between PTG and *well-being* is not the same experience or conceptual underpinning. Findings suggest that the clinical determinants of each reflect different aspects of resilience (e.g., [63]). For instance, PTG can occur in the absence of perceived well-being in patients who are palliative. PTG is thought to strengthen relative homeostasis by reducing personal distress through "transformative" insights and beliefs even in the presence of suffering and advanced disease [64].

PTG and Cognitive Expectation of Clinical Benefit The definitions of PTG and deriving a positive benefit appear to be similar within the context of a potential threat such as cancer. However, cognitive expectations in a future clinical benefit and posttraumatic growth are actually distinct constructs arising from different healing processes [65, 66]. Cognitive beliefs in a future clinical benefit tend to be predicated in previous experiences with medical challenges that resulted in positive clinical outcomes. Conversely, posttraumatic growth emerges from a stress-activated process of *ruminative learning* aimed at finding a meaningful understanding of the cancer experience that leads to a positive change in behavior or thinking with respect to the self, others, or a greater being [7, 67, 68]. Both behaviors may be manifested by individuals with cancer and their caregivers.

5.5 Research Findings among the Key Variables of the Stress Adaptation Coping System of Resilience (Review Part IV Chap. 9)

This section highlights empirically known findings among the key variables of the self-regulating stress-coping system of resilience (Fig. 5.2). It is not meant to be an exhaustive review of interrelationships, but to highlight known moderating, direct, and indirect (mediating) pathways among the key variables across stress-coping studies of varying rigor.

A Meta-Analyses Based on the CSM

A path analysis of the proposed relationships within the common sense model of self-regulation based on studies of the CSM produced support for a dynamic process model in which illness-related representations were shown to have direct effects on coping responses and clinical (illness) outcomes (Fig. 5.2) [14]. For instance, path analyses demonstrated that the illness representation of the threat (i.e., a cancer diagnosis) had direct and negative effects on illness outcomes. Moreover, threat-related beliefs were associated with adaptive and/or maladaptive coping strategies which in turn affected clinical outcomes [14]. Thus, problem- and/or emotion-focused coping strategies mediated the relationship between the illness representation (beliefs) and illness-related outcomes. Secondly, emotion- and/or problem-focused coping strategies also mediated the relationship

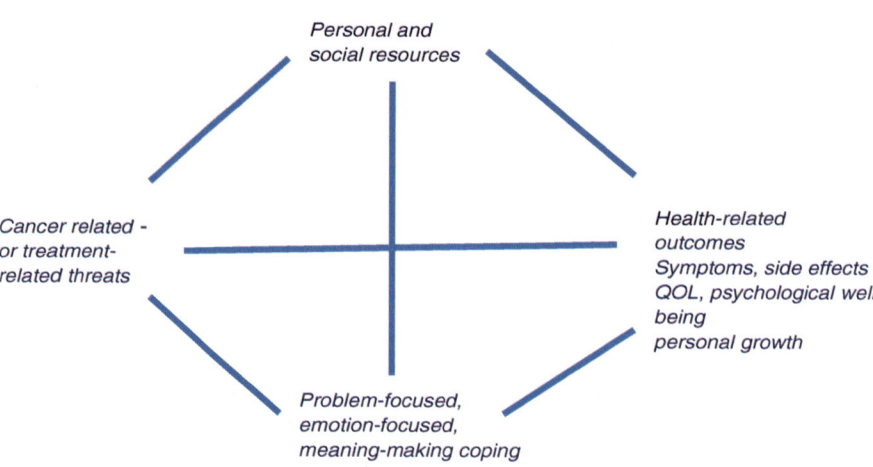

Fig. 5.2 Overall schematic of the evidentiary interrelationships discussed in the sections that follow

between emotional representations of the illness threat (such as fear, distress, and anxiety) and perceived control, and illness-related outcomes and functional well-being [14].

Cognitive representations that reflected a high level of threat (e.g., a cancer diagnosis, with poor treatability and serious life-threatening consequences) were positively associated with emotion-focused coping strategies including denial and expressing emotions [69]. Conversely, the representation of the cancer as "controllable" was associated with positive cognitive reappraisals and problem-solving coping strategies. Thus, clinical efforts to promote resilience and better health-related outcomes must focus not only on the individual's *beliefs or appraisals* about the cancer and treatment-related threats impacting outcomes but also *the coping strategies* mobilized by those beliefs [14]. To summarize, the CSM captures multifaceted attributes of illness- and treatment-related threats to offer a more complex understanding of the myriad factors that may directly or indirectly impact health-related functions and outcomes via problem- or emotion-focused coping efforts [8].

The Stress-Coping Adaptive Process of Resilience (e.g., [6, 13, 14, 16])

Studies that have explored the use of stress-induced coping efforts and health-related outcomes in patients with cancer or their family caregivers tend to be based on stress-coping or meaning-making models of adaptation [7, 10, 13, 16]. In contrast to the CSM model, the stressor such as a cancer diagnosis or a cancer recurrence tends to serve as the unmeasured stressful context for the study of the coping-related interrelationships.

Stress, Coping Strategies, and Health Outcomes
Studies of patients with cancer and caregivers tend to conceptualize the "stressor" in more contextual rather than measurable terms. For instance, the diagnostic phase has served as the stressful context for assessing the use of coping strategies in patients with gastric cancer without including a measure of its stress-inducing characteristics (e.g., [70–72]). Implicitly stressful situations that served as the context for a study of coping efforts included patients in different cancer *stages* or undergoing different forms of anticancer *treatment* [71, 73].

Coping Responses and Health-Related Outcomes Cancer *survivors* who used "adaptive" coping behaviors were shown to experience better quality of life [2, 74, 75]. "Adaptive" or resilient-promoting coping strategies included the use of positive reappraisal, meaning finding, seeking support, problem-solving behaviors, and religiosity [2, 76]. A meta-analysis of 33 studies comprising 3133 patients with prostate cancer showed that those who used active coping efforts such as approach seeking, problem-focused and emotion-focused coping had better psychological and physical health, although the effect size increases were modest for the emotion- and problem-focused coping strategies [77]. Conversely, those who relied on avoidant coping were shown to have poor psychological adjustment and physical health. Because the majority of studies in the meta-analysis were cross-sectional, bidirectional effects cannot be ruled out. In a longitudinal study, patients with advanced, incurable cancer who used emotional support and acceptance as their coping efforts reported higher levels of quality of life and less anxiety and depression at 12 months than those who did not [73].

Patients especially in the advanced stages of cancer have also been shown to use religious/spiritual strategies of coping [78]. A meta-analysis of 101 papers of 32,000 patients with cancer investigated the relationship between religion/spiritual coping and physical health [17]. Religion/spiritual coping measures were divided into affective, behavioral, cognitive, and "other" dimensions. Physical health was categorized as physical well-being, functional well-being, and physical symptoms. The findings showed that overall use of religion/spiritual coping was significantly related to overall physical health, underscoring the importance of considering the religious/spiritual coping needs of patients with cancer.

In a cross-sectional study of 170 patients with advanced terminal cancer, linear regression analyses showed significant relationships between the use of positive religious coping strategies (e.g., item: "I have been looking for a stronger connection with God") and better overall quality of life, including better scores on physical symptoms and the existential subscale (based on the McGill Quality of Life Measure) [75]. The existential subscale referred to meaning, purpose, (goals), and living in the present (everyday is a gift, life is worthwhile and controllable) [79, 80].

Conversely, the use of negative religious coping (e.g., item: "I have been wondering whether God has abandoned me") was significantly related to poorer quality of life and lower scores on existential and psychological QOL subscales. Similarly, meaning-focused coping strategies (positive reappraisals, fostering positive sensory experiences such as enjoying a sunset, or infusing daily life with meaning) were significantly related to psychological well-being in patients, for instance, who had cancer-related surgery [81].

In the main, individuals who have or had cancer and used avoidance, denial, substance use, and self-blame tended to experience increased distress, anxiety, depression, and poor quality of life including poor social, physical, and role functioning [2, 71, 82]. A systematic review also reported a significant, moderate-to-high relationship between "disengaged" coping strategies (such as distancing or avoidance) and psychological distress in individuals with head and neck cancer [83]. The findings underscore the value of patients finding meaning in living with cancer though a sense of the spiritual or of something greater than the self. The findings also highlight the importance of promoting cognitive reappraisal, emotion-focused and problem-focused coping, and supportive relationships to promote emotion regulation in distressed individuals.

Coping Clusters Over Time
Studies highlighted the use of various coping efforts over time. Women with life-threatening, advanced ovarian cancer facing physically difficult treatments and disease recurrence were followed over 12 months in order to assess their use of one or more of three clusters of coping-related items obtained by factor analysis: (a) taking action/framing (included planning, active coping, positive reframing, and humor); (b) social and emotional support (items based on instrumental and emotional support); (c) acceptance/denial [73]. The longitudinal data indicated that the majority of women (89%) relied on the *taking action/framing* set of coping efforts. Use of social and emotional coping efforts tended to decrease over time in 84% of the women suggesting successful adaptation over time, and 26% of the women *accepted reality*, whereas 74% used *"some" denial* at various periods over the course of the year. The findings remind clinicians of the multiple coping efforts that may be used to manage stressors as observed, for instance, among women with ovarian cancer.

Significantly, patients who were highly stable users of the *taking action/framing* set of coping efforts over the 12 months reported significantly less depression at 12 months [73]. Those who *accepted reality* also reported significantly less depression and less anxiety at 12 months. Notwithstanding, 6% ($n = 4$) of the women who were high stable users of *taking action/framing* still reported clinical or subclinical depression levels compared to those women who were not highly stable users. And 8% of the women who were highly stable users of social and emotional support reported a significantly better quality of life. The more positive coping behaviors used by the women (i.e., use of action/framing, social and emotional support and acceptance of reality), the greater their quality of life at 12 months. These findings support Folkman and Greer's [9] theoretical contention that a combination of problem-focused (planning and taking action) and emotion-focused (humor and reframing) coping strategies is used to confront various stressors associated with cancer. Beesley's findings are also consistent with those of Dunkel-Schetter's [16] study in which people with diverse cancers mobilized a range of problem- and emotion-focused coping strategies (seeking support, focusing on the positive, distancing, cognitive escape/avoidance, and behavioral escape/avoidance). These findings highlight the complex use of diverse coping strategies needed to readjust to stressful challenges in order to gradually accept reality or maintain well-being. A one-size-fits-all problem-solving modality does not exist.

Personal Resources
Personal resources, also known as resilient-promoting personal strengths such as self-efficacy and optimism are modifiable depending on the individual's appraisal of the stressor (e.g., [84, 85]). For instance, when a stressor is perceived as manageable, optimism and a sense of self-efficacy are likely to be enhanced. Conversely, individuals experiencing perceived distress are more likely to report low levels of optimism and self-efficacy [33, 86, 87]. In another study, levels of stress and optimism in survivors with breast cancer were observed to fluctuate over 12 months following chemotherapy with differential effects on emotional distress, fatigue, and difficulties with cognition [84]. The environmental context may be a modulating factor on levels of optimism and self-efficacy experienced by patients, signaling the importance of assessing the personal resources of patients and caregivers over the course of the cancer and survival trajectory.

Stress, Personal Resources, and Patient Outcomes An early study of 54 postoperative women with breast cancer showed that optimism appeared to be a moderator of the relationship between stress and immune functioning, as measured by levels of natural killer cell activity (NKCA) and interferon-gamma (IFN-γ) [88]. That is, optimism appeared to buffer the negative effects of stress on NKCA though not on IFN-γ. The findings from the small cross-sectional study suggest the need for a larger sample and more rigorous design. Although the findings from RCTS have shown significant beneficial effects of support, a social resource, on the health outcomes of cancer patients, rigorous studies investigating the buffering and indirect or mediating effects of personal resources on biological indicators of resilience are lacking (e.g., [89, 90]).

Personal Resources and Health-Related Outcomes Optimism and self-efficacy have also shown direct and positive effects on quality of life, and inverse effects on mood disturbance, anxiety, and depressive symptoms in patients with cancer (e.g., [51, 91, 92]). For instance, self-efficacy for coping was significantly related to lower levels of distress and higher quality of life in patients after tumor surgery as well as patients with diverse cancers across stages of the disease including transitioning to survivorship (e.g., [81]). Individuals with a history of adult, adolescent, and childhood cancers who scored high on optimism and support were more likely to experience posttraumatic growth, although Kolokotroni's (2014) review of 11 studies showed contradictory findings (e.g., [68, 93]).

Cross-sectional data from studies of patients with various cancers also suggest positive relationships between resilience (as a personal resource) and quality of life with possible differential findings depending on the type of cancer and phase of treatment [94, 95]. Cross-sectional findings of 276 patients on active treatment showed significant positive relationships between resilience and quality of life in lung cancer patients compared to those individuals with gastric or colorectal cancers [94]. The highest quartile of a measure of resilience (based on the Connor-Davidson Resilience Measure) was also associated with a 64% decrease in the risk of emotional distress compared to the lowest quartile based on an odds ratio analysis. Another cross-sectional study of 343 patients with cancer undergoing chemotherapy, radiotherapy, or chemoradiation treatment showed that resilience especially in older adults was significantly related to less emotional distress and more physical activity based on structural equation modeling [96]. Conversely, long-term survivors of hematopoietic cell transplant with low levels of resilience were significantly more likely to experience emotional distress and experienced the poorest mental health-related quality of life [97]. These findings provide evidence of the important relationship between resilience and health-related outcomes in patients with cancer and provide scientific rationale for nurses to promote and protect the resilience of patients and caregivers throughout the continuum of care. The studies also highlight the important relationships of other personal resources on the health outcomes of patients with cancer.

Personal Resources and Coping Responses Personal strengths appear to influence cognitive and behavioral coping strategies in individuals with diverse stages and treatment phases of cancer [2]. A sense of optimism and self-efficacy were significantly associated with less negative coping appraisals and less avoidant coping behaviors in patients undergoing treatment for advanced-stage cancer [92]. The findings highlight the relationships of sense of optimism and self-efficacy on coping response of patients with cancer [92]. A recent study explored the impact of three "personality" characteristics (distressed, resilient, and normative) on use of coping strategies in patients undergoing chemotherapy for breast, lung, gastrointestinal, and gynecological cancers [98]. Compared to individuals in the normative and resilient categories, the distressed group was reported to favor less use of active coping, less positive reframing, less acceptance, and less emotional support, which are known adaptive resilient-promoting coping approaches. Rather, they preferred the use of denial, emotional venting, behavioral disengagement, and self-blame, that is, maladaptive coping behaviors. The distressed group also scored higher on anxious preoccupation, helplessness, hopelessness, fatalism, and avoidance and lower on fighting spirit compared to the other groups. These findings illustrate the clinical importance of developing interventions that address the patient's beliefs about the cancer-related threat, their consequential emotional distress, as well as their cognitive and behavioral coping responses.

Mediating and Interactional Coping Effects

One cross-sectional study of women, newly diagnosed with gynecological cancers revealed mediating coping effects between *resilience and quality of life* [99].

Mediation analyses suggested that coping strategies of expressing positive emotions, positive reappraisal (of the cancer experience), and developing a sense of meaning and peacefulness accounted for 62.6% of the relationship between resilience and quality of life. Resilient women appeared to have a higher quality of life when they utilized coping strategies that expressed positive emotions, positively reframed the cancer experience and cultivated a sense of meaning in their lives.

Coping- and meaning-focused strategies were also observed to mediate the relationship between self-efficacy and health-related quality of life in individuals following tumor surgery, suggesting that a belief in one's ability to manage stressful situations leads to the use of effective coping strategies resulting in better health-related outcomes (e.g., Fig. 5.2) [81].

A theory-driven path analysis examined the role of meaning in patients undergoing chemotherapy or radiation therapy for gastric cancer [70]. Meaning in life (a measure of global meaning) exerted positive effects on psychological well-being only indirectly via problem-focused, emotion-focused, and meaning-focused coping strategies, consistent with Folkman and Greer's [9] theoretical contention that individuals use a combination of coping efforts to manage stress effects and to maintain well-being. Situational meaning pertaining to the cancer experience was also indirectly related to psychological well-being via the mediating effects of emotion- and meaning-focused coping strategies. However, in this instance, situational meaning led to a reduction in the use of emotion-focused and meaning-focused coping which were subsequently associated with low levels of psychological well-being. Situational meaning refers to the individual's perception of the significance of the cancer as a consequence of its threat to his or her global assumptions about the world and the self which have been challenged by the reality of cancer (Review Part IV, Chap. 10). Conversely, meaning in life in this study may relate to an individual's revised goals and values that have been realigned with clinical reality enabling the use of more effective coping strategies (in which global assumptions about the world and the self were reconciled with situational meanings to produce a new meaning in life). These findings need to be replicated using a longitudinal data set in order to validate the direction of effects suggested by the path analysis.

Interactional Effects on Patient Outcomes A consecutive 28-day study of patient/caregiver dyads following hematopoietic stem cell transplantation indicated *that interactional effects* between daily high levels of "coping" self-efficacy beliefs and emotion-focused coping behaviors (that is use of reframing and acceptance) in patients were associated with a significantly high positive affect within the patient/caregiver dyads [100]. Moreover, interactional effects between the *caregiver's* higher than usual level of self-efficacy and the *patient's* use of instrumental coping (i.e., planning and active coping) were also associated with increased positive affect within the dyad. The findings highlight the extent to which patients and caregivers experience reciprocal behavioral effects and the importance of enhancing both patient and caregiver self-efficacy beliefs through self-management programs or by promoting cognitive and behavioral coping strategies tailored to the daily illness and treatment-related demands of cancer.

Although current knowledge is that personal strengths are susceptible to change as a function of the stress-related context, these studies highlight how important personal resources are for promoting emotion-regulating adaptive coping efforts.

Social Resources (Support) (See Part IV Chap. 11)

Stressors, Support, and Health-Related Outcomes Social support appears to exert direct, mediating, and stress-buffering effects on quality of life, psychological well-being, depression, anxiety, and survival in patients with ovarian and colorectal cancers, and breast cancer survivors (e.g., [49, 101, 102]). For instance, the quality of the patient–partner relationship was found to positively impact the patient's and partner's adjustment to colorectal cancer [103].

In contrast, a perceived lack of support was associated with depression, anxiety, and an increased risk of a shortened life in women with breast cancer, suggesting the clinical importance of screening for support at diagnosis and providing supportive interventions before, during, and after treatment (e.g., [89]). Moreover, in an early study of patients with ovarian cancer, those with self-reported social support were found to have higher levels of natural killer cell cytotoxicity in tumor-infiltrating lymphocytes (TIL) as well as in peripheral blood mononuclear cells (PBMC), controlling for stage of cancer [104]. Conversely, distress was associated with lower levels of NK cytotoxicity in TIL. The findings have been supported by other biobehavioral studies on support [89, 90, 105]. These findings may explain in part why individuals with breast cancer who feel supported by family and/or friends appear to have a lengthened survivorship [35, 106]. Future rigorously designed RCTS with biological and psychosocial clinical endpoints would further inform the relationships between support, health and survivability in patients with cancer and their family caregiver.

Sources of Support Deno and colleagues' (2012) study of emotionally distressed patients with facial disfigurement due to head and neck cancer reported that *the source* of support was an important mediating factor of distress [107]. Whereas family support was unrelated directly or indirectly to a decrease in emotional distress, friend support appeared to improve social distress but not emotional distress. The effects of sources of support may vary depending on patient needs. Given growing evidence of the effects of support on health-related outcomes and survivorship, perceived support should be assessed frequently across disease stages and during the transition to survivorship [108].

Support Changes Over Time Changes in levels of support quantity and quality over the course of the diagnosis, treatment, and/or survivorship show differential effects on emotional well-being and health-related quality of life [109, 110]. For instance, new survivors of breast cancer reported a significant decline in the quantity but not quality of support in the year following the end of treatment [110]. Moreover, a reduction in support quality was a significant predictor of depression, negative affect, and stress [110]. The results were consistent with those obtained from a two-year study of newly diagnosed patients with colorectal cancer who were followed over 2 years [109]. Perceived availability of support decreased following the colorectal diagnosis and treatment in about one-third of the patients. The patients with less support were found to have poorer health-related quality of life. Changes in well-being and quality of life in relation to support over the course of the treatment and survivorship underscore the importance of fostering the patient's personal relationships and family support.

Support and Coping Responses Perceived support, especially emotional/informational, affectionate, and tangible forms of support, was consistently shown to promote adaptive coping efforts in cancer patients and survivors [15, 49, 50]. Similarly, secure attachment was significantly associated with the use of active coping, reappraisals, and religion in cancer survivors [111]. For instance, perceived support among patients with melanoma cancer was associated with significantly less behavioral disengagement (maladaptive coping efforts) and significantly greater use of active coping, positive reframing, planning, acceptance, and humor (adaptive coping strategies) than those reporting lower levels of support [50].

Support from family or friends can have an important and positive effect on the coping responses of cancer patients and survivors by helping patients manage cancer- and treatment-related demands, suggesting emotion-focused, problem-focused, and meaning-making coping strategies [2]. Support can modulate the patient's appraisal of the stress and suggest more effective cognitive and behavioral ways of managing adversity as already noted. These findings underscore the clinical imperative of encouraging the patient and caregiver supportive relationship.

Path analysis using cross-sectional data from patients with diverse cancers revealed that adaptive coping strategies (active coping, planning, and positive reframing) were significant mediators of the relationship between perceived support and PTG, with support showing nonsignificant direct effects on PTG [49]. This finding is consistent with that of another cross-sectional study in which positive reframing and religion appeared to mediate the relationship between secure attachment and posttraumatic growth, although reverse effects are also possible [112]. When both support or attachment and coping efforts were concurrently analyzed in structural modeling equations, support's main effect was to foster adaptive coping efforts that subsequently had direct effects on positive change and personal growth captured by constructs of PTG and psychological well-being [58, 59]. However, prospective data are needed to determine the actual direction of the effects among the variable in the studies.

Support and Personal Resources
Optimism Social support and optimism exert moderating as well as direct and indirect effects on health-related outcomes. Both support and optimism have been independently associated with higher levels of quality of life in patients with cancer [28]. However, optimism was also shown as a moderator of the relationship between

support and anxiety in patients with advanced cancer. That is, greater support was associated with less anxiety in patients with low levels of optimism, demonstrating buffering or protective effects on these patients. Curiously, support was not associated with less anxiety in patients with high optimism. Optimistic patients may attract the support they need, and therefore, in and of itself more support does not alter anxiety levels. Alternatively, the increase in support may signal to the advanced cancer patient that he is in decline causing more anxiety [28]. Studies which have investigated the conditions in which individuals accepted support for emotional distress found that the social context was an important factor to consider clinically, in particular the fit between the support offered and the desired type of support needed [113].

Self-efficacy Bidirectional relationships between self-efficacy and support have been found across several studies. For instance, the effects of the support patients received from family, friends, and health personnel on health-related indicators following surgery for lung cancer was shown to be mediated by the patient's level of self-efficacy [33]. In other words, received support enhanced the patients' self-efficacy which in turn improved health outcomes. These findings are in support of the *enabling hypothesis*.

Other findings support the *cultivation hypothesis* in which the patient's self-efficacy facilitated their receipt of needed support (e.g., [114]). Thus, the clinical context may influence the nature of the directional effects between support and self-efficacy which will also vary over time depending on the individual's source of stress along the continuum and the personal and social resources at their disposal to manage the stress. As we will learn in Part IV Chaps. 9 and 10, an important goal of nursing workshops would involve facilitating self-efficacy coping abilities so that patients may learn how to successfully seek and maintain the support they need as well as to develop other adaptive coping responses.

Resilience In a cross-sectional study of cancer patients, resilience was shown to be positively associated with higher levels of support and lower levels of hopelessness (e.g., [115]). Support was also shown to be a mediator of the relationship between resilience and quality of life in patients with breast cancer [116]. Resilient individuals were better able to attract and maintain support which in turn resulted in better health outcomes (Fig. 5.3).

Conversely, a summary measure of resilience was shown to be a significant mediator of the relationship between perceived support and posttraumatic growth (PTG) in survivors of colorectal cancer (Fig. 5.3) [45]. Although perceived support demonstrated significant but relatively small direct effects on PTG, it exerted significantly larger direct effects on resilience which in turn showed similarly large positive effects on PTG [45]. Resilience here is a personal resource captured at a moment in time and reflective of the individual's overall adaptive capabilities. These findings

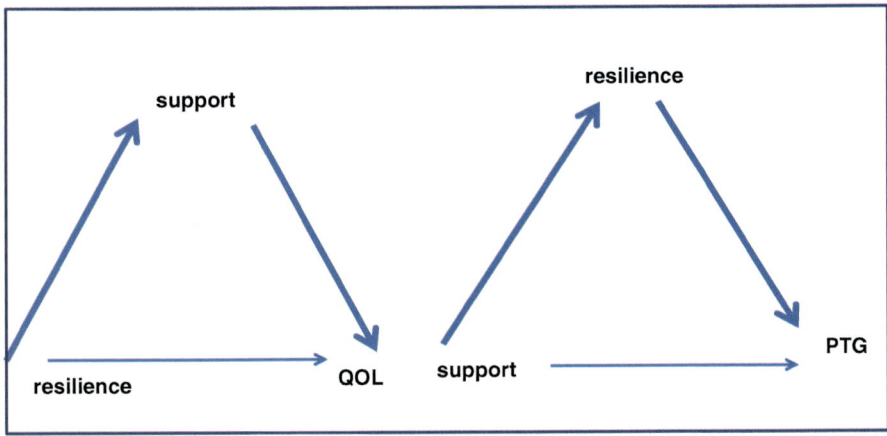

Fig. 5.3 Mediating effects on quality of life (QOL) or posttraumatic growth (PTG) [115, 116]

strongly suggest that nursing interventions must include enhancing the quality of the patient's informal supports which is so vital to strengthening resilience and by extension health and well-being.

5.6 Nursing Implications

Table 5.1 summarizes the important takeaway from the literature review of Sect. 5.5. Emotion-regulating, stress-coping resilience may be said to be the psychosocial complement of the underlying processes of biological resilience, and both mutually interact and are integrally interrelated. Psychological resilience depends on the patient's ability to mobilize effective emotion-regulating cognitive and behavioral coping responses to psychological stress. It also depends on numerous interrelated and mutually regulating personal and social resources that directly or indirectly influence the adaptive processes of stress-coping resilience, serving also as protective buffers depending on the clinical context (e.g., [108]). The intensity, duration, and frequency and controllability of stress exposures, the resilient-promoting/interfering personal and social resources, and the cognitive and behavioral coping responses have a complex interacting impact on psychological resilience and health-related outcomes.

This chapter only presented widely known, clinically relevant, variables associated with the emotion-regulating system of psychological resilience. The chapter offered findings of key personal resources and support that influence coping efforts, suggesting that these resources may be leveraged by nursing interventions in order to promote psychological resilience in patients and caregivers (e.g., [33, 119]). The studies in which a measure of psychological resilience was included as a personal resource suggest that a cumulative index of resilience assessed at one moment in time may be valuable in estimating the patient's overall resilience at different points

Table 5.1 Key takeaways of research findings in the field of psychological adaptive coping resilience

Findings
1. Individuals who feel supported also show higher resilience and quality of life and likely lengthen survival [35, 116]
2. Resilience is an adaptive process and also considered as a personal resource or strength when measured at one moment in time [94, 117]
3. Adaptive coping efforts include taking action, humor, planning, positive reappraisal, meaning found, seeking support, problem-solving strategies, sense of religiosity/spirituality [2, 10, 16]
4. Other coping strategies include fostering sensory experiences (e.g., enjoying a sunset), use of distraction, finding meaning in order, and purpose (e.g., daily life events, routine) [15, 118]
5. Maladaptive coping behaviors include prolonged distancing, escape/avoidance, alcohol/drug use, self-blame associated with poor QOL [16]
6. Individuals with high self-efficacy likely promote active coping and meaning-focused coping behaviors [30]
7. Personal resources such as self-efficacy and optimism are modifiable and impact both coping efforts and health outcomes [84]
8. Support can lead to increased active coping, planning, and positive reframing [49]

of potential vulnerability along the continuum. It would add useful information for developing relevant psychosocial interventions with targeted behavioral and neurophysiological indicators (e.g., Review Table 3.2). Informal support was also found to be a better predictor of patient survivorship than any other form of support, providing evidence for strengthening the patient's quality of supportive relationships with significant "family" members including the informal caregiver as part of nursing's care of patients and caregivers (e.g., [89]). Finally, hope must be nurtured in nursing interventions: It may disappear temporarily as a coping strategy when hope as the patient originally conceived it appears hopeless. But it can reemerge again when the patient has been helped to reorient their hope toward new possibilities within realistic clinical contexts [25, 26].

The stress-coping adaptation system of resilience optimally functions under stressful conditions of short duration in which the individual has learned to adapt or successfully habituate to similarly stressful situations [53]. If patient stress is prolonged, unpredictable, and unregulated (which may be evidenced by individuals with poor coping capabilities in the advanced stages of cancer), allostatic overload may result (that is, evidence of poor resilience), thereby posing a real threat to the individual's health and survivorship (Review Part III Chaps. 6 and 7). It is unclear when psychological resilience converts to maladaptation, but one can assume that newly diagnosed patients with cancer have already been exposed to chronic stress and their resilient capabilities need to be clinically assessed [31].

The evidentiary data in this chapter indicate that a key objective of nursing in cancer care is to reduce emotional distress and secondly to strengthen psychological (and biological) adaptation (i.e., resilience) by encouraging relevant coping-promoting nursing interventions as early as the diagnostic phase and by strengthening informal supportive relationships. The individual's supportive relationship is critical for encouraging positive reappraisals, problem-focused, emotion-focused, and meaning-making coping responses in loved ones facing stressors along the illness and recovery continuum.

References

1. McEwen BS, Gray J, Nasca C. Recognizing resilience: learning from the effects of stress on the brain. Neurobiol Stress. 2015;1:1–11. PubMed PMID: 25506601. Pubmed Central PMCID: PMC4260341. Epub 2014/12/17. Eng.
2. Seiler A, Jenewein J. Resilience in cancer patients. Front Psych. 2019;10:208. PubMed PMID: 31024362. Pubmed Central PMCID: PMC6460045. Epub 2019/04/27. eng.
3. McEwen BS. In pursuit of resilience: stress, epigenetics, and brain plasticity. Ann N Y Acad Sci. 2016;1373(1):56–64. PubMed PMID: 26919273. Epub 2016/02/27. eng.
4. Wang M, Zhao J, Zhang L, Wei F, Lian Y, Wu Y, et al. Role of tumor microenvironment in tumorigenesis. J Cancer. 2017;8(5):761–73. PubMed PMID: 28382138. Pubmed Central PMCID: PMC5381164. Epub 2017/04/07. eng.
5. Kalisch R, Muller MB, Tuscher O. A conceptual framework for the neurobiological study of resilience. Behav Brain Sci. 2015;38:e92. PubMed PMID: 25158686. Epub 2014/08/28. eng.
6. Folkman S, Lazarus RS, Dunkel-Schetter C, DeLongis A, Gruen RJ. Dynamics of a stressful encounter: cognitive appraisal, coping, and encounter outcomes. J Pers Soc Psychol. 1986;50(5):992–1003. PubMed PMID: 3712234. Epub 1986/05/01. eng.
7. Park CL. Making sense of the meaning literature: an integrative review of meaning making and its effects on adjustment to stressful life events. Psychol Bull. 2010;136(2):257–301. PubMed PMID: 20192563. Epub 2010/03/03. eng.
8. Leventhal H, Phillips LA, Burns E. The Common-Sense Model of Self-Regulation (CSM): a dynamic framework for understanding illness self-management. J Behav Med. 2016;39(6):935–46. PubMed PMID: 27515801. Epub 2016/08/16. eng.
9. Folkman S, Greer S. Promoting psychological well-being in the face of serious illness: when theory, research and practice inform each other. Psycho-Oncology. 2000;9(1):11–9. PubMed PMID: 10668055. Epub 2000/02/11. eng.
10. Park C, Folkman S. Meaning in the context of stress and coping. Rev Gen Psychol. 1997;1:115–44.
11. Folkman S, Lazarus RS, Gruen RJ, DeLongis A. Appraisal, coping, health status, and psychological symptoms. J Pers Soc Psychol. 1986;50(3):571–9. PubMed PMID: 3701593. Epub 1986/03/01. eng.
12. Folkman S, Moskowitz J. Positive affect and meaning-focused coping during significant psychological stress. In: Hewstone M, Schut HAW, de Wit JBF, van den Bos K, Stroebe MS, editors. The scope of social psychology: theory and applications. New York: Psychology Press; 2007. p. 193–208.
13. Lazarus R, Folkman S. Stress, appraisal and coping. New York: Springer; 1984.
14. Hagger MS, Koch S, Chatzisarantis NLD, Orbell S. The common sense model of self-regulation: meta-analysis and test of a process model. Psychol Bull. 2017;143(11):1117–54. PubMed PMID: 28805401. Epub 2017/08/15. eng.
15. Park CL, Edmondson D, Fenster JR, Blank TO. Meaning making and psychological adjustment following cancer: the mediating roles of growth, life meaning, and restored just-world beliefs. J Consult Clin Psychol. 2008;76(5):863–75. PubMed PMID: 18837603. Epub 2008/10/08. eng.

16. Dunkel-Schetter C, Feinstein LG, Taylor SE, Falke RL. Patterns of coping with cancer. Health Psychol. 1992;11(2):79–87. PubMed PMID: 1582383. Epub 1992/01/01. eng.
17. Jim HS, Pustejovsky JE, Park CL, Danhauer SC, Sherman AC, Fitchett G, et al. Religion, spirituality, and physical health in cancer patients: a meta-analysis. Cancer. 2015;121(21):3760–8. PubMed PMID: 26258868. Pubmed Central PMCID: PMC4618080. Epub 2015/08/11. eng.
18. Alarcon G, Bowling NA, Khazon S. Great expectations: a meta analytic examination of optimism and hope. Personal Individ Differ. 2013;54:821–7.
19. Snyder C, Harris C, Anderon JR, Holleran SA, Irving IM, Sigmon ST, et al. The wills and the ways: development and validation of an -individual difference measure of hope. J Pers Soc Psychol. 1991;60:570–85.
20. Gum A, Snyder CR. Coping with terminal illness: the role of hopeful thinking. J Palliat Care. 2002;5(6):883–94.
21. Chadwick A, Zoccola PM, Figueroa WS, Rabideau EM. Communication and stress: effects of hope evocation and rumination messages on heart rate, anxiety, anxiety and emotions after a stressor. Health Commun. 2016;31(12):1447–59.
22. Nierop-van Baalen C, Grypdonck M, van Hecke A, Verhaeghe S. Associated factors of hope in cancer patients during treatment: a systematic literature review. J Adv Nurs. 2020;76(7):1520–37. PubMed PMID: 32133663. Epub 2020/03/07. eng.
23. Sinclair S, Pereira J, Raffin S. A thematic review of the spirituality literature within palliative care. J Palliat Med. 2006;9(2):464–79.
24. Brothers BM, Andersen BL. Hopelessness as a predictor of depressive symptoms for breast cancer patients coping with recurrence. Psycho-Oncology. 2009;18(3):267–75. PubMed PMID: 18702065. Pubmed Central PMCID: PMC2743157. Epub 2008/08/15. eng.
25. Duggleby W, Hicks D, Nekolaichuk C, Holtslander L, Williams A, Chambers T, et al. Hope, older adults, and chronic illness: a metasynthesis of qualitative research. J Adv Nurs. 2012;68(6):1211–23. PubMed PMID: 22221185. Epub 2012/01/10. eng.
26. Jacobsen J, Kvale E, Rabow M, Rinaldi S, Cohen S, Weissman D, et al. Helping patients with serious illness live well through the promotion of adaptive coping: a report from the improving outpatient palliative care (IPAL-OP) initiative. J Palliat Med. 2014;17(4):463–8. PubMed PMID: 24579823. Epub 2014/03/04. eng.
27. Temel JS, Greer JA, Muzikansky A, Gallagher ER, Admane S, Jackson VA, et al. Early palliative care for patients with metastatic non-small-cell lung cancer. N Engl J Med. 2010;363(8):733–42. PubMed PMID: 20818875. Epub 2010/09/08. eng.
28. Applebaum AJ, Stein EM, Lord-Bessen J, Pessin H, Rosenfeld B, Breitbart W. Optimism, social support, and mental health outcomes in patients with advanced cancer. Psycho-Oncology. 2014;23(3):299–306. PubMed PMID: 24123339. Pubmed Central PMCID: PMC4001848. Epub 2013/10/15. eng.
29. Sorato DB, Osorio FL. Coping, psychopathology, and quality of life in cancer patients under palliative care. Palliat Support Care. 2015;13(3):517–25. PubMed PMID: 24783996. Epub 2014/05/03. eng.
30. McCorkle R, Ercolano E, Lazenby M, Schulman-Green D, Schilling LS, Lorig K, et al. Self-management: enabling and empowering patients living with cancer as a chronic illness. CA Cancer J Clin. 2011;61(1):50–62. PubMed PMID: 21205833. Pubmed Central PMCID: PMC3058905. Epub 2011/01/06. eng.
31. Fava GA, McEwen BS, Guidi J, Gostoli S, Offidani E, Sonino N. Clinical characterization of allostatic overload. Psychoneuroendocrinology. 2019;108:94–101. PubMed PMID: 31252304. Epub 2019/06/30. eng.
32. Lutgendorf SK, Sood AK, Antoni MH. Host factors and cancer progression: biobehavioral signaling pathways and interventions. J Clin Oncol. 2010;28(26):4094–9. PubMed PMID: 20644093. Pubmed Central PMCID: PMC2940426. Epub 2010/07/21. eng.
33. Banik A, Luszczynska A, Pawlowska I, Cieslak R, Knoll N, Scholz U. Enabling, not cultivating: received social support and self-efficacy explain quality of life after lung cancer surgery. Ann Behav Med. 2017;51(1):1–12. PubMed PMID: 27418357. Epub 2016/07/16. eng.

34. Chirico A, D'Aiuto G, Penon A, Mallia L, De Laurentiis M, Lucidi F, et al. Self-efficacy for coping with cancer enhances the effect of reiki treatments during the pre-surgery phase of breast cancer patients. Anticancer Res. 2017;37(7):3657–65. PubMed PMID: 28668857. Epub 2017/07/03. eng.
35. Andersen BL, Thornton LM, Shapiro CL, Farrar WB, Mundy BL, Yang HC, et al. Biobehavioral, immune, and health benefits following recurrence for psychological intervention participants. Clin Cancer Res. 2010;16(12):3270–8. PubMed PMID: 20530702. Pubmed Central PMCID: PMC2910547. Epub 2010/06/10. eng.
36. Lundman B, Alex L, Jonsen E, Norberg A, Nygren B, Santamaki Fischer R, et al. Inner strength--a theoretical analysis of salutogenic concepts. Int J Nurs Stud. 2010;47(2):251–60. PubMed PMID: 19577237. Epub 2009/07/07. eng.
37. Amstadter AB, Moscati A, Oxon MA, Maes HH, Myers JM, Kendler KS. Personality, cognitive/psychological traits and psychiatric resilience: a multivariate twin study. Personal Individ Differ. 2016;91:74–9. PubMed PMID: 29104336. Pubmed Central PMCID: PMC5667653. Epub 2016/03/01. eng.
38. Carver CS, Antoni MH. Finding benefit in breast cancer during the year after diagnosis predicts better adjustment 5 to 8 years after diagnosis. Health Psychol. 2004;23(6):595–8. PubMed PMID: 15546227. Epub 2004/11/18. eng.
39. Carver CS, Scheier MF. Dispositional optimism. Trends Cogn Sci. 2014;18(6):293–9. PubMed PMID: 24630971. Pubmed Central PMCID: PMC4061570. Epub 2014/03/19. eng.
40. Diehl M, Hay EL. Personality-related risk and resilience factors in coping with daily stress among adult cancer patients. Res Hum Dev. 2013;10(1):47–69. PubMed PMID: 23646033. Pubmed Central PMCID: PMC3640793. Epub 2013/05/07. eng.
41. Bandura A. Self-efficacy: toward a unifying theory of behavioral change. Psychol Rev. 1977;84(2):191–215. PubMed PMID: 847061. Epub 1977/03/01. eng.
42. Chirico A, Serpentini S, Merluzzi T, Mallia L, Del Bianco P, Martino R, et al. Self-efficacy for coping moderates the effects of distress on quality of life in palliative cancer care. Anticancer Res. 2017;37(4):1609–15. PubMed PMID: 28373421. Epub 2017/04/05. eng.
43. Scheier M, Carver CS. Effects of optimism on psychological and physical well being: theoretical overview and empirical update. Cogn Ther Res. 1992;16(2):201–28.
44. Carver CS, Scheier MF. On the self regulation of behavior. Cambridge University Press; 1998.
45. Dong X, Li G, Liu C, Kong L, Fang Y, Kang X, et al. The mediating role of resilience in the relationship between social support and posttraumatic growth among colorectal cancer survivors with permanent intestinal ostomies: a structural equation model analysis. Eur J Oncol Nurs. 2017;29:47–52. PubMed PMID: 28720265. Epub 2017/07/20. eng.
46. Seeman TE, Gruenewald TL, Cohen S, Williams DR, Matthews KA. Social relationships and their biological correlates: Coronary Artery Risk Development in Young Adults (CARDIA) study. Psychoneuroendocrinology. 2014;43:126–38. PubMed PMID: 24703178. Epub 2014/04/08. eng.
47. Seeman TE, McEwen BS, Rowe JW, Singer BH. Allostatic load as a marker of cumulative biological risk. Proc Natl Acad Sci U S A. 2001;98:4770–5.
48. Cohen S, Wills TA. Stress, social support, and the buffering hypothesis. Psychol Bull. 1985;98(2):310–57. PubMed PMID: 3901065. Epub 1985/09/01. eng.
49. Cao W, Qi X, Cai DA, Han X. Modeling posttraumatic growth among cancer patients: the roles of social support, appraisals, and adaptive coping. Psycho-Oncology. 2018;27(1):208–15. PubMed PMID: 28171681. Epub 2017/02/09. eng.
50. Kalbfleisch M, Cyr A, Gregorio N, Nyhof-Young J. Investigating coping strategies and social support among Canadian melanoma patients: a survey approach. Can Oncol Nurs J. 2015;25(1):60–72. PubMed PMID: 26642495. Epub 2015/12/09. eng.
51. Thieme M, Einenkel J, Zenger M, Hinz A. Optimism, pessimism and self-efficacy in female cancer patients. Jpn J Clin Oncol. 2017;47(9):849–55. PubMed PMID: 28591864. Epub 2017/06/08. eng.
52. Mystakidou K, Tsilika E, Parpa E, Gogou P, Panagiotou I, Vassiliou I, et al. Relationship of general self-efficacy with anxiety, symptom severity and quality of life in cancer patients

before and after radiotherapy treatment. Psycho-Oncology. 2013;22(5):1089–95. PubMed PMID: 22615047. Epub 2012/05/23. eng.
53. McEwen BS. Neurobiological and systemic effects of chronic stress. Chronic Stress (Thousand Oaks, Calif). 2017;1:2470547017692328. PubMed PMID: 28856337. Pubmed Central PMCID: PMC5573220. Epub 2017/09/01. eng.
54. Karimi M, Brazier J. Health, health-related quality of life, and quality of life: what is the difference? PharmacoEconomics. 2016;34(7):645–9. PubMed PMID: 26892973. Epub 2016/02/20. eng.
55. Giesinger JM, Kuijpers W, Young T, Tomaszewski KA, Friend E, Zabernigg A, et al. Thresholds for clinical importance for four key domains of the EORTC QLQ-C30: physical functioning, emotional functioning, fatigue and pain. Health Qual Life Outcomes. 2016;14:87. PubMed PMID: 27267486. Pubmed Central PMCID: PMC4897949. Epub 2016/06/09. eng.
56. Pilz MJ, Aaronson NK, Arraras JI, Caocci G, Efficace F, Groenvold M, et al. Evaluating the thresholds for clinical importance of the EORTC QLQ-C15-PAL in patients receiving palliative treatment. J Palliat Med. 2021;24(3):397–404. PubMed PMID: 32835601. Epub 2020/08/25. eng.
57. Ryff CD. Psychological well-being revisited: advances in the science and practice of eudaimonia. Psychother Psychosom. 2014;83(1):10–28. PubMed PMID: 24281296. Pubmed Central PMCID: PMC4241300. Epub 2013/11/28. eng.
58. Ryff CD, Keyes CL. The structure of psychological well-being revisited. J Pers Soc Psychol. 1995;69(4):719–27. PubMed PMID: 7473027. Epub 1995/10/01. eng.
59. Tedeschi RG, Calhoun LG. Posttraumatic growth: conceptual foundations and empirical evidence. Psychol Inq. 2004;15:1–18.
60. Tedeschi RG, Calhoun LG. Beyond the concept of recovery: growth and the experience of loss. Death Stud. 2008;32(1):27–39. PubMed PMID: 18652064. Epub 2008/07/26. eng.
61. Mols F, Vingerhoets AJ, Coebergh JW, van de Poll-Franse LV. Well-being, posttraumatic growth and benefit finding in long-term breast cancer survivors. Psychol Health. 2009;24(5):583–95. PubMed PMID: 20205013. Epub 2010/03/06. eng.
62. Ruini C, Vescovelli F, Albieri E. Post-traumatic growth in breast cancer survivors: new insights into its relationships with well-being and distress. J Clin Psychol Med Settings. 2013;20(3):383–91. PubMed PMID: 23229823. Epub 2012/12/12. eng.
63. Zoellner T, Maercker A. Posttraumatic growth in clinical psychology - a critical review and introduction of a two component model. Clin Psychol Rev. 2006;26(5):626–53. PubMed PMID: 16515831. Epub 2006/03/07. eng.
64. Frankl V. Man's search for meaning. Boston: Beacon Press; 2006.
65. Schulz U, Mohamed NE. Turning the tide: benefit finding after cancer surgery. Soc Sci Med. 2004;59(3):653–62. PubMed PMID: 15144772. Epub 2004/05/18. eng.
66. Pacheco-Lopez G, Engler H, Niemi MB, Schedlowski M. Expectations and associations that heal: immunomodulatory placebo effects and its neurobiology. Brain Behav Immun. 2006;20(5):430–46. PubMed PMID: 16887325.
67. Sears SR, Stanton AL, Danoff-Burg S. The yellow brick road and the emerald city: benefit finding, positive reappraisal coping and posttraumatic growth in women with early-stage breast cancer. Health Psychol. 2003;22(5):487–97. PubMed PMID: 14570532. Epub 2003/10/23. eng.
68. Kolokotroni P, Anagnostopoulos F, Tsikkinis A. Psychosocial factors related to posttraumatic growth in breast cancer survivors: a review. Women Health. 2014;54(6):569–92. PubMed PMID: 24911117. Epub 2014/06/10. eng.
69. Hagger MS, Orbell S. A meta- analytic review of the common sense model of illness representations. Psychol Health. 2003;18(2):141–84.
70. Krok D, Telka E. The role of meaning in gastric cancer patients: relationships among meaning structures, coping, and psychological well-being. Anxiety Stress Coping. 2019;32(5):522–33. PubMed PMID: 31234657. Epub 2019/06/27. eng.

References

71. Nipp RD, El-Jawahri A, Fishbein JN, Eusebio J, Stagl JM, Gallagher ER, et al. The relationship between coping strategies, quality of life, and mood in patients with incurable cancer. Cancer. 2016;122(13):2110–6.
72. Nipp RD, Greer JA, El-Jawahri A, Moran SM, Traeger L, Jacobs JM, et al. Coping and prognostic awareness in patients with advanced cancer. J Clin Oncol. 2017;35(22):2551–7. PubMed PMID: 28574777. Pubmed Central PMCID: PMC5536163. Epub 2017/06/03. eng.
73. Beesley VL, Smith DD, Nagle CM, Friedlander M, Grant P, DeFazio A, et al. Coping strategies, trajectories, and their associations with patient-reported outcomes among women with ovarian cancer. Support Care Cancer. 2018;26(12):4133–42. PubMed PMID: 29948398. Epub 2018/06/28. eng.
74. Park CL, Pustejovsky JE, Trevino K, Sherman AC, Esposito C, Berendsen M, et al. Effects of psychosocial interventions on meaning and purpose in adults with cancer: a systematic review and meta-analysis. Cancer. 2019;125(14):2383–93. PubMed PMID: 31034600. Pubmed Central PMCID: PMC6602826. Epub 2019/04/30. eng.
75. Tarakeshwar N, Vanderwerker LC, Paulk E, Pearce MJ, Kasl SV, Prigerson HG. Religious coping is associated with the quality of life of patients with advanced cancer. J Palliat Med. 2006;9(3):646–57. PubMed PMID: 16752970. Pubmed Central PMCID: PMC2504357. Epub 2006/06/07. eng.
76. Bernard M, Strasser F, Gamondi C, Braunschweig G, Forster M, Kaspers-Elekes K, et al. Relationship between spirituality, meaning in life, psychological distress, wish for hastened death, and their influence on quality of life in palliative care patients. J Pain Symptom Manag. 2017;54(4):514–22. PubMed PMID: 28716616. Epub 2017/07/19. eng.
77. Roesch SC, Adams L, Hines A, Palmores A, Vyas P, Tran C, et al. Coping with prostate cancer: a meta-analytic review. J Behav Med. 2005;28(3):281–93. PubMed PMID: 16015462. Epub 2005/07/15. eng.
78. Park CL, Sherman AC, Jim HS, Salsman JM. Religion/spirituality and health in the context of cancer: cross-domain integration, unresolved issues, and future directions. Cancer. 2015;121(21):3789–94. PubMed PMID: 26258608. Pubmed Central PMCID: PMC4618033. Epub 2015/08/11. eng.
79. Cohen SR, Mount BM, Bruera E, Provost M, Rowe J, Tong K. Validity of the McGill Quality of Life Questionnaire in the palliative care setting: a multi-centre Canadian study demonstrating the importance of the existential domain. Palliat Med. 1997;11(1):3–20. PubMed PMID: 9068681. Epub 1997/01/01. eng.
80. Cohen SR, Mount BM, Tomas JJ, Mount LF. Existential well-being is an important determinant of quality of life. Evidence from the McGill Quality of Life Questionnaire. Cancer. 1996;77(3):576–86. PubMed PMID: 8630968. Epub 1996/02/01. eng.
81. Boehmer S, Luszczynska A, Schwarzer R. Coping and quality of life after tumor surgery: personal and social resources promote different domains of quality of life. Anxiety Stress Coping. 2007;20(1):61–75. PubMed PMID: 17999215. Epub 2007/11/14. eng.
82. Turner-Sack AM, Menna R, Setchell SR, Maan C, Cataudella D. Posttraumatic growth, coping strategies, and psychological distress in adolescent survivors of cancer. J Pediatr Oncol Nurs. 2012;29(2):70–9. PubMed PMID: 22422791. Epub 2012/03/17. eng.
83. Morris N, Moghaddam N, Tickle A, Biswas S. The relationship between coping style and psychological distress in people with head and neck cancer: a systematic review. Psycho-Oncology. 2018;27(3):734–47. PubMed PMID: 28748624. Epub 2017/07/28. eng.
84. Cohen M, Levkovich I, Pollack S, Fried G. Stability and change of postchemotherapy symptoms in relation to optimism and subjective stress: a prospective study of breast cancer survivors. Psycho-Oncology. 2019;28(10):2017–24. PubMed PMID: 31351023. Epub 2019/07/28. eng.
85. Schou I, Ekeberg Ø, Ruland CM. The mediating role of appraisal and coping in the relationship between optimism-pessimism and quality of life. Psycho-Oncology. 2005;14(9):718–27. PubMed PMID: 15669084. Epub 2005/01/26. eng.

86. Grimmett C, Haviland J, Winter J, Calman L, Din A, Richardson A, et al. Colorectal cancer patient's self-efficacy for managing illness-related problems in the first 2 years after diagnosis, results from the ColoREctal Well-being (CREW) study. J Cancer Surviv. 2017;11(5):634–42. PubMed PMID: 28822053. Pubmed Central PMCID: PMC5602065. Epub 2017/08/20. eng.
87. Jacobs JM, Shaffer KM, Nipp RD, Fishbein JN, MacDonald J, El-Jawahri A, et al. Distress is interdependent in patients and caregivers with newly diagnosed incurable cancers. Ann Behav Med. 2017;51(4):519–31. PubMed PMID: 28097515. Pubmed Central PMCID: PMC5513787. Epub 2017/01/18. eng.
88. Von Ah D, Kang DH, Carpenter JS. Stress, optimism, and social support: impact on immune responses in breast cancer. Res Nurs Health. 2007;30(1):72–83. PubMed PMID: 17243109. Epub 2007/01/24. eng.
89. Lutgendorf S, De Geest K, Bender D, Ahmed A, Goodheart M, Dahmoush L, Zimmerman M, et al. Social influences on clinical outcomes of patients with ovarian cancer. J Clin Oncol. 2012;30(23):2885–90.
90. Lutgendorf SK, Andersen BL. Biobehavioral approaches to cancer progression and survival: mechanisms and interventions. Am Psychol. 2015;70(2):186–97. PubMed PMID: 25730724. Pubmed Central PMCID: PMC4347942. Epub 2015/03/03. eng.
91. Hinz A, Friedrich M, Kuhnt S, Zenger M, Schulte T. The influence of self-efficacy and resilient coping on cancer patients' quality of life. Eur J Cancer Care. 2019;28(1):e12952. PubMed PMID: 30334331. Epub 2018/10/20. eng.
92. Sumpio C, Jeon S, Northouse LL, Knobf MT. Optimism, symptom distress, illness appraisal, and coping in patients with advanced-stage cancer diagnoses undergoing chemotherapy treatment. Oncol Nurs Forum. 2017;44(3):384–92. PubMed PMID: 28635986. Epub 2017/06/22. eng.
93. Turner JK, Hutchinson A, Wilson C. Correlates of post-traumatic growth following childhood and adolescent cancer: a systematic review and meta-analysis. Psycho-Oncology. 2018;27(4):1100–9. PubMed PMID: 29096418. Epub 2017/11/03. eng.
94. Zeng J, Hong ZQ, Peng FL, Mu ZL, Zhu YF, Zhen Z, et al. Predicting changes in quality of life and emotional distress in Chinese patients with lung, gastric, and colon-rectal cancer diagnoses: the role of psychological resilience. Psycho-Oncology. 2017;26:829–35.
95. Manne SL, Kissane D, Zaider T, Kashy D, Lee D, Heckman C, et al. Holding back, intimacy, and psychological and relationship outcomes among couples coping with prostate cancer. J Fam Psychol. 2015;29(5):708–19. PubMed PMID: 26192132. Pubmed Central PMCID: PMC5225663. Epub 2015/07/21. eng.
96. Matzka M, Mayer H, Köck-Hódi S, Moses-Passini C, Dubey C, Jahn P, et al. Relationship between resilience, psychological distress and physical activity in cancer patients: a cross-sectional observation study. PLoS One. 2016;11(4):e0154496. PubMed PMID: 27124466. Pubmed Central PMCID: PMC4849643. Epub 2016/04/29. eng.
97. Rosenberg AR, Bradford MC, McCauley E, Curtis JR, Wolfe J, Baker KS, et al. Promoting resilience in adolescents and young adults with cancer: results from the PRISM randomized controlled trial. Cancer. 2018;124(19):3909–17. PubMed PMID: 30230531. Epub 2018/09/20. eng.
98. Langford D, Morgan S, Cooper B, Paul S, Kober K, Wright F, et al. Association of personality profiles with coping and adjustment to cancer among patients undergoing chemotherapy. Psycho-Oncology. 2020;29:1060–7.
99. Manne SL, Myers-Virtue S, Kashy D, Ozga M, Kissane D, Heckman C, et al. Resilience, positive coping, and quality of life among women newly diagnosed with gynecological cancers. Cancer Nurs. 2015;38(5):375–82. PubMed PMID: 25521911. Pubmed Central PMCID: PMC4470889. Epub 2014/12/19. eng.
100. Kroemeke A, Sobczyk-Kruszelnicka M. Salutary effect of daily coping self-efficacy: impact on day-by-day coping to mood effects within dyads following hematopoietic stem cell transplantation. Anxiety Stress Coping. 2019;32(6):728–41. PubMed PMID: 31464139. Epub 2019/08/30. eng.

101. Huang CY, Hsu MC. Social support as a moderator between depressive symptoms and quality of life outcomes of breast cancer survivors. Eur J Oncol Nurs. 2013;17(6):767–74. PubMed PMID: 23623178. Epub 2013/04/30. eng.
102. Costa ALS, Heitkemper MM, Alencar GP, Damiani LP, Silva RMD, Jarrett ME. Social support is a predictor of lower stress and higher quality of life and resilience in brazilian patients with colorectal cancer. Cancer Nurs. 2017;40(5):352–60. PubMed PMID: 27171810. Epub 2016/05/14. eng.
103. Kayser K, Acquati C, Reese JB, Mark K, Wittmann D, Karam E. A systematic review of dyadic studies examining relationship quality in couples facing colorectal cancer together. Psycho-Oncology. 2018;27(1):13–21. PubMed PMID: 27943551. Epub 2016/12/13. eng.
104. Lutgendorf SK, Sood AK, Anderson B, McGinn S, Maiseri H, Dao M, et al. Social support, psychological distress, and natural killer cell activity in ovarian cancer. J Clin Oncol. 2005;23(28):7105–13. PubMed PMID: 16192594. Epub 2005/09/30. eng.
105. Lutgendorf SK, DeGeest K, Dahmoush L, Farley D, Penedo F, Bender D, et al. Social isolation is associated with elevated tumor norepinephrine in ovarian carcinoma patients. Brain Behav Immun. 2011;25(2):250–5. PubMed PMID: 20955777. Pubmed Central PMCID: PMC3103818. Epub 2010/10/20. eng.
106. Andersen BL, Yang HC, Farrar WB, Golden-Kreutz DM, Emery CF, Thornton LM, et al. Psychologic intervention improves survival for breast cancer patients: a randomized clinical trial. Cancer. 2008;113(12):3450–8. PubMed PMID: 19016270. Pubmed Central PMCID: PMC2661422. Epub 2008/11/19. eng.
107. Deno M, Tashiro M, Miyashita M, Asakage T, Takahashi K, Saito K, et al. The mediating effects of social support and self-efficacy on the relationship between social distress and emotional distress in head and neck cancer outpatients with facial disfigurement. Psycho-Oncology. 2012;21(2):144–52. PubMed PMID: 22271534. Epub 2012/01/25. eng.
108. De Leeuw JR, De Graeff A, Ros WJ, Hordijk GJ, Blijham GH, Winnubst JA. Negative and positive influences of social support on depression in patients with head and neck cancer: a prospective study. Psycho-Oncology. 2000;9(1):20–8. PubMed PMID: 10668056. Epub 2000/02/11. eng.
109. Haviland J, Sodergren S, Calman L, Corner J, Din A, Fenlon D, et al. Social support following diagnosis and treatment for colorectal cancer and associations with health-related quality of life: results from the UK ColoREctal Wellbeing (CREW) cohort study. Psycho-Oncology. 2017;26(12):2276–84. PubMed PMID: 29094430. Epub 2017/11/03. eng.
110. Fong AJ, Scarapicchia TMF, McDonough MH, Wrosch C, Sabiston CM. Changes in social support predict emotional well-being in breast cancer survivors. Psycho-Oncology. 2017;26(5):664–71. PubMed PMID: 26818101. Epub 2016/01/29. eng.
111. Schmidt SD, Blank TO, Bellizzi KM, Park CL. The relationship of coping strategies, social support, and attachment style with posttraumatic growth in cancer survivors. J Health Psychol. 2012;17(7):1033–40. PubMed PMID: 22253327. Epub 2012/01/19. eng.
112. Schmidt SD, Blank TO, Bellizzi KM, Park CL. The relationship of coping strategies, social support, and attachment style with posttraumatic growth in cancer survivors. J Health Psychol. 2011;17(7):1033–40. PubMed PMID: 22253327. Epub 2012/01/19. eng.
113. Carolan CM, Smith A, Davies GR, Forbat L. Seeking, accepting and declining help for emotional distress in cancer: a systematic review and thematic synthesis of qualitative evidence. Eur J Cancer Care. 2018;27(2):e12720. PubMed PMID: 28597493. Epub 2017/06/10. eng.
114. Hohl DH, Schultze M, Keller J, Heuse S, Luszczynska A, Knoll N. Inter-relations between partner-provided support and self-efficacy: a dyadic longitudinal analysis. Appl Psychol Health Well Being. 2019;11(3):522–42. PubMed PMID: 31231970. Epub 2019/06/25. eng.
115. Somasundaram RO, Devamani KA. A comparative study on resilience, perceived social support and hopelessness among cancer patients treated with curative and palliative care. Indian J Palliat Care. 2016;22(2):135–40. PubMed PMID: 27162423. Pubmed Central PMCID: PMC4843551. Epub 2016/05/11. eng.

116. Zhang H, Zhao Q, Cao P, Ren G. Resilience and quality of life: exploring the mediator role of social support in patients with breast cancer. Med Sci Monit. 2017;23:5969–79. PubMed PMID: 29248937. Pubmed Central PMCID: PMC5744469. Epub 2017/12/19. eng.
117. McEwen BS. Physiology and neurobiology of stress and adaptation: central role of the brain. Physiol Rev. 2007;87(3):873–904. PubMed PMID: 17615391. Epub 2007/07/07. eng.
118. Park CL, Edmondson D, Hale-Smith A, Blank TO. Religiousness/spirituality and health behaviors in younger adult cancer survivors: does faith promote a healthier lifestyle? J Behav Med. 2009;32(6):582–91. PubMed PMID: 19639404. Epub 2009/07/30. eng.
119. Zhang J, Yin Y, Wang A, Li H, Li J, Yang S, et al. Resilience in patients with lung cancer: structural equation modeling. Cancer Nurs. 2021;44(6):465–72. PubMed PMID: 32618622. Epub 2020/07/04. eng.

Part III

Poor Resilience

Introduction

Part III is designed to examine the progressive neural biological and behavioral impairments that occur throughout the whole person caused by exposure to chronic stress in the absence of protective personal and social resources [1]. If this toxic stress is left unregulated, the growing inability of the person's neural structures, pathways and mediators to flexibly adapt to environmental stress leads to poor resilience, facilitating the development of cancer or another chronic illness depending on the individual's genetic predisposition (eg. [2–6]). Chapter 6 discusses biological and behavioral characteristics of poor resilience in relation to the wide spread corrosive effects of toxic stress on neuro structures, synapses, neural physiological and molecular pathways, DNA and behaviors, and introduces concepts of allostatic load/overload bas (eg. [1–4]). Chapter 7 examines the systemic environmental factors that are conducive to tumorigenesis, cancer progression, and metastases (eg. [7–9]).

References

1. Fava GA, McEwen BS, Guidi J, Gostoli S, Offidani E, Sonino N. Psychoneuroendocrinology 2019;108:94–101.
2. McEwen BS. Neurobiological and systemic effects of chronic stress. Chronic Stress. 2017;1:9:1–11. PubMed PMID: 28856337. Pubmed Central PMCID: PMC5573220. Epub 2017/09/01. eng.
3. McEwen B, Nasca C, Gray JD. Neuripsychopharmacology 2016;41:3–23.
4. McEwen B, Gray JD, Nasca C. Recognizing resilience: Learning from the effects of stress on the brain. Neurobiology of stress 2015;1:1–11.
5. McEwen B, Stellar, E. Stress and the individual. Mechanisms leading to disease. Arch Internal Med 1993;153:2093–101.
6. McEwen BS, Wingfield JC. What is in a name? Integrating homeostasis, allostasis and stress. Horm Behav. 2010;57:105–11.

7. Wang M, Zhao J, Zhang L, Wei F, Lian Y, Wu Y, et al. Role of tumor microenvironment in tumorigenesis. J Cancer. 2017;8(5):761–73. PubMed PMID: 28382138. Pubmed Central PMCID: PMC5381164. Epub 2017/04/07. eng.
8. Kirtonia A, Sethi G, Garg M. The multifaceted role of reactive oxygen species in tumorigenesis. Cell Mol Life Sci. 2020;77(22):4459–83. PubMed PMID: 32358622. Epub 2020/05/03. eng.
9. Lutgendorf SK, Andersen BL. Biobehavioral approaches to cancer progression and survival: mechanisms and interventions. Am Psychol. 2015;70(2):186–97. PubMed PMID: 25730724. Pubmed Central PMCID: PMC4347942. Epub 2015/03/03. eng.

Poor Resilience

6.1 Introduction

The "wear and tear" of repeated or prolonged, stress-related experiences result in widespread psychological, cognitive, behavioral, and neurophysiological impairments of the whole person that threaten overall resilience, and if left unregulated, ultimately leads to genetically predisposed chronic illness [1]. These daily demands and major stressors are made all the more *toxic* when the individual lacks personal and social resources and coping skills that might afford some protective buffer against the corrosive nature of 'chronic activation of the biological stress response system' ([2]).

This chapter explores the concept of poor resilience or maladaptation due to chronic stress in which the individual's ability to cope effectively is lacking. We learn what happens biologically and behaviorally when recurring forms of stress surpass the individual's adaptive neurophysiological stress response system and psychosocial coping responses.

6.2 Objectives

At the end of this chapter, you will be able to:

- Define what is meant by maladaptation and poor resilience
- Discuss oxidative stress and its deleterious effects on the neurobiology of the human organism
- Describe the biological, physical, and psychological effects of chronic psychological stress and the development of systemic inflammation
- Explain the role of various cytokines in the manifestation of symptoms and side effects
- Describe the significance of epigenetic changes, their main causes, and potential effects on the human organism

Clinical Anecdote 6.1
H was hard to miss in the waiting room adjacent to the treatment room. Each time our schedules overlapped, she could be observed just quietly weeping beside her mother who appeared helpless to reassure her. One day while we were both left waiting for our turn to get chemotherapy, H's mother started a conversation. She wondered why it was that so many patients were so calm awaiting chemotherapy. She was distressed because her daughter had a stage 1 diagnosis, and the doctors and nurses had reassured her daughter to no avail of the likelihood of a complete recovery.

6.3 Definitions

Poor Resilience

Poor resilience refers to prolonged environmental challenges that may be characterized as potentially threatening, unpredictable, of variable intensity, frequency and duration causing protracted activation of the stress response system. The consequential effects are widespread systemic damage to neural structures, neural physiological and molecular pathways and processes that result in a lack of biological and behavioral flexibility to successfully adapt to on going stress over the lifespan [1]. Stress-related causes may include an adverse early childhood, acrimonious divorce, death of a loved one, hostile marriage, an aversive work environment, prolonged loneliness, or living with a life-threatening illness. Clinicians often do not give enough clinical significance to the cumulative neural–physiological molecular and behavioral disturbances accrued over a *lifetime of stressful* experiences, which can disrupt biological- resilient capabilities and compromise the adult's ability to effectively adapt to cancer- and treatment-related and other stressors. Poor resilience has been described in terms of allostatic load and allostatic overload.

Allostatic Load (AL) [2–5] (See Table 6.1)

Allostatic load (AL) refers to chronic exposure to stress that causes *impairments* to brain architecture and neural flexibility that also regulates stress induced changes to parametric values associated with neuroendocrinal, cardiac, digestive, and immune mediators and subsequent behavior and behavioral states which eventually limit successful adaptation to life experiences and the ability of the whole person to maintain homeostasis (Table 6.1) (e.g., [2] p.94, [28]). Dysregulated stress effects are *compounded* by inadequate cognitive and behavioral coping skills, personal resources, supportive relationships, and lifestyle behaviors [2]. Unhealthy *lifestyle* behaviors include the use of drugs, excessive alcohol, cigarettes, lack of physical exercise, poor sleep, and an inadequate diet along with sustained anxiety and depressive moods. Thus, the conceptualization of allostatic load/overload consists of biological and behavioral impairments that threaten the resilience of the individual. AL can result either from too much stress and/or too many inadequate behavioral responses to

Table 6.1 Key biological and behavioral indicators to consider in assessing allostatic load and allostatic overload [2, 6–10]

Emotional state
• Emotional distress, existential distress, anxiety, depressed mood, fear.
• Sees illness as a challenge/threat.
Stressor events (e.g., [11, 12])
• Experience of early life adversity
• Sources of current stress
• Short acute stressors or prolonged and chronic (e.g., family, career, financial, cancer, treatment, and partner/spouse)
Coping and support behaviors (e.g., [11, 13, 14])
• Use of positive reappraisal, use of emotion-focused, problem-focused, emotion-focused and meaning-focused coping and behavioral coping strategies, success reaching out and maintaining meaningful informal, and formal supportive relationships
• Use of avoidant behaviors, lacks hope
Personal resources/strengths and supportive relationships (e.g., [15–18])
• For example, optimistic, maintains supportive relationships
Lifestyle behaviors [19]
• Diet, physical activity/exercise, sleep, weight, use of alcohol and drugs, smoking
Stress mediators [2, 20]
• Levels of urinary NOR, cortisol
• Serum measure of DHEA-S
• Inflammatory cytokines (IL-6, IL-2, NK cells, T cells)
• C-reactive protein
Other physiological biomarkers [2, 20]
• Resting systolic and diastolic blood pressure, body mass index, waist-to-hip ratio, high-density lipoproteins (HDL), low-density lipoproteins *(LDL)* fasting glucose
Symptoms/side effects [2, 21]
• Emotional distress, anxiety, fear, sadness, depressive mood, existential distress, pain, nausea, emesis, lack of meaning, purpose, difficulty concentrating, intrusive ideation, loss, fatigue, persistent headache, difficulty sleeping, suppressed cell-mediated immunity, suppressed NK cell activity, loss of appetite, diarrhea/constipation etc.
Distress thermometer ≥4 severe distress; < 4 minimal to small-moderate distress> [22]
Health-related outcomes (e.g., [23–27]) (see Chaps. 5 and 7)
• Cancer, Cancer progression, cancer recurrence
• QOL, psychological Well-being, PTG
Clinical implications
Identifying and managing stress-related exposure/experience along the continuum: diagnosis, presurgery/postsurgery, pre-/post medical treatments, transition to survivorship, and end of life

allostatic challenges [2, 28, 29]. AL sometimes is described in terms of toxic stress, defined as "strong, frequent stressors and/or prolonged activation of the stress response system when personal and social resources are inadequate or limited" [2, 30].

Table 6.2 Measurable terms to describe resilience and poor resilience

Scientific terms to describe stress effects on mind and body	Definition
Allostasis	Neurobiological, social, physical, and behavioral adjustments triggered by manageable environmental stressors of short duration that are restored (healed) to within their normal parametric range when stress ends. Includes good and tolerable forms of stress effects [24] (Review Part II, Chaps. 3 and 4)
Allostatic load (AL)	AL refers to the cumulative chronic effects of daily stresses and moderate-to-major stressful experiences associated with neural structural and systemic – impairments including disruptions to circadian rhythms, damaging lifestyle behaviors such as social isolation, inadequate diet, lack of exercise with inadequate personal and social resources resulting in life experiences that strain the individual's ability to successfully adapt [2], p 94
Allostatic overload (OL)	OL is the result of chronic toxic stress that *exceeds the individual's neural biological and behavioral stress response systems* causing progressive systemic damage to neural physiological and molecular signaling pathways and processes as well as psychosocial, cognitive, and behavioral impairments, ultimately resulting in disease in the absence of personal and social resources [2]. Here chronic stress may refer to "toxic stress that becomes so extreme or unpredictable that the human organism can no longer respond effectively" [31, p. 576]

Fava and colleagues [2] argue that it is also important to assess the stressful impact of seemingly "normal" demands or activities of daily living, which may be experienced by some as being more stressful due to inefficient coping capabilities or supportive resources. Other individuals who appear to be managing at a behavioral level with inadequate coping skills or supportive relationships may, on investigation, reveal a dysregulated neurobiological profile (e.g., Table 6.2). These clinical examples strongly support the need for clinical interventions aimed at providing relevant information about the deleterious effects of stress on the whole being and introducing suggested strategies individuals can use to regulate their emotions, successfully adapt to stressful experiences, and enhance resilience independent of stress starting in the diagnostic phase (Review Parts IV and V).

Allostatic Overload (See Part II Chap. 3)

*Allostatic overloa*d occurs when the ubiquitous stress induced psychosocial–behavioral and neurobiological disturbances surpass the body's biological stress response system's ability to effectively adapt [2]. Allostatic overload is the "chronic, cumulative effects of stressful situations in life experienced by the individual as extremely *taxing or exceeding* his or her coping skills" [2, p. 96]. Here *AO* refers to "stress that becomes so extreme or unpredictable that the human organism can no longer respond effectively" [32, p. 576] Clinical Anecdote 6.1 may be an example of an individual suffering allostatic overload.

The transitional tipping points between a tolerable (allostasis) and *toxic state* (i.e., allostatic load) and between a toxic state (allostatic load) and *allostatic overload* have yet to be identified clinically based on critical prognostic indicators [2, 33]. As observed by the definitions (Table 6.2), a distinction between allostatic load and overload is unclear. However, allostatic overload is conceptualized as an extreme toxic state in which widespread physiological dysregulation is likely to "accelerate" accompanied by increased oxidative stress, leading to chronic disease and even a hastened death, without clinical interventions [24, p. 2]. A cumulative index of biological and behavioral indicators of AL/OL may be said to be a proxy measure of poor resilience, or an inability to adapt effectively to environmental challenges, threatening the individual's health and survival (See Table 6.1).

6.4 The Four Conditions of Chronic Stress

Biological resilience is typically described in terms of the stress-induced activation of the biological stress response system, which is normally maintained for a reasonably short interval, and then efficiently shuts off at the end of stress with the activation of the negative glucocorticoid feedback system, enabling the reemergence of the parasympathetic nervous system and its processes of reparation, healing, and low metabolism at basal levels of physiology.

Conversely, chronic stress may be associated with the following biological conditions:

1. *Inability to Adapt to Similar Stressors.* Failure of the stress-activated HPA axis system to adapt to similar recurring stressors via habituation contributes to the eventual biological strain on the normal stress response system. In normal situations, the *magnitude of the stress response* to the same repeated stressor would *diminish* over time as the individual adapted to the stressors [29], But frequently repeated stress responses can gradually result in the inability of the neural–endocrine stress response system to habituate over time to the same type of stressor. An example might be the reactivation of the stress response to the same elevated level of intensity each time the patient had to receive an intravenous line for chemotherapy.
2. *The Stress Response System Cannot Shut Off in a Timely Manner.* The inability of the stress response system to switch off at the end of stress may be due to a defective negative glucocorticoid feedback system, which would normally induce the stress-activated HPA axis system to shut down, and circulating cortisol levels to be downregulated [29]. Instead, glucocorticoids continue to circulate causing abnormal structural changes, such as fewer neuronal dendrites in the PFC and hippocampus and neuronal death in the gyrus dentate (the site of neurogenesis) of the hippocampus. These structural changes impede executive functioning and cause difficulties in learning and thinking clearly. Conversely, the circulating glucocorticoids cause dendritic propagation in the neurons of the amygdala, resulting in heightened emotional reactivity such as anxiety, fear, or emotional distress [29].

3. *"Inadequate Activation"* of the Biological Stress Response System. In an advanced stage of poor resilience such as allostatic overload, the biological stress response system is only insufficiently *activated* by chronic stress. The impaired HPA axis is associated with elevated circulating glucocorticoids, inflammatory cytokines, and catecholamines, which drive systemic inflammation, immune suppression, and neurostructural, physiological and molecular damage to related pathways and processes that ultimately result in cellular and DNA mutations [29].
4. *The Brain Demonstrates a Consistent Lack of Flexibility* (Review Chap. 4). Chronic stress causes a lack of dynamic neural plasticity in the brain making it difficult for neural remodeling needed to respond appropriately to life experiences (see section "Brain, Neural Circuitry, and Threat to Brain's Plasticity"). Because the brain is the main organ of adaptation to stress, its dynamic capacity for neural structural plasticity in response to stress is critical in coordinating a flexible response throughout the neuroendocrine, metabolic, immune, autonomic, and cardiovascular systems, functions, and behaviors [4, 30]. For instance, a lack of dynamic plasticity throughout the brain's neural circuitry causes not only an impaired biological response but also impaired judgment and emotional responses; it disrupts the individual's cognitive flexibility in finding different adaptive solutions to various future stressors [2, 24]. Neural flexibility is an essential resilient capability as the developing human organism must learn to adapt to new situations by drawing on previous experiences to various stressors that are also associated with new or adaptive neural circuitry that guides subsequent behavior. Factors that contribute to a lack of neural plasticity include chronic stress, early childhood adversity, age, genetic predisposition, and possibly sex differences in how the brain responds to stressors [1].

6.5 Pervasive Neurobiological Maladaptive Disruptions (Review [1, 29])

Significantly, allostatic load/overload suppresses the human's innate capacity to defend him/herself against foreign organisms, detect and eliminate rogue cancer cells, or heal cell tissues and repair damaged DNA, exposing the human to the threat of chronic illnesses, such as cancer, disease progression, and other comorbidities, depending on his or her genetic predisposition [1]. The myriad neural structural and neurobiological disturbances caused by chronic stress, described in the remaining chapter, underscore the threat of allostatic load/overload to homeostasis, internal coherence, overall resilience and health, and survival [1].

Brain, Neural Circuitry, and Threat to Brain's Plasticity

As the central mediating organ of stress, the brain determines what is actually threatening and what physiological, functional, and behavioral responses are required (e.g., [4, 29]). Although other regions of the brain are likely affected by chronic stress, the interconnected neural circuitry of the prefrontal cortex (PFC), hippocampus, and amygdala have been the subject of the majority of stress-related studies. These three regions undergo neural structural plastic alterations in response to acute and chronic stress directed by epigenetic changes and gene expression, which determine the biological adjustments made to the HPA axis, ANS, immune, cardiovascular, gut, and metabolic systems, and nonlinear adjustments made to interrelated mediators, which in turn influence behavior [24].

Stress innervates the HPA axis and SNS, resulting in the release of stress-related hormones such as cortisol and noradrenaline (NOR). When stress is overly prolonged, these circulating hormones transform from initially protective to toxic effects on various neural cell structures and pathways. Neural plastic remodeling occurs, with a reduction in the spinal densities and excrescences at neural synapses, increased pruning and shrinkage of neural dendrites, and less neural growth, all of which now impede the normal flow of neural physiological communication throughout the human organism [29]. Neural imaging shows that the stress-induced volume size of the PFC and hippocampus tends to be smaller than normal, and neurogenesis in the hippocampus is suppressed. Conversely, the volume size of the amygdala is increased [29].

Although biological alterations are generally *reversible* following stressful episodes of *short* duration, these changes become more long-lasting and progressively damaging when subjected to chronic stress—especially when the intensity and duration of the stress coincide with the prenatal, neonatal, childhood, and adolescent years [32]. These developmental phases are known to be particularly sensitive to positive but also adverse experiences that result in maladaptation. When childhood experiences are toxic and long-lasting, the brain's altered neural structures are less amenable to adaptive plasticity in response to future stressors, resulting in biological and behavioral impairments, which may be observed as increased impulsivity, emotional reactivity, impaired judgment, and a lack of cognitive flexibility to find adaptive solutions to demands and challenges in adulthood [1]. This will become clearer as the effects of biological impairments on the behavioral functions of these brain regions are highlighted.

Prefrontal Cortex (PFC)

This brain region regulates executive cognitive functions, goal-directed and self-regulating behaviors, attention, working memory, and cognitive flexibility [29, 34, 35]. Chronic stress impedes cognitive capabilities such as reasoning, effective problem-solving, and attention-focused behaviors. Underlying *these impaired behaviors is significant volume shrinkage* due to loss of dendritic complexity in the prelimbic medial PFC. In contrast, the neurons in the orbitofrontal PFC, which typically promote the affective component of cognitive behavior, show a stress-induced increase in dendritic complexity with larger dendritic spines, suggesting greater emotional responsiveness or interference with cognition.

Amygdala

This brain region is associated with emotions, aggression, and affect-based learning, especially "fear conditioning." Chronic stress causes neuronal hypertrophy in the basal–lateral region of the amygdala (BLA). The increase in the number of dendritic spines along synapses significantly increases the magnitude of the behavioral response of the amygdala to emotionally inducing environmental stimuli, such as a cancer diagnosis [32]. At the same time, chronic stress downregulates the normally controlling functions of the PFC over the amygdala, thereby enabling amplified emotional reactions combined with a diminished capacity for cognitive thinking and decision making. This phenomenon is frequently observed, usually temporarily, in patients receiving a cancer diagnosis which understandably may arouse emotions that temporarily reduce cognitive abilities to concentrate on the doctor's feedback. But in individuals who have been chronically stressed, an emotionally reactive response may persist, impeding their ability to make plans, problem solve effectively, and contribute to clinical decisions concerning their treatment, or even to proactively engage in health-promoting behaviors relevant to their survival.

Hippocampus

This region is involved in memory formation, specifically episodic, declarative, contextual and spatial memory, learning, and mood (e.g., [36]). The region of the dentate gyrus of the hippocampus is specifically associated with keeping memories intact and appears to be involved in memory retrieval and recall. The hippocampus also plays a role in moderating the stress response of the HPA axis [36]. Numerous experimental findings indicate that chronic stress produces long-term spatial memory impairments due to the well-known damaging effects on the CA3 pyramidal neurons of the hippocampus and the dentate gyrus. The CA3 pyramidal neurons play an important role in processing memory, including encoding spatial representations and episodic memories [37]. For instance, pattern separation is the process by which different but related memories may be created from similar inputs [38]. When a patient is distressed during conversation with the physician about the upcoming cancer-related treatment and various issues surrounding the course of chemotherapy, two different but related issues may be conflated or confused in the patient's mind.

The Dentate Gyrus and Neurogenesis Adult neurogenesis or the production of new adult-born neurons occurs throughout life in the sub-granular layer of the dentate gyrus (within the hippocampus) [38]. Adult-born neurons contribute to learning and episodic memory formation and spatial navigational learning, particularly during the maturational phase when they are known for their unusual excitability and plasticity and are responsive to extensive stimuli [39]. However chronic or prolonged psychological stress manifested as protracted anxiety, emotional distress, depression, or fear, for instance, about dying or a cancer recurrence, can suppress adult neurogenesis due to the chronically elevated and corrosive effects of circulating glucocorticoids (e.g., [40]).

Suppressing neurogenesis has been shown to affect long-term memory and context-dependent memory, especially within a fearful context (see Gonçalves et al. [39] for comprehensive review). Suppressing neurogenesis makes the process of adaptation through learning more difficult. Consider the situation where the dietician suggests that the patient modify a mainly carbohydrate diet and consume more green vegetables and berries which requires learning new recipes and dishes. A suppressed neurogenesis may make normally easy behavioral transitions more difficult.

6.6 Impaired HPA Axis, ANS, and Immune Functioning

Chronic unregulated psychological stress damages the normal functioning of the stress response system consisting mainly of the central brain, HPA axis, SAM, PNS, and immune systems with deleterious consequences such as a cancer diagnosis and or its progression [41]. Chronic stress destabilizes the dynamic balance between the SNS and PNS with excess activation of the SNS and SAM systems which suppress the healing and reparative systems of the PNS (cholinergic) and dopaminergic systems [29]. As chronic stress persists, HPA axis hyperactivity eventually *subsides to basal levels,* whereas cortisol levels may remain high due in part to the damaged negative feedback inhibition system that would normally shut down the flow of cortisol at the end of a stressful event (e.g., [42]).

Evidence of chronic stress may be *observed* in low heart rate variability (that is the oscillations are small, irregular, and chaotic amplitudes), and the lack of synchronization among circadian rhythms such as the sleep–wake cycle, the body temperature cycle, and other time-ordered cellular and physiological functions among biological constituents throughout the human organism. The body requires synchrony among its complex interrelated systems and subsystems to ensure biological coherence, conservation of energy, and homeostasis (see Sect. 6.9 below) [43, 44]. The time-ordered, self-limiting "on/off" modulating switches of key stress mediators and other mechanisms of resilience become dysregulated (e.g., [45]).

Impaired Negative Feedback Inhibition System and Damaged Glucocorticoid (GR) Receptors

Chronic stress causes a physiological condition known as *glucocorticoid resistance,* which disrupts normal functioning of the *negative feedback inhibition system.* Three different glucocorticoid signaling dysfunctions have been identified: (1) downregulation (such as reduction of glucocorticoid receptors) due to persistent hypercortisol flow, (2) an impaired GR characterized by decreased sensitivity to its ligand (cortisol), which interferes with normal ligand–receptor binding. The third potential problem involves potential changes in genetic structure, including epigenetic modifications associated with chronic stress [46–48]. For instance, damaged glucocorticoid receptors (GRs) are unable to transfer cortisol from the cell cytoplasm to the nucleus where it would normally *stimulate IkB gene expression which suppresses the activation of* the "master" pro-inflammatory transcription factor, nuclear factor kappa B (NFKB) [49]. Glucocorticoid resistance ultimately disrupts the normal, rapid activation of the stress response system resulting in persistently elevated circulating cortisol which damages cell structures, pathways, and DNA [45]. Impaired glucocorticoid receptor signaling leads to an imbalance between mineralocorticoid and glucocorticoid receptor (MR and GR) signaling, which has been implicated in the development of chronic illnesses.

Impaired PNS Healing Processes

Chronic elevation of circulating cortisol in particular but also norepinephrine and pro-inflammatory cytokines has been implicated in the *downregulation* (i.e., suppression) of the parasympathetic nervous system (PNS) due to chronic stress. The PNS is the central healing system of the human organism. Its myriad reparative functions at normal levels of physiology include maintaining biorhythms and vital signs within normal parameters, modulating the excitability of the SNS, and wound healing [43, 50]. A suppressed PNS has been associated with unregulated chronic hyperactivity of the locus coeruleus noradrenergic system, resulting in chronic anxiety and even cardiovascular and other chronic illnesses [43]. An inhibited PNS has been associated with dysregulated biorhythms, suppression of cell-mediated immunity, and slower wound healing time [30, 51–54].

Dysregulated Immune System

The immune system has a reciprocal relationship with the central nervous system and, significantly, the stress response system involving the brain and HPA axis (e.g., [41, 52, 55]). Stress hormones such as NOR (from the SAM) and glucocorticoids (from the adrenal cortex) bind with leukocyte (WBC) cell surface receptors to first activate, and then, as stress persists, suppress B- and T-lymphocyte proliferation and antibody production [52, 56]. Significantly, chronic stress inhibits the activity, counts, and functions of innate natural killer cells (NKC), interferon-gamma (IFN-γ), and cytotoxic T-lymphocytes that are so essential for cancer cell surveillance and for eliminating cancer cells and protecting the human organism from viral and bacterial invasion (e.g., [52]). Immune impairments are largely mediated by increased circulating glucocorticoids due to epigenetic modifications associated with chronic stress [47, 48].

Leukocytes also release cytokines and neuropeptides that are conveyed to the cell surface receptors of the hypothalamus–limbic system which maintains the elevated cortisol levels, further disrupting immune functioning. In this way, bidirectional reinforcing patterns of dysfunctional activity are maintained [57, 58]. Because immune dysregulation impedes the individual's ability to defend against and eliminate cancer cells, viruses, and bacteria, the individual's risk of chronic illness, comorbidity, and/or cancer progression in patients with cancer is increased.

6.7   Other Dysregulated Mediators

Among the numerous mediators negatively affected by chronic stress and a suppressed PNS are brain-derived neurotrophic factor (BDNF), neural cell adhesion molecule (NCAM), dopamine, gamma-aminobutyric acid (GABA), and glutamate (e.g., [59–61]). For instance: *BDNF* suppression in some brain areas such as the PFC and CA3 of the hippocampus has been shown to impair normal functions such as neuronal growth, maturation and differentiation of nerve cells, synaptic plasticity, repair, and negatively impact cognitive learning [62]. Conversely, chronic stress increases *BDNF mRNA* expression in the basal lateral amygdala contributing to dendritic growth which is manifested behaviorally by intensified emotional reactions such as prolonged anxiety and distress.

GABA is an inhibitory amino acid neurotransmitter which *normally calms excitable nervous impulses* between neurons in the brain, and is associated with relaxing effects (NIH-Genetics Home Reference. https://ghr.nim.nih.gov/gene/BDNF. Accessed Sept 2018). An early experimental study showed that early life stress impaired the development of GABA receptor systems in the brain with future consequences seen in the manifestation of excessive fearfulness in adulthood [63]. GABA and glutamate serve complementary functions that regulate synaptic transmissions and neural plasticity involved in maintaining neural structures [64]. Chronic stress leads to GABA dysfunction and excessive glutamate excitability.

Glutamate is an excitatory amino acid that plays a critical role in regulating synaptic transmissions and neural plasticity by activating key ionotropic (NMDA and AMPA) and metabotropic glutamate receptors [65]. Glutaminergic synapses typically consist of presynaptic terminals that are associated with postsynaptic terminals (i.e., dendritic spines) in contrast to synapses at which monoaminergic neurotransmitters are released (for instance, dopamine, norepinephrine, adrenaline and histamine, serotonin, and histamine) [65]. The number of receptors available at synapses is critical for enabling excitatory synaptic efficacy.

During acute and chronic stress, elevated circulating glucocorticoids (via endocannabinoid signaling) trigger changes in glutamate neural transmissions in the PFC, frontal cortex, amygdala, and hippocampus. Unregulated flow of glutamate during chronic stress may lead to permanent neuronal loss and dendritic shrinkage in the CA3, dentate gyrus neurons of the hippocampus, medial amygdala, and PFC, thereby disrupting normal neuronal intercommunications. Stress-induced NMDA dendritic remodeling observed in the mPFC is associated with depressive behavior according to animal research findings [1].

NCAMs are adhesion molecules involved in cell recognition and cell–cell adhesion. Cell–cell adhesion is important for cell communication and regulation, and for normal tissue development and maintenance. Cell adhesion refers to the ability of a cell to adhere to another cell or the extracellular matrix which regulates cell behavior and functions [66]. Cell adhesion is generally dysregulated, while the PNS remains suppressed, and it has also been found to be suppressed in patients with cancer [66, 67].

Dopamine which is normally activated by cognitive expectation of a benefit (reward) has been shown to be suppressed by chronic stress [68]. Chronic stress has a negative impact on dopamine levels in the mesolimbic dopamine system. One explanation for the inability of cognitive expectations to induce a clinical benefit in patients with a history of chronic stress is likely low levels of dopamine which predispose these individuals to depression (Review Part IV Chap. 12).

6.8 The Impaired Dopaminergic Reward System

Chronic unexpected stress disrupts the neurobiological pathways associated with dopaminergic structures in the mesolimbic system, specifically the crucial dopamine-releasing ventral tegmental area (VTA) and nucleus accumbens [69]. Aversive neuroplastic changes to dendritic spines and dendrites at excitatory/inhibitory synapses of the reward circuitry contribute further impairments that likely compromise the healing-inducing effects of cognitive expectations (to be discussed in Part IV Chap. 12 [70]. Dopaminergic impairments have also been implicated in a *compromised immune system*, in depression, obesity, and other abnormal clinical outcomes as part of complex interrelated biological processes that involve many systems including the stress response mechanism [71].

6.9 Dysregulated Circadian Rhythm

Prolonged dysregulated flow of glucocorticoids impairs the suprachiasmatic nucleus (SCN), which is the master circadian pacemaker for the brain and the body [72]. An impaired circadian rhythm is associated with poor resilience and well being, disrupting homeostatic systems and resulting in health-related conditions such as sleep disorders, obesity, and insulin resistance [73]. It contributes to a lack of biological coherence imposing a greater metabolic burden on the body's ability to maintain homeostasis.

An impaired SCN disrupts normal diurnal circadian rhythms located throughout the brain, neurons, peripheral tissues, and organs at cellular–molecular levels [74]. This is typically reflected by a more flattened circadian rhythm, characterized by lower morning and higher evening cortisol levels. When prolonged, the cumulative deleterious effects may be devastating to the individual's health [72]. A significant reduction in sleep has been associated with an increase in body mass, decrease in parasympathetic regulation over sympathetic effects, elevated cortisol and insulin levels in the evening, and an increase in inflammatory cytokines as well as other bodily dysfunctions, seriously compromising the individual's resilience.

6.10 Chronically Stress-Induced Epigenetic Changes

Stress-induced epigenetic changes are a function of stressor-genome interactions mediated by stress mediators that alter the selection of genes to be transcribed and expressed (without altering the DNA sequence). These stress-induced epigenetic changes favor those genes that promote a pro-inflammatory internal environment [47, 75]. Dysregulated circulating glucocorticoids, neuropeptides, neurotransmitters, and hormones interact with the genome to induce epigenetic changes (e.g., via DNA methylation and histone acetylation), which impair normal gene expression ([76], e.g., [77]). Chronic stress-induced epigenetic changes create neurobiological and functional impairments throughout the whole organism resulting in poor biological and behavioral resilience [76]. These changes not only favor gene expression of inflammatory cytokines, but of myriad chemokines, neurotransmitters, and hormonal and transcription factors such as the master inflammatory transcription factor, NFKB, that contribute to chronic systemic inflammation. A history of early childhood stress has been known to permanently alter patterns of gene expression for instance in the hippocampus or prefrontal cortex, which may help to explain why some individuals in adulthood continue to experience difficulty adapting to stress [32].

6.11 Systemic Inflammation

Whereas inflammation is normally an essential, highly regulated, self-limited, and ordered phase of the healing process, chronic systemic inflammation refers to a complex, microenvironment of unregulated biochemical, hormonal, and molecular disturbances. It can include potential DNA/RNA damage emanating from impaired cellular structures, functions, and pathways caused by a dysregulated stress response system and the production of excessive reactive oxygen species (ROS) due to increased metabolic demands (see Sect. 6.12 below) (e.g., [2]). Cytokines such as Il-8, IL-6, IL-1, Il-12, IL-1B, and TNF-α as well as inflammatory-stimulating factors such as prostaglandin E2, interferon, C-reactive protein (acute phase proteins), and chemokines, macrophages, and eosinophils all contribute to systemic inflammation [23, 78].

As discussed, prolonged distress disrupts the flow of cortisol and impairs its normally anti-inflammatory functions and the body's circadian rhythm. Because of the impaired functions of cortisol, the I_KB protein that maintains an inert NFkB within the cell cytoplasm now degenerates, releasing NFkB, which now moves into the cell nucleus where it binds to specific DNA sequences that start the transcription of multiple inflammatory pathways that negatively impact cancer cell survival, proliferation, progression, and metastases [78, 79]. NFkB is a key transcription factor in the development of inflammatory-based chronic illnesses, and many cancers. Stress has also been found to downregulate or shut down P53, an important tumor suppressor gene [80].

Prolonged elevation of the circulating stress mediators leads to an *ANS imbalance*, dysregulated immune system, metabolic stress, oxidative damage, and a damaged negative feedback inhibition system that culminates in chronic systemic inflammation and poor resilience (maladaptation). The presence of chronic unregulated systemic inflammation increases the likelihood of developing chronic illnesses, such as diabetes, depression, cardiovascular disease, and cancer [67, 78, 79].

Systemic Inflammation and Sickness Behaviors Systemic inflammation drives the manifestation of symptoms or so-called sickness behaviors seen in chronic illness and cancer [21, 81]. Stress-induced inflammatory cytokines access the brain, via different peripheral neural pathways, which activate *"sickness" behaviors* such as depression, fatigue, impaired sleep, cognitive dysfunction, and/or increased sensitivity to pain. These sickness behaviors are associated with elevated circulating pro-inflammatory innate cytokines, IFN-alpha (interferon), TNF (tumor necrosis factor), pro-inflammatory transcription signaling pathways (e.g., NFkB and p53 MAPK), and various hormones (e.g., CRH, noradrenaline, and cortisol) [79, 82–84]. Elevated pro-inflammatory cytokines, such as interleukin-6 (IL-6), interleukin-IL-1A (IL-1A), interleukin-1B (IL-1B), and tumor necrosis factor (TNF-α) are associated with anxiety, depressed mood, fatigue, pain, and difficulty sleeping, *sickness behaviors* that often present in clusters [81, 85]. IL-6 has been associated with fatigue, cognitive dysfunction, and impaired sleep [86]. Corticotropin-releasing hormone (CRH) has been associated with depression, anxiety, impaired sleep, anorexia, and decreased activity [21].

Increased flow of IL-6, IL-1, TNF-α, impaired cortisol levels, and NFkB have also been associated with dysregulated sleep patterns, depression, anxiety, lack of appetite, and cognitive difficulty in cancer patients [81, 86]. These behavioral symptoms exacerbate the person's allostatic load. The bidirectional effects among various dysregulated physiological mediators within a systemic inflammatory environment and behavioral symptoms signal an increased risk or presence of chronic disease, including cancer [2].

6.12 Metabolic Oxidative Stress

The compensatory neurobiological changes throughout the human organism in response to chronic stress exert an excessive metabolic burden on the ability to provide sufficient energy resources to maintain homeostasis. This physiological effort culminates in oxidative stress, which is an imbalance between the production of reactive oxygen species (ROS), a by-product of oxidative metabolism, *and* the ability of the body to detoxify the free radicals with antioxidants [28].

ROS consists of free radicals that seek stability by gaining electrons from protein and the molecules of tissues, cells, and even DNA and RNA. In doing so, ROS causes widespread neural structural damage to cell and DNA components including lipids, proteins, and RNA, affecting gene expression, signaling pathways, body regulation systems and telomere length which predispose the individual to chronic illnesses, including cancer [23, 87]. For example, DNA-coded "scripts" direct how cells and other dynamic processes of the person must operate to maintain health, resilience, and healing capabilities. When ROS damages DNA by causing mutations or by impairing a tumor *suppressor* gene, the chances for cancer to develop are seriously enhanced [88].

Oxidative stress may be more likely to occur in individuals who sustain an *acutely stressful event* such as a cancer diagnosis *and* have a history of previous chronic stress compared to newly diagnosed patients without such a history [28]. Aschbacher and colleagues' experimental study [28] reported that even the *anticipation of something* "bad" may be worse than the actual stressor event itself, triggering oxidative stress. The anticipation may be influenced by memories of a previous period of chronic stress. Anticipatory stress is evoked by emotional fears and cognitive beliefs about what one imagines will happen (a nocebo effect) as opposed to what actually is experienced. That finding underscores the clinical imperative of taking the time to clarify the patient's assumptions that may be rooted in previously stressful experiences. Part of this intervention would include discussing coping skills and mindful practices they can use to downregulate distress and promote their resilience (Review Chaps. 9, 10, 12 and 13).

6.13 Weakened Bioelectromagnetic Field

Chronic stress causes widespread impairments throughout the various structures, functions, and processes associated with the psychoneuroendocrine and immune network, which is thought to lead to a weakened bioelectromagnetic field [44, 89, 90]. This dynamic field is involved in all biological activities including maintaining homeodynamic equilibrium.

Bernardi and colleagues [44] showed that the normal biorhythmic amplitudes of the heart, respiration, blood pressure, and mid-cerebral activity tend to become more chaotic and irregular with age or even mild distress. Chronic stress from depression, posttraumatic stress, and chronic anxiety have been associated with prolonged SNS arousal and a reduction in heart rate variations (HRV) that is also coincident with the surplus of circulating pro-inflammatory cytokines and cortisol [43, 91]. These increasingly chaotic variations in the various biorhythms of the body mind reflect an increasingly inefficient use of potential energy and metabolic resources that ultimately lead to a shortened life. It is thought that complementary therapies such as acupuncture and healing touch or reiki are aimed at restoring a healthier bioelectromagnetic magnetic field [92].

6.14 Behavioral Indicators of Poor Resilience [11, 48] (Review Part II Chaps. 3–5)

Individuals with poor resilience tend to manifest a number of telling indicators across psychosocial and behavioral dimensions: For instance: *psychological indicators* include *prolonged* emotional distress, heightened anxiety, intrusive ideation, depressed mood, lack of energy, fatigue, sense of helplessness, and difficulty concentrating. *Dysfunctional emotion-regulating coping skills* include poor reappraisal capability, poor self-regulation, problem-solving, and overdependence on avoidance, denial, and self-blame. *A lack of personal resources* may be shown by a poor sense of self-efficacy, personal control, and sense of hopelessness, despair, and demoralization. *Inadequate social resources* are suggested by problematic relationships and loneliness. *Poor lifestyle behaviors* include a lack of exercise, excessive smoking, alcohol use, drug use, difficulty sleeping, obesity, poor nutrition, diet, and eating habits. This information may be obtained via a nursing assessment (see Table 6.1 above) during stressful situations of short and prolonged duration. In essence, these behaviors are the likely external manifestation of the underlying widespread deleterious biological consequences of chronic stress (e.g., [2]).

6.15 Nursing Implications

Poor resilience or allostatic load/overload (AL) suggests a potential failure of the individual's biology and behavior to adapt to chronic stress (Review Part II Chap. 3). One growing trend in the clinical/research literature on resilience is the use of a cumulative index based on stress and resilient-related psychosocial–behavioral (including lifestyle), neurophysiological, biochemical, metabolic, immune, and even molecular indicators (i.e., biological and behavioral markers) in order to provide an overall measure of allostatic load/overload in the whole person. Such an index might identify particular areas of biological and behavioral vulnerability that could be targets of proposed multimodal multitargeted interventions (ALs) (e.g., [2, 48, 93]).

As a practical matter, until a reliable and validated cluster of biological and behavioral indicators is established (which may also vary as a function of the type of cancer), it seems more useful to select from stress mediators, the biomarkers that are relevant to the patient's medical condition as well as emotional state and behavioral indicators which can inform the nurse's overall assessment of the patient's state of resilience. This information can help to determine the appropriate multimodal, multitargeted interventions. The assessment may include measuring blood pressure, pulse, heart rate, C-RP, IL-6 cortisol, LDL, HDL, NOR and epinephrine levels, lymphocytes, presence of side effects and symptoms, lifestyle behaviors, coping strategies, and support. These clinical indicators may be used to monitor a patient's clinical status over time and to evaluate the efficacy of a therapeutic approach.

For instance, C-reactive protein (CRP) levels >3.0 mg/L plus high cortisol levels over time may be indicative of glucocorticoid resistance. High CRP, being a measure of systemic inflammation, may also indicate an increased risk of disease progression. High NOR levels, high heart rate, and low heart rate variability (less variability in heart beats) may signify a suppressed PNS and signal allostatic load/overload. Chronic stress leads to increased levels of low-density lipoproteins (bad cholesterol) and triglycerides, and decreased levels of high-density lipoproteins (HDL) or good cholesterol, placing the individual at risk for comorbid conditions such as cardiac problems. A cumulative index of relevant behavioral and biological markers can offer critical insight into the resilient status or health of the whole person.

Emotional distress refers to subjective emotions that convey an inability to cope effectively. These include prolonged anxiety, fear, and/or intrusive ideation. The distress thermometer with follow-up clinical questions provides an excellent screening tool to assess the individual's level of emotional distress, appraisal of the identified stressors, and use of coping responses [22]. An important aspect of the nursing assessment includes the key components of an emotion-regulating adaptive coping system, that is, coping efforts and use of personal and social resources (Review Part II Chap. 5). Prolonged emotional distress may also be indicative of metabolic exhaustion and increased ROS due to widespread physiological disturbances throughout the individual, reflective also of poor resilience [23, 87].

An Unhealthy Lifestyle A clinical assessment of indicators of potential poor resilience would cover the amount and type of daily exercise, nutrition and diet, fatness or obesity, alcohol consumption, drug use as well as sleep habits, appetite, and binge eating. Chronic stress has been significantly related to infrequent physical activity and exercise [94], to greater obesity, and a shortened survival, for instance, in patients with breast cancer [95, 96]. The lack of daily physical activity alone has been significantly related to an increased cancer risk in patients with bladder, colon, endometrial, esophageal adenocarcinoma, renal and gastric, and breast cancer [9, 97, 98]. Obesity carries its own dangers as well. Research has shown that obesity impairs CD8+ T-lymphocyte cell functioning in the tumor microenvironment, which facilitates tumor growth [99].

Whereas "*overnutrition*," which refers to consuming more nutrients than needed, results in obesity and is associated with systemic inflammation, "*undernutrition*," or inadequate receipt of nutrients due to a poor diet or lack of appetite, is associated with immunosuppression. The individual's daily dietary intake and physical activity have a direct bearing on the individual's resilient capability and by extension the risk of allostatic load [100].

Final Thoughts
Research suggests that it may be possible to improve biological resilience in individuals with a history of chronic psychological stress [24]. Not all persons who have experienced early childhood adversity experience later chronic illness or cancer. Early life adversity is context-driven and its toxic effects may be mitigated by a nurturing individual or a genetic predisposition to resilience, or by specifically tailored mind–body interventions that may improve the brain's plasticity (flexibility) (e.g., [1]). The fact that the brain's architecture continues to be remodeled throughout life (at least to some extent) via underlying epigenetic changes provides further support for the use of targeted psychosocial interventions to promote healing and resilient capabilities in all patients and caregivers. Notwithstanding, individuals exposed to prolonged stress *as adults* may be more likely to make a greater resilient recovery in the aftermath of a major stressor event such as cancer compared to adults *who were first exposed to an early life history* of significant adversity. It is clear that patients and caregivers with any history of chronic distress need targeted nursing interventions to enhance resilient capabilities [2, 28].

The significance of prolonged stress-induced biological and behavioral impairments regarding the potential for future resilience, has yet to be fully understood. Whatever healing may occur when stress ceases, as ascertained by the individual's subsequent behavior, may still mask an underlying altered and potentially more *vulnerable* neural circuitry that places the person at greater risk for illness in the future—*notwithstanding the behavioral appearances of resilience* [24].

Animal research has shown that even when behaviors are restored to normal functioning following a period of chronic stress, the *altered neural structures and pattern of gene expression* are not restored exactly to prestress baseline levels; they have a *similar but different* neural–structural circuitry [24, 59]. As observed also in humans with a history of chronic adversity the animal research demonstrated that exposure to future stressors tended to elicit a more heightened reactive response. This may relate to the stress-induced changes in neural circuitry and/or patterns of gene expression that do not return to prestress baseline patterns, compared to the controls without a chronically stressed period. The epigenetic changes that occurred during the protracted period of chronic stress may have precluded a more measured and cognitively flexible response to environmental challenges [24, 59, 101].

These human and animal findings suggest that past and even current chronic stress-related experiences may continue to play a modulating influence on an individual's adaptive capability in the face of cancer. A uni-item measure of either psychological, biological, and/or physical well-being will not capture the extent of underlying biological disturbances that may persist. It is for this reason that clinical measures of allostatic load/overload are increasingly recommended to identify chronically stressed individuals with cancer who are at risk for developing comorbid conditions and/or a poorer future health (Review Part II Chap. 3).

To summarize, individuals with cancer and persistent levels of emotional distress and/or a history of severe, unpredictable, and chronic stress need appropriate multimodal multitargeted interventions that target as much as possible biological and psychological endpoints, starting at diagnosis, and including individuals from stage 1 to stage 4 cancer.

References

1. McEwen BS. Neurobiological and systemic effects of chronic stress. Chronic Stress (Thousand Oaks, Calif). 2017;1:2470547017692328. PubMed PMID: 28856337. Pubmed Central PMCID: PMC5573220. Epub 2017/09/01. eng.
2. Fava GA, McEwen BS, Guidi J, Gostoli S, Offidani E, Sonino N. Clinical characterization of allostatic overload. Psychoneuroendocrinology. 2019;108:94–101. PubMed PMID: 31252304. Epub 2019/06/30. eng.
3. McEwen BS. Stress, adaptation, and disease. Allostasis and allostatic load. Ann N Y Acad Sci. 1998;840:33–44. PubMed PMID: 9629234. Epub 1998/06/18. eng.
4. McEwen BS, Nasca C, Gray JD. Stress effects on neuronal structure: hippocampus, amygdala, and prefrontal cortex. Neuropsychopharmacology. 2016;41(1):3–23. PubMed PMID: 26076834. Pubmed Central PMCID: PMC4677120. Epub 2015/06/17. eng.

5. McEwen BS. Allostasis and allostatic load: implications for neuropsychopharmacology. Neuropsychopharmacology. 2000;22(2):108–24. PubMed PMID: 10649824. Epub 2000/01/29. eng.
6. Dunkel-Schetter C, Feinstein LG, Taylor SE, Falke RL. Patterns of coping with cancer. Health Psychol. 1992;11(2):79–87. PubMed PMID: 1582383. Epub 1992/01/01. eng.
7. McEwen BS. Biomarkers for assessing population and individual health and disease related to stress and adaptation. Metab Clin Exp. 2015;64(3 Suppl 1):S2–S10. PubMed PMID: 25496803. Epub 2014/12/17. eng.
8. Dunkel-Schetter C, Folkman S, Lazarus RS. Correlates of social support receipt. J Pers Soc Psychol. 1987;53(1):71–80. PubMed PMID: 3612494. Epub 1987/07/01. eng.
9. WCRF/AICR. Diet, Nutrition, physical activity and cancer: a global perspective. Continuous update project expert report. dietandcancerreport.org: 2018.
10. Park CL. Making sense of the meaning literature: an integrative review of meaning making and its effects on adjustment to stressful life events. Psychol Bull. 2010;136(2):257–301. PubMed PMID: 20192563. Epub 2010/03/03. eng.
11. Leventhal H, Phillips LA, Burns E. The Common-Sense Model of Self-Regulation (CSM): a dynamic framework for understanding illness self-management. J Behav Med. 2016;39(6):935–46. PubMed PMID: 27515801. Epub 2016/08/16. eng.
12. Vehling S, Philipp R. Existential distress and meaning-focused interventions in cancer survivorship. Curr Opin Support Palliat Care. 2018;12(1):46–51. PubMed PMID: 29251694. Epub 2017/12/19. eng.
13. Cao W, Qi X, Cai DA, Han X. Modeling posttraumatic growth among cancer patients: the roles of social support, appraisals, and adaptive coping. Psycho-Oncology. 2018;27(1):208–15. PubMed PMID: 28171681. Epub 2017/02/09. eng.
14. Folkman S, Lazarus RS, Gruen RJ, DeLongis A. Appraisal, coping, health status, and psychological symptoms. J Pers Soc Psychol. 1986;50(3):571–9. PubMed PMID: 3701593. Epub 1986/03/01. eng.
15. McCorkle R, Ercolano E, Lazenby M, Schulman-Green D, Schilling LS, Lorig K, et al. Self-management: enabling and empowering patients living with cancer as a chronic illness. CA Cancer J Clin. 2011;61(1):50–62. PubMed PMID: 21205833. Pubmed Central PMCID: PMC3058905. Epub 2011/01/06. eng.
16. Alarcon G, Bowling NA, Khazon S. Great expectations: a meta analytic examination of optimism and hope. Personal Individ Differ. 2013;54:821–7.
17. Cohen M, Levkovich I, Pollack S, Fried G. Stability and change of postchemotherapy symptoms in relation to optimism and subjective stress: a prospective study of breast cancer survivors. Psycho-Oncology. 2019;28(10):2017–24. PubMed PMID: 31351023. Epub 2019/07/28. eng.
18. Sumpio C, Jeon S, Northouse LL, Knobf MT. Optimism, symptom distress, illness appraisal, and coping in patients with advanced-stage cancer diagnoses undergoing chemotherapy treatment. Oncol Nurs Forum. 2017;44(3):384–92. PubMed PMID: 28635986. Epub 2017/06/22. eng.
19. World Cancer Research Fund AIfcr. Diet, nutrition, physical activity and cancer: a global perspective. Summary of 3rd expert report. Continuous update project expert report.: dietandcancerreport.org; 2018.
20. Seeman TE, McEwen BS, Rowe JW, Singer BH. Allostatic load as a marker of cumulative biological risk. Proc Natl Acad Sci U S A. 2001;98:4770–5.
21. Miller AH, Ancoli-Israel S, Bower JE, Capuron L, Irwin MR. Neuroendocrine-immune mechanisms of behavioral comorbidities in patients with cancer. J Clin Oncol. 2008;26(6):971–82. PubMed PMID: 18281672. Pubmed Central PMCID: 2770012.
22. Riba MB, Donovan KA, Andersen B, Braun I, Breitbart WS, Brewer BW, et al. Distress management, version 3.2019, NCCN clinical practice guidelines in oncology. J Natl Compr Canc Netw. 2019;17(10):1229–49. PubMed PMID: 31590149. Pubmed Central PMCID: PMC6907687. Epub 2019/10/08. eng.

23. Kirtonia A, Sethi G, Garg M. The multifaceted role of reactive oxygen species in tumorigenesis. Cell Mol Life Sci. 2020;77(22):4459–83. PubMed PMID: 32358622. Epub 2020/05/03. eng.
24. McEwen BS, Gray J, Nasca C. Recognizing resilience: learning from the effects of stress on the brain. Neurobiol Stress. 2015;1:1–11. PubMed PMID: 25506601. Pubmed Central PMCID: PMC4260341. Epub 2014/12/17. Eng.
25. Tedeschi RG, Calhoun LG. Beyond the concept of recovery: growth and the experience of loss. Death Stud. 2008;32(1):27–39. PubMed PMID: 18652064. Epub 2008/07/26. eng.
26. Giesinger JM, Kuijpers W, Young T, Tomaszewski KA, Friend E, Zabernigg A, et al. Thresholds for clinical importance for four key domains of the EORTC QLQ-C30: physical functioning, emotional functioning, fatigue and pain. Health Qual Life Outcomes. 2016;14:87. PubMed PMID: 27267486. Pubmed Central PMCID: PMC4897949. Epub 2016/06/09. eng.
27. Ryff CD. Psychological well-being revisited: advances in the science and practice of eudaimonia. Psychother Psychosom. 2014;83(1):10–28. PubMed PMID: 24281296. Pubmed Central PMCID: PMC4241300. Epub 2013/11/28. eng.
28. Aschbacher K, O'Donovan A, Wolkowitz OM, Dhabhar FS, Su Y, Epel E. Good stress, bad stress and oxidative stress: insights from anticipatory cortisol reactivity. Psychoneuroendocrinology. 2013;38(9):1698–708. PubMed PMID: 23490070. Epub 2013/03/16. eng.
29. McEwen BS. Physiology and neurobiology of stress and adaptation: central role of the brain. Physiol Rev. 2007;87(3):873–904. PubMed PMID: 17615391. Epub 2007/07/07. eng.
30. McEwen BS. In pursuit of resilience: stress, epigenetics, and brain plasticity. Ann N Y Acad Sci. 2016;1373(1):56–64. PubMed PMID: 26919273. Epub 2016/02/27. eng.
31. Karatsoreos IN, McEwen BS. Psychobiological allostasis: resistance, resilience and vulnerability. Trends Cogn Sci. 2011;15(12):576–84. PubMed PMID: 22078931. Epub 2011/11/15. eng.
32. Karatsoreos IN, McEwen BS. Annual Research Review: the neurobiology and physiology of resilience and adaptation across the life course. J Child Psychol Psychiatry. 2013;54(4):337–47. PubMed PMID: 23517425. Epub 2013/03/23. eng.
33. McEwen B. Central effects of stress hormones in health and disease: understanding the protective and damaging effects of stress and stress mediators. Eur J Pharmacol. 2008;583:174–85.
34. McEwen BS, Gianaros PJ. Stress- and allostasis-induced brain plasticity. Annu Rev Med. 2011;62:431–45. PubMed PMID: 20707675. Epub 2010/08/17. eng.
35. McEwen BS, Morrison JH. The brain on stress: vulnerability and plasticity of the prefrontal cortex over the life course. Neuron. 2013;79(1):16–29. PubMed PMID: 23849196. Pubmed Central PMCID: PMC3753223. Epub 2013/07/16. eng.
36. Eiland L, McEwen BS. Early life stress followed by subsequent adult chronic stress potentiates anxiety and blunts hippocampal structural remodeling. Hippocampus. 2012;22(1):82–91. PubMed PMID: 20848608. Epub 2010/09/18. eng.
37. Cherubini E, Miles R. The CA3 region of the hippocampus: how is it? What is it for? How does it do i? Front Cell Neurosci. 2015;9:1–3.
38. Johnston ST, Shtrahman M, Parylak S, Gonçalves JT, Gage FH. Paradox of pattern separation and adult neurogenesis: a dual role for new neurons balancing memory resolution and robustness. Neurobiol Learn Mem. 2016;129:60–8. PubMed PMID: 26549627. Pubmed Central PMCID: PMC4792723. Epub 2015/11/10. eng.
39. Gonçalves JT, Schafer ST, Gage FH. Adult neurogenesis in the hippocampus: from stem cells to behavior. Cell. 2016;167(4):897–914. PubMed PMID: 27814520. Epub 2016/11/05. eng.
40. McEwen BS. Stress, sex, and neural adaptation to a changing environment: mechanisms of neuronal remodeling. Ann N Y Acad Sci. 2010;1204(Suppl):E38–59. PubMed PMID: 20840167. Pubmed Central PMCID: PMC2946089. Epub 2010/09/25. eng.
41. Lutgendorf SK, Andersen BL. Biobehavioral approaches to cancer progression and survival: mechanisms and interventions. Am Psychol. 2015;70(2):186–97. PubMed PMID: 25730724. Pubmed Central PMCID: PMC4347942. Epub 2015/03/03. eng.

42. Danese A, McEwen BS. Adverse childhood experiences, allostasis, allostatic load, and age-related disease. Physiol Behav. 2012;106(1):29–39. PubMed PMID: 21888923. Epub 2011/09/06. eng.
43. Thayer JF, Sternberg E. Beyond heart rate variability: vagal regulation of allostatic systems. Ann N Y Acad Sci. 2006;1088:361–72. PubMed PMID: 17192580.
44. Bernardi L, Sleight P, Bandinelli G, Cencetti S, Fattorini L, Wdowczyc-Szulc J, et al. Effect of rosary prayer and yoga mantras on autonomic cardiovascular rhythms: comparative study. BMJ. 2001;323(7327):1446–9. PubMed PMID: 11751348. Pubmed Central PMCID: 61046.
45. Raison CL, Miller AH. When not enough is too much: the role of insufficient glucocorticoid signaling in the pathophysiology of stress-related disorders. Am J Psychiatry. 2003;160(9):1554–65. PubMed PMID: 12944327. Epub 2003/08/29. eng.
46. Juruena MF, Agustini B, Cleare AJ, Young AH. A translational approach to clinical practice via stress-responsive glucocorticoid receptor signaling. Stem Cell Invest. 2017;4:13. PubMed PMID: 28275643. Pubmed Central PMCID: PMC5334557. Epub 2017/03/10. eng.
47. Mathews HL, Konley T, Kosik KL, Krukowski K, Eddy J, Albuquerque K, et al. Epigenetic patterns associated with the immune dysregulation that accompanies psychosocial distress. Brain Behav Immun. 2011;25(5):830–9. PubMed PMID: 21146603. Pubmed Central PMCID: PMC3079772. Epub 2010/12/15. eng.
48. Mathew A, Doorenbos AZ, Li H, Jang MK, Park CG, Bronas UG. Allostatic load in cancer: a systematic review and mini meta-analysis. Biol Res Nurs. 2021;23(3):341–61. PubMed PMID: 33138637. Epub 2020/11/04. eng.
49. de Quervain D, Schwabe L, Roozendaal B. Stress, glucocorticoids and memory: implications for treating fear-related disorders. Nat Rev Neurosci. 2017;18(1):7–19. PubMed PMID: 27881856. Epub 2016/11/25. eng.
50. Thayer JF, Sternberg EM. Neural aspects of immunomodulation: focus on the vagus nerve. Brain Behav Immun. 2010;24(8):1223–8. PubMed PMID: 20674737. Pubmed Central PMCID: PMC2949498. Epub 2010/08/03. eng.
51. Wilson ER, Wisely JA, Wearden AJ, Dunn KW, Edwards J, Tarrier N. Do illness perceptions and mood predict healing time for burn wounds? A prospective, preliminary study. J Psychosom Res. 2011;71(5):364–6. PubMed PMID: 21999981. Epub 2011/10/18. eng.
52. Webster Marketon JI, Glaser R. Stress hormones and immune function. Cell Immunol. 2008;252(1–2):16–26. PubMed PMID: 18279846.
53. Kiecolt-Glaser J, Marucha P, Malarkey W, Mercado A, Glaser R. Slowing of wound healing by psychological stress. Lancet. 1995;346:1–3.
54. McEwen BS. Sleep deprivation as a neurobiologic and physiologic stressor: allostasis and allostatic load. Metab Clin Exp. 2006;55(10 Suppl 2):S20–3. PubMed PMID: 16979422.
55. McEwen BS. Protective and damaging effects of stress mediators. N Engl J Med. 1998;338(3):171–9. PubMed PMID: 9428819.
56. Glaser R, Kiecolt-Glaser JK. Stress-induced immune dysfunction: implications for health. Nat Rev Immunol. 2005;5(3):243–51. PubMed PMID: 15738954.
57. Watkins AD. Perceptions, emotions and immunity: an integrated homeostatic network. QJM. 1995;88(4):283–94. PubMed PMID: 7796079.
58. Rossman ML, Shrock D. Mind-body medicine in integrative cancer care. In: Abrams DL, Weil A, editors. Integrative oncology. New York: Oxford University Press; 2009. p. 244–57.
59. Gray JD, Milner TA, McEwen BS. Dynamic plasticity: the role of glucocorticoids, brain-derived neurotrophic factor and other trophic factors. Neuroscience. 2013;239:214–27. PubMed PMID: 22922121. Pubmed Central PMCID: PMC3743657. Epub 2012/08/28. eng.
60. Ninan I. Synaptic regulation of affective behaviors; role of BDNF. Neuropharmacology. 2014;76:684–95. PubMed PMID: 23747574. Pubmed Central PMCID: PMC3825795. Epub 2013/06/12. eng.
61. Magarinos AM, Li CJ, Gal Toth J, Bath KG, Jing D, Lee FS, et al. Effect of brain-derived neurotrophic factor haploinsufficiency on stress-induced remodeling of hippocampal neurons. Hippocampus. 2011;21(3):253–64. PubMed PMID: 20095008. Pubmed Central PMCID: PMC2888762. Epub 2010/01/23. eng.

62. Bennett MR, Lagopoulos J. Stress and trauma: BDNF control of dendritic-spine formation and regression. Prog Neurobiol. 2014;112:80–99. PubMed PMID: 24211850. Epub 2013/11/12. eng.
63. Caldji C, Francis D, Sharma S, Plotsky PM, Meaney MJ. The effects of early rearing environment on the development of GABAA and central benzodiazepine receptor levels and novelty-induced fearfulness in the rat. Neuropsychopharmacology. 2000;22(3):219–29. PubMed PMID: 10693149. Epub 2000/02/29. eng.
64. Duman RS, Sanacora G, Krystal JH. Altered connectivity in depression: GABA and glutamate neurotransmitter deficits and reversal by novel treatments. Neuron. 2019;102(1):75–90. PubMed PMID: 30946828. Pubmed Central PMCID: PMC6450409. Epub 2019/04/05. eng.
65. Popoli M, Yan Z, McEwen BS, Sanacora G. The stressed synapse: the impact of stress and glucocorticoids on glutamate transmission. Nat Rev Neurosci. 2011;13(1):22–37. PubMed PMID: 22127301. Pubmed Central PMCID: PMC3645314. Epub 2011/12/01. eng.
66. Khalili AA, Ahmad MR. A review of cell adhesion studies for biomedical and biological applications. Int J Mol Sci. 2015;16(8):18149–84. PubMed PMID: 26251901. Pubmed Central PMCID: PMC4581240. Epub 2015/08/08. eng.
67. Wang M, Zhao J, Zhang L, Wei F, Lian Y, Wu Y, et al. Role of tumor microenvironment in tumorigenesis. J Cancer. 2017;8(5):761–73. PubMed PMID: 28382138. Pubmed Central PMCID: PMC5381164. Epub 2017/04/07. eng.
68. Baik JH. Stress and the dopaminergic reward system. Exp Mol Med. 2020;52(12):1879–90. PubMed PMID: 33257725. Pubmed Central PMCID: PMC8080624. Epub 2020/12/02. eng.
69. Bissonette GB, Roesch MR. Development and function of the midbrain dopamine system: what we know and what we need to. Genes Brain Behav. 2016;15(1):62–73. PubMed PMID: 26548362. Pubmed Central PMCID: PMC5266527. Epub 2015/11/10. eng.
70. Russo SJ, Nestler EJ. The brain reward circuitry in mood disorders. Nat Rev Neurosci. 2013;14(9):609–25. PubMed PMID: 23942470. Pubmed Central PMCID: PMC3867253. Epub 2013/08/15. eng.
71. Ouakinin SRS, Barreira DP, Gois CJ. Depression and obesity: integrating the role of stress, neuroendocrine dysfunction and inflammatory pathways. Front Endocrinol. 2018;9:431. PubMed PMID: 30108549. Pubmed Central PMCID: PMC6079193. Epub 2018/08/16. eng.
72. McEwen BS, Karatsoreos IN. Sleep deprivation and circadian disruption: stress, allostasis, and allostatic load. Sleep Med Clin. 2015;10(1):1–10. PubMed PMID: 26055668. Epub 2015/06/10. eng.
73. Karatsoreos IN, Bhagat S, Bloss EB, Morrison JH, McEwen BS. Disruption of circadian clocks has ramifications for metabolism, brain, and behavior. Proc Natl Acad Sci U S A. 2011;108(4):1657–62. PubMed PMID: 21220317. Pubmed Central PMCID: PMC3029753. Epub 2011/01/12. eng.
74. Rosenwasser AM, Turek FW. Neurobiology of circadian rhythm regulation. Sleep Med Clin. 2015;10(4):403–12. PubMed PMID: 26568118. Epub 2015/11/17. eng.
75. Bhasin MK, Dusek JA, Chang BH, Joseph MG, Denninger JW, Fricchione GL, et al. Relaxation response induces temporal transcriptome changes in energy metabolism, insulin secretion and inflammatory pathways. PLoS One. 2013;8(5):e62817. PubMed PMID: 23650531. Pubmed Central PMCID: PMC3641112. Epub 2013/05/08. eng.
76. Schuebel K, Gitik M, Domschke K, Goldman D. Making sense of epigenetics. Int J Neuropsychopharmacol. 2016;19(11):1–10.
77. Maze I, Noh KM, Allis CD. Histone regulation in the CNS: basic principles of epigenetic plasticity. Neuropsychopharmacology. 2013;38(1):3–22. PubMed PMID: 22828751. Pubmed Central PMCID: PMC3521967. Epub 2012/07/26. eng.
78. Kaulmann A, Bohn T. Carotenoids, inflammation, and oxidative stress-implications of cellular signaling pathways and relation to chronic disease prevention. Nutr Res. 2014;34(11):907–29. PubMed PMID: 25134454. Epub 2014/08/20. Eng.
79. DiDonato JA, Mercurio F, Karin M. NF-κB and the link between inflammation and cancer. Immunol Rev. 2012;246(1):379–400. PubMed PMID: 22435567. Epub 2012/03/23. eng.

80. Feng Z, Liu L, Zhang C, Zheng T, Wang J, Lin M, et al. Chronic restraint stress attenuates p53 function and promotes tumorigenesis. Proc Natl Acad Sci U S A. 2012;109(18):7013–8. PubMed PMID: 22509031. Pubmed Central PMCID: PMC3345015. Epub 2012/04/18. eng.
81. Rosenblat JD, Cha DS, Mansur RB, McIntyre RS. Inflamed moods: a review of the interactions between inflammation and mood disorders. Prog Neuro-Psychopharmacol Biol Psychiatry. 2014;53:23–34. PubMed PMID: 24468642. Epub 2014/01/29. Eng.
82. Bower JE, Ganz PA, Irwin MR, Kwan L, Breen EC, Cole SW. Inflammation and behavioral symptoms after breast cancer treatment: do fatigue, depression, and sleep disturbance share a common underlying mechanism? J Clin Oncol. 2011;29(26):3517–22. PubMed PMID: 21825266. Pubmed Central PMCID: 3179252.
83. Dantzer R. Cytokine-induced sickness behavior: mechanisms and implications. Ann N Y Acad Sci. 2001;933:222–34. PubMed PMID: 12000023. Epub 2002/05/10. eng.
84. Dantzer R, Kelley KW. Twenty years of research on cytokine-induced sickness behavior. Brain Behav Immun. 2007;21(2):153–60. PubMed PMID: 17088043. Pubmed Central PMCID: PMC1850954. Epub 2006/11/08. eng.
85. Irwin MR. Inflammation at the intersection of behavior and somatic symptoms. Psychiatr Clin North Am. 2011;34(3):605–20. PubMed PMID: 21889682. Pubmed Central PMCID: PMC3820277. Epub 2011/09/06. eng.
86. Miller AH, Maletic V, Raison CL. Inflammation and its discontents: the role of cytokines in the pathophysiology of major depression. Biol Psychiatry. 2009;65(9):732–41. PubMed PMID: 19150053. Pubmed Central PMCID: PMC2680424. Epub 2009/01/20. eng.
87. Sillar JR, Germon ZP, DeIuliis GN, Dun MD. The role of reactive oxygen species in acute myeloid leukaemia. Int J Mol Sci. 2019;20(23):6003. PubMed PMID: 31795243. Pubmed Central PMCID: PMC6929020. Epub 2019/12/05. eng.
88. Gidron Y, Russ K, Tissarchondou H, Warner J. The relation between psychological factors and DNA-damage: a critical review. Biol Psychol. 2006;72(3):291–304. PubMed PMID: 16406268. Epub 2006/01/13. eng.
89. Kučera O, Cifra M. Radiofrequency and microwave interactions between biomolecular systems. J Biol Phys. 2016;42(1):1–8. PubMed PMID: 26174548. Pubmed Central PMCID: PMC4713408. Epub 2015/07/16. eng.
90. Jaross W. Hypothesis on interactions of macromolecules based on molecular vibration patterns in cells and tissues. Front Biosci (Landmark Ed). 2018;23:940–6. PubMed PMID: 28930582. Epub 2017/09/21. eng.
91. Thayer JF, Smith M, Rossy LA, Sollers JJ, Friedman BH. Heart period variability and depressive symptoms: gender differences. Biol Psychiatry. 1998;44(4):304–6. PubMed PMID: 9715364.
92. Reeve K, Black PA, Huang J. Examining the impact of a Healing Touch intervention to reduce posttraumatic stress disorder symptoms in combat veterans. Psychol Trauma. 2020;12(8):897–903. PubMed PMID: 33346680. Epub 2020/12/22. eng.
93. Walker FR, Pfingst K, Carnevali L, Sgoifo A, Nalivaiko E. In the search for integrative biomarker of resilience to psychological stress. Neurosci Biobehav Rev. 2017;74(Pt B):310–20. PubMed PMID: 27179452. Epub 2016/05/18. eng.
94. Stults-Kolehmainen MA, Sinha R. The effects of stress on physical activity and exercise. Sports Med (Auckland, NZ). 2014;44(1):81–121. PubMed PMID: 24030837. Pubmed Central PMCID: PMC3894304. Epub 2013/09/14. eng.
95. Cortesi L, Sebastiani F, Iannone A, Marcheselli L, Venturelli M, Piombino C, et al. Lifestyle intervention on body weight and physical activity in patients with breast cancer can reduce the risk of death in obese women: the EMILI study. Cancers. 2020;12(7):1709. PubMed PMID: 32605075. Pubmed Central PMCID: PMC7407899. Epub 2020/07/02. eng.
96. Tomiyama AJ. Stress and obesity. Annu Rev Psychol. 2019;70:703–18. PubMed PMID: 29927688. Epub 2018/06/22. eng.
97. McTiernan A, Friedenreich CM, Katzmarzyk PT, Powell KE, Macko R, Buchner D, et al. Physical activity in cancer prevention and survival: a systematic review. Med Sci Sports Exerc.

2019;51(6):1252–61. PubMed PMID: 31095082. Pubmed Central PMCID: PMC6527123. Epub 2019/05/17. eng.
98. Lahart IM, Metsios GS, Nevill AM, Carmichael AR. Physical activity, risk of death and recurrence in breast cancer survivors: a systematic review and meta-analysis of epidemiological studies. Acta Oncol (Stockholm, Sweden). 2015;54(5):635–54. PubMed PMID: 25752971. Epub 2015/03/11. eng.
99. Ringel AE, Drijvers JM, Baker GJ, Catozzi A, García-Cañaveras JC, Gassaway BM, et al. Obesity shapes metabolism in the tumor microenvironment to suppress anti-tumor immunity. Cell. 2020;183(7):1848–66.e26. PubMed PMID: 33301708. Pubmed Central PMCID: PMC8064125. Epub 2020/12/11. eng.
100. Alwarawrah Y, Kiernan K, MacIver NJ. Changes in nutritional status impact immune cell metabolism and function. Front Immunol. 2018;9:1055. PubMed PMID: 29868016. Pubmed Central PMCID: PMC5968375. Epub 2018/06/06. eng.
101. Gray JD, Rubin TG, Hunter RG, McEwen BS. Hippocampal gene expression changes underlying stress sensitization and recovery. Mol Psychiatry. 2014;19(11):1171–8. PubMed PMID: 24342991. Epub 2013/12/18. Eng.

Cancer   7

7.1 Introduction

Prolonged, unregulated stress leads to widespread, patho-physiological disturbances that exhaust energy resources needed to maintain homeostasis and psycho-biological coherence. Early child adversity and/or a history of prolonged distress that exceed personal and supportive resources and coping capabilities tend to predispose the individual to the development of chronic illness(es), including many cancers. This chapter presents a basic overview of the main pathophysiological characteristics of carcinomas, the tumor microenvironment, and pro-inflammatory tumor-promoting pathways.

7.2 Objectives

At the end of the chapter, you will be able to:

1. Identify the principal features of cancer
2. Describe the main characteristics of the tumor microenvironment (TME)
3. Gain understanding of the characteristics of the TME in relation to cancer initiation, progress, and invasion
4. Identify potential biomarkers and psychological markers that may serve as part of the evaluation of clinical interventions aimed at promoting resilience in patients

Clinical Anecdote 7.1
One evening, while doing some exercises, I discovered a lump. By virtue of its size and solidity, I was very sure it was a tumour, and was also shocked for not having previously detected its presence. In retrospect I had made the wildest miscalculation

that I could handle anything life pitched in my direction- pursue graduate work, continue to work, take care of two young school-aged children. I was so caught up keeping up with everything 'on my plate' that I apparently ignored tell-tale cues -the constant fatigue, weight gain, mild shortness of breath, eating too many carbohydrates, exercising less and less, a gnawing sensation of anxiety. It was a huge mistake with cold consequences.

7.3 Chronic Illness

Chronic illness is the leading cause of death worldwide, representing an estimated 71% of all deaths [1]. Whereas worldwide definitions vary, one working definition is from the Australian Institute for Health and Welfare (2016) which refers to chronic illness in terms of (1) complex multifactorial causes, (2) a protracted developmental phase, possibly without symptoms, (3) a prolonged illness that may be accompanied by other health-related complications, (4) functional impairments or disability [2]. Clinical examples include rheumatoid arthritis, cardiovascular disease, diabetes, neurological disease, and many cancers [1]. Clinical detection often occurs only after the disease has advanced sufficiently to manifest various symptoms. For newly diagnosed patients, cancer is frequently an unforeseen event.

Whereas normal acute inflammatory processes associated with physical healing are ordered and self-limiting, chronic illnesses emerge from a progressively systemic inflammatory environment manifested by neurostructural impairments and progressive pathophysiological alterations due to unregulated chronic psychological stress [3–6]. Although the process is biologically complex and related to numerous intrinsic and extrinsic factors, ROS-induced cellular, RNA, and/or DNA structural damage appears to be implicated in the development of chronic illnesses [7, 8]. The type manifested is thought to be linked to the person's genetic predisposition, epigenetic changes, and/or DNA mutations.

7.4 Cancer

Cancer is an insidious disease, a silent predator, and the leading cause of death worldwide, with almost 10 million deaths in 2020 [9]. The most common causes of death worldwide in descending order of prevalence are as follows: breast ($n = 2.26$ million (M), lung ($n = 2.21$ M), colon and rectum ($n = 1.93$ M), prostate ($n = 1.41$ M), skin (nonmelanoma) ($n = 1.20$ M), and stomach ($n = 1.09$ M). One third of cancer deaths are attributed to tobacco and alcohol use, high body mass index, inadequate intake of fruits and vegetables, and insufficient physical activity.

Definition

Cancer refers to a group of related diseases that are characterized by the unregulated, uncontrollable division of abnormal cells that are capable of invading nearby

Table 7.1 10 major characteristics of cancer [10]

1. Uncontrollable cellular replication	6. Enables proliferative signaling pathways
2. Evades or inactivates genes that suppress cancer growth	7. Uncontrolled cell energy use
3. Enables invasion and metastases	8. Avoids immune destruction
4. Withstands/inhibits cellular apoptosis	9. Genome instability and mutation
5. Triggers angiogenesis	10. Tumor-enhanced inflammation

tissues, "breaking off," and traveling to other body locations via the blood and lymph systems in order to develop another cancer site (Table 7.1). There are many types of cancers, generally identified by the region of the body in which they originated. Carcinomas, the most common type of cancer, are developed in the epithelial cells that line body surfaces [11].

Types of carcinomas include breast, lung and bronchus cancer, prostate, colon, and rectum. Other forms of cancer include sarcomas, leukemias, lymphomas, and myelomas. Sarcomas are a cancer of connective tissues and develop in mesenchymal cells that create bones and soft tissues. Whereas osteosarcoma refers to cancer of bone, cartilage, and blood vessels, soft tissue sarcoma occurs in fat, muscle, nerves, fibrous tissues, blood or lymph, and deep skin tissues. Leukemia is a cancer of the bone marrow and other blood-generating organs that are manifested in the blood system as abnormal leukocytes. Lymphoma and myeloma are cancers of the immune system. Because carcinomas are the most prevalent, and most studied from a nonpharmacological perspective, this chapter draws mainly on various carcinomas to illustrate the pathophysiology of the disease [11].

7.5 Factors Conducive to the Development of Cancer

Theories about the potential causes of cancer abound. Inherited genetic mutations, as well as prolonged exposure to toxic social or physical environmental factors, are thought to enhance the risk of developing various cancers [12]. Toxins associated with tobacco smoke, air pollution, industrial and agricultural chemicals, asbestos, and radiation are strongly posited to pose important threats. Other factors include the types, quality and quantity of food groups consumed, and lifestyle choices related to body weight (obesity) physical activity, alcohol consumption, and smoking [1, 12].

Chronic stress characterized by allostatic load and oxidative stress are important conditions in tumorigenesis [13]. In addition, the behaviors of endogenous bacteria and viruses have been implicated in tumorigenesis and cancer progression of various tumors [14, 15]. Viral infections are thought to account for more than 10% of human cancers [14, 15]. Because a dysregulated microbiome is strongly associated with a cancer-inducing inflammatory environment and suppressed immune functioning, this chapter will first highlight its role in enhancing the risk of cancer, in recognition of the microbiome as an endogenous contextual layer that also influences the development of cancer. What follows is a simplified overview that will hopefully contribute to an overall clinical understanding of cancer, providing a meaningful context for proposing nursing interventions in the care of patients with cancer and their caregivers.

The Microbiome

The microbiome refers to the trillions of microorganisms and their genomes that live throughout the human body with the largest numbers concentrating in the gut, genital tract, and other mucosal surfaces [16]. These mainly symbiotic microorganisms (also known as microbiota) consist mostly of bacteria, as well as smaller numbers of viruses, and even fewer eukaryotes and archaea [17]. The microbiome also has been referred to as the "genes and genomes of the microbiota as well as the products of microbiota and the host environment" [16].

Billions of pervasive microorganisms along the mucosa and surfaces of the respiratory tract, gut, and genitourinary tract cohabit symbiotically with the human body. This microbiome which develops from birth with contributions from maternal microbiota and the external environment varies in composition between individuals. Hormone-like biological constituents and bacterial metabolites mediate the relationship between bacteria and the human body [16]. For instance, gut bacteria communicate with the brain; gut bacteria also communicate with the hormonal and immune systems of the human body [18].

Disturbances to the microbiome are associated with various diseases, including cancer [16, 18]. A disrupted microbiome may cause cancer by promoting mucosal inflammation or systemic dysregulation. It can interfere with anticancer immune functioning and metabolism, and, in so doing, promotes the cancerogenic process. A disturbed microbiota also can reduce the efficacy of cancer therapy (see [16] review). Moreover, pathogenic bacteria can mimic parts of the biological communication pathways so that a host/pathogen communication system is now carcinogenic.

Bacterial Infection and Human Mitochondria An estimated 20% of all cancers are now thought to be associated with microbial infection (see [18] review). Mitochondria, the working organelle of the cell is responsible for a number of important cellular functions: regulating apoptosis, innate immune responses, and the production of adenosine 5' triphosphate (ATP) via oxidative phosphorylation in which chemical energy from food is converted into ATP, another form of energy. It is also implicated in the synthesis of cellular elements such as amino acids, nucleotides, and lipid metabolism. Scientific data strongly suggest that endogenous bacteria, similar to *many viruses, can* damage mitochondrial DNA (mtDNA) increasing the individual's risk of developing cancer. Exogenous factors like smoking and chemical pollution contribute to mitochondrial DNA mutations which are linked to greater mtDNA replication errors, underscoring the critical imperative of healing damaged DNA or mutations [18].

Bacteria have been observed in tumors and in normal tissue surrounding the tumor [16]. Pathogenic bacteria induce mutations within the mtDNA of human

Table 7.2 Nuclear pathways associated with DNA repair

6 major nuclear repair pathways [18]
1. Direct reversal
2. Nucleotide excision repair (NER)
3. Base excision repair (BER)
4. Mismatch repair (MMR)
5. Recombination repair (RER)
6. Translesion synthesis (TLS)

mitochondria, reducing its oxidative phosphorylation capabilities, dysregulating related pathways such as the electron transport chain, and ultimately reducing the body's ability to carry out normal cellular functions. During early initiation and growth, the tumor cells are driven by an accelerated and unregulated growth associated with DNA mutations which direct at an epigenetic level the switch from an oxygen source of energy (i.e., mtDNA oxidative phosphorylation) to a glucose energy source via glycolysis, or glucose-dependent pathways which provide greater amounts of energy in order to maintain the accelerated rate of proliferation of the tumor [19, 20]. The finding suggests that glucose should be reduced in the diets of patients with cancer.

Bacteria from the microbiome and pathogenic bacteria also impair the normal cell's ability to repair DNA damage and target mitochondrial intrinsic apoptotic pathways for further dysregulation (Table 7.1) [18]. Apoptosis is a highly controlled cell mechanism needed for orderly cellular growth and development, tissue homeostasis, and immune defense activities against foreign agents (bacteria, viruses, and cancer cells). In essence, the normal reparative process for 5/6 major nuclear pathways (with the exception of the TLS pathway) must induce apoptosis or rapid cell death when damaged cellular functions are detected (see Table 7.2). This process involves detecting the damaged part and degrading it through a number of steps that culminate in the mutated part being "marked" for phagocytosis (eliminated). And then, the cell's complex nuclear reparative pathways can restore the DNA helix. These restorative pathways have also been observed in mitochondrial DNA. Unrepaired damage to nuclear and mitochondrial DNA coupled with an inability to carry out efficient reparative activities leads to further replication mutations, cell dysfunctions, and uncontrollable cell proliferation [21].

Consequently, the bacteria's anti-apoptotic effects are strongly associated with an increased risk of a cancer onset. Anti-apoptotic effects provide a survival benefit for cancer cells and also contribute to chemotherapeutic resistance. Although the proposed links are not completely delineated scientifically, many dysregulated elements of the mitochondrial apoptotic pathways have been observed in cancer.

7.6 The Development of Cancer

Cancer is a metabolic and genetic disease caused by inherited and reactive oxygen species (ROS)-induced genetic mutations responsible for altering signaling pathways associated with various growth factors, hormones, and survival-related defense systems that enable undifferentiated growth, proliferation, and metastasis of the tumor [13]. The development of cancer consists of multiple steps: It involves the normal cell or stem cell which accumulates a critical number of cellular mutations so that the cell now reflects the essential attributes of a cancer cell or cancer stem cell. These characteristics include sustained angiogenesis, the ability to elude apoptosis, avoid tumor suppressors (anti-growth factors), sustain dysregulated growth, limitless proliferation, and differentiation within the tumor (at an unregulated and rapid pace compared to normal cells), and possess invasive metastatic capability [22].

Against the backdrop of a highly stress-sensitive and reactive endogenous microbiome that can play a role in promoting cancer, we now pivot to an extremely simplified description of (1) the characteristics of a cancer cell and the role of cancer stem cells, (2) key ROS-induced alterations that transform a normal cell to a tumor cell, (3) the role of systemic inflammation, and (4) the tumor microenvironment in promoting cancer progression and metastases [10, 13, 23]. Systemic inflammation, oxidative stress, and reactive oxygen species/reactive nitrogen species (ROS/RNS), cancer stem cells, the tumor microenvironment, cancer-associated fibroblasts (CAFs), and immune suppression are among the key biological mediators in the relationship between chronic stress and cancer.

Cancer Stem Cells (CSCs)

Normal stem cells are an integral part of multicellular organisms, such as humans, and divide by mitosis to produce new stem cells or differentiate into mature cells of a specific tissue. In contrast, the origins of CSCs are still being clarified: Genetic mutations are hypothesized to transform normal stem cells into cancer stem cells (CSCs), which are also referred to as cancer-initiating stem cells [22, 23]. CSCs may also arise from progenitor cells located in adult tissues. CSCs also are formed by a process known as *epithelial–mesenchymal transition* (EMT): differentiated cells with oncogenic mutations transition to a de-differentiated state of cancer stem cell-like phenotypes and/or cancer stem cells that meet the developmental requirements of a growing cancer (see section "Epithelial-to- Mesenchymal Transition (EMT) in Tumor Progression and Recurrence"). This process is thought to be facilitated by various signaling pathways such as Notch, nuclear factor kappa beta (NFkB) a transcription factor, and a cytokine called transforming growth factor-beta (TGF-B) [23, 24].

CSCs and cancer cells are distinguished from normal cells by a number of morphological and cell function alterations (Table 7.3). CSCs comprise only a small portion of the cancer cells within the tumor and have unlimited and indefinite self-replication capabilities and produce all the heterogeneous cells of the original tumor [22–24]. This suggests that stem cells drive the growth and proliferation of the tumor. Cancer stem cells have the same metabolic capabilities, similar signaling pathways, and cell cycling activities as normal stem cells, albeit with abnormal regulation.

7.6 The Development of Cancer

Table 7.3 Distinguishing features between normal stem cells and cancer stem cells [22–24]

Normal stem cells	Cancer cell stem cells
1. Unlimited proliferation potential within the requirements of the biological system	1. Unlimited proliferation potential, resulting in failure to regulate tissue growth
2. Tissue-specific stem cell types	2. Resist apoptosis
3. Constitutes small portion of given cell tissues	3. Consist of small portion of cancer tissue
4 Built-in ability for apoptosis	4. Escape anti-growth chemical signals
5. Does not destroy immune cells	5. Escape immune surveillance and anticancer cell activities
6. Contributes to cell and tissue regeneration	6. Increase cellular motility needed for metastasis
7. Capable of migrating to the organ of their origin	7. Change phenotypes without genetic mutation

The Role of ROS in Tumorigenesis and Cancer Progression (Review [13, 22])

The transformation from normal cells into the "tumorigenic state" involves a number of ROS-induced genetic mutations that alter critical cellular signaling pathways resulting in malignant properties characterized by changes in cell morphology and functions that enable undifferentiated growth (Table 7.4) [13]. ROS plays an essential role not only in the initiation, but also in the angiogenesis, progression, and metastases of cancer. Normal cell functions depend on redox homeostasis in which oxidants and antioxidants maintain a relative homeostatic balance. *Oxidative stress* alters that balance, favoring circulating ROS that exceed the body's antioxidant capacity to neutralize or eliminate the reactive molecules. Under these conditions, ROS interact with cell molecules and their DNA, causing DNA damage and oncogenic mutations within normal cells and critically adult stem cells, altering the genes that control cell growth and differentiation, thereby transforming these normal cells into tumorigenic cancer cells and cancer stem cells [13, 22].

ROS interacts with the normal genes of cells to convert proto-oncogenes into activated oncogenes that trigger oncogenic signaling pathways, block normal functioning of tumor suppressors, enable escape from immune cells, promote angiogenesis, and facilitate the development of the *microenvironment*. *ROS* unleashes unregulated and undifferentiated proliferation of cells with all the main characteristics of a tumor cell and cancer stem cell [22, 25, 26]. Other critical genes of normal cells that are transformed by mutations caused by interactions with elevated levels of cellular ROS include DNA repair and cell cycle genes [13]. These oncogenic transformations alter the cell's normal's signaling pathways. A signaling pathway refers to a set of biochemical reactions in which a number of molecules cooperate together to modulate a cell function such as apoptosis or cell division. Oncogenic transformations dysregulate these pathways so that their functions take on the characteristics of a cancer cell.

Table 7.4 ROS-induced impairments to normal gene expression of various cellular functions [13, 22]

Critical genes dysregulated by ROS interactions	Descriptions
1. Proto-oncogenes	Normal genes encoding for proteins responsible for stimulating cell division (normal growth) and inhibiting cell differentiation. These genes can be converted into oncogenes (that cause cancer cell growth) through mutations which dysregulate various growth factors, such as epidermal growth factor receptor (EGFR), platelet-derived growth factor receptor (PDGFR), endothelial growth factor receptor (VEGFR), and human epithelial growth factor receptor2 (HER2/neu)
2. Tumor suppressor genes	These genes code for a protein that normally functions to limit cell growth and division, or even promote apoptosis
3. DNA repair genes	Genes to maintain genome integrity: Identifying and removing DNA lesions, DNA damage, and correcting replication errors
4. Cell cycle genes	Normal cell genes encoding for proteins responsible for the progression of one or more phases of the cell cycle
5. Immune escape	The immune system's capacity to get rid of transformed precancer cells or cancer cells no longer functions, and reflects a failure of immune surveillance

As illustrated by Kirtonia (2020), one such pathway, known as MAPK, is required for normal cell growth, differentiation, and survival. But ROS *oxidizes and deactivates* the MAPK phosphatases while *activating* epithelial growth factor receptor (EGFR) and platelet-derived growth factor receptor (PDGFR) signaling pathways (i.e., RAS and ERK), thereby promoting dysregulated cellular growth. In another example, the P13k/AKT/mTOR intracellular signaling pathway in the healthy cell has a natural inhibitor, PTEN, which normally controls or regulates signal transduction and

biological processes such as cellular proliferation, apoptosis, metabolism, and angiogenesis, thereby helping to prevent cancer. However, ROS (specifically O_2^- and H_2O_2) deactivates or degrades PTEN, a tumor suppressor gene, via oxidation (i.e., removing electrons associated with its phosphatase protein product) enabling dysregulated biological processes that result in cancer. A dysregulated PTEN is observed in breast, glioblastomas, melanomas, prostate, and endometrial cancers [13].

In summary, unregulated ROS alter normal cellular pathways needed for healthy cellular functioning, transforming these normal cells into cancer cells that are fueled by ROS. ROS becomes the significant regulator of impaired signal pathways involved in angiogenesis, metastases, immune escape, and an altered microbiome, which drives the initiation of tumorigenesis, cancer progression and metastasis [13, 27]. The inflammatory environment facilitates the process of transforming a normal cell to a cancer cell.

Cancer and Antioxidant Capabilities

Cancer cells are characterized by a state of oxidant/antioxidant redox imbalance favoring an increase in oxidants (ROS) within the cancer cell [13, 28]. This characteristic of the cancer cell induces dysregulated signaling pathways within itself that promote cancer cell growth and progression. Cancer cells *also produce antioxidant* capabilities, albeit only to a certain level in order to "detoxify" the *deleterious effects of ROS* while enabling the cancer cells to continue to benefit from an oxidant milieu which enables cancer development and ensures its survival [28]. This antioxidant capability is thought to be associated with cancer resistance to some anticancer therapies and is the focus of oncological strategies to overcome this resistance in part by increasing oxidative stress within cancer cells *above their preferred toxicity threshold* [28].

The Tumor Microenvironment (TME)

The tumor microenvironment is the "ecosystem" that surrounds the cancer cell to facilitate tumor growth, progression, and metastases [10]. It consists of normal stromal cells, vascular cells, fibroblasts, and inflammatory cytokines such as growth factors, chemokines, transcription factors (e.g., NFkB), and inflammatory cytokines, which play essential roles in promoting tumorigenesis and growth and proliferation.

Cancer cells are also surrounded by an extracellular matrix (ECM) and tumor stromal cells along with pro-inflammatory molecules and pathways (see Table 7.5). Stress-induced epigenetic changes modulate gene expression in support of *pro-inflammatory* interrelated systems and signaling pathways that secrete myriad inflammatory cytokines. These include interleukin-1 (IL-1), IL-1B, IL-2, IL-6, tumor necrosis factor-alpha (TNF-α) and interferon-y' (IFN-y'); chemokines, transcription factors, growth factors, and stress-related hormones, such as NOR and cortisol [30]. TNF-α in particular has been identified as one of the complex pro-inflammatory cytokines due to its dual functions depending on the cellular context [13, 27, 31]. For instance, TNF-α has been known to inhibit tumor progression yet within the TME, TNF-α has also been implicated in every phase of breast cancer development, including tumor progression, metastases, and the acquisition of drug resistance.

In addition to neuroendocrine and inflammatory immune cells that are present in the TME, there are also cellular and noncellular constituents that are thought to drive the formation of cancer cells. These include the extracellular matrix, myofibroblasts, fibroblasts, adipose cells, blood and lymphatic vascular network, reactive oxygen species (ROS), inducible nitric oxide synthase (iNOS), prostaglandins, NFkB, and various cancer-inducing growth factors such as VEGF [10, 27]. It is important to note that adipose cells in the TME secrete more than 50 types of cytokines, chemokines, and hormone-like factors, which are thought to support the onset of myriad forms of cancer [10]. Interactions between cancer cells and components in the stroma, especially the activated fibroblasts, play a vital role in initiating and promoting cancer cell growth [10, 29].

The TME is also fueled by tumors and cancer cells that secrete inflammatory factors [29]. The TME plays an important role in the clinical status of the cancer patient and his or her prognosis due to its potential for enhancing chemoresistance, for promoting cancer's survival via angiogenesis, for facilitating metastases via the process of epithelial–mesenchymal transition (see below), and by causing various

Table 7.5 Key elements in a tumor-producing microenvironment

Terms	Description
1. Extracellular matrix (ECM)	Binds cells together; regulates cell functions such as adhesion, cell-to-cell communication, migration, proliferation, differentiation, and cell invasion, metastatic capacities; secretes all cytokines, growth factors [29]
2. Stromal cells	Nonmalignant cells surrounding cancer cells; can differentiate into different cell types; support cell functions critical to tissue functions; secrete hormones. Changes within the inflammatory TME to support cancer growth [29]
3. Tumor	Consists of cancer cells and stromal cells; many tumors secrete vascular endothelial growth factor (VEGF) to create angiogenesis for nutrients [10]
4. Tumor stromal cells	Made up of fibroblasts, vascular endothelial cells, immune cells, and ECM; may promote tumorigenesis by interfering with drug delivery [10]
5. Cancer-associated fibroblasts (CAFs)	Constantly activated fibroblasts from tumor stroma interact with molecular pathways to increase cancer initiation, proliferation, and invasion; controls tumor angiogenesis by secreting vascular endothelial growth factor (VEGF); secretes other growth factors (e.g., transforming growth factor-beta (TGF-beta), platelet-derived growth factor (PDGF), cytokines including IL-22, IL-6 that promote cancer initiation, degradation of ECM proteins; and chemoresistance [10]
6. Epithelial-to-mesenchymal transition (EMT)	Inflammation-induced transformation of cancer cells from epithelial-to-mesenchymal properties that enable migration to evade cancer treatment and embed in distal regions with invasive properties to enable tumor recurrence and metastases [23]
7. Adipocytes	Cells (tissue), normally maintain energy in form of lipids; associated with hypoxia which creates an increased inflammatory environment; secretes more than 50 cytokines, chemokines, and hormone-like factors [10]
8. Chemoresistance	Drug resistance is associated with genetic and epigenetic changes, and also CAFs [10]
9. Certain cytokines	Certain cytokines are thought to promote tumorigenesis: It includes IL-6, TNF-α, TBF-ß [10]

stress-inducing symptoms such as fatigue, depression, anorexia, weight loss, and anemia [24, 32].

Cancer-Associated Fibroblasts (CAFs) (See Table 7.5 for Definitions)

Cancer-associated fibroblasts (CAFs) are instrumental in the initiation of tumor cells and their growth [10]. CAFs refer to *stress-activated fibroblasts from the tumor's stroma,* which do not turn off in a timely manner, thereby facilitating cancer growth. Whereas activated fibroblasts normally occur at the site of an injury and are inactivated *with healing,* cancer-associated fibroblasts remain continuously activated at the original site of the lesion or injury, secreting various cytokines (such as IL-6, which promotes the secretion of VEGF).

The tumor microenvironment interacts with CAFs in the initiation and propagation of tumor cells [33]. CAFs are involved in *remodeling* the extracellular matrix (ECM) within the TME to support cancer progression. The ECM, which normally helps to bind cells together and regulate cell proliferation, now appears to promote cancer cell growth and proliferation, when remodeled by activated CAFs. CAFs also interact with various neuroendocrine cells, cytokines, and other immune cells within the TME to promote cancer progression and metastasis, as well as cancer cell initiation [10, 29].

CAFs, for example, secrete chemokines and growth factors such as transforming growth factor-beta (TGF-ß), platelet-derived growth factor (PDGF), and galectin-1, a small protein with carbohydrate-binding capabilities, which are implicated in a number of cancer-promoting activities. Studies indicate that CAFs play an important role in modulating tumor-promoting angiogenesis, facilitating drug resistance to diverse treatments of various cancers, and damaging proteins of the extracellular matrix [26]. CAFs are found in many types of tumors including breast, pancreatic, lung, prostate, gastric, colorectal cancers, and cholangiocarcinoma. In contrast, when the microenvironment is in a healthy state and not flooded by various inflammatory and hormonal factors, it tends to provide bio-physiological protection *against* tumorigenesis [10]. This finding suggests that clinical interventions that reduce emotional distress and potentially systemic inflammation, and strengthen overall biological and psychological resilience especially *starting* in the diagnosis phase may be clinically therapeutic. It may help to modify, even modestly the internal milieu so that it is potentially less predisposed to cancer growth and proliferation.

Immune Evasion
Cell-mediated immunity is not as effective in eliminating cancer within the TME as outside it [4, 10]. Due in part to the inflammatory TME, the suppressed immune functions mean that cancer cells do not have to contend with activated immune cells within the TME seeking to destroy them *before* they embed themselves within the TME, which facilitates cancer cell proliferation and survivability [4, 10]. For example, cancer stem cells in the TME can also change their cell surface receptors and suppress nearby immune functions by interfering with their cell signaling capabilities and as a consequence evade detection by anticancer cells [4, 10, 23]. Stress-induced immune suppression also enables the overexpression of inflammatory cytokines that facilitate cancer cell development [4, 10, 23].

7.7　Progression, Invasion, and Metastases

Research findings show that not only chronic psychological stress but also the *growing tumor itself*, as well as *chemotherapy*, *surgery*, and *radiation*, contribute to systemic inflammation by producing countless inflammatory cytokines and chemokines and other pro-inflammatory factors [29, 32]. The deleterious impact of cancer treatments (albeit temporarily) in addition to the tumor itself contributes to the suppression of immune defenses and overproduction of reactive oxygen species (ROS), enabling cancer progression and metastases [13]. Whereas cancer-related treatment targets rapidly proliferating cancer cells, it is inefficient against the more slowly replicating cancer stem cells.

Chemoresistance

Chemoresistance is an important cause of treatment failure associated with chemo-, radiation, and even immunotherapy due to multiple factors, but in particular the role of cancer stem cells (CSCs) in treatment resistance, tumor recurrence, and metastases [13]. In order to eliminate cancer, treatments must target the cancer stem cells, which are capable of launching a huge multi-targeted defense to protect the tumor. This results in therapy-related resistance.

Whereas chemoradiation therapy is mainly efficacious against actively proliferating cancer cells, CSCs tend to replicate more slowly than cancer cells, thereby potentially evading the toxic effects of a given anticancer treatment. In addition, some cancer cells become *dormant* evading the toxic effects of therapy by utilizing epithelial-to-mesenchymal transition (EMT) and its reverse mechanism mesenchymal-to-epithelial transition (MET) [23] (see section "Epithelial-to-Mesenchymal Transition (EMT) in Tumor Progression and Recurrence"). Tumor cell dormancy refers to tumor cell populations that remain undetectable until clinical evidence of disease emerges [23].

Cancer stem cells also have been shown to circumnavigate cancer treatments in other effective ways. For instance, these cells are capable of drug efflux. CSCs can increase the expression of multidrug resistance transporters that in effect transport cytotoxic chemotherapies *out of the cancer cell* thereby contributing to chemoresistance [23]. The CSCs interact with cancer cells and the extracellular matrix (ECM) in the TME to facilitate angiogenesis, metastasis, and resistance to antitumor treatments [34].

Excess levels of ROS in normal cells lead to activation of cell death (apoptosis). Conversely cancer stem cells are characterized by low levels of ROS although the oxidant to antioxidant ratio still favors cancer progression (eg 28). This feature of CSCs reduces the likelihood of ROS-induced apoptosis caused for instance by chemotherapy [23]. Studies of leukemic stem cells have shown that low ROS levels in CSCs facilitate their ability to withstand the effects of chemotherapeutic agents [13]. Finally, resistance to cancer therapy is also mediated by cancer cells' ability to repair their DNA [23]. Notwithstanding, anticancer treatments are generally aimed at inducing cancer cell death either by directly or indirectly damaging cancer DNA [35].

Epithelial-to-Mesenchymal Transition (EMT) in Tumor Progression and Recurrence

CSCs and cancer cells may evade anticancer treatment via the complex process of epithelial-to-mesenchymal transition (EMT) [23]. EMT refers to a "cellular process in which (differentiated) epithelial cells gain mesenchymal (de-differentiated) properties due to the downregulation (i.e., suppression) of epithelial properties. The EMT de-differentiation of cancer stem cell phenotypes enables cells to evade the toxic effects of treatment, and to migrate to distal regions, taking hold undetected until invasive capacities may be triggered, and new cancer colonies (metastases) established" [36].

EMT is induced by biochemical signals that epithelial cancer cells or cancer stem cells receive emanating from the TME. Subsequent changes in gene expression cause the suppression of epithelial characteristics and the uptake of mesenchymal characteristics. The epithelial properties of the cancer cell tend to be characterized by stable epithelial cell–cell functions, polarity, and interactions with its basement membrane. The *differentiated epithelial cells* can transition from epithelial-to-mesenchymal phenotypes and acquire cancer stem cell-like properties, which include de-differentiation, migratory capabilities, and metastasis [24].

Some research has also suggested that mesenchymal-to epithelial transitions (METs) also occur [24, 36]. For instance, the transition from epithelial to a mesenchymal state tends to produce significant diversity of phenotypic manifestations. The process is characterized by a hybrid intermediate E/M state that results in a range of transient de-differentiated cancer stem-like cells with capabilities of self-renewal of needed differentiated cell types (epithelial components) [24, 36]. In other words, once mesenchymal-like cancer stem cells or cancer cells have translocated to a distal region, they transition back to a more epithelial "identity" through the process of mesenchyme-to-epithelial transition (MET) in order to restore their proliferative capabilities.

The process of EMT with respect to cancer cells and stem cells displays considerable "plasticity": diverse intermediate states of hybrid E/M may be found across the EMT spectrum although their significance has yet to be fully understood. EMT processes are regulated by transcription factors that also modulate changes to chromatin and subsequent gene expression [24, 36]. In cancer, similar processes of transitional capability occur in nonepithelial cancers such as leukemia or melanoma [36]. EMT occurs across numerous cellular processes that are still under investigation. These include during normal embryonic development, later development, adult wound healing, and in tissue fibrosis and cancer as described in the EMT process above [36].

Metastases

EMT is deeply involved in the metastatic process as outlined in section "Epithelial-to-Mesenchymal Transition (EMT) in Tumor Progression and Recurrence". The first step is for epithelial cancer cells to escape the primary tumor by relaxing cell–cell adhesion, degrading the basement membrane of the epithelium and ECM so that escape from the primary tumor site and the invasion of nearby tissues is possible. Tumor cells enter the circulatory system by crossing the endothelium and invading vascular and/or lymphatic vessels. Only a small number of tumor cells can withstand immune attacks or programmed cell death which occurs as a consequence of separating from the ECM. Some cells, however, may infiltrate nearby tissues or migrate to tissues (parenchyma) of distal organs. Safe within these new environments a small number seed or establish a foothold and proliferate into fully functioning secondary (metastatic) tumors that become clinically detectable and life-threatening [36].

7.8 Nursing Implications

This chapter has focused on tumor initiation, progression, and invasion in which evidence has illuminated some of the complex processes by which cancerous tumors seem to take hold and proliferate within an inflammatory microenvironment caused by chronic stress. Knowledge of these biological processes even in simplified form unmasks some of the mystery surrounding how epithelial tumors may be initiated and progress unimpeded when endogenous conditions created by chronic stress are met.

There is growing evidence that:

1. Deleterious effects of unregulated, stress-induced reactive oxygen species (ROS) and reactive nitrogen species (RNI) on cell structures cause DNA mutations that contribute to tumorigenesis.
2. Chronic stress-induced brain remodeling directed by epigenetic changes and gene expression, if left unabated, leads to widespread impaired neurophysiological and immune processes and functions that produce a systemic inflammatory milieu consisting of cumulative inflammatory cytokines that together with an extracellular matrix, fibroblasts, and stromal cells surround fledgling cancer cells and cancer stem cells to constitute the tumor microenvironment which interacts with the cancer stem cells and cancer cells to support their growth and proliferation.
3. Cancer cells have a number of strategies to evade anticancer treatments such as the bidirectional EMT process and drug efflux.
4. Within the inflammatory TME, cancer cells are protected by immunosuppression. Cancer stem cells can evade immune detection by changing their cell surface receptors and by interfering with immune cell signaling capabilities. As a consequence, cancer cells can evade detection by anticancer cells.
5. Conversely, cell-mediated immune surveillance is more effective in tracking down and eliminating cancer cells present in the vascular and lymphatic vessels than within the tumor microenvironment. Residual cancer cells are more likely to travel these pathways in the aftermath of surgery as they seek distal locations in which to colonize. That finding highlights the clinical importance of mounting clinical interventions in the pre/post treatment phases such as surgery in order to reduce emotional distress and strengthen immune functioning (eg [37, 38]).

This chapter provides a simplified description of the etiology, development, proliferation, and metastases of epithelial tumors. Hopefully, it may inform the clinical context within which to consider therapeutic interventions that may help the whole person. For example, the first objective may be to reduce emotional distress in the hope that it may attenuate the expression of inflammatory molecules that sustain an inflammatory environment. Reducing emotional distress may enable the reemergence of healing processes to strengthen innate and cell-mediated immunity, especially during vulnerable intervals along the treatment trajectory, for instance, before and especially after surgery during which residual cancer cells migrate to distal regions, unimpeded until the start of chemotherapy Embedded in distal regions these cancer cells can produce metastases years after the end of treatment. Healing-promoting interventions are discussed in Part IV.

References

1. WHO. WHO Health statistics and information systems. 2016.
2. Bernell S, Howard SW. Use your words carefully: what is a chronic disease? Front Public Health. 2016;4:159. PubMed PMID: 27532034. Pubmed Central PMCID: PMC4969287. Epub 2016/08/18. eng.
3. McEwen BS. Allostasis and allostatic load: implications for neuropsychopharmacology. Neuropsychopharmacology. 2000;22(2):108–24. PubMed PMID: 10649824. Epub 2000/01/29. eng.
4. Lutgendorf SK, Andersen BL. Biobehavioral approaches to cancer progression and survival: mechanisms and interventions. Am Psychol. 2015;70(2):186–97. PubMed PMID: 25730724. Pubmed Central PMCID: PMC4347942. Epub 2015/03/03. eng.
5. McEwen BS. Protective and damaging effects of stress mediators: central role of the brain. Dialogues Clin Neurosci. 2006;8(4):367–81. PubMed PMID: 17290796. Pubmed Central PMCID: PMC3181832. Epub 2007/02/13. eng.
6. McEwen BS. Neurobiological and systemic effects of chronic stress. Chronic Stress. 2017;1:9. PubMed PMID: 28856337. Pubmed Central PMCID: PMC5573220. Epub 2017/09/01. eng.
7. Sillar JR, Germon ZP, DeIuliis GN, Dun MD. The role of reactive oxygen species in acute myeloid leukaemia. Int J Mol Sci. 2019;20:23. Pubmed Central PMCID: PMC6929020. Epub 2019/12/05. eng.
8. Balzan S, Lubrano V. LOX-1 receptor: a potential link in atherosclerosis and cancer. Life Sci. 2018;198:79–86. PubMed PMID: 29462603. Epub 2018/02/21. eng.
9. (WHO) WHO. Cancer. 2021.
10. Wang M, Zhao J, Zhang L, Wei F, Lian Y, Wu Y, et al. Role of tumor microenvironment in tumorigenesis. J Cancer. 2017;8(5):761–73. PubMed PMID: 28382138. Pubmed Central PMCID: PMC5381164. Epub 2017/04/07. eng.
11. (NCI) NCI. What is cancer. 2020.
12. World Cancer Research Fund AIfcr. Diet, nutrition, physical activity and cancer: A global perspective. Summary of 3rd expert report. Continuous update project expert report. dietandcancerreport.org; 2018.
13. Kirtonia A, Sethi G, Garg M. The multifaceted role of reactive oxygen species in tumorigenesis. Cell Mol Life Sci. 2020;77(22):4459–83. PubMed PMID: 32358622. Epub 2020/05/03. eng.
14. Gaglia MM, Munger K. Editorial overview: viruses and cancer. Curr Opin Virol. 2019;39:3. PubMed PMID: 31732371. Epub 2019/11/17. eng.
15. Stern J, Miller G, Li X, Saxena D. Virome and bacteriome: two sides of the same coin. Curr Opin Virol. 2019;37:37–43. PubMed PMID: 31177014. Pubmed Central PMCID: PMC6768692. Epub 2019/06/10. eng.
16. Picardo SL, Coburn B, Hansen AR. The microbiome and cancer for clinicians. Crit Rev Oncol. 2019;141:1–12. PubMed PMID: 31202124. Epub 2019/06/16. eng.
17. Ursell LK, Metcalf JL, Parfrey LW, Knight R. Defining the human microbiome. Nutr Rev. 2012;70(1):38–44. PubMed PMID: 22861806. Pubmed Central PMCID: PMC3426293. Epub 2012/08/17. eng.
18. Strickertsson JAB, Desler C, Rasmussen LJ. Bacterial infection increases risk of carcinogenesis by targeting mitochondria. Semin Cancer Biol. 2017;47:95–100. PubMed PMID: 28754330. Epub 2017/07/30. eng.
19. Benny S, Mishra R, Manojkumar MK, Aneesh TP. From Warburg effect to Reverse Warburg effect; the new horizons of anti-cancer therapy. Med Hypotheses. 2020;144:110216. PubMed PMID: 33254523. Epub 2020/12/02. eng.

20. Tekade RK, Sun X. The Warburg effect and glucose-derived cancer theranostics. Drug Discov Today. 2017;22(11):1637–53. PubMed PMID: 28843632. Epub 2017/08/28. eng.
21. Larsen NB, Rasmussen M, Rasmussen LJ. Nuclear and mitochondrial DNA repair: similar pathways? Mitochondrion. 2005;5(2):89–108. PubMed PMID: 16050976. Epub 2005/07/30. eng.
22. Bose B, Shenoy S. Stem cell versus cancer and cancer stem cell: Intricate balance decides their respective usefulness or harmfulness in the biological system. J Stem Cell Res. 2014;4(2):1–9.
23. Steinbichler TB, Dudás J, Skvortsov S, Ganswindt U, Riechelmann H, Skvortsova. Therapy resistance mediated by cancer stem cells. Semin Cancer Biol. 2018;53:156–67. PubMed PMID: 30471331. Epub 2018/11/25. eng.
24. Wang H, Unternaehrer JJ. Epithelial-mesenchymal transition and cancer stem cells: at the crossroads of differentiation and dedifferentiation. Dev Dyn. 2019;248(1):10–20. PubMed PMID: 30303578. Epub 2018/10/12. eng.
25. del Pilar Sosa Idelchik M, Begley U, Begley T, Melendez J. Mitochondrial ROS control of cancer. Semin Cancer Biol. 2017;47:57–66.
26. Shiga K, Hara M, Nagasaki T, Sato T, Takahashi H, Takeyama H. Cancer-associated fibroblasts: their characteristics and their roles in tumor growth. Cancer. 2015;7(4):2443–58. PubMed PMID: 26690480. Pubmed Central PMCID: PMC4695902. Epub 2015/12/23. eng.
27. Landskron G, De la Fuente M, Thuwajit P, Thuwajit C, Hermoso MA. Chronic inflammation and cytokines in the tumor microenvironment. J Immunol Res. 2014;2014:149185. PubMed PMID: 24901008. Pubmed Central PMCID: PMC4036716. Epub 2014/06/06. eng.
28. Panieri E, Santoro MM. ROS homeostasis and metabolism: a dangerous liason in cancer cells. Cell Death Dis. 2016;7(6):e2253. PubMed PMID: 27277675. Pubmed Central PMCID: PMC5143371. Epub 2016/06/10. eng.
29. Greten FR, Grivennikov SI. Inflammation and cancer: triggers, mechanisms, and consequences. Immunity. 2019;51(1):27–41. PubMed PMID: 18281672. Pubmed Central PMCID: 2770012.
30. Miller AH, Ancoli-Israel S, Bower JE, Capuron L, Irwin MR. Neuroendocrine-immune mechanisms of behavioral comorbidities in patients with cancer. J Clin Oncol. 2008;26(6):971–82. PubMed PMID: 31900901. Epub 2020/01/05. eng.
31. Cruceriu D, Baldasici O, Balacescu O, Berindan-Neagoe I. The dual role of tumor necrosis factor-alpha (TNF-α) in breast cancer: molecular insights and therapeutic approaches. Cell Oncol. 2020;43(1):1–18. PubMed PMID: 31315034. Pubmed Central PMCID: PMC6831096. Epub 2019/07/18. eng.
32. Macciò A, Madeddu C. Inflammation and ovarian cancer. Cytokine. 2012;58(2):133–47. PubMed PMID: 22349527. Epub 2012/02/22. eng.
33. DiDonato JA, Mercurio F, Karin M. NF-κB and the link between inflammation and cancer. Immunol Rev. 2012;246(1):379–400. PubMed PMID: 22435567. Epub 2012/03/23. eng.
34. López de Andrés J, Griñán-Lisón C, Jiménez G, Marchal JA. Cancer stem cell secretome in the tumor microenvironment: a key point for an effective personalized cancer treatment. J Hematol. 2020;13(1):136. PubMed PMID: 33059744. Pubmed Central PMCID: PMC7559894. Epub 2020/10/17. eng.
35. Li LY, Guan YD, Chen XS, Yang JM, Cheng Y. DNA repair pathways in cancer therapy and resistance. Front Pharmacol. 2020;11:629266. PubMed PMID: 33628188. Pubmed Central PMCID: PMC7898236. Epub 2021/02/26. eng.
36. Yang J, Antin P, Berx G, Blanpain C, Brabletz T, Bronner M, et al. Guidelines and definitions for research on epithelial-mesenchymal transition. Nat Rev Mol Cell Biol. 2020;21(6):341–52. PubMed PMID: 32300252. Pubmed Central PMCID: PMC7250738. Epub 2020/04/18. eng.
37. Cohen L, Parker PA, Vence L, Savary C, Kentor D, Pettaway C. et al. Presurgical stress management improves post operative immune function in men with prostate cancer undergoing radical prostatectomy. Psychosomatic Medicine, 2011;73:218–25.
38. Andersen BL, Yang Hae-Chung, Farrar WB, Golden-Kreutz DM, Emery CF, Thornton LM et al. Psychologic intervention improves survival for breast cancer patients. Cancer 2008;113:3450–8.

Part IV

Fostering Healing and Resilience

1.1 Introduction

Facilitating healing in nursing practice has to do with making an individual feel whole, usually experienced as an overall sense of well-being. Healing may be conceptualized in different interrelated ways. In the first half of this book, we learned about the role of healing in biological and psychological resilience. In Part IV, healing is addressed in terms of diverse psychosocial interventions that may be mobilized by the nurse to foster innate and self-induced processes of healing in order to strengthen, protect, or restore the individual's resilient capabilities. Each chapter addresses a specific therapeutic approach and its respective role in influencing processes of healing and resilience. We examine ways that nurses may leverage scientific theory and evidence to offer relevant healing or resilient-strengthening strategies.

Chapter 8 discusses the key elements within the quality of the nurse–patient relationship that are conducive to creating a healing environment. These include the nurse's competence, effective skills of communication, and sense of compassion, strengthened by a shared understanding that the patient is known by the nurse and his or her healthcare team (e.g., [1]).

Chapter 9 discusses psychosocial nursing strategies that promote emotion-regulating coping capabilities of resilience. Nursing strategies that facilitate healing by encouraging more positive or neutral reappraisals of the cancer- and treatment-related threats, adapting relevant cognitive and behavioral coping skills, and using goal-oriented problem-solving strategies to manage the clinical consequences of the cancer or its treatment are reviewed [2–4]. Personal and social resources or strengths that may be leveraged by the nurse to foster more effective coping capabilities in the face of adversity are also discussed.

Chapter 10 focuses on psychosocial interventions to foster meaning in patients and caregivers who are struggling to find meaning in the face of a cancer diagnosis or a shortened life (e.g., [5, 6]). The concept of meaning is approached from a theoretical and evidentiary perspective that serves as the predicate for suggesting relevant therapeutic approaches [6–8]. It reviews ways that the individual may come to terms with a diagnosis of cancer and/or find new meaning in the experience through the process of realigning beliefs and assumptions about the world and the self as a function of clinical realities.

Chapter 11 has to do with ways to strengthen supportive relationships with close family members, as exemplified by the family caregiver. Research findings strongly suggest that patients heal when they are socially attached to loved ones who provide the support they need [9, 10].

Chapter 12 addresses the potential clinical outcomes of patients holding either positive or negative treatment-related expectations [11, 12]. Theoretical underpinnings, experimental research, and some controlled studies serve as the scientific predicate for proposing a number of psychosocial interventions to promote positive expectations for a clinical outcome and to counter the potential consequential effects of holding negative treatment-related expectations [13]. Social and physical factors of the clinical environment that may interfere with the goals of treatment by inadvertently suppressing healing effects are also highlighted, and suggested strategies to counteract these potential ill effects are examined.

Chapter 13 discusses the self-induced healing strategies of mindful meditation and the relaxation response technique that downregulates the stress response and promotes the reemergence of biological healing or reparative processes (e.g., [14, 15]). Chapter 14 presents the therapeutic role of physical touch and Reiki and therapeutic touch in inducing healing-related outcomes especially in patients with terminal disease and caregivers [16, 17] (Table 1). Whereas the field of healthy lifestyle behaviors exceeds the scope of this book, relevant findings and suggested nursing interventions are included in each chapter of Part V.

Table 1 Definitions of healing

Healing Processes
• *Innate, self-induced* capabilities of a patient that can restore, improve psychological, biological, social, emotional, and physical *wholeness*. In so doing, the person cognitively processes different clinical, biological, behavioral, and spiritual facets, and processes and functions of the self into a reintegrated whole (eg [14])
• *Psychological* healing refers to the process of transforming emotional distress into a state of well-being via strategies such as emotion regulation, beliefs about wellness, hope, development of self-efficacy, and the use of behavioral strategies such as the relaxation response, physical exercise, or yoga (eg [12, 18, 19])
• *Cognitive healing* refers to processes of reappraisal, such as clarifying cognitive distortions and perspective-taking leading to learning, coming to terms with new clinical realities, and personal growth [18, 20]
• *Physical healing* refers to the regenerative cellular processes associated with wound healing [21]
In Interaction With
• *Biological healing* reversal of neural and physiological alterations caused by stress especially throughout the HPA axis, SAM, and immune system
– Interrelated with the dopamine pathways associated with the neural reward circuitry [22]
– Restoration of neural structures, pathways, functions, and normal variation in the pattern of interrelationships among biological factors at basal levels [23]

References

1. Durkin J, Usher K, Jackson D. Embodying compassion: a systematic review of the views of nurses and patients. J Clin Nurs. 2019;28(9-10):1380–92; PubMed PMID: 30485579. Epub 2018/11/30. eng.
2. Jassim GA, Whitford DL, Hickey A, Carter B. Psychological interventions for women with non-metastatic breast cancer. Cochrane Database Syst Rev. 2015;5:CD008729; PubMed PMID: 26017383. Epub 2015/05/29. eng.
3. Antoni MH. Psychosocial intervention effects on adaptation, disease course and biobehavioral processes in cancer. Brain Behav Immun. 2013;30 Suppl:S88–98; PubMed PMID: 22627072. Pubmed Central PMCID: PMC3444659. Epub 2012/05/26. eng.
4. Dunkel-Schetter C, Feinstein LG, Taylor SE, Falke RL. Patterns of coping with cancer. Health Psychol. 1992;11(2):79–87; PubMed PMID: 1582383. Epub 1992/01/01. eng.
5. Lee V, Cohen SR, Edgar L, Laizner AM, Gagnon AJ. Meaning-making and psychological adjustment to cancer: development of an intervention and pilot results. Oncol Nurs Forum. 2006;33(2):291–302; PubMed PMID: 16518445. Epub 2006/03/07. eng.
6. Vehling S, Philipp R. Existential distress and meaning-focused interventions in cancer survivorship. Curr Opin Support Palliat Care. 2018;12(1):46–51; PubMed PMID: 29251694. Epub 2017/12/19. eng.
7. Park C, Folkman S. Meaning in the context of stress and coping. Rev General Psychol. 1997;1:115–44.
8. Folkman S, Moskowitz J. Positive affect and meaning-focused coping during significant psychological stress. In: Hewstone M, Schutt HAW, de Wit JBF, van den Bos K, Stroebe MS, editors. The scope of social psychology: theory and applications. New York, NY: Psychology Press; 2007. p. 193–208.
9. Antoni MH, Lutgendorf SK, Blomberg B, Carver CS, Lechner S, Diaz A, et al. Cognitive-behavioral stress management reverses anxiety-related leukocyte transcriptional dynamics. Biol Psychiatry. 2012;71(4):366–72; PubMed PMID: 22088795. Pubmed Central PMCID: PMC3264698. Epub 2011/11/18. eng.
10. Lutgendorf S, De Geest K, Bender D, Ahmed A, Goodheart M, Dahmoush L, Zimmerman M, et al. Social influences on clinical outcomes of patients with ovarian cancer. J Clin Oncol. 2012;30(23):2885–90.
11. Colloca L, Barsky AJ. Placebo and Nocebo Effects. N Engl J Med. 2020;382(6):554–61; PubMed PMID: 32023375. Epub 2020/02/06. eng.
12. Benson H, Stark M. Timeless healing: the power and biology of belief. New York: Simon & Schuster; 1997.
13. Petrie KJ, Rief W. Psychobiological mechanisms of placebo and nocebo effects: pathways to improve treatments and reduce side effects. Annu Rev Psychol. 2019;70:599–625; PubMed PMID: 30110575. Epub 2018/08/16. eng.
14. Carlson LE. Mindfulness-based interventions for coping with cancer. Ann N Y Acad Sci. 2016;1373(1):5–12; PubMed PMID: 26963792. Epub 2016/03/11. eng.
15. Bhasin MK, Dusek JA, Chang BH, Joseph MG, Denninger JW, Fricchione GL, et al. Relaxation response induces temporal transcriptome changes in energy metabolism, insulin secretion and inflammatory pathways. PLoS One. 2013;8(5):e62817; PubMed PMID: 23650531. Pubmed Central PMCID: PMC3641112. Epub 2013/05/08. eng.
16. Jakubiak BK, Feeney BC. Affectionate touch to promote relational, psychological, and physical well-being in adulthood: a theoretical model and review of the research. Pers Soc Psychol Rev. 2017;21(3):228–52; PubMed PMID: 27225036. Epub 2016/05/27. eng.
17. Post-White J, Kinney ME, Savik K, Gau JB, Wilcox C, Lerner I. Therapeutic massage and healing touch improve symptoms in cancer. Integr Cancer Ther. 2003;2(4):332–44; PubMed PMID: 14713325. Epub 2004/01/10. eng.
18. Folkman S, Lazarus RS, Dunkel-Schetter C, DeLongis A, Gruen RJ. Dynamics of a stressful encounter: cognitive appraisal, coping, and encounter outcomes. Journal of personality and social psychology. 1986;50(5):992–1003. PubMed PMID: 3712234. Epub 1986/05/01. eng.

19. Leventhal H, Philliips LA, Burns E. The common sense model of self regulation (CSM): a dynamic framework for understanding illness self management. J Behav Med 2016;39:935–46.
20. Meichenbaum D. A clinical handbook for assessing and treating adults with post-traumatic stress disorder (PTSD). Waterloo, Ontario: Institute Press; 1994.
21. Guo S and DiPietro LA. Factors affecting wound healing. J Dent Res 2010;89:219–29.
22. Pacheco-Lopez G, Engler H, Niemi M-B, Schedlowski M. Expectations and associations that heal: Immunomodulatory placebo effects and its neurobiology. Brain, behavior, and immunity. 2006;20:430–46.
23. McEwen B Physiology and neurobiology of stress and adaptation: Central role of the brain. Physiol Rev 2007;87:873–904.

The Quality of the Nurse–Patient Relationship

8

It's quite simple: one sees clearly only with the heart
Antoine de St Exupery, The Little Prince

8.1 Introduction

The clinical environment within which healing and resilience may be facilitated has at its core the quality of the nurse–patient relationship. Indisputably, one of the most essential therapeutic activities of a nurse is to establish a meaningful relationship with the patient and caregiver so that processes of healing and resilience may be optimized and psychosocial and other interventions may be further enabled. A therapeutic nurse–patient relationship offers a safe, healing environment within which self-reflection and new strategies to manage the illness, treatment, and recovery may be fostered [1]. Arguably, the quality of the nurse–patient relationship depends on at least four main factors: competence, communication skillfulness, compassion, and a sense of connectedness with the patient and family caregiver. It is popular to describe the relationship of the nurse with the patient as a therapeutic alliance with patients on mental health units [2]. Yes, but to be therapeutic requires that the individual feels known by the nurse, and for that reason I prefer the quality of the nurse–patient relationship in describing its therapeutic characteristics. This chapter is devoted to the quality of the nurse–patient relationship and the essential attributes that influence patient healing and resilience.

8.2 Objectives

At the end of the chapter, you will be able to:

a. Describe the essential cognitive, behavioral, and emotional attributes of the nurse–patient relationship
b. Discuss the concept of support within the nurse–patient relationship
c. Discuss strategies used to develop a sense of connectedness with the patient
d. Analyze the key attributes of competence, communication skillfulness, compassion, and a sense of connectedness within the context of the nurse–patient (and/or caregiver) relationship(s)

Clinical Anecdote 8.1
Feeling cared for as a patient came in many guises. It was experienced each time the administrative assistant made a point of greeting me by name at the treatment centre and engaging in a few words of informal banter- as if to tell me "I see you, I know you." Although I was never assigned to a primary nurse, a small coterie of clinic nurses usually cared for me, and imparted their caring in different ways: sometimes with a small joke (e.g. we have missed you around here) but mainly by engaging me in personal conversation: How had I been feeling since the last chemo, how was my family managing: Tell me about your work, even though everyone knew that I was now on leave. One nurse cooked dumplings from time to time which she gave to her patients to encourage them to eat, but also to enable patients to take a couple of nights off from cooking. All their greetings in clinic sent the clear message that I was a person in my own right. One nurse from this precious group however went further: In a moment of self doubt regarding my clinical status midway through treatment, this nurse had the gift of compassionate awareness, and in a quiet unassuming way slipped into a chair beside me, and started a conversation that allowed me to express my worries which had clearly been evident by the expression on my face. She quietly listened, assessed how I had been doing since the last treatment, and suggested alternative explanations to account for the elevated lab results. I knew what she was doing, but nonetheless it provided comfort and re assurance that she further amplified by seeking more information from the oncologist who in a timely way also dropped by the clinic to see me.

8.3 Why Patients Need a Quality Relationship with the Nurse

Because most patients with cancer feel vulnerable when faced with a life-threatening disease, the importance of placing the patient, according to Nightingale, "in the best possible condition to promote healing" is a clinical imperative [3]. A life-threatening illness such as cancer causes "a physical, social, emotional, and psychological assault on the whole person" [4]. The effects of active disease combined with anti-cancer therapies compromise resilient capabilities such as energy, immunity, and physical strength. In fact, the very presence of cancer is arguably a manifestation of the mind's and body's diminished ability over time to effectively withstand stress.

Along with a new or recurring diagnosis are the ofttimes painful and/or disfiguring medical treatments (surgery, radiation, chemotherapy), the interminable tests, other comorbid and traumatizing cancer-related threats, and constant uncertainty: each one of which may temporarily *overwhelm* the patient's biological and behavioral abilities to cope. The majority of patients and their family caregivers experience periodic distress along the continuum [5]. There may be distress of actual or impending loss and the mourning that may ensue for a former healthy life, intact body image, and a productive career. The person may initially feel overwhelmed and helpless to know what might be done to improve the chances for survival. Some lose faith in their own ability to rally, or they may feel that the effort is hopeless. Indeed, they may just feel defeated, too tired, and lacking in energy to kick start their own self-healing.

Whereas most patients recognize the invaluable contribution of medicine in the treatment of their illness, most do not realize that of equal importance is learning HOW to live with cancer in a way that promotes their innate healing and resilient capabilities. Establishing a meaningful nurse–patient relationship creates a safe and trusted space within which the patient and family caregiver may share deeply held thoughts and feelings, find support, comfort, and encouragement. It is also where information and purposeful discussion can overcome emotional resistance and new coping skills may be adopted that can enhance current and future resilient capabilities.

8.4 Definition

Peplau 1988 described the nurse's relationship with the patient (and caregiver) as the therapeutic *process* of communication dependent on the cultivation of interpersonal skills [29]. More recently, the *quality* of the nurse–patient relationship has been referred to as a therapeutic relationship, a therapeutic alliance, a therapeutic engagement, and a helping relationship. It is responsive to the thoughts, feelings, and behaviors of the patient and caregiver while also using scientific knowledge and skills to proactively protect and buffer the individual from unnecessary pain and suffering [30].

An integrative review identified the components of a therapeutic engagement between the nurse and patient in acute mental health care which can be applicable to all nurses and patients in cancer care [30]. These included facilitating growth, understanding the patient from his or her experiential perspective, and selecting the relevant therapeutic approach. A cross-sectional study of patient perceptions of quality nursing care on an acute in-patient unit in Australia identified the perceived caring behaviors by nurses as a critical component of the relationship [27]. Essential attributes of a committed and meaningful nurse–patient relationship included the nurse's ability to proactively listen and understand the patient's perspective, the ability to convey feelings such as compassion toward the patient and family, as well as to respond emotionally and proactively to their suffering [27, 31]. Other key elements include competence (that is evidence-based practice) and a sense of connectedness between the nurse and patient and caregiver [10, 14, 32]. Thus, the quality of the nurse–patient relationship (Sect. 8.5) may be characterized by competence, compassion, communication, and a sense of connectedness to be discussed further in the sections that follow.

8.5 The Quality of the Nurse–Patient Relationship

Table 8.1 summarizes the essential components of a quality nurse–patient (or caregiver) relationship. The quality of this relationship may be observed in the extent to which the patient and nurse trust, understand, engage, and experience an affinity toward one another for the shared purpose of promoting the patient's health. The nurse–patient relationship is distinguished by the nurse's warmth and nonjudgmental openness toward the patient and caregiver, timely presence, a sensitive, compassionate, and respectful approach; a heightened awareness of a shared humanity, even a shared appreciation for the spiritual. Anchoring this therapeutic relationship is the quality of affective connectedness and commitment which facilitates the patient's sense of *being known* by the nurse, leading to opportunities that Buber has described as *momentary healing-inducing "encounters"* [12]. Further contributing to the quality of this relationship is the nurse's compassion, competence, and communication skills which will be discussed below. These characteristics delineate the key attributes of a therapeutic relationship between patient and nurse and/or caregiver and nurse.

This relationship is influenced by one another's values, attitudes, beliefs, behaviors, assumptions about wellness, and philosophy of life [15, 17]. But as an expert nurse, it is less about having the same or similar perspectives and more about the nurse's understanding of the full measure of the whole human being who lives with cancer and the nurse's ability to engage in a "totality of being" with that person [12]. It is about the nurse's ability to draw on all senses in the moment and to possess the clinical expertise to respond on multiple levels including a transcendent level that can foster healing within what Buber has described as "momentary encounters." Ultimately, the ability of the nurse to foster healing will depend on the "fit" between what the nurse offers of her/himself to the patient and/or caregiver and what the whole patient needs (i.e., in terms of her/his biopsychosocial being) [22].

Table 8.1 Quality of the nurse–patient relationship: key components

1. Evidenced-based knowledge and clinical skills [6–8]
2. Communication skills [9–11])
3. A shared sense of mutual connection [12–14]
4. A partnership committed to mutually agreed health-related goals [15–17]
5. Ability to convey compassion and understanding [18–20]
6. Established regular nurse's presence [14, 21, 22]
7. Conveys support and feelings of being cared for [23, 24]
8. Sensitive evaluations of clinical concerns, and the effect of nursing practice on patient and caregiver clinical outcomes [25]
9. Patient-centered whole person care [22, 26–28]

Clinical Research

A Heideggerian hermeneutical study explored the meanings and feelings associated with caring for critically ill patients within the context of the nurse–patient relationship through multiple interviews with 12 intensive care nurses [22]. Although most critically ill patients were unable to communicate verbally with their nurses, the nurses experienced profound feelings of empathy, caring, and even love which also impacted how they made sense of the world and the self. According to the nurses, the relationship experienced between nurse and patient was mutually affective and dependent on one another.

A systematic review of 5 qualitative studies and four quantitative studies examined patient perceptions of their relationship with the nurse in the oncology outpatient clinic [10]. The data showed that the quality of the nurse–patient relationship was central to patient satisfaction with their care. Specifically, it was key to the patients' ability to cope with daily life, the cancer, and treatment. Patients also expressed the opinion that the quality of the relationship impacted their attitudes toward treatment and side effects and their ability to reduce feelings of distress and obtain the information they needed about the treatment and side effects to feel emotionally in control. In this regard, patients highly valued the ability to experience meaningful communications with their nurse. Patients also expressed the need to have hope and to maintain a positive mood both of which were appreciatively nurtured by the nurse. Finally, patients preferred the same nurse at the clinic visits which patients perceived as important for establishing a meaningful relationship within which the ability to cope could be facilitated.

Nurse–Patient Relationship on Patient Outcomes Randomized controlled studies that have investigated the effects of the nurse–patient therapeutic relationship on patient outcomes is a relatively recent and much needed development of the nursing literature. A systematic review and meta-analysis of 13 eligible randomized controlled trials showed small-to-moderate effects across individual studies [16]. Based on a random-effects model, the overall effect size estimate was small albeit significant, suggesting that the quality of the nurse–patient relationship has at least a small impact on the patients' health care outcomes. Given the paucity of RCTS on this topic in the research literature, including cancer care, there is a clinical need to develop more rigorous RCT trials to investigate the effect of the nurse–patient relationship on healing and resilience as well as health in cancer care.

8.6 Relational Characteristics of the Nurse–Patient Relationship

Essential characteristics of the nurse–patient relationship to be discussed further include: (1) the nurse's presence, (2) competence in scientific knowledge and healing-promoting skills, (3) communication skills, (4) compassion, and (5) a sense of connectedness with the patient and family caregiver.

Being Present

Along with *doing* for the patient, there is *being* with the patient emotionally, physically, and cognitively [33]. It is a prerequisite for establishing a compassionate and connected therapeutic relationship [33, 34]. Being present is a proactive behavior in which the nurse gives full attention to the individual's emotional distress, concerns, and/or need to be understood and known [18, 20]. It means the nurse reorienting his/her thoughts, intents, and purposes to the individual(s) the nurse is engaged with, and drawing on all senses to establish a heightened and present awareness of the whole human being. It is about listening, paying attention so that the individuals' thoughts, feelings, and behaviors may be accurately interpreted, reflected back, and mutually understood.

Finding an efficient strategy to eliminate intrusive personal or work-related thoughts that would impede being fully present to the individual is a necessary precondition for engaging with the patient and/or family caregiver. This can be challenging when working in a stressful clinical environment. But it is not impossible, if, for example, the nurse takes a few deep breaths to center her/himself before entering the patient's room.

Being fully present is facilitated by "carving out" a confidential space with the patient, for instance, by pulling up a chair and sitting down opposite, eye to eye, in order to observe, interpret, and discuss concerns face to face, the chair being close enough to the individual or enable a nurse's touch. These behavioral actions demonstrate the intent to be fully present, that is, fully engaged in what the individual and family caregiver discuss with the nurse or convey by facial expression. A confidential space also facilitates being fully present in reflective silence with the patient and family caregiver, for instance, during periods of distress or existential suffering.

Being present means opening one's self through all the senses to the patient in a manner that draws the nurse toward a deeper understanding of the patient's experience in its totality. Specifically, consciously "opening one's heart" to the patient's reality and suffering is an essential step along a compassionate path to fostering the patient's healing [35, 36]. According to the biophysicist Oschman [37], learning to *open our hearts* to our patients emits energy which is perceived by the other as "caring and warmth." This capability has been beautifully captured in The Little Prince, by Antoine de St Exupery, and by a caption, also quoted by Servan-Schreiber: " Here is my secret" said the fox. "It's quite simple: one sees clearly only with the heart." And that ability depends on the quality of the nurse's presence. As we will discuss further below, an active presence is necessary for communication, compassion, and a sense of connectedness, all essential prerequisites for creating a healing nurse–patient relationship.

Clinical Anecdote 8.2

As a third year history student, I volunteered to work in a fishing village along the Labrador coast with the Grenfell Mission. My summer job was to help the nurse in the Nursing Station while her colleague was on summer break. One of my first assignments was to care for a young woman S, who was 36 years old with end stage cancer.

The hospital consisted of two small wards of 4 beds each, one for the men, the other, for the women. S was the only patient hospitalized during my stay. We did not talk very much, but every morning and evening I used to roll her bed between the windows facing east and west, respectively so that S could enjoy the sunrises and sunsets. And in between we would sometimes sing together, or more usually, she would just fall asleep as I strummed the strings of a guitar. Being quietly with S, I learned something about the healing effects of presence. And sharing M's love of nature, each rising and setting of the sun lifted both our spirits toward the blazing horizon.

Communication

The ability to communicate effectively in nursing practice is a clinical imperative. It is fundamental to establishing a meaningful relationship with the patient and family caregiver, and starts with the ability of the nurse to accurately identify the patient's emotional cues [25, 38]. Communication skills underlie the nurse's ability to understand the patient and caregiver's needs and sources of distress. These skills also are the essential means for engaging in emotionally laden, difficult topics regarding the patient's illness, prognosis, treatment, end-of-life concerns, and existential suffering [38, 39]. Communication skills facilitate explorations of the patient's and caregiver's deepest thoughts and feelings. These skills enable the initiation of a conversation when the patient's news is "bad," as well as engage the patient and caregiver in a therapeutic partnership to alleviate pain and suffering, anger and fear, or to reorient the patient and caregiver toward more effective coping strategies and supportive behaviors. These skills are needed to facilitate emotion-regulating coping strategies and to help the patient and caregiver make sense of the changes in their lives and or find new meanings. Communication effectiveness lies at the heart of promoting effective patient and caregiver decision making around the treatment and illness that incorporates their preferences, mediated by a deep sensitivity to their level of health literacy [38, 40].

Skills of Communication (Table 8.2)

The nurse is in a privileged position to be privy to the personal thoughts, feelings, beliefs, attitudes, and behaviors the patient may hold about himself, including beliefs and assumptions about the world and his/her place in it. Deploying cognitive strategies such as active listening, reflected feedback, reframing, clarifying, providing relevant information, deconstructing generalizations and distorted meanings, summarizing, and normalizing are all necessary strategies dependent upon communication skills in any clinic setting but particularly in oncology (Review Part IV, Chaps. 9–11). Effective communication is also shaped by a warm and compassionate approach, the ability to sensitively discern or interpret spoken or unspoken patient cues, knowing when to reach out and touch the patient in shared understanding [20, 25]. These skills also communicate the nurse's desire to understand, to correctly interpret, and ultimately to know and support the patient and his or her family caregiver.

Whereas nurses with effective communication skills appear to positively influence patient satisfaction and well-being [44], a lack of effective communication skills results in patient and family distress and reluctance to share feelings and thinking with the nurse and, critically, only inhibits the ability to get the help they need (Table 8.2) [45].

Table 8.2 A few simple suggestions to enhance communication skills [41–43]

The do's
1. Be aware of your body language
2. At the start of any interaction, clarify the goals of the meeting and desired outcomes, so everyone is on the same page. It may be as simple as "Just wanted to check in with you, see how you are feeling and doing, and if there is anything, I can do to help"
3. Invite the individual to share his story, "To help me help you, would you be open to sharing what happened in this situation?" "I would like to follow up on a few things you have shared to deepen my understanding of your experience. Is that ok?" (Ask permission)
4. Listen to the individual, ask open-ended exploratory questions as needed
5. Summarize what the patient/caregiver has said and also share your *perception* of *the emotional* impact of the situation on the individual. This conveys active listening by acknowledging what has been said and emotionally experienced which validates the individual as well as ensuring your understanding of the situation
6. Reflect on the gathered information in terms of possible explanations and interpretations (generate hypotheses). For instance, *"My understanding* of what you have just shared goes something like this..." "I *feel* the emotional impact of what you are sharing with me" rather than *"you are getting* quite emotional"
7. Ask the individual for their interpretation—what do they think is most troubling, most worrisome, what could also be improved or changed—and their proposed strategies. For instance, "I am wondering now that you can hear your thoughts out loud, whether this may have led you to think about the situation in a different way"
8. Share relevant facts (information) for discussion, in which the individual ideally is encouraged to generate their own decisions based on the information; make suggestions as the situations calls for "I am wondering whether you have considered..." as a strategy for facilitating decision making
9. Use open-ended questions, reflective feedback, clarifications, paraphrasing techniques, and even relevant metaphors such as "It ain't over till it's over"
10. Convey compassion with a soft tone of voice, eye-to-eye contact, and the appropriate use of physical touch (Chap. 14)
11. Be present with an open heart and focus all of your attention on the whole person Be aware of the individual's body movements, what he says, and respectful of silences; be appropriately responsive in a timely fashion
12. Use "collective" words like *"Let's* work on this issue together." Convey that you and the patient are a partnership with the same hopes and *share* the same health-related goals. They are not alone
The don'ts
1. Do not interrupt
2. Do not challenge health-related beliefs that you do not agree with
3. Do not give advice
4. Do not unwittingly challenge the patient's hope by offering ambiguous comments such as "You have lived longer than anyone else with your kind of cancer"
5. Never scold or accuse, for example, "You always get angry." Rather reframe as "I am concerned that something may be troubling you"

Although the nurse is the one healthcare provider who spends the most time with the patient and family caregiver, many nurses express difficulty communicating effectively to meet the various psychosocial and emotional needs of their patients and families. Many hesitate to discuss a distressing change in care or prognosis or to broach decision-making matters surrounding end-of-life and spiritual matters [9, 15, 38]. Others lack skills in communicating compassion or even empathy [9, 15, 38]. Yet, nurses in oncology *rarely* receive formal learning in advanced communication skills particularly with respect to difficult clinical situations within their professional purview of practice. A meta-analysis suggests that years of clinical experience in caring for patients with cancer do not improve healthcare provider communication expertise; and formal training even after graduation in advanced practice nurses is a clinical imperative [46].

Facilitating Personal Narratives
One of the simplest and most meaningful strategies for building a meaningful relationship with the patient and family is through storytelling or eliciting personal narratives [38]. Through narratives, the patient (and/or the caregiver) can become known to the nurse, and both may become more connected with the nurse through sharing of personal thoughts and feelings, values, priorities, and beliefs that have guided life experiences, as well as hopes for treatment and future wellness or fears about death and dying.

Patient narratives may be encouraged when a nurse seeks to learn about the patient's or caregiver's life experiences before and since cancer. The content may be shaped by the nature of the nurse's inquiry or the patient's own initiative. These narratives enable the patient to temporarily forget the stressful implications of the disease or treatment and even find a degree of personal acceptance and comfort by reconnecting with that part of the self that is about a meaningful life. Narratives are also an important strategy in meaning making, to be discussed in Chap. 10.

Clinical Research
A meta-analysis of 17 clinical trials assessed communication skills programs for nurses, physicians, and other healthcare providers caring for cancer patients and family caregivers mainly in ambulatory care settings [46]. The main findings were that healthcare providers who received communication skills training were: (a) more apt to use open-ended questioning afterward with patients, compared to controls, (b) more likely to show empathy toward patients and their caregivers, and (c) less inclined to simply provide the facts of the clinical situation, but rather tailor the delivery with an empathic approach to the patient or caregiver. Conversely, no differences between the groups were detected in relation to eliciting patient concerns and providing relevant information. The Cochrane review did not address whether these communication programs discussed specific strategies for communicating with compassion during very emotional and difficult conversations with respect to stopping treatment, cancer progression, cancer recurrence, death and dying, and or existential suffering of patients and caregivers. Nor did the analysis lead to recommendations concerning the content of these programs.

In order to be truly effective, nurses must be trained in communication skills that will enable compassionate and effective interactions with patients and family caregivers [9, 45]. These training programs should be designed around specific topics identified by the nurse attendees to ensure their learning needs are met. Memorial Sloan Kettering Cancer Centre offers such a program to nurses and other healthcare providers [9, 45].

Compassion

Compassion is a core component of a therapeutic nurse–patient relationship [47]. It is a highly valued attribute of health care yet has been difficult to define [18, 20, 47]. Compassion, as a concept of practice and as a moral virtue, has been identified as one of five nursing values and is formally recognized as a fundamental component of the profession [48]. Core components of compassion include the *virtuous motivation* of the nurse who first recognizes and then is compelled *to act* in response to a suffering patient in order to alleviate that suffering in some way. *Virtuous* refers to feelings of love, kindness, and beneficence. *Taking action* refers to an altruistic act, reacting to patient needs in a timely manner, and even constitutes conscious inaction, for instance, when a nurse sensitively assesses the patient's need to be alone or nontalkative. Yet a clear nursing (or healthcare) definition of its core attributes to guide practice is a work in progress [18, 20, 48].

Clinical Research
A qualitative study of 10 patients' experiences of compassionate nursing care identified three characteristics: *knowing* the patient and giving the patient time; understanding the patient's perspective; and thirdly, effective communication [49]. Patients also wondered whether compassion could be taught. Studies of nurses' and patients' perceptions of compassion have highlighted the lack of a consistent definition of compassion [20, 49]. Compassion expressed by nurses was often most evident within the context of a critically ill or suffering patient [20, 22]. Nurses conveyed compassion through their physical, emotional, and cognitive presence with the patient (time together), their ability to "engage" in or experience the patient's suffering, and the quality of their communications and support [18, 20].

Patients experienced the nurse's compassion through awareness and receipt of the nurse's "virtuous" desire to respond to their distress. Moreover, the nurses' virtues were understood by the patient in terms of love, beneficence, and kindness. Compassion was seen to take place within the nurse's therapeutic relationship with the sufferer. Defining attributes of compassion were a meaningful connection with the patient, the quality of nonverbal and verbal communication, the nurse's presence and taking meaningful action [20]. In a secondary analysis of 12 narrative interviews, Durkin and colleagues found that compassion was also expressed through the nurse's act of touch which was so perceived by the patient. Touch was used to convey an "authentic connection" between the nurse and the patient. According to the authors, the nurse that avoids touching the patient at relevant moments denies the patient their need for compassion [20].

8.6 Relational Characteristics of the Nurse–Patient Relationship

Durkin further investigated compassion through the perspectives of nine seasoned researchers based on a modified Delphi approach. The consensus of the nurse experts was that compassion similarly involved (a) being aware of the patient's emotional state, (b) having the desire to alleviate suffering, (c) and then taking meaningful action. Compassion is enabled through the nurse's presence, her verbal and nonverbal communication skills, and a meaningful nurse–patient relationship, distinguished by a shared connection and expressed in part, by what the nurse and patient do together on behalf of the patient. However, the expert researchers also agreed that whereas the nurse should be sensitive to the suffering of a patient, it is not essential to emotionally share that suffering in order to convey compassion [18].

In summary, compassion involves conscious awareness of the patient's emotional state [50], a motivation to alleviate the observed suffering [51], and a response with meaningful action [52]. The deeply felt call to action resulting in a meaningful response is thought to distinguish compassion from empathy or sympathy in which the individual may understand and feel badly for another person's suffering but may not act to relieve it [47].

A Sense of Connectedness with Patients and Family Caregivers

At the epi-center of a therapeutic nurse–patient relationship lies the sense of connectedness the nurse experiences with her/his patient and family caregiver (Table 8.3). This refers to the sense of mutual affinity, shared understanding, trust, and regard between the nurse and the patient and/or caregiver. Essential attributes of connectedness include patient-centered care (and/or family caregiver), the patient being *"known"* to the nurse, and the nurse's ability to sensitively modulate social and physical factors in the patient–nurse environment in order to enhance healing opportunities and reduce the risk of clinical situations that may undermine healing (See Chap. 12) [54, 55].

Einstein's theory of energy equals mass times the speed of light squared; that is, $E = MC^2$ [56]. This theory posits that energy and mass are transmutable at subatomic levels, suggesting that all forms of organic connectedness may be experienced by the self at the level of subatomic particles where matter and energy are continuously exchanged and accordingly, may be potentially experienced as profound knowing of another being, from which a deep sense of solace and emotional comfort may be derived. In an analogous sense, we may derive comfort from Tennyson's words, "I am a part of everything I have met" (Ulysses, Tennyson 1842). Patients have a need for such depth of human, and spiritual and organic forms of connection to help make sense of their existential being; it is a need exemplified by some people in their connectedness to something greater than the self, whether that is the universe or a spiritual entity, nature, or loved ones [4, 12]. (see Part IV Chap. 10).

This innate drive for human connectedness is evident in the attachment bonds of infancy through adolescence and adulthood through which emotional regulation, human development, resilience, and healing capabilities are fostered [57] Individuals strive to reproduce this seminal connection in meaningful, supportive relationships

Table 8.3 Attributes of a nurse–patient connection [10, 17, 25, 43, 50, 53]

Purpose
• To create a mutual understanding and regard with the patient
• Create *a sense of connectedness* similar to attachment bonds, essential for growth, development, resilience, and healing
Cognitive strategies to enhance connectedness include the following
• Presence, active listening, encourage storytelling
• Normalize patient feelings
• Acknowledge patient beliefs
• Convey relevant information about the disease and treatment
• Convey compassionate understanding regarding the emotional impact of the disease, treatment, and uncertainty in the patient's life
• Demonstrate proactive response to patient concerns
Clinical implications
• Establishes patient trust and emotional security
• Facilitates patient sharing of his deepest thoughts and feelings
• Establishes basis for meaningful dialog around issues of major concern to the patient
• Fosters the sense of *being known* in a patient
• Facilitates *momentary* healing-inducing encounters

with partners, family, and friends. The nurse–patient relationship may be viewed as a particular form of this human connection, a special kind of attachment borne in a health crisis and shaped by the specific characteristics and needs of the individual with cancer [58]. Inherent within these attachment bonds are feelings of trust and security, of being known, and emotionally supported that have been shown to foster growth, resilient capabilities, healing, and a sense of overall well-being [59].

Conversely, the lack of a shared connection between nurse and patient can undermine the patient's sense of security, hope, and ability to cope. Consider the following clinical encounter with the surgeon.

Clinical Anecdote 8.3

Karen was sitting in the examination room anxiously awaiting her results when the doctor entered rather brusquely, without acknowledging her presence; his behaviour distracted, his mind elsewhere. Opening the chart, his head still bowed, he told her, "You have cancer, it has spread-though this should be no surprise to you given the size of the tumour..." Karen remained calm, or maybe was in profound shock at the diagnosis and how it was transmitted. But she said nothing. So he continued, "I will have the secretary add your name to the surgery roster, and you will be contacted." At this point Karen found her voice, "When do you suppose I might have the surgery?" to which he replied, "Give me a break. You may not realize it but I am extremely busy with other patients as well." And that was that; Karen left the examination room without another word, without a plan, completely deflated, and now truly distressed and fearful about her prospects for survival. And she immediately changed doctors.

This anecdote sadly illustrates how a lack of emotional connectedness with patients can influence our professional interactions. It can profoundly worsen a patient's already fragile emotional equanimity. This physician's complete lack of empathy exacerbated Karen's already high level of distress. Low perceived support has been shown to increase biological markers for angiogenesis, inflammation, and a dysregulated innate immunity [60]. For example, patients with ovarian cancer and poor perceived support have shown high levels of noradrenaline within the tumor site as well as fewer natural killer cytotoxic cells in tumor-infiltrating lymphocytes; the physiological indicators suggested that distress (that is, elevated noradrenaline) was driving cancer growth unimpeded by a weakened cellular immunity [59, 61]. To many patients and their loved ones, the doctor and nurse represent the patient's best hope to survive. Having failed to connect on any level with Karen, this doctor had left a sense of hopelessness and helplessness in his wake [62]. Although this health professional displayed a woeful lack of compassion, one has to believe that he was suffering from burnout and had little of his whole self to offer his patients with potentially devastating consequences (Chap. 19). As health professionals we have no idea to what extent an off handed remark, an inadvertent look away from the patient can contribute to the patient's distress.

Clinical Implications The nurse's ability to *meaningfully connect with* the patient and caregiver enable discussions of the spiritual or of nature or something meaningful to the patient, that can be deeply therapeutic particularly in the advanced stages of the disease. Through conversation, the patient's existential suffering or distress may be linked to something greater than the self. It can stimulate the patient's thinking about different kinds of meaning that may be discovered within the experience of cancer [63]. A spiritual-oriented discussion may lead the patient to make his or her own connection with the human cycle of life and death, health and suffering, thereby potentially embedding the patient's subjective experience within a more meaningful universal context [4]. And that connected understanding of our shared humanity may bring a kind of acceptance and comfort (Chap. 18).

Being Known

Establishing a meaningful connection with a patient or family caregiver involves acknowledging the individual's need to be *known* by his or her healthcare provider (Table 8.4). A meaningful connection reassures the patient that he or she will not be "forgotten" and will be treated in a timely and thorough way with all needed resources mobilized to achieve an optimal clinical benefit [14]. Being known emanates from an authentic, deeply felt nurse–patient connection of mutual regard and respect and likely emerges at the level of a shared belief system or the nurse's profound respect for the patient's beliefs about health, illness, and future wellness even when those beliefs may differ from the nurse's beliefs.

The patient's perception that he or she is *known* as an individual with cancer is only possible when the nurse goes beyond discussions about treatment and procedures to embrace the patient as an individual with his or her unique perspective on life, health, illness, and future wellness which are all driven by a system of beliefs, desires, and intents [17, 64]. The first goal of the nurse is to "see" the world from

Table 8.4 Characteristics of being known [12, 14, 15, 17, 53] (Chaps. 10 and 12)

Being known
• Emanates from an authentic connection with a significant other
• *Shared belief system* that shapes the person's cognitive expectations about health, illness, and future wellness
• Shared nurse and patient goals for treatment and hoped for outcomes
Effects of being known
• Patient belief that he or she will be optimally cared for and treated in a timely, comprehensive fashion
• Downregulates the stress response to allow healing processes to reemerge
• Enhances potential for *momentary healing* encounters

the patient's perspective in order to gain deeper insight into his or her needs, desires, and clinical expectations. For that to occur, an egalitarian relationship of mutual regard, trust, and sharing must exist. These conditions must be met in order for meaningful, open (vulnerable), and genuine dialog to flow.

Thus, being known is about the nurse *knowing* the individual living with cancer rather than the cancer patient. The sense of b*eing known* by the nurse is fostered by *knowing* the person's care and treatment preferences, *possessing* the scientific and clinical knowledge to contribute to whole person care and as previously stated *knowing* the individual's unique emotional needs, values, and beliefs, such as their philosophy of life, their beliefs about healing, and health-related experiences. And finally, it involves possessing sensitive and personalized communication skills that convey compassion and understanding of the individual and his or her needs.

Clinical Anecdote 8.4
Although I knew the oncologist very well, it had been years since we had had any kind of meaningful conversation. As I answered his intake questions, it became apparent from the way I responded that I knew more about cancer, healing approaches and medical treatments than he had initially assumed. He put down the pen and looked right at me. "What do you need to know and what can I do to make that happen ...." And so we discussed the nature of my cancer, the lack of an obvious treatment protocol, the latest research findings, and his proposed plan of action which included consulting not only with the members of the tumour board, but with other medical colleagues working across Canada and the US. He then shared his intention to review some of the latest research findings based on my particular cancer type during the weekend. Would I like to review those articles, and then meet the following Tuesday to discuss the results together? The oncologist had stopped seeing me as only a patient. I became an individual with cancer, someone it is true he had once known well. But I left that meeting feeling comforted by the fact that I was known by my oncologist in ways that I believed were imperative for my future well being.

Being known by the nurse can provide the patient with a sense of security and trust *to explore the clinical implications of the illness* in relation to personal needs, hopes, changing roles, and beliefs and expectations about the future with the nurse. This process of exploratory self-reflection may be replete with different possibilities for healing nurtured by the nurse who has established a meaningful connection with the thoughts, feelings, and actions of the patient.

Being known is a multilayered healing-promoting springboard from which the patient and nurse can meaningfully examine important connections from the person's past and current life. Sharing one's story about the past can reconnect the patient with those illness-related experiences that, if positive, may enhance his or her future expectations for wellness, and re-activate relevant healing-promoting neurophysiological pathways (See Chap. 12) [55, 65].

Momentary Encounters

It is within the context of a deeply shared connection between two beings that *momentary*, healing-inducing encounters may be optimized [12]. Although this momentary convergence of the minds is not essential for healing to occur within the nurse–patient relationship, these encounters can bring the patient profound momentary relief from his or her conscious awareness of cancer-related stresses. These encounters are fleeting, cannot be "forced" and dissipate at the moment of self-awareness. At their core appears to be restorative processes and special sources of healing experienced as a shared "transcendent sense of wholeness" within the dyad.

Momentary encounters may be cultivated through mutual and deeply concentrated exchanges of thoughts and feelings around issues of utmost relevance to the patient. Buber has written about these moments, when the level of communication is so heightened, that all awareness of time and place is temporarily rendered insensate by an intense communion of simultaneous thoughts, mutual understandings, and feelings which deeply affect both the patient and the nurse. In these genuine, meaningful encounters, healing processes are activated [21, 66].

Once either person becomes aware of this transcendent experience, the moment evaporates. Yet Buber and others have speculated that it is within these unique cognitively coincident parameters that healing is optimized. In these moments, there is a complete synchrony of human relatedness causing an electromagnetic current of authentic understanding [12]. Today, scientists hypothesize that the existence of a biofield, an electromagnetic field, around each person may synergistically overlap and exchange energy or information at the particle level of communication [67, 68]. Evidence of this energy field comes from in vitro and human studies that have shown the healing effects of therapeutic touch or Reiki on various cell lines, human immune cells, and human emotions [69, 70] (Review Part IV, Chap. 14).

Clinical Anecdote 8.5
One afternoon while sitting in my hospital bed, recovering from a surgical procedure, and contemplating what would happen next medically, a family friend, a physician in supportive care, dropped by to see me. As he entered the room he said hello, grabbed a chair and brought it alongside my bed, so that we sat eye- to-eye. It happened to be a sunny day with dust drenched rays that shimmered across the room, endless sparkles of life and hope. We watched silently for a minute, and then

he said, This reminds me of music from...With the passage of time I am unsure, but think it was Ma Vlast because that moment is vividly connected to images of the Moldau river coursing its way through Prague. And something in that image of that river moving so majestically to that music recalled the transfigurative nature of all things, and the infinite connections with each other, and with the universe. It was a momentary "time-out" that had been made possible by his knowing me. Since then I have wondered at all the other clinical moments in which such a therapeutic encounter might have healed the human spirit.

Enhancing Support (See Part IV, Chap. 11)
Intrinsic to the experience of feeling connected and being known is feeling cared for and supported. The potential impact of the nurse's support cannot be underestimated. As with attachment bonds, emotionally supportive relationships help to alleviate emotional distress and the potential perceived estrangement of patients with cancer from the world of the living [71]. Patients with *higher perceived informal support* (that is from loved ones) show lower levels of inflammatory markers, such as interleukin-6, vascular endothelial growth factor (VEGF), and matrix metalloproteinase-9 (MMP-9) especially within the tumor microenvironment. They also have higher natural killer cell cytotoxicity in peripheral blood mononuclear cells (PBMC) as well as greater tumor-infiltrating T- lymphocytes, according to studies of patients with ovarian cancer [61, 72]. The quality of the nurse–patient relationship is enhanced by the nurse's provision of emotional and informational support and by physical comfort activities which in turn also strengthen the patient's feelings of connectedness with the nurse [71]. Maunsell's et al. [73] study has shown that survival was longest in patients who identified either a doctor or nurse as a confidant. Other studies have found no such predictive data when support was measured in terms of the *quantity* of available members of the social network, suggesting that it is the quality of the support rather than quantity of members that makes a significant difference in the patient's potential for healing and resilience [74].

In providing a caring and emotionally supportive relationship, clinical research suggests that the nurse's compassionate and competent behaviors can protect and buffer the individual from stress-related processes that drive cancer growth and shorten survival [75]. This support may be all the more invaluable to the patient's resilience when it includes helping the patient and caregiver strengthen the quality of their supportive relationship. Supportive relationships provide direct and buffering effects that protect as well as nurture the individual's resilient potential in adverse conditions such as cancer [71, 75–78].

Evidence-Based Practice (EBP) (Review Part V, Chap. 19)

The quality of the nurse–patient relationship ultimately depends on an evidence-based nursing practice [2, 79–82]. Scientific knowledge and expert clinical skills are the essential prerequisites for developing a meaningful nurse–patient relationship.

According to the clinical nursing literature, however, clinical nurses continue to struggle to acquire an evidence-based practice beyond the implementation of medically driven techniques and procedures as well as symptom management. There is a paucity of standardized psychosocial interventions [7, 32, 81, 83]. Findings from a pretest/posttest online educational module to improve evidence-based practice skills of registered nurses revealed positive attitudes toward EBP, but perceptions of their practice, knowledge, and skills were reported to be significantly lower [46]. Significantly, these perceptions did not vary according to the nurses' education or years of experience. Although clinical experience certainly has a role to play in developing clinical expertise however, given the complexity of healthcare practices today, it is no longer sufficient.

The main challenge to evidence-based practice is that the majority of clinic nurses lack knowledge of the principles of research methodology and critical analytic skills to meaningfully review nursing research and incorporate relevant findings into their clinical practice. For example, nursing has a critical mass of nurse scholars involved in nursing research [84–88]. Within cancer care, nurse-led randomized controlled trials have provided findings of the effectiveness of self-management interventions on the clinical outcomes of patients and/or caregivers with promising results. These studies were developed by nurse scholars; advanced practice clinical nurses *were trained* in the self-management strategies to be evaluated by the clinical trial [85–87, 89, 90]. Yet these findings are likely to have a minimal impact on clinical nurses in general who care for patients with cancer every day without the benefit of comparable clinical "training" workshops, supported by a conceptual nursing model, providing a scientific rationale for incorporating this intervention in their practice.

In a systematic review of 31 RCTS evaluating nurse-led interventions for patients with breast cancer during treatment and survivorship, teaching, guidance, counseling and case management were shown to be effective in managing symptoms although none improved the patients' HQOL [83]. These interventions followed a strict written protocol (as would be expected in a RCT), which also strongly suggested that the nurses in these RCTS also participated in some pretrial education, although only 16 studies described the actual preparatory training. Yet again, it is not enough to train nurses to implement an intervention to meet the requirements of a randomized clinical trial, if the profession does not find some way to disseminate the acquisition of these skills to clinical nurses working in cancer care.

The fact that only a paucity of randomized controlled trials in the nursing literature has evaluated psychosocial interventions to promote the resilience of persons with cancer might be partly redressed by introducing a conceptual model of the whole person that directs nurse researchers and clinicians to relevant concepts of the person, providing the clinical context for identifying patient and caregiver concerns that would benefit from relevant psychosocial interventions. Is it possible that the lack of a conceptual model of whole person care that articulates nursing goals and desired patient outcomes as well as key concepts to guide the acquisition of relevant scientific knowledge and skills may account in part for the finding of a systematic meta-review of 25 *systematic review*s which reported that clinical guidelines were often met with resistance by nursing staff due to a number of factors [91] including the perceived lack of clinical applicability, which suggests the absence of a clear vision of nursing practice.

Because the quality of the nurse–patient relationship is not only a core value but also the key cornerstone of nursing practice, it behooves the nursing profession to do a reset and take stock of where we are headed into the twenty-first century, especially regarding the quality of the nurse patient/caregiver relationship powered by evidence-based competence, communication skills, compassion, and a sense of shared connectedness across clinical settings. This professional imperative necessitates that all arms of the discipline work together toward delineating the overarching goals, foundational concepts, and desired outcomes of the profession.

This chapter has identified a number of distinguishing features of the quality of the nurse–patient relationship that can make a therapeutic difference in the lives of patients and their caregivers. One of the challenges regarding the nurse's competence relates to evidence-based nursing practice and its defining characteristics, goals, desired outcomes, and evidentiary content. A conceptual nursing model of the *whole person* directs nursing's primary clinical focus to the whole person with cancer and their family caregiver. The focus on the whole person serves as the delineating context within which the key concepts relevant to the care of the whole person are identified.

In the absence of a whole person perspective, an "evidence-based" practice tends to reflect medically driven technical knowledge and skills, the management of physical symptoms, the delivery of treatment, and a paucity of randomized controlled trials that evaluate relevant psychosocial nursing interventions of the whole person (with cancer). Procedures and symptom management are essential aspects of the patient's care which *complement* but do not define the nurses' biopsychosocial care of the whole person.

References

1. McAndrew S, Chambers M, Nolan F, Thomas B, Watts P. Measuring the evidence: reviewing the literature of the measurement of therapeutic engagement in acute mental health inpatient wards. Int J Ment Health Nurs. 2014;23(3):212–20. PubMed PMID: 24103061. Epub 2013/10/10. eng.
2. Moreno-Poyato AR, Delgado-Hito P, Leyva-Moral JM, Casanova-Garrigós G, Montesó-Curto P. Implementing evidence-based practices on the therapeutic relationship in inpatient psychiatric care: a participatory action research. J Clin Nurs. 2019;28(9-10):1614–22. PubMed PMID: 30588686. Epub 2018/12/28. eng.
3. Skretkowicz V. Florence Nightingale's notes on nursing and notes on nursing for the labouring classes. New York: Springer; 2010.
4. Mount BM, Boston PH, Cohen SR. Healing connections: on moving from suffering to a sense of well-being. J Pain Symptom Manag. 2007;33(4):372–88. PubMed PMID: 17397699. Epub 2007/04/03. eng.
5. Riba MB, Donovan KA, Andersen B, Braun I, Breitbart WS, Brewer BW, et al. Distress management, version 3.2019, NCCN clinical practice guidelines in oncology.

References

JNCCN. 2019;17(10):1229–49. PubMed PMID: 31590149. Pubmed Central PMCID: PMC6907687. Epub 2019/10/08. eng.
6. Grossman M, Hooton M. The significance of the relationship between a discipline and its practice. J Adv Nurs. 1993;18(6):866–72. PubMed PMID: 8320379. Epub 1993/06/01. eng.
7. Stannard D. A practical definition of evidence-based practice for nursing. J Perianesth Nurs. 2019;34(5):1080–4. PubMed PMID: 31582131. Epub 2019/10/05. eng.
8. Lehane E, Leahy-Warren P, O'Riordan C, Savage E, Drennan J, O'Tuathaigh C, et al. Evidence-based practice education for healthcare professions: an expert view. BMJ Evid-Based Med. 2019;24(3):103–8. PubMed PMID: 30442711. Pubmed Central PMCID: PMC6582731. Epub 2018/11/18. eng.
9. Banerjee SC, Manna R, Coyle N, Penn S, Gallegos TE, Zaider T, et al. The implementation and evaluation of a communication skills training program for oncology nurses. Transl Behav Med. 2017;7(3):615–23. PubMed PMID: 28211000. Pubmed Central PMCID: PMC5645276. Epub 2017/02/18. eng.
10. Prip A, Møller KA, Nielsen DL, Jarden M, Olsen MH, Danielsen AK. The patient-healthcare professional relationship and communication in the oncology outpatient setting: a systematic review. Cancer Nurs. 2018;41(5):11–22. PubMed PMID: 28753191. Pubmed Central PMCID: PMC6259679. Epub 2017/07/29. eng.
11. Thorne S, Hislop TG, Kim-Sing C, Oglov V, Oliffe JL, Stajduhar KI. Changing communication needs and preferences across the cancer care trajectory: insights from the patient perspective. Support Care Cancer. 2014;22(4):1009–15. PubMed PMID: 24287506. Epub 2013/11/30. eng.
12. Buber M. I thou. New York: Simon & Schuster; 1970.
13. Hartley S, Raphael J, Lovell K, Berry K. Effective nurse-patient relationships in mental health care: a systematic review of interventions to improve the therapeutic alliance. Int J Nurs Stud. 2020;102:103490. PubMed PMID: 31862531. Pubmed Central PMCID: PMC7026691. Epub 2019/12/22. eng.
14. Thorne SE, Kuo M, Armstrong EA, McPherson G, Harris SR, Hislop TG. 'Being known': patients' perspectives of the dynamics of human connection in cancer care. Psycho-Oncology. 2000;14(10):887–98; discussion 99–900. PubMed PMID: 16200520. Epub 2005/10/04. eng.
15. Benson H, Friedman R. Harnessing the power of the placebo effect and renaming it "remembered wellness". Annu Rev Med. 1996;47:193–9. PubMed PMID: 8712773.
16. Kelley JM, Kraft-Todd G, Schapira L, Kossowsky J, Riess H. The influence of the patient-clinician relationship on healthcare outcomes: a systematic review and meta-analysis of randomized controlled trials. PLoS One. 2014;9(4):e94207. PubMed PMID: 24718585. Pubmed Central PMCID: PMC3981763 Chairman of Empathetics, LLP. This does not alter the authors' adherence to all the PLOS ONE policies on sharing data and materials. Epub 2014/04/11. eng.
17. Benson H, Stark M. Timeless healing: the power and biology of belief. New York: Simon & Schuster; 1997.
18. Durkin J, Jackson D, Usher K. Defining compassion in a hospital setting: consensus on the characteristics that comprise compassion from researchers in the field. Contemp Nurse. 2020;56(2):146–59. PubMed PMID: 32420794. Epub 2020/05/19. eng.
19. Durkin J, Jackson D, Usher K. The expression and receipt of compassion through touch in a health setting: a qualitative study. J Adv Nurs. 2021;77:1980–91.
20. Durkin J, Usher K, Jackson D. Embodying compassion: a systematic review of the views of nurses and patients. J Clin Nurs. 2019;28(9):1380–92. PubMed PMID: 30485579. Epub 2018/11/30. eng.
21. Erickson HL. Modeling and role-modeling: a view from the client's world. 2006.
22. Vouzavali FJ, Papathanassoglou ED, Karanikola MN, Koutroubas A, Patiraki EI, Papadatou D. 'The patient is my space': hermeneutic investigation of the nurse-patient relationship in critical care. Nurs Crit Care. 2011;16(3):140–51. PubMed PMID: 21481116. Epub 2011/04/13. eng.
23. House JS. Measures and concepts of social support. New York: Academic; 1985.
24. House JS, Landis KR, Umberson D. Social relationships and health. Science. 1988;241(4865):540–5. PubMed PMID: 3399889. Epub 1988/07/29. eng.

25. Blanch-Hartigan D. An effective training to increase accurate recognition of patient emotion cues. Patient Educ Couns. 2012;89:274–80.
26. Blasini M, Peiris N, Wright T, Colloca L. The role of patient-practitioner relationships in placebo and nocebo phenomena. Int Rev Neurobiol. 2018;139:211–31. PubMed PMID: 30146048. Pubmed Central PMCID: PMC6176716. Epub 2018/08/28. eng.
27. Edvardsson D, Watt E, Pearse F. Patient experiences of caring and person-centeredness are associated with perceived nursing care quality. J Adv Nurs. 2017;73:217–27.
28. Hutchinson T. Whole person care. New York: Springer; 2010.
29. Nelson S. Theories focused on interpersonal relationships. In: Rich JB, editor. Philosophies and theories for advanced nursing practice. Sudbury: Jones & Bartlett Learning; 2011. p. 271–311.
30. McAllister S, Robert G, Tsianakas V, McCrae N. Conceptualising nurse-patient therapeutic engagement on acute mental health wards: an integrative review. Int J Nurs Stud. 2019;93:106–18. PubMed PMID: 30908958. Epub 2019/03/26. eng.
31. Moreno-Poyato AR, Montesó-Curto P, Delgado-Hito P, Suárez-Pérez R, Aceña-Domínguez R, Carreras-Salvador R, et al. The therapeutic relationship in inpatient psychiatric care: a narrative review of the perspective of nurses and patients. Arch Psychiatr Nurs. 2016;30(6):782–7. PubMed PMID: 27888975. Epub 2016/11/28. eng.
32. Chapman EJ, Edwards Z, Boland JW, Maddocks M, Fettes L, Malia C, et al. Practice review: evidence-based and effective management of pain in patients with advanced cancer. Palliat Med. 2020;34(4):444–53. PubMed PMID: 31980005. Epub 2020/01/26. eng.
33. van der Cingel M. Compassion in care: a qualitative study of older people with a chronic disease and nurses. Nurs Ethics. 2011;18(5):672–85. PubMed PMID: 21642333. Epub 2011/06/07. eng.
34. Sinclair S, McClement S, Raffin-Bouchal S, Hack TF, Hagen NA, McConnell S, et al. Compassion in health care: an empirical model. J Pain Symptom Manag. 2016;51(2):193–203. PubMed PMID: 26514716. Epub 2015/10/31. eng.
35. Servan-Schreiber D. Anticancer: a new way of life. New York: Viking; 2008.
36. Servan-Schreiber D. The instinct to heal. Stuttgart: Holtzbrinck Publishers; 2004.
37. Oschman J. Energy and the healing response. J Bodyw Mov Ther. 2005;9:9–15.
38. Wittenberg E, Reb A, Kanter E. Communicating with patients and families around difficult topics in cancer care using the COMFORT communication curriculum. Semin Oncol Nurs. 2018;34(3):264–73. PubMed PMID: 30100368. Pubmed Central PMCID: PMC6156926. Epub 2018/08/14. eng.
39. Moore PM, Rivera S, Bravo-Soto GA, Olivares C, Lawrie TA. Communication skills training for healthcare professionals working with people who have cancer. Cochrane Database Syst Rev. 2018;7(7):CD003751. PubMed PMID: 30039853. Pubmed Central PMCID: PMC6513291 known. Camila Olivares: none known. Theresa A Lawrie: none known. Epub 2018/07/25. eng.
40. Chang HL, Li FS, Lin CF. Factors influencing implementation of shared medical decision making in patients with cancer. Patient Prefer Adherence. 2019;13:1995–2005. PubMed PMID: 31819381. Pubmed Central PMCID: PMC6885555. Epub 2019/12/11. eng.
41. Meichenbaum D. A clinical handbook for assessing and treating adults with post-traumatic stress disorder (PTSD). Waterloo: Institute Press; 1994.
42. Jacobsen J, Kvale E, Rabow M, Rinaldi S, Cohen S, Weissman D, et al. Helping patients with serious illness live well through the promotion of adaptive coping: a report from the improving outpatient palliative care (IPAL-OP) initiative. J Palliat Med. 2014;17(4):463–8. PubMed PMID: 24579823. Epub 2014/03/04. eng.
43. Benson H, Stuart E. The wellness book: the comprehensive guide to maintaining health and treating stress-related illness. New York: Simon and Schuster; 1992.
44. McCarthy B. Patients' perceptions of how healthcare providers communicate with them and their families following a diagnosis of colorectal cancer and undergoing chemotherapy treatment. Eur J Oncol Nurs. 2014;18(5):452–8. PubMed PMID: 24954770. Epub 2014/06/24. eng.

45. Meystre C, Bourquin C, Despland JN, Stiefel F, de Roten Y. Working alliance in communication skills training for oncology clinicians: a controlled trial. Patient Educ Couns. 2013;90(2):233–8. PubMed PMID: 23158787. Epub 2012/11/20. eng.
46. Moore L. Effectiveness of an online educational module in improving evidence-based practice skills of practicing registered nurses. Worldviews Evid-Based Nurs. 2017;14(5):358–66. PubMed PMID: 28267902. Epub 2017/03/08. eng.
47. Sinclair S, Beamer K, Hack TF, McClement S, Raffin Bouchal S, Chochinov HM, et al. Sympathy, empathy, and compassion: a grounded theory study of palliative care patients' understandings, experiences, and preferences. Palliat Med. 2017;31(5):437–47. PubMed PMID: 27535319. Pubmed Central PMCID: PMC5405806. Epub 2016/08/19. eng.
48. McCaffrey G, McConnell S. Compassion: a critical review of peer-reviewed nursing literature. J Clin Nurs. 2015;24(19-20):3006–15. PubMed PMID: 26216380. Epub 2015/07/29. eng.
49. Bramley L, Matiti M. How does it really feel to be in my shoes? Patients' experiences of compassion within nursing care and their perceptions of developing compassionate nurses. J Clin Nurs. 2014;23(19-20):2790–9. PubMed PMID: 24479676. Pubmed Central PMCID: PMC4263156. Epub 2014/02/01. eng.
50. Dewar B, Nolan M. Caring about caring: developing a model to implement compassionate relationship centred care in an older people care setting. Int J Nurs Stud. 2013;50(9):1247–58. PubMed PMID: 23427893. Epub 2013/02/23. eng.
51. Dewar B, Pullin S, Tocheris R. Valuing compassion through definition and measurement. Nurs Manag. 2011;17(9):32–7. PubMed PMID: 21473217. Epub 2011/04/09. eng.
52. Strauss C, Lever Taylor B, Gu J, Kuyken W, Baer R, Jones F, et al. What is compassion and how can we measure it? A review of definitions and measures. Clin Psychol Rev. 2016;47:15–27. PubMed PMID: 27267346. Epub 2016/06/09. eng.
53. Fricchione G. Separation-attachment theory in illness and the role of the healthcare practitioner. In: Hutchinson T, editor. Whole person care. New York: Springer; 2010. p. 45–58.
54. Pacheco-Lopez G, Doenlen R, Krugel U, Arnold M, Wirth T, Riether C, et al. Neurobehavioural activation during peripheral immunosuppression. Int J Neuropsychopharmacol. 2013;16(1):137–49. PubMed PMID: 22217400. Epub 2012/01/06. eng.
55. Pacheco-Lopez G, Engler H, Niemi MB, Schedlowski M. Expectations and associations that heal: immunomodulatory placebo effects and its neurobiology. Brain Behav Immun. 2006;20(5):430–46. PubMed PMID: 16887325.
56. Gron O. Introduction to Einstein's theory of relativity. 2nd ed. Cham: Springer; 2020.
57. Mikulincer M, Shaver PR. Attachment orientations and emotion regulation. Curr Opin Psychol. 2019;25:6–10. PubMed PMID: 29494853. Epub 2018/03/02. eng.
58. Fricchione GL. Illness and the origin of caring. J Med Humanit. 1993;14(1):15–21. PubMed PMID: 11612936. Epub 1993/04/01. eng.
59. Lutgendorf S, De Geest K, Bender D, Ahmed A, Goodheart M, Dahmoush L, Zimmerman M, et al. Social influences on clinical outcomes of patients with ovarian cancer. J Clin Oncol. 2012;30(23):2885–90.
60. Wang M, Zhao J, Zhang L, Wei F, Lian Y, Wu Y, et al. Role of tumor microenvironment in tumorigenesis. J Cancer. 2017;8(5):761–73. Pubmed Central PMCID: PMC5381164. Epub 2017/04/07. eng.
61. Lutgendorf SK, Sood AK, Anderson B, McGinn S, Maiseri H, Dao M, et al. Social support, psychological distress, and natural killer cell activity in ovarian cancer. J Clin Oncol. 2005;23(28):7105–13. PubMed PMID: 16192594. Epub 2005/09/30. eng.
62. Robinson S, Kissane DW, Brooker J, Burney S. A systematic review of the demoralization syndrome in individuals with progressive disease and cancer: a decade of research. J Pain Symptom Manag. 2015;49(3):595–610. PubMed PMID: 25131888. Epub 2014/08/19. eng.
63. Frankl V. Man's search for meaning. Boston: Beacon Press; 2006.
64. Park CL. Making sense of the meaning literature: an integrative review of meaning making and its effects on adjustment to stressful life events. Psychol Bull. 2010;136(2):257–301. PubMed PMID: 20192563. Epub 2010/03/03. eng.

65. Colloca L, Barsky AJ. Placebo and nocebo effects. N Engl J Med. 2020;382(6):554–61. PubMed PMID: 32023375. Epub 2020/02/06. eng.
66. Erickson HL. Philosophy and theory of holism. Nurs Clin North Am. 2007;42(2):139–63. PubMed PMID: 17544676.
67. Jaross W. Hypothesis on interactions of macromolecules based on molecular vibration patterns in cells and tissues. Front Biosci. 2018;23:940–6. PubMed PMID: 28930582. Epub 2017/09/21. eng.
68. Kučera O, Cifra M. Radiofrequency and microwave interactions between biomolecular systems. J Biol Phys. 2016;42(1):1–8. PubMed PMID: 26174548. Pubmed Central PMCID: PMC4713408. Epub 2015/07/16. eng.
69. Reeve K, Black PA, Huang J. Examining the impact of a healing touch intervention to reduce posttraumatic stress disorder symptoms in combat veterans. Psychol Trauma. 2020;12(8):897–903. PubMed PMID: 33346680. Epub 2020/12/22. eng.
70. Van der Zee EA, Boersma GJ, Hut RA. The neurobiology of circadian rhythms. Curr Opin Pulm Med. 2009;15(6):534–9. PubMed PMID: 19710613. Epub 2009/08/28. eng.
71. Cohen S, Wills TA. Stress, social support, and the buffering hypothesis. Psychol Bull. 1985;98(2):310–57. PubMed PMID: 3901065. Epub 1985/09/01. eng.
72. Costanzo ES, Lutgendorf SK, Sood AK, Anderson B, Sorosky J, Lubaroff DM. Psychosocial factors and interleukin-6 among women with advanced ovarian cancer. Cancer. 2005;104(2):305–13. PubMed PMID: 15954082. Epub 2005/06/15. eng.
73. Maunsell E, Brisson J, Deschenes L. Social support and survival among women with breast cancer. Cancer. 1995;76(4):631–7. PubMed PMID: 8625157.
74. Cousson-Gélie F, Bruchon-Schweitzer M, Dilhuydy JM, Jutand MA. Do anxiety, body image, social support and coping strategies predict survival in breast cancer? A ten-year follow-up study. Psychosomatics. 2007;48(3):211–6. PubMed PMID: 17478589. Epub 2007/05/05. eng.
75. Nausheen B, Gidron Y, Peveler R, Moss-Morris R. Social support and cancer progression: a systematic review. J Psychosom Res. 2009;67(5):403–15. PubMed PMID: 19837203. Epub 2009/10/20. eng.
76. Andersen BL, Yang HC, Farrar WB, Golden-Kreutz DM, Emery CF, Thornton LM, et al. Psychologic intervention improves survival for breast cancer patients: a randomized clinical trial. Cancer. 2008;113(12):3450–8. PubMed PMID: 19016270. Pubmed Central PMCID: PMC2661422. Epub 2008/11/19. eng.
77. Costa ALS, Heitkemper MM, Alencar GP, Damiani LP, Silva RMD, Jarrett ME. Social support is a predictor of lower stress and higher quality of life and resilience in Brazilian patients with colorectal cancer. Cancer Nurs. 2017;40(5):352–60. PubMed PMID: 27171810. Epub 2016/05/14. eng.
78. Lutgendorf SK, Andersen BL. Biobehavioral approaches to cancer progression and survival: mechanisms and interventions. Am Psychol. 2015;70(2):186–97. PubMed PMID: 25730724. Pubmed Central PMCID: PMC4347942. Epub 2015/03/03. eng.
79. Bayer V, Amaya B, Baniewicz D, Callahan C, Marsh L, McCoy AS. Cancer immunotherapy: an evidence-based overview and implications for practice. Clin J Oncol Nurs. 2017;21(2):13–21. PubMed PMID: 28315552. Epub 2017/03/21. eng.
80. Upton D, Upton P. Development of an evidence-based practice questionnaire for nurses. J Adv Nurs. 2006;53(4):454–8. PubMed PMID: 16448488. Epub 2006/02/02. eng.
81. Hagmann C, Cramer A, Kestenbaum A, Durazo C, Downey A, Russell M, et al. Evidence-based palliative care approaches to non-pain physical symptom management in cancer patients. Semin Oncol Nurs. 2018;34(3):227–40. PubMed PMID: 30120000. Epub 2018/08/19. eng.
82. Morgan B, Tarbi E. The role of the advanced practice nurse in geriatric oncology care. Semin Oncol Nurs. 2016;32(1):33–43. PubMed PMID: 26830266. Epub 2016/02/03. eng.
83. Chan RJ, Teleni L, McDonald S, Kelly J, Mahony J, Ernst K, et al. Breast cancer nursing interventions and clinical effectiveness: a systematic review. BMJ Support Palliat Care. 2020;10(3):276–86. PubMed PMID: 32499405. Epub 2020/06/06. eng.
84. Denlinger CS, Sanft T, Baker KS, Broderick G, Demark-Wahnefried W, Friedman DL, et al. Survivorship, version 2.2018, NCCN clinical practice guidelines in oncology.

JNCCN. 2018;16(10):1216–47. PubMed PMID: 30323092. Pubmed Central PMCID: PMC6438378. Epub 2018/10/17. eng
85. Dionne-Odom JN, Taylor R, Rocque G, Chambless C, Ramsey T, Azuero A, et al. Adapting an early palliative care intervention to family caregivers of persons with advanced cancer in the rural deep south: a qualitative formative evaluation. J Pain Symptom Manag. 2018;55(6):1519–30. PubMed PMID: 29474939. Pubmed Central PMCID: PMC5951755. Epub 2018/02/24. eng.
86. Bakitas MA, Tosteson TD, Li Z, Lyons KD, Hull JG, Li Z, et al. Early versus delayed initiation of concurrent palliative oncology care: patient outcomes in the ENABLE III randomized controlled trial. J Clin Oncol. 2015;33(13):1438–45. PubMed PMID: 25800768. Pubmed Central PMCID: PMC4404422 online at www.jco.org. Author contributions are found at the end of this article. Epub 2015/03/25. eng.
87. Dionne-Odom JN, Azuero A, Lyons KD, Hull JG, Prescott AT, Tosteson T, et al. Family caregiver depressive symptom and grief outcomes from the ENABLE III randomized controlled trial. J Pain Symptom Manag. 2016;52(3):378–85. PubMed PMID: 27265814. Pubmed Central PMCID: PMC5023481. Epub 2016/06/07. eng.
88. Lee V, Cohen SR, Edgar L, Laizner AM, Gagnon AJ. Meaning-making and psychological adjustment to cancer: development of an intervention and pilot results. Oncol Nurs Forum. 2006;33(2):291–302. PubMed PMID: 16518445. Epub 2006/03/07. eng.
89. Bakitas M, Lyons KD, Hegel MT, Balan S, Brokaw FC, Seville J, et al. Effects of a palliative care intervention on clinical outcomes in patients with advanced cancer: the Project ENABLE II randomized controlled trial. JAMA. 2009;302(7):741–9. PubMed PMID: 19690306. Pubmed Central PMCID: PMC3657724. Epub 2009/08/20. eng.
90. Dionne-Odom JN, Azuero A, Lyons KD, Hull JG, Tosteson T, Li Z, et al. Benefits of early versus delayed palliative care to informal family caregivers of patients with advanced cancer: outcomes from the ENABLE III randomized controlled trial. J Clin Oncol. 2015;33(13):1446–52. PubMed PMID: 25800762. Pubmed Central PMCID: PMC4404423. Epub 2015/03/25. eng.
91. Correa VC, Lugo-Agudelo LH, Aguirre-Acevedo DC, Contreras JAP, Borrero AMP, Patiño-Lugo DF, et al. Individual, health system, and contextual barriers and facilitators for the implementation of clinical practice guidelines: a systematic metareview. Health Res Policy Syst. 2020;18(1):74. PubMed PMID: 32600417. Pubmed Central PMCID: PMC7322919. Epub 2020/07/01. eng.

Promoting Emotion-Regulating Coping Resilience

9

> *So never lose an opportunity of urging a practical beginning, however small, for it is wonderful how often in such matters the mustard-seed germinates and roots itself*
>
> Florence Nightingale

9.1 Introduction

Patients and caregivers are called upon to manage stressful aspects of the cancer and treatment experience, for which they may feel understandably ill-prepared [1]. The stresses over the continuum can at times exceed the individual's ability to cognitively, emotionally, and/or functionally cope, thereby negatively impacting their normal resilient capabilities [2–4].

This chapter (and the one that follows on meaning making) covers nursing strategies to facilitate effective cognitive and behavioral emotion-regulating coping adaptive responses in patients and caregivers. These strategies comprise the nurse's essential psychosocial "tool kit" for relieving emotional distress by sensitively redirecting the patient or caregiver toward more effective coping responses, at the bedside, in clinic, and at home prior, during, and after treatment. Many of these coping behaviors have been incorporated into formalized cognitive–behavioral stress management (CBSM) programs for group workshops [5] (Appendix in this chapter). But they are also meant to be used more informally as the nurse assesses the clinical need to proactively respond to the patient's or caregiver's distress or alternatively, to strengthen their current repertoire of resilient-promoting coping efforts.

This chapter also reviews the essential components of self-management interventions (SMI) based on coping's problem-solving steps [6]. SMI has been implemented with patients and caregivers in survivorship [7], during treatment [8], and throughout the palliative phase, with promising results [9] (Review Part V; Appendices A and B).

9.2 Objectives

At the end of the chapter, you will be able to:

1. Describe and distinguish the use of reframing, reappraisal and cognitive restructuring as nursing strategies to reduce emotional distress
2. Knowledgeably discuss nursing strategies that may be particularly relevant for promoting resilience at different phases across the diagnosis, treatment, survival, and end-of-life continuum
3. Discuss the purpose and main components of self management strategies

Clinical Anecdote 9.1
We cannot predict how we would handle a cancer diagnosis. We can only hope that being tested we are able to draw on the resilient resources and coping capabilities acquired over our lifetime so that life's challenges may be managed with some grace. I have seen patients in tears quietly overflowing in sadness at each scheduled treatment, their loving relatives unable to comfort them despite their concerted efforts to offer solace and help.

I was unprepared for the effect those words, 'You have cancer' would have (once again) during my first appointment with the oncologist. As the oncologist spoke I was focused on a very glacial sensation that had permeated my whole being. The emotional morass was so unpleasant that I tried to distract myself with a flow of " What next" questions. I wanted to know the prognosis (very bad) and the treatment plan (there was no known protocol), and how the oncologist planned to proceed (team approach). I even wanted to know what the latest clinical research findings indicated- I was coping by trying to assert a sense of personal control over my medical care, but really to control my anxiety.

I willed myself to concentrate on gathering relevant information so that I could envision a path forward toward health. It made me feel that I was doing something. And I was facilitated in this task by a very perceptive and sympathetic oncologist. He seemed to understand that this new found determination helped to displace my anxiety and make room for a growing calmness and sense of purpose.

9.3 Definitions: The Emotion/Self-Regulating Coping System of Psychological Resilience (Review Part II, Chaps. 4 and 5; Appendix in this Chapter and Appendices A and B)

Psychological resilience is the ability of the human organism to adapt or effectively cope in the face of environmental challenges [10]. Incorporating fundamental elements from the stress-coping model [4, 11], meaning-making model [12, 13], and the common sense model of self-regulation [14], the *therapeutic nursing goals of the emotion-regulating* coping system of resilience are to (1) reduce emotional distress, (2) promote emotion regulation, (3) enable healing, (4) strengthen overall resilience, and (5) enhance well-being and quality of life in the aftermath of a psychological threat, through the facilitation of the patient's and caregiver's cognitive and behavioral coping efforts.

Generally cognitive coping efforts refer to emotion-focused, meaning-focused and problem-focused strategies to manage a stressful event. Strategies may include cognitive reappraisal, deliberate rumination, perspective-taking, planning, positive refocusing, analyzing, storytelling and use of problem solving. Cognitive strategies may also include unhelpful coping strategies such as blaming, catastrophizing, or prolonged use of denial and avoidance [4, 11, 15].

Emotion-focused coping efforts have to do with strategies used to reduce emotional distress caused by the stressful situation [11, 14] (see Part II Chap. 5). An example is the use of distraction to take one's mind off the knowledge that the cancer is advancing.

Meaning-making coping efforts refer to strategies involving the cognitive reappraisal of the stressor in a way that may enhance psychological well-being, acceptance, or personal growth [12, 13, 16].

Clinical Anecdote 9.2
Mrs. X was emotionally distressed, tormented by a misguided belief that her diagnosis was a "death sentence" even though the cancer was stage 1, and she had every reason to believe that she would survive. Yet, nothing the nurses said could convince her otherwise. She was holding on to her catastrophizing belief. Mrs. X's coping response conveyed a sense of helplessness and despair. By succumbing to that despair, she had effectively suppressed her potential cognitive capabilities that might have enabled her to consider other, more effective, less physiologically damaging coping options. Her helplessness suggested that Mrs. X did not see herself as possessing either personal strengths such as self efficacy beliefs, effective coping skills, or the support she needed to successfully manage the reality of the cancer.

Problem-focused coping efforts are defined as the strategies used to manage the stressor or threat, for example, when a patient has just been diagnosed with cancer and immediately generates a list of things he must ask the doctor at his first appointment to learn about the disease and the doctor's approach.

Problem-focused coping efforts also have to do more specifically with the acquisition of self-management strategies (see section "Facilitating Self-Management Strategies") to enhance self-efficacy beliefs by learning to manage practical problems associated with the consequences of cancer and/or treatment [1, 17]. Key elements of a self-management program typically include helping the individual to define the problem, set the goal, desired outcome and develop a detailed action plan and evaluation criteria. The nurse provides relevant practical education (for eg. teaching patient or caregiver how to give a medication by injection), information about the cancer and/or treatment; and use of resource materials tailored to the needs of the patient and caregiver [18]. The nurse also draws on strategies such as breaking down perceived threats into component parts to determine what aspects of the threat can or cannot be acted upon.

Behavioral coping skills refer to physical activities which have, as the intended goal, reducing emotional distress. These activities typically include exercise, mindfulness behaviors such as Benson's relaxation response technique [19], Carlson's mindfulness-based cancer recovery program [20], and Kabat Zinn's mindful meditation [21], discussed as relevant throughout Part V. Other mindful activities may include qi gong and gentle yoga (Review Chap. 14).

9.4   Randomized Controlled Intervention Studies (RCTs): Enhancing Coping Efforts (Appendix in this Chapter, Appendix in Chaps. 10, 11, 13, and 14, and Appendices A–C)

Here is a brief summary of psychosocial coping-related interventions that can be incorporated into nursing practice to strengthen the resilience of patients and caregivers.

Cognitive–Behavioral Strategies (CBS) (Review Appendix in this Chapter)

Meta-analyses and clinical trials consistently show that CBS result in significant improvements in quality of life, pain, fatigue, anxiety, and depressive mood as assessed mainly in patients with breast cancer and prostate cancer and/or their caregivers [5, 22, 23]. Cognitive and behavioral strategies have been incorporated into multimodal intervention programs with demonstrated clinical benefits, for instance, in women with nonmetastatic breast cancer [24]; Appendix in this chapter). The common sense model (CSM) of self-regulation [2, 14], cognitive behavioral stress management (CBSM) interventions [25], and mindfulness-based cancer recovery interventions [20] are the most well-known cognitive and behavioral coping-promoting interventions shown to effectively improve the lives of individuals with cancer. Behavioral coping strategies are also discussed further in Part V (see also Appendix in Chap. 13 and Appendix C).

Self-Management Interventions (SMI) (Appendix A)

Self-management interventions have been implemented mainly with survivors of cancer [7, 26, 27], patients during tumor-related treatment [28], as well as patients [29] and family caregivers [30] in palliative phases of cancer with mixed results.

Cancer Survivors A systematic review identified content, mode of delivery, composition of sessions, and SM skills in 12 studies that met the inclusion criteria, followed by meta-analysis of 9 RCTS with 2804 participants [27]. The qualitative synthesis showed that the majority of SMI interventions occurred with survivors of breast cancer. SMI content covered medical, behavioral, and emotional management with educational and information-related components and relied mostly on a Web-based delivery mode. The frequently assessed clinical outcomes were depression, quality of life, and self-efficacy. The meta-analysis showed a medium effect size improvement in health-related quality of life as well as a large effect size reduction in levels of fatigue bordering on significance [27]. A systematic review of 41 studies of self-management interventions also highlighted the preponderance of breast cancers, characterized by variability in the structure, content and outcomes for cancer survivors across the studies [31].

Palliative Care Patients and Caregivers A RCT demonstrated that SMIs improved survival rates in patients who received early palliative care compared to later palliative care [29]. A systematic review of 11 studies assessed the effects of SMI in patients with solid tumors as well as hematological malignancies. Five of the 9 studies showed that the SMI produced a significant effect in reducing psychological distress in adults with cancer. The four studies in which SMI produced nonsignificant findings involved patients with hematological cancers, suggesting that this under studied population requires further clinical studies [28].

Family Caregivers A systematic review of 11 studies investigated the effects of psychosocial ($n = 2$), educational ($n = 4$), or psychoeducational ($n = 6$) interventions on family caregivers of patients being cared for at home [30]. SMIs appeared to reduce emotional distress, caregiving burden, and improve quality of life, self-efficacy, and competence in family caregivers caring for patients with advanced disease at home, although the content of the interventions varied across studies. For instance, a RCT investigated the effects of a SMI in 122 caregivers–patients in palliative care. Caregivers were randomized to either receive the intervention in the early palliative phase (shortly after diagnosis) or delayed phase (3 months after a new palliative diagnosis) [18]. The results showed a between-group difference at 3 months with a significant effect size reduction in depression scores favoring the early group over the delayed group. No significant differences at 3 months were found for quality of life, burden, stress, and demand. Between-group differences in *a terminal phase decline analysis* did show that the early group was significantly less depressed than the delayed group and experienced significantly less stress burden. But there were no significant differences between groups for quality of life, objective burden, and demand burden. These findings suggested that nursing interventions need to be more flexible and more tailored to caregiver needs, with more face-to-face meetings [18, 32]. Last, randomized pilot studies of a self-management intervention for couples dealing with head and neck cancer and survivors of colorectal and lung cancer demonstrated promising results [7, 33].

9.5 Suggested Nursing Approaches

Resilient individuals tend to possess personal strengths and social supports that enable their ability to cope with health-related challenges [34]. Notwithstanding, resilient people may also initially falter in the face of a cancer-related threat because the cognitive and behavioral coping responses previously relied on to successfully manage stressful experiences may not be as applicable in the current clinical context [35].

Promoting relevant coping strategies and self-management skills depends on characteristics of the patient or caregiver, clinical context, personal and social resources, individual coping-related capabilities, symptom burden, the stated problem(s), and their beliefs about the cancer-/treatment-related threats and emotional response. A cancer threat that is perceived as *changeable*, controllable, and "coherent" tends to lead to effective problem-focused coping efforts [2, 36].

In contrast, a cancer threat that is perceived *as uncontrollable* may be associated with high emotional distress and emotion-focused and or meaning-focused coping efforts may be helpful [11, 12, 14]. Lazarus and Folkman [4] cautioned that the appropriate selection of coping strategies must be context-driven: Encouraging the use of problem-focused coping strategies to further the patient's pursuit of a cure is detrimental when no cure exists. In contrast, engaging the newly diagnosed, highly distressed patient and/or caregiver in meaning-focused coping efforts to reduce emotional distress can enhance a sense of personal control, purpose, and hope for a quality life (Part IV Chap. 10; Review Appendix in this chapter and Appendix in Chap. 10 and Appendix B).

Finally, resilient individuals who are treated as outpatients during treatment or during the transition to survivorship or at home in the terminal phase of life may benefit from a *nurse-supported* self-management intervention to increases their sense of self-efficacy with respect to handling basic clinical demands emanating from the treatment or stage of the cancer [18, 29, 37] (Appendix in this chapter and Appendix A). The quality of the nurse–patient and caregiver relationships lies at the core of successfully engaging patient and caregiver in healing enhancing, coping-promoting interventions (Part IV, Chap. 8).

Nursing Assessment

Emotional Distress
The first objective of a nursing assessment is to examine the potential presence of threats or stressor events being experienced by the patient and/or caregiver and its impact on their roles, functions, relationships, and overall well-being. An individual's level of emotional distress may quickly be assessed with the screening tool of the distress thermometer which includes perceived causes for the distress [38]; Part II, Chap. 3). But to gain further clinical understanding of the significance of a cancer- or treatment-related stressor, it may be useful to conceptualize these threats in terms of *the individual's cognitive representations* of *the illness-related* and

treatment-related threat(s) and the corresponding emotional representations (i.e., affective responses) [14] (Table 9.1). Part of this stress assessment is to explore past stressors and their effects on the individual in terms of the intensity, duration, frequency, and context (usually in relation to their coping efforts).

In assessing the individual's sources of stress, it is important to explore related concerns that may touch on feelings of loss regarding their former life, changes in their roles and responsibilities, family relationships, and uncertainty about the future [39].

Reducing negative emotional reactions is key to enabling neurophysiological healing processes to reemerge, so that the prefrontal cortex and hippocampus, which regulate executive decision-making and memory-related capabilities, may be reactivated and the amygdala's activities reduced, enabling critical thinking, decision making, cognitive flexibility, and more adaptive coping efforts subsequently to be mobilized [10, 40] (Review Part II, Chaps. 4 and 5). Thus, the first nursing goal is to assess the intensity, frequency, and past and current causes associated with distress in order to enable the subsequent development of appropriate multimodal coping interventions.

Coping Efforts (Review Appendix B)

The second objective is to assess the types, diversity, and flexible use of various coping efforts that have been used to manage identified stressors past and present (Table 9.2). In principle, this typically refers to three sets of cognitive efforts: problem-focused, emotion-focused, and meaning-making; elements of all three may be identified in the coping clusters of patients managing a particular stressor and its negative emotional reactions [11, 12, 14]. (Meaning-making efforts are examined further in Chap. 10). Meaning making has to do with the global assumptions and beliefs individuals hold about the world in relation to the self which are typically challenged by the patient's and caregiver's perception of the threat and situational meaning(s) they have created about the threatening event, such as the

Table 9.1 Cognitive attributes of the illness-related threat [14]

Attributes	Definitions
1. Identity (health threat)	The medical diagnosis, disease type, and symptoms
2. Consequences (threat)	Current and future implications of the disease or treatment on one's (1) personal life (family and career roles) and (2) whole being (cognitively, socially, behaviorally, physically), symptoms and side effects, quality of life, and health
3. Timeline (potential threat)	Expected/unexpected onset, duration, intensity, frequency
4. Causes	Genetics, diet, lack of exercise, stress, early childhood adversity, other exacerbating factors
5. Illness coherence	Patient's overall integrated understanding of the illness which corresponds to clinical reality and consistent with healthcare explanations
6. Perceived control	Extent to which disease is perceived by the patient as controllable/uncontrollable

cancer diagnosis [13, 42]. Strategies typically used by the individual include reappraisals of the threat in a way that finds new meanings and hope. Chapter 10 discusses a more complex process that nurses may consider to promote meaning making which can lead to personal growth and acceptance [43, 44].

Behavioral efforts typically involve activities that downregulate the stress response system: examples include relaxation exercises, mindful meditation, or physical activities such as walking. Personal and social resources such as self-efficacy beliefs and optimism and social support influence the individual's use of various coping strategies and need to be considered in a clinical assessment [45–47].

Not All Coping Efforts Are Adaptive Some coping efforts may prolong and exacerbate the experience of stress (Table 9.3). The use of escape avoidance, venting, self-blaming, thought suppression, persistent meaning seeking, denial and incessant unregulated rumination come to mind. *Escape-avoidant* behaviors, for instance, may be utilized by patients during the initial threat of a traumatic diagnosis, but long term, its use is associated with poor psychological well-being and reduced physical, role, and social functioning [16]. Emotionally laden negative appraisals of the illness (such as, catastrophizing beliefs) exert direct negative effects on well-being and role functioning and positive effects on distress [16, 55]. When prolonged and in the absence of other more resilient-promoting strategies, these strategies result in poor resilience and psychopathological outcomes.

Ineffective coping efforts interfere with the cognitive ability to more positively reappraise the cognitive threat so that emotional distress may be reduced [2, 5]. From McEwen's work with biological and psychological resilience, maladaptive coping reduces cognitive judgment and executive thinking [56]. Maladaptive coping efforts over time are associated with persistent emotional stress causing suppressed cell-mediated immune functions, compromising the potential for a lengthened survivorship [57, 58].

Self-Management Interventions

The third area of a nursing assessment pertains to the patient or caregiver's potential or actual self-management capabilities. Individuals who are assessed as fundamentally resilient, with stress levels that are a normal reflection of the cancer-related experience, and who draw on appropriate cognitive and behavioral coping strategies

Table 9.2 Examples of cognitive coping efforts [11, 16, 39, 41]

Cognitive reappraisal	Seeking and maintaining support
Avoidance short term	Hope
Distraction	Acceptance
Emotional venting as part of more effective coping efforts	Meaning making
Problem-focused activities	Spiritual/religious coping (also part of meaning)
Focus on the positive	A fighting spirit

9.5 Suggested Nursing Approaches

Table 9.3 Examples of maladaptive coping behaviors and health-related outcomes

Behaviors	Health-related outcomes
Escape/avoidance	Depressive symptoms [48, 49]
Thought suppression	Depression risk [50]
Emotion suppression	Depression, anxiety risk [51, 52]
Rumination	Anxiety risk [53, 54]
Catastrophizing	Anxiety, depression [6, 54]
Negative appraisals	Depressive symptoms [49]
Self-blaming	
Continuous venting	

to maintain emotional regulation are appropriate candidates for learning self-management strategies. Because cancer may progress and over time caregivers assume a greater caregiver burden, self-management activities that may have been previously assumed by patients and/or caregivers must be regularly assessed across the continuum.

Other Relevant Contextual Patient and Caregiver Information to Assess

As part of the coping assessment, gather patient information about:
1. Past versus current experiences with serious illness or life-threatening events and coping responses, including history of early childhood adversity (Part II Chap. 3)
2. Current symptoms and side effects
3. Personal and social resources, in particular, sense of self-efficacy and quality of supportive relationships (Review Part II Chap. 6; to be discussed in Part IV Chap. 14)
4. Patient beliefs and cognitive expectations about their treatment and future wellness based on past experiences with serious illness, treatments, and memories of the care they received (Part IV Chap. 12). These beliefs are also a form of coping efforts that have been shown to be associated with clinical benefits.

Summary Cognitive and behavioral coping strategies can either be resilient-promoting or maladaptive, depending on the clinical context, strategies used, and availability of personal and supportive resources. Some patients focus on problem solving and are determined to actively "fight" the cancer; others prefer to take a more accepting, "genteel" approach; and most combine emotion-, problem-, and meaning-focused coping strategies [59].

A Clinical Assessment Strategy: Patient/Caregiver Narratives (Also Review Patient Narratives in Part IV Chap. 10, Section "Cognitive Restructuring and Distorted Beliefs" and Table 10.2)

Eliciting the patient's narrative is a well-known therapeutic nursing strategy that provides invaluable information about what matters to the patient and caregiver. For the nurse during an assessment, it serves as an often effective way into the individual's world that can provide an important perspective within which the individual's emotional distress, coping strategies, and personal and social capabilities and supports are revealed and potential patient vulnerabilities may be exposed [60, 61].

Retelling of the distressing event during a nursing assessment is often therapeutic and may even temporarily relieve feelings of anxiety by facilitating cognitive processing of the stressor event [53]. As will be discussed further in Chap. 10 on facilitating meaning, a patient's narrative may be shaped around different themes depending on the therapeutic intent (see Chap. 10, section "Cognitive Restructuring and Distorted Beliefs"). In the telling, it can facilitate the patient's ability to organize the different, interrelated facets of his main concerns, fears, or threats into a reintegrated more coherent whole that may facilitate the process of making sense of what has happened and/or further to come to terms with it.

Nursing Interventions: Promoting Emotion-Regulating Coping Efforts (Review Part IV Chap. 10; Appendix in this Chapter and Appendix B)

Psychological resilience depends on the individual's ability to successfully adjust their cognitive and behavioral coping efforts to a stressful situation in order to cope more effectively. Nursing strategies are aimed at facilitating the individual's effective coping responses to a threat via the tailored adoption of problem-focused, emotion-focused, and meaning-making coping efforts [6, 62] as well as behavioral coping strategies. Self-management strategies, discussed in section "Facilitating Self-Management Strategies", are typically utilized to enhance the self-efficacy and problem-solving capabilities in managing the practical consequences of the cancer or treatment

Meaning-making nursing interventions involve the use of reframing, perspective-taking, use of alternative interpretations/explanations, providing contextual information, facilitating reappraisal, deliberate rumination (see Part IV Chap. 10), and use of cognitive restructuring. Because meaning is so important to facilitating patient healing and resilience, it is addressed in depth in Chap. 10 from theoretical and empirical perspectives, accompanied by suggested nurse strategies.

Emotionally oriented nursing interventions encourage the use of emotion-focused coping efforts to reduce or contain negative emotional reactions. These strategies may include normalizing the situation, reframing, encouraging use of distraction such as engaging in a pleasant activity, hobby and/or being with friends, a present-oriented focus, positive self-talk, and using positive affirmations.

Problem-solving nursing interventions promote the patient's ability to find the appropriate solution or plan of action to address practical problems arising from the cancer or its treatment [6, 14] (see section "Facilitating Self-Management Strategies"). Problem-solving interventions involve the patient and/or caregiver with the support of the nurse to generate the plan of action based on a series of steps that include evaluating its effect. A problem-solving coping approach is typically

9.5 Suggested Nursing Approaches

part of self-management programs. Before the nurse and patient can generate a plan of action, the nurse may need to use strategies such as cognitive restructuring, reducing generalized patient metaphors to help the patient define the problem.

Behavioral strategies (Review Part IV Chap. 16; Part V). The majority of cognitive coping efforts include a behavioral component to reduce the intensity of emotional distress, including feelings of uncertainty, fear of recurrence, loss of control and symptoms of depression, anxiety, fatigue, and insomnia [63]. These behavioral interventions may include relaxation exercises, mindful meditation, the relaxation response technique, or engaging in daily physical exercise [64], for instance, suggesting physical exercise such as daily walks depending on the individual's clinical status to increase endorphin levels and stimulate immune cells to fight the cancer [65]. Benson's relaxation response technique and other mindfulness activities such as meditation invite the practitioner to focus on a word, mantra, prayer, or the breath as a strategy for *distancing the individual's emotions* from intrusive beliefs [66].

The Nurse's Essential "Resilient-Promoting Toolbox"

What follows is a closer look at a number of coping-promoting nursing interventions. (See also Appendix in this chapter, Appendix in Chaps. 10, 11, 13, and 14, and Appendices A and B).

Reframing [6]
This frequently used nurse strategy offers alternative more positive perspectives, interpretations, and explanations to account for an individual's distressing situation. For instance, a family caregiver's statement that "caregiving is too distressing" should be first acknowledged, and the reasoning for this belief also explored. But in addition, the nurse might consider reframing the act of caregiving as a "heartfelt gift" from one human being to another [67]. But what if the nurse's comment was made without prior knowledge of the nature of the patient–caregiver relationship. What if the caregiver's stress-related comments had to do with the patient's continuous displays of acrimonious behavior toward the caregiver, unbeknownst to the nurse. Reframing the caregiver's feelings in this manner might have a further exacerbating negative effect. Reframing *is only effective once* an in-depth understanding of the patient/caregiver context has been achieved and is typically one of a number of strategies the nurse may use to help people shift their thinking toward a more positive or at least neutral reappraisal of the challenging situation.

Cognitive Restructuring and Distorted Beliefs [6, 67]
Cognitive restructuring is a common strategy that is used by healthcare providers, including nurses to transform *inaccurate, unrealistic, or irrational* beliefs into more accurate, balanced, and rational thoughts so that emotional distress may be reduced [67, 68]. Irrational thoughts may be "generated" in response to a cancer threat when we feel personally helpless to alter its consequences. These distortions interfere

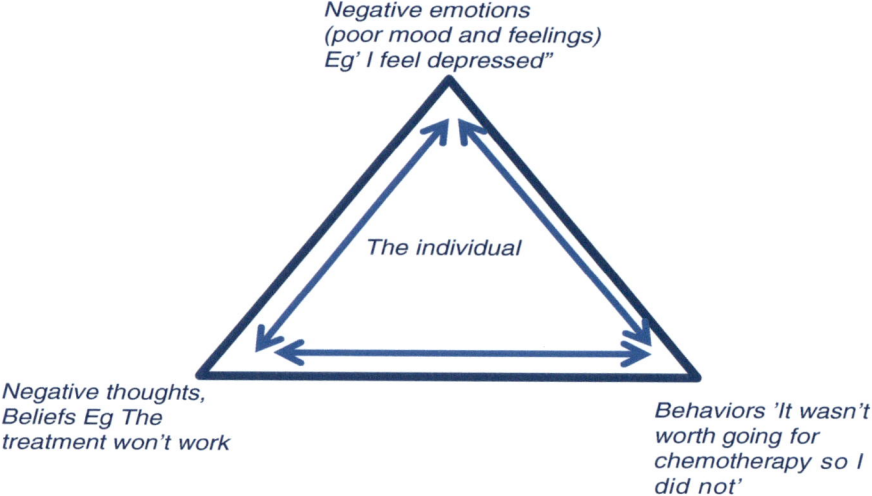

Fig. 9.1 Impact of negative thoughts/distorted beliefs

with the individual's ability to use coping strategies that help to reduce distress and protect resilience and health potential. Typical distorted thinking include catastrophizing, overgeneralizing, overpersonalizing, and seeing things as black or white.

The overall nursing goal is to facilitate the individual's ability to replace the distorted thought or belief with other thoughts rooted in facts and clinical reality that can reduce stress and enable a better adjustment. Cognitive restructuring is based on a simple hypothesis that there are bidirectional relationships among thoughts/beliefs, emotions (mood and feelings), and behaviors (e.g., Fig. 9.1). Its primary nursing strategy is use of Socratic questioning. Socratic questioning stimulates the individual's ability to think critically about the thoughts (beliefs), emotions, and behaviors that have an important bearing on his well-being and health-related outcomes.

Cognitive Restructuring Steps Typically Involve [6, 67]

Identifying Distorted Beliefs

Cognitive distortions include catastrophizing (i.e., I am as good as dead), overgeneralizing (everyone gets sick on chemo), misguided myths (you go into the hospital and never come out), all or nothing statements (e.g., I will try this once, and if it doesn't work, I'm done!), self-blaming (it is my fault that I have cancer), and significantly the tendency to dismiss the positive in one's illness, such as the *positive significance* of a stage 1 cancer diagnosis. These cognitive distortions lead to poor psychological well-being, role dysfunction, and enhanced distress [2]. Maladaptive coping efforts over time become energy-depleting, potentially compromising the patient's ability to live as long as possible with cancer or as a potential survivor. Nurses may identify distorted beliefs through the patient's narrative.

9.5 Suggested Nursing Approaches

Help the Person Distinguish between a Belief and a Fact
- Distinguish between a belief and a fact, and explain how beliefs are assumptions, untethered to actual facts, yet they influence our emotions and behavioral choices, if we allow them. For instance, you might say something like "A fact is that you are currently ill and doctors have scientific evidence that favors the use of a specific chemotherapy in order to eliminate your type of cancer." Conversely, a misguided belief is that "you are doomed."
- Examine patient/caregiver "evidence" for the belief versus the fact? i.e., What are the origins of this belief? Ask whether there other possible reasons to account for the belief. And/or,
- "What information has led you to this way of thinking?".
- How often do you think and feel this way? Is the belief an automatic thought (i.e., just pops unwanted into your mind), what are its triggers, when did it start, and what gave rise to this belief (previous experience, an inaccurate fact, what someone told you?).
- What is your expectation for the treatment. What led you to this *opinion*?
- How do you imagine your future? How did this belief come about?
- Introduce relevant information and facts that counter or dispel the individual's cognitive distortions or irrational thinking.

Link Thoughts to Emotions (and to Behaviors)
- Draw the patient/caregiver's attention to *the impact of the negative beliefs/thoughts* on his emotional state, behaviors, and physical condition. For example, the patient who says "the diagnosis is hopeless" may be asked whether the doctor stated it was hopeless or is that what the patient took away from the discussion.
- If the patient/caregiver agrees it is his belief, then connect the belief to the patient/caregiver's *emotional state*: How does your belief that the diagnosis is hopeless affect your mood? (depressed, sad, fearful).
- Then, connect the negative emotional state *to his behavior*: How does your depressed mood impact your behavior (I cannot get out of bed these days. I do not feel like eating very much).
- Also link the effects of his negative emotional state *to his physical health*. "Is this affecting your physical health in any way (I seem to have a lot more pain, fatigue, lack of energy)." You might want to point out that a distorted belief that is not a fact has the "power" to make one miserable, when it has no basis in reality. (Note: Keep in mind that a patient with cancer may have actual pain that causes a depressed or distressed mood which must be ruled out first).
- Now, ask the patient/caregiver *to think* about a favorite person or place—how does it make him feel? or describe the emotions that surface when he thinks that his medical treatment will make him better. *The important message is that by changing the thought you can change the feeling and experience a sense of personal control over the situation.*
- Ask the individual to *monitor* his own thoughts and when the distorted belief (It is hopeless) emerges, to counter it with factual *self-talk* such as "the diagnosis is

very hopeful because the cancer is at the very earliest stage and I am on the right treatment." Or say "Finally, I know why I have been tired and now we are doing something about it!" Or "The oncologist is very hopeful so I am too!". Encourage the patient to keep up the self-talk. Ask the patient to avoid using "I *should*" or "*I would*" and use instead, "I *want to/or will* use facts in my self-talk to change my thoughts and feelings."

The therapeutic intent is to help the patient recognize the bidirectional effects among thoughts, feelings, behaviors, and physical symptoms, and significantly his ability to break that emotionally distressing cycle. By changing his thoughts, for instance, by thinking about a favorite person or place, he can change his mood and behaviors.

Conversely, point out that when the patient/caregiver *repeatedly* reinforces a "negative" belief with feelings of depression or despair, it becomes a *perceived* truth rather than what it is just a belief that can be changed.

Another Use of Cognitive Restructuring (for Illustrative Purposes)

Explore the Patient's Assumptions and Beliefs about the World and Self
- Identify the assumptions behind the belief (i.e., cancer has always meant death; it makes me feel helpless). Explore all possible patient explanations for his beliefs (my mother's sister died from cancer at a young age). You might respond with: "I am sorry to learn about your aunt, so many years ago. But medical science has improved tremendously since then. There are new agents produced every year that are significantly more effective than in the past... Thanks to these major advances cancer is increasingly considered a chronic illness."
- Provide facts and information within which the patient can reappraise his beliefs.

Explore the Emotional and Behavioral Costs Versus Benefits of Holding onto a Distorted Belief (Review Chap. 12)
- For example, let us look at what the *effect* of holding onto to this belief has had on your life—You say that your diagnosis is "hopeless" and everyday you feel more depressed and unable to function, yet you also state that you begin chemotherapy at the end of the week and that the oncologists feel you have a curative cancer. *How do you reconcile holding onto a negative belief that is in your power to change,* with *these very hopeful treatments?*
- Provide information about the potential effects of holding negative beliefs on treatment efficacy (See Chap. 12) [69–71].
- Consider sharing research findings showing that positive beliefs activate our biological reward system which can enhance immune functioning that is essential in tracking down and eradicating roving cancer cells [72, 73].
- Similarly, ask "What are the costs to your health in continuing with an observed pattern of maladaptive behavior (e.g., missed treatments), thinking (it is all useless), and feeling (despair)".

9.5 Suggested Nursing Approaches

Clinical Anecdote 9.3

It was E's second visit to see the nurse since being officially discharged from all treatment. As part of the new transition to survivorship program the nurse was following a few individuals who seemed to be hesitating to embrace their "new normal" life. This was despite the all clear medical consensus and having participated in a group workshop that was aimed at addressing the common concerns of new survivors and their family caregivers. The nurse welcomed E with a "How goes it, E?" a warm, open- ended introduction. It was their second visit. "Well not much really. Just watching a bit of TV and trying to read."

The nurse—"And trying to read. Most days or just today."
E Shrugs
N It sounds like you are having difficulty concentrating.
E I think so—I have all these thoughts in my mind, and I just go with them
N What kind of thoughts
E It's silly.
N: Mmm How do these thoughts make you feel?
E Fearful,
N That doesn't sound silly to me. And what do you do then
E I just sit there in my thoughts.
N Would you mind sharing those thoughts with me?
E Well I won't know when the cancer comes back. It will just pop up, and it will be too late to do anything about it.
N: It sounds like your beliefs about cancer are weighing heavily on your thoughts and your ability to detect the cues and act in a timely way. Would that be fair to say?
E nods.
N Let me just say that your fears of cancer coming back tend to be a normal experience right after treatment so long as these worries do not continue to take charge of your feelings and your ability to enjoy life.
Silence and the nurse continues;
Would you be open to examining these fears a bit more and we could try some coping strategies together that you might use during the week? A plan of action for the week, until we meet again!
E nods.
N Can we start by sorting out together these fearful thoughts?

Based on This Clinic Anecdote, the Nurse May Consider Many Clinical Strategies

- Explore the reasoning, meaning, and etiology associated with these maladaptive fears. Ask: Do these fears make sense? What would be the consequences of letting these fears persist?
- Distinguish between a belief and a fact. How do the facts impact these intrusive thoughts?
- Ask the individual to consider the impact of *facts* on her emotions and behaviors such as her ability to promote a healthy lifestyle; see friends

- Reassure the individual that experiencing these fears is *normal* so long as this strategy is *short-lived*! [74]
- Provide clinical information that increases feelings of self-efficacy and personal control: a) the *clinical* cues that require a return to *the clinic;* b) health-promoting behaviors and their positive effect on enhancing survival [1]. For instance, use of daily exercise not only promotes physical fitness and effective immune functioning but also reduces emotional distress [75, 76].
- Other options to reduce emotional stress might include using behavioral strategies: the relaxation response technique and mindful meditation which may also be helpful in decreasing the intensity of negative thoughts on emotions and behaviors [77]

Summary of Coping-Promoting Strategies
Strategies include the use of Socratic questioning, distinguishing between a fact and a belief, encouraging patient self-monitoring and self-talk to modulate negative thoughts and to identify potential triggers, use of relevant information and reframing.

Break Down Generalizations into Smaller Manageable Components
(Fig. 9.2) [6]
This is a useful strategy to help an individual effectively reappraise a generalized belief such as "I am a coward" by breaking the thought down into more *manageable* parts (Fig. 9.2). These smaller parts may then be examined with the individual in

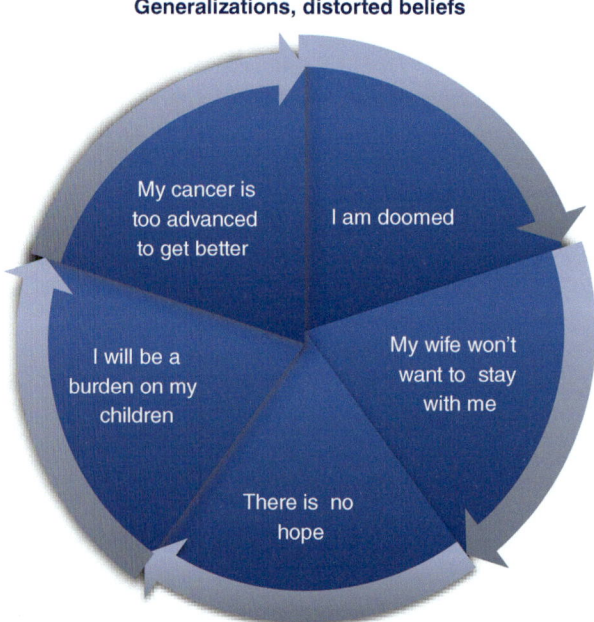

Fig. 9.2 Reducing generalizations into smaller, manageable parts [6]

terms of whether each component is changeable or not; even a persistent threat once broken into smaller parts can become manageable and render a greater sense of personal control to the individual [6]. The following steps are for illustrative purposes:

1. When the patient uses a cognitive distortion such as, "I am doomed," ask what he means by doomed. He might (for illustrative purposes) respond with more specific statements such as (a) I cannot work because of my illness (He may be worried about finances), (b) my wife cannot care for me at home (I cannot care for myself alone), (c) my doctor says my treatment does not follow a protocol (he is afraid he cannot be cured).
2. The nurse and patient now divide and prioritize those parts into (a) changeable or manageable and (b) unchangeable based on the discussion of each component.
3. Together nurse and patient decide how to address each concern via a problem-solving approach (see section "Facilitating Self-Management Strategies"). The patient might propose inviting his wife to the next meeting in order to "brainstorm" together to find reasonable solutions for the patient's "controllable" concerns.
4. The core immutable issue, "achieving a cure," might be addressed through other context-driven options. For arguments sake, the nurse acknowledges the fact that there may be no cure, but provides an alternative option for a quality of life with cancer as a chronic illness and strategies to enhance his resilience, including his immune function and overall health. Many patients fear cancer because they do not realize that given new anticancer therapies, cancer has become a chronic illness for more and more patients, and by adopting healthy lifestyle behaviors they can strengthen their resilience and health (PartV; Part III, Chap. 7).

Living with a chronic illness might lead to a further discussion with the patient and his spouse (family caregiver or significant other) about emotion-regulating and health-promoting lifestyle behaviors as well as the importance of supportive relationships. All enable a better healthier quality of life that can support current treatment and help keep a cancer recurrence at bay. In other clinical contexts, it may be helpful to mention to some highly distressed and reluctant-to-change patients that when we must confront things that cannot be changed, we are still given the opportunity to change how we respond to these life challenges with clear therapeutic benefits such as psychological well-being and acceptance [78].

Use Metaphors and Literary or Music-Related References
Metaphors and aphorisms can be very effective in conveying an important perspective. For instance, "Every cloud has a silver lining," or "it ain't over till it's over" or "no one knows when we are going to die" can come in handy in order to draw a distressed person back from a downward spiral in the conversation. Conversely, a patient may express that "bad things happen to bad people," when in life we know that bad things happen to good people. Through using various metaphors, the nurse can contextualize the individual's experience of cancer toward a more universal human playing field in which we all must learn to deal with the "life we have been

dealt with" in order to find emotional equanimity. Quoting from poetry such as the line in the poem Ulysses by A Tennyson that "we are part of all that we have met" may offer comfort or serve as a segue into existential conversations about the human condition, the spiritual, and our connectedness to all living things and the world. These sayings can foster a shift in thinking toward more positive cognitive reappraisals and deeper more insightful meanings and possibilities in the present life. Using metaphors is often a useful way of talking about a frightening topic; many metaphors have a universal resonance and message that the patient is free to consider without feeling somehow labeled as dysfunctional.

Encourage Positive Affirmations [6, 67]

An affirmation is a positive, meaningful expression in the present tense that enhances emotional well-being or reaffirms a behavioral capability. For instance, an individual on the morning of cancer surgery may use an affirmation, repeatedly to strengthen resolve and capability. "I can do this" or "Just keep going one step at a time." The affirmation is usually made in response to a goal or emotionally charged problem.

Commendations [6, 67]

A commendation is a statement that recognizes the individual's positive changes or evidence of personal growth. For instance, as the individual begins to shift toward a more positive reappraisal of his treatment, the *nurse may offer a commendation* by reviewing the positive changes he has made and the positive impact it has had on his quality of life [67].

Protecting Patient Hope (See Part II, Chap. 5; Part V Chap. 18)

Hope may be defined as "positive expectations for goal attainment" or "beliefs about possibilities for the future" [79]. Hope is a dynamic coping strategy, context-driven that ebbs and flows as a function of changes in the meanings that are attributed, for instance, to cancer-related threats [80]. A qualitative study of hope and healing in patients living with lung cancer revealed the resilience of hope with the identification of four main themes: (1) shattered hope, for instance, when confronting a life-threatening diagnosis, (2) tentative steps toward new hope captured by three subthemes: wanting to return to their former healthy life, pulling themselves out of the "morass" (i.e., due to a lack of hope and exhaustion worrying about the diagnosis), and (3) finding reasons to hope by "imposing order and purpose" in their life that enabled other hoped for possibilities [81].

Hope is a critical strategy for mitigating threats and uncertainty and for maintaining a sense of wholeness especially when patients are facing a life-threatening illness [81]. When patient hopes are inadvertently dashed, the patient may succumb to a sense of despair and hopelessness or existential distress associated with suppressed immune functioning, and an increased inflammatory environment favoring cancer progression that may ultimately lead to a hastened death [82, 83]. Even when hope is unrealistic from a medical perspective, caution must be taken. Unrealistic hope according to Folkman is what most patients may initially experience and indeed even require in order to come to terms with their clinical reality; it rarely becomes an issue of extreme denial [84]. The goal is to acknowledge the patient's hopes allowing him to progress at his own pace in realigning his hopes to functional capabilities and growing understanding of his clinical condition. Thus, the patient must be sensitively redirected in a timely fashion as a function of patient readiness toward clinical realities [74, 85, 86]. Protecting hope may involve drawing on different strategies across phases of the illness. A nurse can help the patient and caregiver to reconceptualize what to hope for as a function of the patient's clinical reality.

Suggested Strategies A patient with a primary tumor and a good prognosis may need the nurse's encouragement *by emphasizing* the likely benefits of the medical treatment be it chemotherapy, surgery, and/or radiation, especially in the early phase of the illness so that the patient's hope for a clinical benefit (Benson's remembered wellness) is nurtured, enabling the mind to activate healing-promoting physiological pathways that may support, in principle, the patient's treatment (see Part IV, Chap. 15 on the Healing Placebo Pathways).

Of course, supporting hope is easy to do when hope is congruent with the clinical expectations of treatment. But even when uncertainty is great, making "room" for the patient's hope is essential [87]. Phrases such as "it is never over till it's over" can provide a leveling perspective that may be hopeful to the patient. When a patient declares that he "hopes for a cure," align your response to his fervent hope with a *supportive phrase* such as "I am wishing you feel better too so let us focus on doing just that" [84].

As cancer progresses, the nurse's interventions may involve reframing the *temporal* context within which hope may still flourish such as "hope for a good day, or week within which the individual can expect to see valued family, great friends, go for a walk during the day or engage in a beloved hobby."

A patient may reject an oncologist's terminal diagnosis leading to a refusal to enter a supportive care program that might in fact prolong his life. "If I acknowledge that the illness is terminal, I will lose all hope." In this example, the nurse may acknowledge the patient's hope to live *"as long as possible"* and discuss how a palliative care program has been shown to do exactly that [88]. In certain contexts, the nurse may choose to gently recognize the patient's desire for hope by referencing hope within the context of life's uncertainties, for instance, by reciting a modified aphorism such as "In life we hope for the best but also plan for the unexpected" suggesting to the patient that uncertainty in life is a shared human condition that allows us to hold two diametrically opposing ideas at the same time that can still provide comfort [84].

Individuals with advanced or terminal cancer hold on to hope even as shifting clinical conditions increasingly alter the hopes they express. With advancing disease hope becomes progressively telescoped by diminishing physical and functional parameters. Ultimately hope is embedded in the most fundamental human behaviors: the presence of loved ones, a last goodbye, or the desire for a peaceful death. One of the most hopeful gifts my oncologist gave to me was stating that we could work together on my getting better: He would focus on eliminating the tumor, while I would focus on staying calm to prevent exacerbating the tumor's growth. He would monitor my treatment while I would take 30-minute daily walks as much as possible to strengthen my overall health to fight the cancer or live well with it. It was a very powerful message of hope even though we *both knew* how advanced my cancer was! The nurse's or oncologist's stated intent to collaborate with the patient toward realizing a shared clinical goal is not only empowering but embeds a sense of security that protects the patient's sense *of hope*.

Promote a Sense of Personal Control
The patient's need for personal control is a coping strategy that is often severely challenged by his changing clinical status or treatment. Some patients feel most comfortable when the HCP is completely in charge of the treatment and clinical decision making. Other patients experience difficulty yielding complete control for their health to the team. A working hypothesis is to always invite the patient to take the lead, for instance, during coping-promoting interventions. You might ask: "Would you be comfortable sharing your story about the events leading up to your diagnosis or cancer recurrence, sharing only as much as you wish." In the section on cognitive restructuring interventions, perhaps also preface your questions about the patient's beliefs by asking permission, such as *"Would it be okay* to explore where these thoughts come from." Insightful practitioners will also explore with a patient the extent to which they would like to be involved in clinical decisions about the course of the treatment or preferences surrounding supportive care interventions.

Astin's [89] research findings suggest that a combination of coping strategies regarding personal control may result in better resilient outcomes. Women who were able to balance their high desire for personal control with acceptance of the need to yield control over some health-related matters had the best psychological outcomes; those with a high desire for personal control and high resistance to letting go of control fared the worst psychologically, as measured by quality of life, depression, and anxiety. It seems that the optimal situation is to enable patients with cancer through a process of negotiation and relevant information, to toggle between their own personal capabilities and those of the healthcare team responsible for their care and treatment.

While it is incumbent upon the nurse whenever possible to support the person's need to maintain personal control over his or her medical treatment, it may become a clinical challenge when the patient's desire for personal control over all aspects of his or her treatments interfere with the timing of medical versus other preferred treatment

Clinical Anecdote 9.4
R was a First Nations mother and grandmother who had lived her whole life on a reservation outside the city. When she was diagnosed with cancer, she was extremely reluctant to begin chemotherapy, strongly believing that a mixture of medicinal herbs passed down through her culture and traditions was a better option for maintaining

her wellness. Conversely the treating oncologist was reluctant to start chemotherapy if R was planning to pursue herbal treatment. At a stalemate, the nurse met with R. By sharing their respective philosophies for getting better, they arrived at a shared belief that both treatment modalities working together could be better than either one alone. And they came to a clinical decision in which herbs would be taken between chemotherapy sessions, leaving a window of no treatment for 48 h on either side of chemotherapy, to avoid the possibility of interactional effects.

Within a nonjudgmental, supportive, and information sharing nurse–patient relationship, patients may be facilitated to embrace new possibilities without personal cost to their self-worth. By valuing the shared health goals of *both* medical traditions while explaining the need to avoid interactional medicinal effects that can occur if both are given at the same time, it was possible to find a win–win solution.

Acceptance

Acceptance as a coping strategy is associated with less anxiety and depression and greater quality of life in noncancer and cancer populations [90]. The process of arriving at *acceptance* of one's clinical reality may involve distinguishing between a situation that cannot be realistically altered and acting on those elements within the stressful situation that can be changed, such as one's emotional responses to the terminal phase of cancer [78, 91]. Ultimately, it may come down to the personal realization that a choice between continuing to suffer psychologically or accepting the clinical circumstances is a matter of personal choice [78].

Relevant information, use of reframing, and a supportive caregiver (family) and healthcare provider (nurse)–patient relationship may facilitate acceptance. Often a meaning-making intervention such as a life review (see Part IV Chap. 10) can facilitate the process of acceptance. This involves exploration of the patient's global, situational, and self-related assumptions and beliefs though the process of directed narratives or storytelling (see Part IV Chap. 10). Part of this exploration has to do with discovering new goals and purposes in meaningful relationships, spiritual connections, hobbies, or work [61, 92].

Facilitating Self-Management Strategies [1, 14]

Patient care and treatments for cancer increasingly occur in outpatient clinics necessitating greater participation by the patient and caregiver in managing their care between treatments. Similarly, patients with advanced or terminal cancer may prefer to receive palliative care at home. Resilient patients and caregivers may be encouraged to actively engage with the nurse in learning how to better manage current and future practical health-related care issues or problems associated with the cancer or treatment to facilitate a sense of self-efficacy and managerial competence, starting even in the diagnostic phase (Table 9.4).

For instance, the nurse may support the patient and caregiver in acquiring new skills to manage the changes in his or her life roles, patient symptoms, assessing physical wounds, and changing dressings at home [14]. The steps involved in problem solving are consistent across clinical concerns and are aimed at finding effective solutions. The nurse helps the patient and caregiver merely to tailor that process to

Table 9.4 Examples of SMI: psychosocial, educational, and/or psychoeducational content [14, 30]

Content areas
1. Provide emotional care, suggested resources, 24/7 telephone support [93]
2. Psychoeducational: For example, provide information on indicators of caregiver stress and burnout, strategies to manage negative emotions such as frustration and anticipatory grief as well as self-care suggestions to protect or enhance caregiver health [94]
3. Educational/informational: regarding symptom management, information about SMI role, nutrition, physical exercise and relaxation response based on patient and caregiver needs [29, 88, 95, 96]
4 Psychoeducational information tailored to caregiver needs, in order to improve psychological well-being, identify positive aspects of role, and prepare for the effects of patient's passing (bereavement) [97]
5. Dyadic approach to reduce stress, maintain hope, and meet information needs: focused on family involvement, optimistic attitude, coping strategies, reducing uncertainty, managing symptoms [18, 32, 98]

the specific demands of the clinical issue. Promoting self-management skills in patients and caregivers can enhance a sense of self-efficacy, and provide better symptom management and utilization of relevant health resources that also facilitate emotion regulation. The ability of the individual to manage practical problems occurs within a family context as much as possible, but is always embedded within a collaborative nurse–patient and/or caregiver partnership oriented toward optimizing the wellness of patient and caregiver [1].

Core SMI Content

Problem-solving strategies are used for different contexts and concerns [6, 67]. One nursing objective has to do with providing generally resilient patients and caregivers with the knowledge and skills to successfully manage practical cancer- or treatment-related concerns. SMIs are designed around conventional problem-solving coping strategies and consist of the following steps:

1. a well-defined practical problem
2. defined goal, desired outcome(s), and steps to get there
3. relevant information about the disease, treatment, and healthcare resources, for instance, how to detect prodromal cues of nausea or pain
4. partnerships with healthcare providers, in this instance, the nurse,
5. skills to develop detailed *action plans*. An action plan is usually the outcome of a clinically related practical problem requiring a purposeful plan of action. The plan will only work if its purpose is in keeping with the person's beliefs about its clinical benefits
6. implementation, evaluation, and modifications as needed

7. regular support and reassurance with nurse-initiated telephone contacts
8. counseling as needed

Desired outcomes include enhanced self-efficacy, health-related quality of life, and appropriate utilization of health resources. One example of a practical problem arising from changing life roles is a caregiver's increased responsibilities for caregiving and in this specific instance learning to administer narcotics to manage patient pain at home in the terminal phase of the illness.

Example of an Action Plan
An action plan is the detailed response to a specific problem tailored to successfully manage it within the context of a nurse/patient/or caregiver partnership. An action plan specifies:

1. The *goal: A behavioral objective* (e.g., to take your prechemotherapy and postchemotherapy antinausea medication.
2. *When* (the action is to occur): For instance, the evening and morning prior to and for 3 days after treatment, specifically, before going to bed and the following morning after breakfast with a glass of water or juice.
3. *Where:* In the kitchen.
4. *Delineate set of clinical expectations*: You should not experience either nausea or vomiting before, during, and after the chemotherapy.
5. *Simple written instructions developed by the patient or caregiver with the nurse's support and reviewed* a final time altogether.
6. *Patient feedback:* Finally, the individual is asked to provide feedback after its implementation within a prespecified time frame such as 24 h later (to increase a sense of personal accountability). What were the experienced benefits to the patient and caregiver? What were the problems?

9.6 Final Thoughts

Perhaps, one of the most important things a nurse can do for a patient and the family caregiver is to anticipate the clinical moments likely to increase emotional distress across the illness, treatment, transition to survivorship, and end-of-life phases and to *proactively act* to provide needed knowledge and skills in order to help manage these moments of vulnerability. Each stressful phase may require an involved nurse to support the patient and loved one in acquiring effective cognitive and behavioral coping strategies. In the next chapter, we focus on meaning which pervades all aspects of effective coping.

Appendix: Psychosocial Interventions—Cognitive–Behavioral Therapy/Cognitive–Behavioral Stress Management Interventions/Self-Efficacy

Author	Purpose/intervention	Study design	Sample/phase of disease	Outcomes
Greer et al. [99]	Assess efficacy of *cognitive–behavioral intervention* on anxiety 6 weekly sessions: (setting goals, education on anxiety, relaxation and coping skills, planning, pacing)	Pilot RCT RA to: (a) CBT (b) Waitlist controls	$N = 40$ terminally ill patients with cancer	(1) Large treatment effects with significant reduction in anxiety
Lau et al. [22] (Part I)	Compared efficacy of *cognitive–behavioral therapy (CBT)* with *integrative mind-body-spirit (IBMS)* intervention in *PATIENTS* based on patient-caregiver parallel groups. (This paper reported patient findings) See Xiu et al. [100] below for description of interventions	RCT RA: (a) CBT ($n = 81$) (b) IBMS ($n = 76$) No control group Patient assessments at baseline, 1, 8, 16 weeks postintervention	$N = 157$ dyads of patients with lung cancer in Hong Kong	(1) CBT showed significantly larger reduction in emotional vulnerability than IBMS (2) IBMS showed larger increase in QOL and spiritual self-care, and greater reduction in depression than CBT (3) Patients in both groups improved in physical, emotional, spiritual but not social areas of QOL

| Jassim et al. [24] | Effectiveness of psychological interventions (24 CBT trials) and (4 psychotherapy trials) on psychological morbidities, quality of life, and *survival in women* with nonmetastatic breast cancer

Interventions
(a) CBT (24/28) aimed at changing thoughts and behaviors about a stressor. Focuses on problem-solving and changing dysfunctional thoughts (beliefs), behaviors, and emotions that interfere with adaptation to a stressor; also other modalities such as progressive muscle relaxation and mindfulness mediation to reduce emotional distress
(b) 4 studies based on psychotherapy | Cochrane library meta-analysis using 28 RCTS ($n = 3940$) participants | $N = 3940$ women with cancer | (1) Pooled standardized mean differences from baseline showed significantly less depression ($P = 0.02$)
(2) 7 studies ($n = 637$) with poor evidence of quality ($I^2 = 95\%$) improved anxiety ($P = 0.0006$)
(3) 8 studies ($n = 776$) with low quality evidence ($I^2 = 64\%$) improved mood disturbance ($P = 0.0003$)
(4) 8 studies ($n = 1536$) showed moderate ($I^2 = 47\%$) quality evidence for the *cognitive–behavioral group rather than the control group*
(5) Only one individually delivered CB intervention significantly enhanced quality of life compared to controls ($P = 0.03$)
(6) Pooled data from 2 group studies showed a nonsignificant overall survival benefit using a CB intervention compared to controls ($P = 0.62$) and with low quality evidence ($I^2 = 0.84\%$)

Conclusion Compared to controls, findings suggest that CBT interventions led to significant decreases in anxiety, depression, and mood disturbances especially when delivered to groups of women. Suggests that what patients want are practical coping-related strategies to address anxiety and depressed mood |

(continued)

Appendix (continued)

Author	Purpose/intervention	Study design	Sample/phase of disease	Outcomes
Xiu et al. [100] (Part II)	Compared efficacy of *cognitive–behavioral therapy (CBT)* with integrative mind-body-spirit (IBMS) intervention in *CAREGIVERS* based on patient-caregiver parallel groups. (This paper reported caregiver findings) *Description of interventions*: *CBT*: relaxation techniques, identify negative thoughts, dysfunctional ways/patterns of coping, used cognitive/behavioral strategies to reduce anxiety and depressed mood; develop strategies to change "dysfunctional" attitudes, values, and implement pleasurable plans *IMBS* Participants learned about holistic well-being, acupressure, qigong, MM, life review	RCT RA (a) CBT ($n = 81$) b) IBMS ($n = 76$) No control group Patient assessments at baseline, 1, 8, 16 weeks postintervention	Caregivers from $N = 157$ dyads of patients and caregivers with lung cancer in Hong Kong	(1) Family caregivers in both groups showed significant moderate effect size improvement in QOL postintervention and follow-up assessments (2) Improvement in insomnia at T1 for both groups that decreased at follow-up (3) Both groups decreased anxiety and perceived stress at follow-up (4) NS in domains of family caregiver burden and depression

Antoni et al. [5]	To evaluate the effects of a *cognitive–behavioral stress management (CBSM)* intervention on negative affect and cognition on anxiety-related transcriptional changes in women during primary treatment for breast cancer. *Intervention* CBSR is a 10-week intervention focused on (a) reducing anxiety (b) increasing coping skills (c) *cognitive restructuring of distorted beliefs*; (d) and relaxation exercises with imagery, didactic explanations, role playing, communication skills, home assignments (such as practicing relaxation and keeping written record of perceived stresses during the week).	RCT RA to (a) CBSM group—10 weeks (b) Psycho-educational intervention—1 day Assessments at baseline, 6 and 12 month follow-ups *Plus:* 79 patients provided peripheral blood leukocyte samples for genome-related transcriptional profiling	199 women with stage 1-111 breast cancer during treatment	(1) *Baseline high negative affect was associated with >50% expression of 201 leukocyte transcripts that include activated expression of pro-inflammatory and metastases-related genes* (2) 10-week CBT intervention *reversed* anxiety-related upregulation of pro-inflammatory gene expression in circulating leukocytes (e.g., IL1A, IL-6, TNF, COX2) (3) Increased Th1 cytokines such as Il-2, IL12, IFN-γ (against pathogens and cancer control) (4) Findings demonstrated molecular signaling pathways by which behavioral interventions can affect physical health by downregulating peripheral inflammatory processes such as NFKB/rel, factors, COX2 and other pro-inflammatory cytokines
Antoni et al. [101]	Effects of a cognitive–behavioral stress management (CBSM) intervention on cancer-specific anxiety, general symptoms of anxiety, serum cortisol, and in vitro Th1 and Th2 cytokine production in women after surgery during treatment *Intervention* See Antoni et al. [5]	RA to (a) CBSM group—10 weeks (b) Psycho-educational group—1 day	Substudy of larger study: 97/199 women with stage 0-111 breast cancer during treatment who had complete data on cortisol and anxiety; and 85 provided immune data	(1) The CBSM group showed significantly (a) reduced levels of cancer-specific anxiety and interviewer rated general anxiety, (b) lower cortisol, and (c) higher production of Th1 cytokines (IL-2, interferon-γ and a IL-2/IL-4 ratio, compared to controls) (2) The effects on anxiety and cortisol held across 12 months (3) The TH-1 changes held only for the first 6 months *Comment:* Th-1 cytokines stimulate development of cell-mediated immune responses against viruses and tumor cells

(continued)

Appendix (continued)

Author	Purpose/intervention	Study design	Sample/phase of disease	Outcomes
Cohen et al. [102]	To assess whether a pre-/postsurgical stress management (SM) intervention improves immune functions in men undergoing surgery for prostate cancer *Intervention* (a) CBT consisted of (1) *2-session presurgical intervention* Info about prostate cancer and surgery, discussed concerns about surgery; taught diaphragmatic breathing, guided imagery, relaxation skills (2) *session 2*—imagined what the surgery would be like; learned problem-solving coping skills, support seeking behaviors, realistic expectations (3) booster sessions on the morning of surgery, and 48 h postsurgery to boost problem-solving approaches, and use of relaxation exercises (b) Supportive attention (SA) (1) 2 sessions provided empathy, detailed psychosocial interview, reflective listening skills, discussed patient concerns (2) Brief boosters on the morning of surgery, 48 h postsurgery	159 RA to (a) stress management (SM) (b) supportive attention (SA) (c) standard care (SC)	Men with early-stage prostate cancer	*The SM intervention* (1) SM group showed significantly higher levels of NK cell cytotoxicity ($p = 0.04$) (2) Increased levels of circulating pro-inflammatory cytokines (IL-12p70) ($p = 0.02$); IL-1b ($p = 0.02$); TNF-α ($p = 0.05$) compared to SA *group* 48 h postsurgery (3) SM group had higher levels of NK cell cytotoxicity ($p = 0.02$) and IL-1B ($p = 0.05$) compared to SC (4) Immune parameters increased for SM group; but decreased or stayed the same for SA and SC groups (5) SM group had significantly better mood scores than SC group ($p = 0.006$) (6) Changes in mood were not related to immune outcomes *Conclusion* Results show potential psychological and immune benefits of presurgical SM intervention. Although findings were statistically significant, they may not have been clinically significant No reference to blinding; inclusion criteria did not target only distressed individuals; findings may change in patients with late-stage prostate cancer

| Kwekkeboom et al. [103] | To investigate (1) effect of cognitive behavioral strategies on symptom cluster burden of pain, fatigue, and sleep disturbances, (2) moderating effects of a number of symptoms or imaging capability on the intervention's impact on outcomes of distress, symptom cluster severity and interference of pain, fatigue and sleep disturbances with daily life (i.e., Interference subscale from MD Anderson Symptom Inventory), (3) mediating effects | RCT 9-week intervention RA to (1) intervention of imagery, relaxation, and distraction strategies (2) cancer education using recordings (attention control) Assessments at: baseline, 3, 6, 9 weeks Interventions by trained nurses, psychologists using a manualized intervention | 164 patients with advanced cancer and on chemotherapy | (1) The CBS intervention was effective in reducing distress from symptom cluster at week 6 only compared to recording condition ($M = 1.82$ vs 2.15, $p < 0.05$) (2) Fewer concurrent symptoms were associated with the CBS intervention being effective in controlling symptom cluster interference (Week 6: $F_{9(1,126)} = 3.88$; $p = 0.03$; Week 9: $F_{(1,126)} = 4.47$, $p = 0.02$) (3) Mediating effects significant at weeks 6 and 9 Regarding: (a) change in stress due to the intervention at week 9 was a significant mediator that significantly reduced symptom cluster severity, distress, and interference (see p. 13) (b) change in outcome expectancy from the intervention at week 6 and week 9 was a significant mediator that significantly reduced symptom cluster interference (p. 13) (c) change in perceived control was a significant mediator that reduced all three outcome measures of symptom cluster severity, distress, and interference Conclusions Although the effectiveness of the intervention showed only modest improvement at week 6, the mediating effect analyses revealed insights into the therapeutic effects of the intervention which in turn significantly improved patient outcomes compared to the control condition |

(continued)

Appendix (continued)

Author	Purpose/intervention	Study design	Sample/phase of disease	Outcomes

Guarino et al. [104]	To assess efficacy of CBT, supportive expressive therapy (SET) and psychoeducational therapy (PET) for women with breast cancer
	(1) CBT ($K = 17$)
	  (a) Focus on ↑affective state and coping with cancer by modifying maladaptive mental schema and ↓ distress, ↓intrusive ideation
	(2) SET ($K = 4$)
	  (a) Cognitive-emotional focused therapy aimed at ↑ development of social support (SS) and emotional expression and examines existential concerns
	(3) Psychoeducation (PET) ($K = 4$) interdisciplinary approach includes
	  (a) Provide education regarding disease, treatments
	  (b) Provide affective, cognitive skills related to coping with experience of illness
		Systematic review/meta-analysis of 25 studies	7834/8472 Women with breast cancer who completed pre-/postassessments	1. QOL
				  a. Meta-analysis based on all 3 interventions ($k = 13$) showed a nonsignificant improvement in QOL based on a medium effect size (0.38, 95% CI, −0.07 to 0.84) $I^2 = 98\%$
				  Subanalyses
				  b. CBT ($k = 8$) improved QOL life based on the highest effect size although not significant ($d = 0.55$ (−0.25 to 1.35) $I^2 = 0.99\%$
				  c. SET ($k = 1$) decreased quality of life with a small nonsignificant effect size ($d = 0.11$ (−0.15 to −0.07)
				2. Anxiety
				  a. Meta-analysis with 10 studies showed anxiety was reduced posttreatment with a medium effect size that was nonsignificant ($d = −0.39$ (−0.91 to 0.14) $I^2 = 98\%$
				  b. PET ($K = 1$) showed medium posttreatment reducing effects for anxiety that were significant ($d = −0.45$ (−0.49 to −0.40)
				  c. SET ($K = 1$) showed a small increased effect posttreatment in anxiety that was significant ($d = 0.10$ (0.02–0.18)
				3. Depression
				  a. Meta-analysis with 12 studies showed a significant medium posttreatment effect that reduced depression $d = −0.35$ (−0.79 to −0.10) $I^2 = 98\%$
				  b. CBT ($k = 10$) showed a medium effect size reduction in depression that was not significant ($d = −0.42$ (−0.06 to 0.12)
				  c. SET ($k = 2$) showed a nonsignificant small effect size decrease in depression ($d = −0.10$ (−2.18 to 2.16) $I^2 = 0.98\%$
				4. Mood ($K = 10$)
				  a. Meta-analysis with 10 studies produced a nonsignificant small effect reduction in mood (i.e., improved mood) $d = −0.17$ (−0.41 to 0.06)
				  b. PET ($K = 3$) showed a nonsignificant medium effect reduction for mood ($d = −0.34$ (−1.05 to 0.36) $I^2 = 97\%$

References

1. McCorkle R, Ercolano E, Lazenby M, Schulman-Green D, Schilling LS, Lorig K, et al. Self-management: enabling and empowering patients living with cancer as a chronic illness. CA Cancer J Clin. 2011;61(1):50–62. PubMed PMID: 21205833. Pubmed Central PMCID: PMC3058905. Epub 2011/01/06. eng.
2. Hagger MS, Koch S, Chatzisarantis NLD, Orbell S. The common sense model of self-regulation: meta-analysis and test of a process model. Psychol Bull. 2017;143(11):1117–54. PubMed PMID: 28805401. Epub 2017/08/15. eng.
3. Chirico A, Lucidi F, Merluzzi T, Alivernini F, Laurentiis M, Botti G, et al. A meta-analytic review of the relationship of cancer coping self-efficacy with distress and quality of life. Oncotarget. 2017;8(22):36800–11. PubMed PMID: 28404938. Pubmed Central PMCID: PMC5482699. Epub 2017/04/14. eng.
4. Lazarus R. Stress, appraisal and coping. New York: Springer; 1984.
5. Antoni MH, Lutgendorf SK, Blomberg B, Carver CS, Lechner S, Diaz A, et al. Cognitive-behavioral stress management reverses anxiety-related leukocyte transcriptional dynamics. Biol Psychiatry. 2012;71(4):366–72. PubMed PMID: 22088795. Pubmed Central PMCID: PMC3264698. Epub 2011/11/18. eng.
6. Meichenbaum D. A clinical handbook for assessing and treating adults with post-traumatic stress disorder (PTSD). Waterloo: Institute Press; 1994.
7. Reb A, Ruel N, Fakih M, Lai L, Salgia R, Ferrell B, et al. Empowering survivors after colorectal and lung cancer treatment: pilot study of a self-management survivorship care planning intervention. Eur J Oncol Nurs. 2017;29:125–34. PubMed PMID: 28720259. Pubmed Central PMCID: PMC5539921. Epub 2017/07/20. eng.
8. Badr H, Smith CB, Goldstein NE, Gomez JE, Redd WH. Dyadic psychosocial intervention for advanced lung cancer patients and their family caregivers: results of a randomized pilot trial. Cancer. 2015;121(1):150–8. PubMed PMID: 25209975. Pubmed Central PMCID: PMC4270818. Epub 2014/09/12. eng.
9. Haun MW, Estel S, Rucker G, Friederich HC, Villalobos M, Thomas M, et al. Early palliative care for adults with advanced cancer. Cochrane Database Syst Rev. 2017;6:CD011129. PubMed PMID: 28603881. Pubmed Central PMCID: PMC6481832. Epub 2017/06/13. eng.
10. McEwen BS, Gianaros PJ. Stress- and allostasis-induced brain plasticity. Annu Rev Med. 2011;62:431–45. PubMed PMID: 20707675. Pubmed Central PMCID: PMC4251716. Epub 2010/08/17. eng.
11. Dunkel-Schetter C, Feinstein LG, Taylor SE, Falke RL. Patterns of coping with cancer. Health Psychol. 1992;11(2):79–87. PubMed PMID: 1582383. Epub 1992/01/01. eng.
12. Park C, Folkman S. Meaning in the context of stress and coping. Rev Gen Psychol. 1997;1:115–44.
13. Park CL. Making sense of the meaning literature: an integrative review of meaning making and its effects on adjustment to stressful life events. Psychol Bull. 2010;136(2):257–301. PubMed PMID: 20192563. Epub 2010/03/03. eng.
14. Leventhal H, Phillips LA, Burns E. The common-sense model of self-regulation (CSM): a dynamic framework for understanding illness self-management. J Behav Med. 2016;39(6):935–46. PubMed PMID: 27515801. Epub 2016/08/16. eng.
15. Folkman S, Lazarus RS, Gruen RJ, DeLongis A. Appraisal, coping, health status, and psychological symptoms. J Pers Soc Psychol. 1986;50(3):571–9. PubMed PMID: 3701593. Epub 1986/03/01. eng.
16. Folkman S, Lazarus RS, Dunkel-Schetter C, DeLongis A, Gruen RJ. Dynamics of a stressful encounter: cognitive appraisal, coping, and encounter outcomes. J Pers Soc Psychol. 1986;50(5):992–1003. PubMed PMID: 3712234. Epub 1986/05/01. eng.
17. McCorkle R, Strumpf NE, Nuamah IF, Adler DC, Cooley ME, Jepson C, et al. A specialized home care intervention improves survival among older post-surgical cancer patients. J Am Geriatr Soc. 2000;48(12):1707–13. PubMed PMID: 11129765. Epub 2000/12/29. eng.

18. Dionne-Odom JN, Azuero A, Lyons KD, Hull JG, Tosteson T, Li Z, et al. Benefits of early versus delayed palliative care to informal family caregivers of patients with advanced cancer: outcomes from the ENABLE III randomized controlled trial. J Clin Oncol. 2015;33(13):1446–52. PubMed PMID: 25800762. Pubmed Central PMCID: PMC4404423 online at www.jco.org. Author contributions are found at the end of this article. Epub 2015/03/25. eng.
19. Bhasin MK, Dusek JA, Chang BH, Joseph MG, Denninger JW, Fricchione GL, et al. Relaxation response induces temporal transcriptome changes in energy metabolism, insulin secretion and inflammatory pathways. PLoS One. 2013;8(5):e62817. PubMed PMID: 23650531. Pubmed Central PMCID: PMC3641112. Epub 2013/05/08. eng.
20. Carlson LE, Tamagawa R, Stephen J, Drysdale E, Zhong L, Speca M. Randomized-controlled trial of mindfulness-based cancer recovery versus supportive expressive group therapy among distressed breast cancer survivors (MINDSET): long-term follow-up results. Psycho-Oncology. 2016;25(7):750–9. PubMed PMID: 27193737. Epub 2016/05/20. eng.
21. Kabat ZJ. Full catastrophe living: using the wisdom of your body and mind to face stress, pain and illness. New York: Delacourt; 1990.
22. Lau BH, Chow AY, Ng TK, Fung YL, Lam TC, So TH, et al. Comparing the efficacy of integrative body-mind-spirit intervention with cognitive behavioral therapy in patient-caregiver parallel groups for lung cancer patients using a randomized controlled trial. J Psychosoc Oncol. 2020;38(4):389–405. PubMed PMID: 32146876. Epub 2020/03/10. eng.
23. Antoni MH. Psychosocial intervention effects on adaptation, disease course and biobehavioral processes in cancer. Brain Behav Immun. 2013;30:88–98. PubMed PMID: 22627072. Pubmed Central PMCID: PMC3444659. Epub 2012/05/26. eng.
24. Jassim GA, Whitford DL, Hickey A, Carter B. Psychological interventions for women with non-metastatic breast cancer. Cochrane Database Syst Rev. 2015;5:CD008729. PubMed PMID: 26017383. Epub 2015/05/29. eng.
25. Antoni MH, Carrico AW, Duran RE, Spitzer S, Penedo F, Ironson G, et al. Randomized clinical trial of cognitive behavioral stress management on human immunodeficiency virus viral load in gay men treated with highly active antiretroviral therapy. Psychosom Med. 2006;68(1):143–51. PubMed PMID: 16449425. Epub 2006/02/02. eng.
26. Huang J, Han Y, Wei J, Liu X, Du Y, Yang L, et al. The effectiveness of the internet-based self-management program for cancer-related fatigue patients: a systematic review and meta-analysis. Clin Rehabil. 2020;34(3):287–98. PubMed PMID: 31793340. Epub 2019/12/04. eng.
27. Kim SH, Kim K, Mayer DK. Self-management intervention for adult cancer survivors after treatment: a systematic review and meta-analysis. Oncol Nurs Forum. 2017;44(6):719–28. PubMed PMID: 29052663. Epub 2017/10/21. eng.
28. Goldberg JI, Schulman-Green D, Hernandez M, Nelson JE, Capezuti E. Self-management interventions for psychological distress in adult cancer patients: a systematic review. West J Nurs Res. 2019;41(10):1407–22. PubMed PMID: 31007160. Epub 2019/04/23. eng.
29. Bakitas MA, Tosteson TD, Li Z, Lyons KD, Hull JG, Li Z, et al. Early versus delayed initiation of concurrent palliative oncology care: patient outcomes in the ENABLE III randomized controlled trial. J Clin Oncol. 2015;33(13):1438–45. Pubmed Central PMCID: PMC4404422 online at www.jco.org. Author contributions are found at the end of this article. Epub 2015/03/25. eng.
30. Ahn S, Romo RD, Campbell CL. A systematic review of interventions for family caregivers who care for patients with advanced cancer at home. Patient Educ Couns. 2020;103(8):1518–30. PubMed PMID: 32201172. Pubmed Central PMCID: PMC7311285. Epub 2020/03/24. eng.
31. Cuthbert CA, Farragher JF, Hemmelgarn BR, Ding Q, McKinnon GP, Cheung WY. Self-management interventions for cancer survivors: a systematic review and evaluation of intervention content and theories. Psycho-Oncology. 2019;28(11):2119–40. PubMed PMID: 31475766. Epub 2019/09/03. eng.
32. Dionne-Odom JN, Taylor R, Rocque G, Chambless C, Ramsey T, Azuero A, et al. Adapting an early palliative care intervention to family caregivers of persons with advanced can-

cer in the rural deep South: a qualitative formative evaluation. J Pain Symptom Manag. 2018;55(6):1519–30. Pubmed Central PMCID: PMC5951755. Epub 2018/02/24. eng.
33. Badr H, Herbert K, Chhabria K, Sandulache VC, Chiao EY, Wagner T. Self-management intervention for head and neck cancer couples: results of a randomized pilot trial. Cancer. 2019;125(7):1176–84. PubMed PMID: 30521075. Pubmed Central PMCID: PMC6420382. Epub 2018/12/07. eng.
34. McEwen BS, Gray J, Nasca C. Recognizing resilience: learning from the effects of stress on the brain. Neurobiol Stress. 2015;1:1–11. PubMed PMID: 25506601. Pubmed Central PMCID: PMC4260341. Epub 2014/12/17. Eng.
35. Eicher M, Matzka M, Dubey C, White K. Resilience in adult cancer care: an integrative literature review. Oncol Nurs Forum. 2015;42(1):3–16. PubMed PMID: 25542332. Epub 2014/12/30. eng.
36. Hagger MS. A meta-analytic review of the common sense model of illness representations. Psychol Health. 2003;18(2):141–84.
37. Bakitas M, Lyons KD, Hegel MT, Balan S, Brokaw FC, Seville J, et al. Effects of a palliative care intervention on clinical outcomes in patients with advanced cancer: the Project ENABLE II randomized controlled trial. JAMA. 2009;302(7):741–9. PubMed PMID: 19690306. Pubmed Central PMCID: PMC3657724. Epub 2009/08/20. eng.
38. Riba MB, Donovan KA, Andersen B, Braun I, Breitbart WS, Brewer BW, et al. Distress management, version 3.2019, NCCN clinical practice guidelines in oncology. JNCCN. 2019;17(10):1229–49. PubMed PMID: 31590149. Pubmed Central PMCID: PMC6907687. Epub 2019/10/08. eng.
39. Folkman S, Greer S. Promoting psychological well-being in the face of serious illness: when theory, research and practice inform each other. Psycho-Oncology. 2000;9(1):11–9. PubMed PMID: 10668055. Epub 2000/02/11. eng.
40. Karatsoreos IN, McEwen BS. The neurobiology and physiology of resilience and adaptation across the life course. J Child Psychol Psychiatry. 2013;54(4):337–47. PubMed PMID: 23517425. Epub 2013/03/23. eng.
41. Jim HS, Pustejovsky JE, Park CL, Danhauer SC, Sherman AC, Fitchett G, et al. Religion, spirituality, and physical health in cancer patients: a meta-analysis. Cancer. 2015;121(21):3760–8. PubMed PMID: 26258868. Pubmed Central PMCID: PMC4618080. Epub 2015/08/11. eng.
42. Park CL. Meaning making in the context of disasters. J Clin Psychol. 2016;72(12):1234–46. PubMed PMID: 26900868. Epub 2016/02/24. eng.
43. Lee V. The existential plight of cancer: meaning making as a concrete approach to the intangible search for meaning. Support Care Cancer. 2008;16(7):779–85. PubMed PMID: 18197427. Epub 2008/01/17. eng.
44. Lee V, Cohen SR, Edgar L, Laizner AM, Gagnon AJ. Meaning-making and psychological adjustment to cancer: development of an intervention and pilot results. Oncol Nurs Forum. 2006;33(2):291–302. PubMed PMID: 16518445. Epub 2006/03/07. eng.
45. Cao W, Qi X, Cai DA, Han X. Modeling posttraumatic growth among cancer patients: the roles of social support, appraisals, and adaptive coping. Psycho-Oncology. 2018;27(1):208–15. PubMed PMID: 28171681. Epub 2017/02/09. eng.
46. Dunkel-Schetter C, Folkman S, Lazarus RS. Correlates of social support receipt. J Pers Soc Psychol. 1987;53(1):71–80. PubMed PMID: 3612494. Epub 1987/07/01. eng.
47. Sumpio C, Jeon S, Northouse LL, Knobf MT. Optimism, symptom distress, illness appraisal, and coping in patients with advanced-stage cancer diagnoses undergoing chemotherapy treatment. Oncol Nurs Forum. 2017;44(3):384–92. PubMed PMID: 28635986. Epub 2017/06/22. eng.
48. Holahan CJ, Moos RH, Holahan CK, Brennan PL, Schutte KK. Stress generation, avoidance coping, and depressive symptoms: a 10-year model. J Consult Clin Psychol. 2005;73(4):658–66. PubMed PMID: 16173853. Pubmed Central PMCID: PMC3035563. Epub 2005/09/22. eng.

49. Bigatti SM, Steiner JL, Miller KD. Cognitive appraisals, coping and depressive symptoms in breast cancer patients. Stress Health. 2012;28(5):355–61. PubMed PMID: 22888085. Pubmed Central PMCID: PMC4105002. Epub 2012/08/14. eng.
50. Wenzlaff RM, Wegner DM. Thought suppression. Annu Rev Psychol. 2000;51:59–91. PubMed PMID: 10751965. Epub 2001/02/07. eng.
51. Gross JJ. Antecedent- and response-focused emotion regulation: divergent consequences for experience, expression, and physiology. J Pers Soc Psychol. 1998;74(1):224–37. PubMed PMID: 9457784. Epub 1998/02/11. eng.
52. Hofmann SG, Asmundson GJG. Acceptance and mindfulness-based therapy: new wave or old hat? Clin Psychol Rev. 2008;28(1):1–16. PubMed PMID: 17904260. Epub 2007/10/02. eng.
53. Creamer M, Burgess P, Pattison P. Reaction to trauma: a cognitive processing model. J Abnorm Psychol. 1992;101(3):452–9. PubMed PMID: 1500602. Epub 1992/08/01. eng.
54. Müller F, Hagedoorn M, Soriano EC, Stephenson E, Smink A, Hoff C, et al. Couples' catastrophizing and co-rumination: dyadic diary study of patient fatigue after cancer. Health Psychol. 2019;38(12):1096–106. PubMed PMID: 31580128. Epub 2019/10/04. eng.
55. Hopman P, Rijken M. Illness perceptions of cancer patients: relationships with illness characteristics and coping. Psycho-Oncology. 2015;24(1):11–8. PubMed PMID: 24891136. Epub 2014/06/04. eng.
56. McEwen BS. Physiology and neurobiology of stress and adaptation: central role of the brain. Physiol Rev. 2007;87(3):873–904. PubMed PMID: 17615391. Epub 2007/07/07. eng.
57. Andersen BL, Farrar WB, Golden-Kreutz DM, Glaser R, Emery CF, Crespin TR, et al. Psychological, behavioral, and immune changes after a psychological intervention: a clinical trial. J Clin Oncol. 2004;22(17):3570–80. PubMed PMID: 15337807. Pubmed Central PMCID: PMC2168591. Epub 2004/09/01. eng.
58. Andersen BL, Yang HC, Farrar WB, Golden-Kreutz DM, Emery CF, Thornton LM, et al. Psychologic intervention improves survival for breast cancer patients: a randomized clinical trial. Cancer. 2008;113(12):3450–8. PubMed PMID: 19016270. Pubmed Central PMCID: PMC2661422. Epub 2008/11/19. eng.
59. Beesley VL, Smith DD, Nagle CM, Friedlander M, Grant P, DeFazio A, et al. Coping strategies, trajectories, and their associations with patient-reported outcomes among women with ovarian cancer. Support Care Cancer. 2018;26(12):4133–42. PubMed PMID: 29948398. Epub 2018/06/28. eng.
60. Petraglia J. Narrative intervention in behavior and public health. J Health Commun. 2007;12(5):493–505. PubMed PMID: 17710598. Epub 2007/08/22. eng.
61. Kruizinga R, Hartog ID, Jacobs M, Daams JG, Scherer-Rath M, Schilderman JB, et al. The effect of spiritual interventions addressing existential themes using a narrative approach on quality of life of cancer patients: a systematic review and meta-analysis. Psycho-Oncology. 2016;25(3):253–65. PubMed PMID: 26257308. Epub 2015/08/11. eng.
62. Antoni MH, Lechner SC, Kazi A, Wimberly SR, Sifre T, Urcuyo KR, et al. How stress management improves quality of life after treatment for breast cancer. J Consult Clin Psychol. 2006;74(6):1143–52. PubMed PMID: 17154743. Epub 2006/12/13. eng.
63. Carlson LE, Zelinski E, Toivonen K, Flynn M, Qureshi M, Piedalue KA, et al. Mind-body therapies in cancer: what is the latest evidence? Curr Oncol Rep. 2017;19(10):67. PubMed PMID: 28822063. Epub 2017/08/20. eng.
64. World Cancer Research Fund. Diet, nutrition, physical activity and cancer: a global perspective. Summary of 3rd expert report. Continuous update project expert report. dietandcancer-report.org; 2018.
65. Idorn M, Thor SP. Exercise and cancer: from "healthy" to "therapeutic"? Cancer Immunol Immunother. 2017;66(5):667–71. PubMed PMID: 28324125. Pubmed Central PMCID: PMC5406418. Epub 2017/03/23. eng.
66. Benson H. The relaxation response. New York: HarperCollins; 2000.
67. Benson H, Stuart E. The wellness book: the comprehensive guide to maintaining health and treating stress-related illness. New York: Simon and Schuster; 1992.

68. Rico-Blázquez M, García-Sanz P, Martín-Martín M, López-Rodríguez JA, Morey-Montalvo M, Sanz-Cuesta T, et al. Effectiveness of a home-based nursing support and cognitive restructuring intervention on the quality of life of family caregivers in primary care: a pragmatic cluster-randomized controlled trial. Int J Nurs Stud. 2021;120:103955. PubMed PMID: 34051585. Epub 2021/05/30. eng.
69. Colloca L, Miller FG. The nocebo effect and its relevance for clinical practice. Psychosom Med. 2011;73(7):598–603. PubMed PMID: 21862825. Pubmed Central PMCID: PMC3167012. Epub 2011/08/25. eng.
70. Colloca L, Barsky AJ. Placebo and nocebo effects. N Engl J Med. 2020;382(6):554–61. PubMed PMID: 32023375. Epub 2020/02/06. eng.
71. Bingel U. Avoiding nocebo effects to optimize treatment outcome. JAMA. 2014;312(7):693–4. PubMed PMID: 25003609. Epub 2014/07/09. eng.
72. Ben-Shaanan TL, Schiller M, Azulay-Debby H, Korin B, Boshnak N, Koren T, et al. Modulation of anti-tumor immunity by the brain's reward system. Nat Commun. 2018;9(1):2723. PubMed PMID: 30006573. Pubmed Central PMCID: PMC6045610. Epub 2018/07/15. eng.
73. Ben-Shaanan TL, Azulay-Debby H, Dubovik T, Starosvetsky E, Korin B, Schiller M, et al. Activation of the reward system boosts innate and adaptive immunity. Nat Med. 2016;22(8):940–4. PubMed PMID: 27376577. Epub 2016/07/05. eng.
74. Jacobsen J, Kvale E, Rabow M, Rinaldi S, Cohen S, Weissman D, et al. Helping patients with serious illness live well through the promotion of adaptive coping: a report from the improving outpatient palliative care (IPAL-OP) initiative. J Palliat Med. 2014;17(4):463–8. PubMed PMID: 24579823. Epub 2014/03/04. eng.
75. Campbell JP, Turner JE. Debunking the myth of exercise-induced immune suppression: redefining the impact of exercise on immunological health across the lifespan. Front Immunol. 2018;9:648. Pubmed Central PMCID: PMC5911985. Epub 2018/05/02. eng.
76. Campbell KL, Winters-Stone KM, Wiskemann J, May AM, Schwartz AL, Courneya KS, et al. Exercise guidelines for cancer survivors: consensus statement from international multidisciplinary roundtable. Med Sci Sports Exerc. 2019;51(11):2375–90. PubMed PMID: 31626055. Epub 2019/10/19. eng.
77. Carlson LE. Mindfulness-based interventions for coping with cancer. Ann N Y Acad Sci. 2016;1373(1):5–12. PubMed PMID: 26963792. Epub 2016/03/11. eng.
78. Frankl V. Man's search for meaning. Boston: Beacon Press; 2006.
79. Gum A, Snyder C. Coping with terminal illness: the role of hopeful thinking. J Palliat Med. 2002;5:883–94.
80. Folkman S. Stress, coping and hope. Psycho-Oncology. 2010;19:901–8.
81. Eustache C, Jibb E, Grossman M. Exploring hope and healing in patients living with advanced non-small cell lung cancer. Oncol Nurs Forum. 2014;41(5):497–508. PubMed PMID: 25158655. Epub 2014/08/28. eng.
82. Kissane DW. Psychospiritual and existential distress. The challenge for palliative care. Aust Fam Physician. 2000;29(11):1022–5. PubMed PMID: 11127057. Epub 2000/12/29. eng.
83. Vehling S, Philipp R. Existential distress and meaning-focused interventions in cancer survivorship. Curr Opin Support Palliat Care. 2018;12(1):46–51. PubMed PMID: 29251694. Epub 2017/12/19. eng.
84. Jacobsen J, Brenner K, Greer JA, Jacobo M, Rosenberg L, Nipp RD, et al. When a patient is reluctant to talk about it: a dual framework to focus on living well and tolerate the possibility of dying. J Palliat Med. 2018;21(3):322–7. PubMed PMID: 28972862. Epub 2017/10/04. eng.
85. Trevino KM, Prigerson HG, Epstein RM, Duberstein PR. Reply to Hope, optimism, and the importance of caregivers in end-of-life care. Cancer. 2019;125(23):4330–1. PubMed PMID: 31381145. Epub 2019/08/06. eng.
86. Mount BM, Boston PH, Cohen SR. Healing connections: on moving from suffering to a sense of well-being. J Pain Symptom Manag. 2007;33(4):372–88. PubMed PMID: 17397699. Epub 2007/04/03. eng.
87. Sevan SD. Not the last good bye: on life, death, healing and cancer. London: Scribe; 2011.

88. Temel JS, Greer JA, Muzikansky A, Gallagher ER, Admane S, Jackson VA, et al. Early palliative care for patients with metastatic non-small-cell lung cancer. N Engl J Med. 2010;363(8):733–42. PubMed PMID: 20818875. Epub 2010/09/08. eng.
89. Astin JA, Anton-Culver H, Schwartz CE, Shapiro DH Jr, McQuade J, Breuer AM, et al. Sense of control and adjustment to breast cancer: the importance of balancing control coping styles. Behav Med. 1999;25(3):101–9. PubMed PMID: 10640223. Epub 2000/01/20. eng.
90. Chabowski M, Polanski J, Jankowska-Polanska B, Lomper K, Janczak D, Rosinczuk J. The acceptance of illness, the intensity of pain and the quality of life in patients with lung cancer. J Thorac Dis. 2017;9(9):2952–8. PubMed PMID: 29221267. Pubmed Central PMCID: PMC5708453. Epub 2017/12/10. eng.
91. Aldao A, Nolen-Hoeksema S, Schweizer S. Emotion-regulation strategies across psychopathology: a meta-analytic review. Clin Psychol Rev. 2010;30(2):217–37. PubMed PMID: 20015584. Epub 2009/12/18. eng.
92. Krok D, Telka E. The role of meaning in gastric cancer patients: relationships among meaning structures, coping, and psychological well-being. Anxiety Stress Coping. 2019;32(5):522–33. PubMed PMID: 31234657. Epub 2019/06/27. eng.
93. McDonald J, Swami N, Hannon B, Lo C, Pope A, Oza A, et al. Impact of early palliative care on caregivers of patients with advanced cancer: cluster randomised trial. Ann Oncol. 2017;28(1):163–8. PubMed PMID: 27687308. Epub 2016/10/01. eng.
94. Leow M, Chan S, Chan M. A pilot randomized, controlled trial of the effectiveness of a psychoeducational intervention on family caregivers of patients with advanced cancer. Oncol Nurs Forum. 2015;42(2):63–72. PubMed PMID: 25806893. Epub 2015/03/26. eng.
95. Kavalieratos D, Corbelli J, Zhang D, Dionne-Odom JN, Ernecoff NC, Hanmer J, et al. Association between palliative care and patient and caregiver outcomes: a systematic review and meta-analysis. JAMA. 2016;316(20):2104–14. PubMed PMID: 27893131. Pubmed Central PMCID: PMC5226373. Epub 2016/11/29. eng.
96. Temel JS, Greer JA, Admane S, Gallagher ER, Jackson VA, Lynch TJ, et al. Longitudinal perceptions of prognosis and goals of therapy in patients with metastatic non-small-cell lung cancer: results of a randomized study of early palliative care. J Clin Oncol. 2011;29(17):2319–26. PubMed PMID: 21555700. Epub 2011/05/11. eng.
97. Hudson P, Trauer T, Kelly B, O'Connor M, Thomas K, Zordan R, et al. Reducing the psychological distress of family caregivers of home based palliative care patients: longer term effects from a randomised controlled trial. Psycho-Oncology. 2015;24(1):19–24. PubMed PMID: 25044819. Pubmed Central PMCID: PMC4309500. Epub 2014/07/22. eng.
98. Northouse LL, Mood DW, Schafenacker A, Kalemkerian G, Zalupski M, LoRusso P, et al. Randomized clinical trial of a brief and extensive dyadic intervention for advanced cancer patients and their family caregivers. Psycho-Oncology. 2013;22(3):555–63. PubMed PMID: 22290823. Pubmed Central PMCID: PMC3387514. Epub 2012/02/01. eng.
99. Greer JA, Traeger L, Bemis H, Solis J, Hendriksen ES, Park ER, et al. A pilot randomized controlled trial of brief cognitive-behavioral therapy for anxiety in patients with terminal cancer. Oncologist. 2012;17(10):1337–45. PubMed PMID: 22688670. Pubmed Central PMCID: PMC3481900 indicated no financial relationships. Section Editors: Eduardo Bruera: None; Russell K. Portenoy: Arsenal Medical Inc., Pfizer, Grupo Ferrer, Transcript Pharma, Xenon (C/A); Allergan, Ameritox, Boston Scientific, Covidien Mallinckrodt Inc., Endo Pharmaceuticals, Forest Labs, K-Pax Pharmaceuticals, Medtronics, Otsuka Pharma, ProStrakan, Purdue Pharma, Salix, St. Jude Medical (RF) Reviewer "A": None Reviewer "B": None. Epub 2012/06/13. eng.
100. Xiu D, Fung YL, Lau BH, Wong DFK, Chan CHY, Ho RTH, et al. Comparing dyadic cognitive behavioral therapy (CBT) with dyadic integrative body-mind-spirit intervention (I-BMS) for Chinese family caregivers of lung cancer patients: a randomized controlled trial. Support Care Cancer. 2020;28(3):1523–33. PubMed PMID: 31280363. Epub 2019/07/08. eng.
101. Antoni MH, Lechner S, Diaz A, Vargas S, Holley H, Phillips K, et al. Cognitive behavioral stress management effects on psychosocial and physiological adaptation in women undergo-

ing treatment for breast cancer. Brain Behav Immun. 2009;23(5):580–91. PubMed PMID: 18835434. Pubmed Central PMCID: PMC2722111. Epub 2008/10/07. eng.
102. Cohen L, Parker PA, Vence L, Savary C, Kentor D, Pettaway C, et al. Presurgical stress management improves postoperative immune function in men with prostate cancer undergoing radical prostatectomy. Psychosom Med. 2011;73(3):218–25. PubMed PMID: 21257977. Epub 2011/01/25. eng.
103. Kwekkeboom K, Zhang Y, Campbell T, Coe CL, Costanzo E, Serlin RC, et al. Randomized controlled trial of a brief cognitive-behavioral strategies intervention for the pain, fatigue, and sleep disturbance symptom cluster in advanced cancer. Psycho-Oncology. 2018;27(12):2761–9. PubMed PMID: 30189462. Pubmed Central PMCID: PMC6279506. Epub 2018/09/07. eng.
104. Guarino A, Polini C, Forte G, Favieri F, Boncompagni I, Casagrande M. The effectiveness of psychological treatments in women with breast cancer: a systematic review and meta-analysis. J Clin Med. 2020;9(1):209. PubMed PMID: 31940942. Pubmed Central PMCID: PMC7019270. Epub 2020/01/17. eng.

Fostering Meaning Making 10

10.1 Introduction

Meaning is sought or found in almost everything we experience that resonates with our inner self—a walk in nature, personal relationships, work, planning a life of service to others, reconciling with a traumatic event. The search for meaning is a human impetus driven by our need to make sense of the world and our place in it and for most the desire to give purpose to our existence [1–3]. Precipitated by cancer-related threats, meaning making can become *an essential coping response* in order to reduce emotional distress and facilitate psychological adaptation to a new reality in the face of shattered global assumptions about the world and our place in it [4, 5].

This chapter is an extension of Chap. 9 on facilitating coping in that seeking and finding meaning are an integral part of the adaptive stress-coping system of resilience. This chapter examines the elements of meaning and how a nurse may foster meaning in patients who are in existential crisis and who feel that life is hardly meaningful with a disease like cancer.

10.2 Objectives

At the end of this chapter, you will be able to

1. Define meaning in life and its potential role in promoting resilience in patients with cancer
2. Describe meaning in life in relation to an individual's assumptions and beliefs about the world and the self
3. Compare the potential effects of situational meaning versus meaning in life and their respective impacts on quality of life

4. Clinically, explore the use of various strategies to facilitate meaning and purpose in patients
5. Distinguish between the concepts of seeking meaning, meaning making, and meaning made in relation to psychological adjustment and personal growth

Clinical Anecdote 10.1
Having cancer can provide a new lease on life, even for a life replete with meaning. It gave me permission to step back from my daily life, and to reacquaint my self with my deepest sense of self in a quest to discover what really made me happy, how I actually wanted to live the rest of my life. I knew that I was fortunate to be able to indulge in this pursuit. But I also realized that I had not paid enough attention to what really counted in life, and having cancer led to some important changes that have given me a deep sense of fulfillment.

10.3 Definitions

Meaning is a complex and dynamic construct of global and situational meaning-making cognitive systems which lies at the core of psychological adaptation in the face of a traumatic event [6]. Within the context of cancer, meaning making (i.e., search for meaning) has to do with the *quest for meaning*, whereas meaning found refers to coming to terms with an incomprehensible, traumatizing, and emotionally distressing event [2]. Meaning made (or found meaning or meaning found) is the outcome of adaptive coping processes that result in meaningful interpretations of a traumatic event for better or worse [6]. Found meaning has to do with making sense of the world and one's place in it, given the stresses one has experienced [4]. It implies that the person's global meanings have accommodated the stress-provoking situational context in order to create a reconstituted meaning in life (meaning made) that is consistent with current reality [2]. Meaning made has to do with establishing an adjusted order and purpose in life distinguished by different goals resulting in a sense of fulfillment and/or acceptance [2, 7].

Found meaning signifies that the individual has made needed adjustments to the stressful circumstances and has regained relative emotional equanimity [5]. Found meaning tends to induce a positive affect that may even coexist alongside a negative mood in patients with cancer [8, 9]. It is an essential coping response that underlies all other coping responses, providing in essence an essential cognitive link between the person and the environment.

Clinical Anecdote 10.2
Since her divorce, Anna had drifted through months and years, seemingly unable to discover new purposes to fill her life or greet challenges as new possibilities. Retreating from the world to devote herself full time to raising her children, left her listless, as she wafted through an emotional void; Her children's achievements of which she was tremendously proud, only underscored the lack of meaning in her own life. When Anna was diagnosed with cancer, it was a wake- up call. All of a sudden her existence which she had perceived as meaningless was now also an uncertainty,

She was a fragile life, blowing in the wind that urgently needed to be tethered to reconsidered meanings in light of the significance of the disease to her very being.

10.4　Emotional and Existential Distress (See Part II Chap. 3)

Patients with cancer and their loved ones often endure periods of considerable distress during treatment, the transition to supportive care, and even to survivorship [10]. Resilient neural–endocrine circuitry, adaptive cognitive–behavioral coping efforts, and personal and social resources accrued over a lifetime of experience enable the majority of cancer patients, to successfully confront cancer-related threats with calm resolve [11, 12]. The ability to make these adaptive cognitive adjustments involves the process of meaning making. Some patients, however, are in existential distress, questioning the meaning of their life which impedes their ability to find acceptance or to make peace with the health-related changes in their life [13, 14].

Both emotional distress and existential distress are human responses to an existential stressor, such as cancer [15]. Although conceptualizations for each are generally distinguishable albeit with overlapping elements, both tend to trigger the search for meaning and have the potential for personal growth and mastery over their distress [16].

Emotional Distress

An estimated 25–52% of cancer patients experience emotional distress at some time across the stages of the disease and transition to survivorship [10]. The National Comprehensive Cancer Network (NCCN) defines cancer-related distress as a negative experience of "a psychological (cognitive, behavioral, emotional), social, spiritual, and/or physical nature that interferes with the ability to cope effectively with cancer, its physical symptoms and its treatment" [10]. Emotional distress is conceptualized along a continuum that extends from "feelings of vulnerability, sadness, and fear to problems that become disabling such as depression, anxiety, panic, social isolation, to existential and spiritual crisis" with no clear clinical threshold to demarcate emotional from existential distress [17]. A traumatic event can cause a sense of personal vulnerability, sadness, anxiety, and fears, often accompanied by intrusive, uncontrollable negative ideation [4].

Existential Distress

Existential distress occurs when a life-threatening event, such as cancer, upends normally self-protective assumptions of security, optimism, hope, controllability, certainty, and trust in one's global meaning of the world, often leading to existential questions about life and death [15, 18]. An estimated 13–25% of patients with cancer experience symptoms of existential distress, such as death anxiety, fear of death, demoralization (feelings of helplessness and hopelessness, the desire for a hastened death), powerlessness, profound loneliness, pointlessness, dignity-related distress, loss, and human grief [15, 19, 20]. These existential symptoms may oscillate, but if sustained over time existential distress is likely present.

A systematic review of 25 studies reported that demoralization, a key component of existential suffering, was prevalent in an estimated 15% of patients with progressive disease and cancer [21]. Poorly controlled physical and psychological symptoms and decreased social functioning were among the factors contributing to the demoralized state of patients. The number of physical problems (such as fatigue, pain, mobility impairments, and sleep disturbances) was also predictive of significantly higher demoralization and depression [22].

Both emotionally distressed and existentially distressed patients may express uncertainty about the future and fear of a cancer recurrence; they are likely to demonstrate maladaptive coping behaviors (such as avoidance). These factors contribute to a state of demoralization that if unaddressed also lead to hopelessness and a loss of purpose [21]. A person whose fear of a cancer recurrence results in intense distress for more than two weeks and is unable to respond adaptively to proposed interventions to reduce distress and/or make effective coping adjustments may be manifesting symptoms of existential distress that threaten their resilience and health [17].

These findings underscore the need for clinical interventions that maintain meaning or facilitate meaning found in at risk patients with cancer and survivors so that psychological well-being may be enhanced [23]. Because physical and psychological symptoms appear to exacerbate feelings of demoralization, interventions must also address these co-occurring symptoms.

10.5 Conceptual Underpinnings

Park's meaning-making model describes two main interrelated forms of meaning: global meaning-oriented systems and situation-specific meanings [2, 23] The model also distinguishes between the search for meaning and meaning made.

Global Meaning-Orienting System

This refers to core beliefs or assumptions about the world and the self [2, 14]. Perceived global meanings shape our world views about fundamental concepts such as predictability, causality, coherence, ethics, and justice as well as our views of the self and our place and purpose in the world in terms of goals for our family and self and future plans [3].

Global goals have to do with "internal representations of desired processes, events, and outcomes" that we already possess, want to maintain, and/or desire in the future [2]. These *global goals* generally relate to health, relationships, work, knowledge, achievement, and religion [24]. For instance, a father in a moment of self-reflection may observe "I am in the prime of my life, blessed with health, a wife, family and a career I had always hoped for." Global meaning addresses the question: What makes my life meaningful [25]?

Situational Meaning

Illness cognitions assigned to cancer are situational beliefs or meanings triggered by the cancer threat. These beliefs typically relate to the extent of the perceived threat to the self, the duration, controllability, consequences, and timing which severely challenge global assumptions about the predictability, order, purpose, goals, and controllability of the world and the self [26, 27]. For instance, a new colorectal cancer diagnosis is likely to be a severe threat to a person's sense of self when it is completely at odds with global assumptions about himself (i.e., there is no prior history of colorectal cancer in his family, he has faithfully adhered to a healthy lifestyle, and he is thriving in his career). According to the meaning-making model, situational meanings diverge from and challenge the person's global meaning goals and beliefs, causing distress [23, 28].

Context-driven situational meanings are predicated on the person's assessment of whether the threatening situation is controllable, why it occurred, and its impact on his or her future. A two-year study of the illness cognitions (or situational meanings) of patients with head and neck squamous cancer showed that strong beliefs about the cancer, the magnitude of negative perceived consequences, a chronic time line, and self-blame for the cancer made a small but significant contribution to a subsequent poor quality of life [29]. Individuals who did not hold strong beliefs about their role in causing the cancer or its consequences were found to have better global health and functioning. Beliefs about the negative consequences and duration of the cancer and the scope of its disruption on the person's life are indicative of situational meanings that are associated with poor adjustment, signaling the need for clinical support. The *extent* to which the situational meaning departs from the global meaning orientation is reflected by the individual's level of distress.

Search for Meaning: Adjusted Global and Situational Meanings

Park's model of meaning making distinguishes between meaning making (search for meaning) and meaning made (i.e., found meaning) [2, 3]. The discrepancy between an individual's perceived global and situational meanings causes emotional distress which triggers *the search for meaning*. This process may involve the person having to modify aspects of his or her global assumptions and/or stress-related situational meanings (for instance, regarding the threat) in order to reconcile the discrepancy between the two and find some measure of meaning or purpose in the situation. The distressed person may rely on reappraisal, problem-focused, emotion-focused, and meaning-focused coping efforts [6, 23].

Most cancer survivors achieve a sense of psychological adaptation by shifting/altering some global meaning components in order to establish relative coherence between situational and global meanings which leads to new meaning and purpose in life [30]. Tomich and Helgeson's case–control study of 328 women survivors 5 years after being diagnosed with breast cancer showed that the survivors tended to perceive the world as generally less controllable and more random compared to women without a history of cancer, although personal control over their daily life was comparable to healthy women and was significantly related to their quality of life [30].

A longitudinal study of 763 women survivors of breast cancer revealed that positive meaning in life (i.e., found meaning based on their positive relationships, and changes in priorities, and outlook on life) as well as a sense of vulnerability (i.e., the world is also a dangerous place and fear of cancer recurrence) coexisted in women survivors as long as 10 years after a breast cancer diagnosis [31]. Whereas positive meaning was related to concurrent and long-term levels of positive affect, a sense of vulnerability was similarly related to negative affect in the same individual. Neither meaning was related to long-term mental or physical health. In another study, women who had lost a relative to breast cancer showed that finding positive meaning was significantly related to an increase in natural killer cell count activity, which is an essential immune capability in tracking down and eliminating roving cancer cells [32, 33].

The results suggest that cancer can be a life-threatening event that triggers a shift in global meanings from a predictable to a more unpredictable world reflected by a greater sense of vulnerability or wariness about the world and one's place in it. And at the same time, the cancer-related perceived threat appears to induce a shift in the individual's values, beliefs, and priorities which enables the individual to find a meaningful life albeit with a different world perspective. Thus, the individual is capable of experiencing both positive and negative effects at the same time [34]. Significant factors such as age at cancer diagnosis, lingering physical symptoms, marital status, and education all contribute to a person's perceived meaning in life and sense of vulnerability. But importantly both global and situational shifts in meaning lead to a more realistic view of the world and the person's place in it.

Cognitive Processing: Assimilation and Accommodation

The search for meaning may occur through intrusive ideations which are a signal of the mind's struggle to process or integrate the cancer-related threat into the person's current global assumptions and beliefs. Cognitive processing involves complementary innate processes of assimilation and accommodation [35]. Assimilation refers to repeated cognitive efforts to alter situational (meaning-based) data to fit into the individual's global meaning representations [2]. Accommodation strives to modify the global representations that already exist. These stress-induced dynamic *cognitive interactions* give rise to adaptive meanings that restore a sense of emotional equilibrium so long as the process is not prolonged or indefinite in duration [2].

Clinical Anecdote 10.3
Mr. G was a young man in his early 40's, just married, good career who had every reason to believe he would fulfill his last main goals of a carefully crafted life, his desire to have a family and a couple of kids. These expectations were completely upended when he learned he had advanced pancreatic cancer. Despite his efforts to use distraction, go cycling, intrusive ideation followed him everywhere. He was exhausted with his inability to fall asleep or remain asleep. A combination of the relaxation response technique, where he learned to acknowledge these unwelcome thoughts but not react emotionally along with anxiolytics and the therapeutic touch technique helped his hyperbolic stress response system to down regulate as he successfully processed these thoughts into his reintegrated whole being [36].

According to the meaning-making model, a *continuous* prolonged search to make sense of a traumatic event is associated with poor adjustment [2]. A case–control study of the search for meaning and meaning found in 72 women 18 months or more after treatment for breast cancer reported that continuous searches for meaning were unrelated to found meaning but were associated with high negative affect levels [37]. When the cognitive gap between the situational stressor and the global-oriented meaning persists, the *unresolved search for meaning over time results in maladaptation*. Individuals who continue to search for meaning during survivorship are likely experiencing senseless rumination and distress and may benefit from a meaning-making intervention.

Among survivors of breast cancer with low global meaning, a positive relationship between intrusive ideation and distress was shown, whereas no association between high global meaning and either intrusive ideation or distress was found, suggesting that high global meaning eliminated the need for cognitive processing (to make sense of what happened) [38]. High global meaning with its goals and core beliefs about the self appears to influence the process of finding benefit in the cancer experience.

Clinical Benefit and Intrusive Ideation A *meta*-analysis of 87 cross-sectional studies reported that clinical benefit was associated with positive intrusive and avoidant behaviors, which was suggestive of cognitive processing efforts [35]. Benefit finding appeared to be associated with psychological adjustment in diverse threatening-related situations including breast cancer and heart disease [39]. For instance, benefit finding showed a large effect size on positive well-being and was also related to less depression. Unexpectedly, finding benefit in a stressful situation was *unrelated* to anxiety, global distress, quality of life, and perceived physical health. Finding benefit through the cancer experience may reflect the positive consequences of a traumatic event rather than a lack of distress [40].

The fact that benefit finding was positively associated with intrusive and avoidant thoughts supports the theoretical contention that intrusive ideation is an innate cognitive process for coming to terms with the impact of the stressor on a person's life. Cognitive processing strives to incorporate the stressor effects within a reintegrated self via processes of assimilation and accommodation (so long as it does not persist) [35]. Finding benefit does not in itself necessarily reconcile the cognitive discrepancy between the individual's global and situational meanings, but it does suggest that finding benefit and positive well-being may co-occur with other clinical outcomes such as global distress, anxiety or a poor quality of life [8, 9].

The Search for Meaning Can Fail

Not all meaning-making efforts prevail. Some patient searches may need supportive assistance *in accepting what does not make sense* by helping these individuals to reappraise and redirect their nonactualized perseverations toward more meaningful goals, priorities, and activities that are possible in their current lives [6, 34]. In these circumstances, nurses can help patients to identify the potential opportunities and possibilities that exist as a consequence of living in the present with cancer [1].

Found Meaning or Meaning Made

Found meaning has to do with making sense of the world and one's place in it, given the stresses one has experienced (Table 10.1) [4]. It implies that the person's global meanings have accommodated the situational context in order to create a reconstituted meaning in life (meaning made) that is consistent with current reality [2]. Meaning made refers to the acquisition of an adjusted order and purpose in life distinguished by different goals, a sense of fulfillment and/or acceptance [2, 7]. Finding meaning can occur anytime; for instance, a religious person may ascertain a greater purpose in the diagnosis. A nonreligious person may accept the diagnosis having lived a long and fulfilled life. Or meaning found may emerge over time through a process of deliberate rumination in which the stressful situation is reappraised, reframed, and ultimately reconciled either by adjusting one's global and/or situational meaning representations [2, 7, 23, 26]. A meaning-made solution results in strengthened resilience or successful adaptation frequently driven by resilient-promoting coping and meaning-focused psychological processes.

A meta-analysis of 62 studies of patients with various cancers showed inverse and significant relationships between meaning in one's life and distress and between sense of coherence (SOC) (a related variable of meaning) and distress [41]. Because the magnitude of the inverse relationship between SOC and distress appeared to be greater than that of meaning in life, the researchers suggested that elements of SOC such as perceived manageability of life's current situation be incorporated into meaning-making clinical interventions. However, as the patients consisted of diverse cancers across all stages from diagnosis to end of life, it is also conceivable that the patients were at varying phases in the process of adjusting their global meaning to a reintegrated meaning in life, which would account for the smaller magnitude in the negative relationship between meaning in life and distress.

A longitudinal study of 270 patients with cancer used hierarchical regression analyses to show that a *strong sense of global meaning* was a significant predictor of less depression and a less demoralized state [18]. Acceptance of death also predicted significantly less anxiety. In contrast, consistent with meaning theory, goal *seeking* predicted greater depression, anxiety, and demoralization. Using secondary analysis of the same data, Vehling et al. [22] also found a risk of existential distress across all stages of the disease in patients with cancer, notwithstanding the buffering effects of global meaning, due to the diversity of existential stressors patients must confront along the continuum.

Table 10.1 Examples of demonstrated meaning made [2]

1. Individual is able to make sense of a stressful situation
2. Experiences a sense of personal growth or demonstrates positive life changes
3. Positive reappraisal of cancer-related threat (situational meaning) and/or changes in global beliefs and goals (global meaning) that are better aligned with clinical reality
4. Conveys acceptance signifying a coming to terms with the trauma event
5. Expresses a renewed sense of meaning and purpose aligned to current realities
6. Makes *causal attributions* that make sense to the individual (review section "A Word About Causal Attributions")

Clinical research suggests that *global meanings may be modified* as a function of the cancer experience. More than 5 years after being diagnosed with breast cancer, women perceived the world as more "random" and "less controllable" compared to women who had never been diagnosed with cancer, suggesting that previous global meaning assumptions about the predictability and controllability of the world had been modified by the cancer experience, although their sense of personal control in their daily life remained similar to that of healthy women [30].

Meaning-Made and Physiological Outcomes

Found meaning has been associated with biological healing, as suggested by a very small number of meaning-related studies that included physiological indicators of resilience [32, 42]. For instance, HIV-seropositive men who engaged in cognitive processing and found meaning in the aftermath of the death of a loved one were shown to have a slower reduction in CD4 T-lymphocytes over time, with lower rates of AIDS-related mortality [42]. CD4 helper T cells are white blood cells that signal other immune cells such as CD8 killer cells to destroy specific targets. Similarly, women who were mourning the loss of a loved one and developed *positive, meaning-related* goals produced a significant increase in natural killer cell cytotoxicity ($r = 0.33$, $p < 0.05$) [32]. These findings offer preliminary evidence that a meaning made perspective reduces emotional distress which is associated with improved immune functioning. The findings are consistent with Wolgast's experimental findings in which positive reappraisal and acceptance were associated with physiological measures of less emotional reactivity according to skin conductance levels (SCL) and facial electromyography (EMG). Positive cognitive reappraisal also appears to reduce brain activity in the regions related to stress-induced emotions such as the amygdala, insula, and striatum due to increased signaling from the prefrontal cortical areas where cognitive appraisals and critical thinking functions occur [43, 44].

Thus, the ability to find meaning in adversity may have protective physiological and immune as well as psychological and cognitive effects. Future controlled studies on the neuroimmunological aspects of found meaning would contribute to a more comprehensive understanding of the therapeutic benefits of meaning on healing and resilient processes in patients with cancer and their family caregivers [45].

Meaning-Made and Posttraumatic Growth

One indicator of found meaning is personal growth [46]. Tedeschi and Calhoun's model of posttraumatic growth identifies key elements of the posttraumatic experience associated with positive changes or posttraumatic growth: (a) the severity of the stressor event, (b) automatic rumination (intrusive ideation), (c) coping efforts, and (d) social support. Posttraumatic growth refers to positive changes that occur as a consequence of having to confront distressing experiences of life [47, 48].

A review of quantitative studies of the psychosocial factors and processes involved in developing posttraumatic growth were consistent with Tedeschi and Calhoun's model of posttraumatic growth [49]. Support facilitated reappraisals of the stressor event, shifted intrusive rumination toward deliberate ruminations by encouraging patient narratives through which new meanings could emerge; the narrative gave rise to a new order, purpose, and changes in global assumptions, priorities, and goals. Consistent with cognitive theory of stress and coping- and meaning-focused strategies, deliberate rumination is a resilient-promoting strategy which involves a process of assessing resources, weighing coping strategies, and reappraisals of the trauma event, producing new meanings that enable the traumatic event to be successfully processed within a reintegrated self [49–51].

In summary, finding meaning through the cancer experience appears to be associated with better resilience, psychological well-being, quality of life, and often personal growth [52–55]. As the review has highlighted, coping- and meaning-focused cognitive efforts lie at the core of psychological adaptive processes of resilience. Finding meaning is central to the individual's ability to understand and accept current clinical realities in order to subsequently develop the strategies required to handle the clinical implications of the cancer and treatment. Thus, the individual's positive adjustment depends on meaning-making strategies aided by a supportive relationship that facilitate their ability to view the traumatic event and their suffering in a more positive meaningful light [56]. Potential nursing interventions include use of narrative or storytelling, deliberate rumination, and encouraging supportive relationships that facilitate the patient's positive reappraisal of stressful events. Other potential nursing interventions will emerge in the following sections of the review, to be discussed further in Nursing Approaches (Sect. 10.7).

Moderators and Mediators of Meaning

Coping-Related Mediators

Meaning made is usually the outcome of adaptive coping processes that result in meaningful interpretations of a traumatic event for better or worse [6]. A study based on path analysis of cross-sectional data from 187 patients with gastric cancer showed that meaning in life (derived from one's global meaning) and situational meanings (meaning associated with a threatening event) indirectly impacted psychological well-being via their direct effects on different coping efforts [28]. Specifically, meaning in life (global meaning) triggered indirect and positive effects on psychological well-being via its positive direct effects on *use of* problem-focused (e.g., acting to manage the problem), emotion-focused (e.g., use of distraction to regulate negative emotions), and meaning-focused (use of reframing or positive reappraisal) coping efforts. The findings indicated that when these coping efforts were included in the path model, the direct effect of meaning in life (MIL) on psychological well-being (PWB) was not significant (beta = 0.09, $p > 0.05$). Problem-focused, emotion-focused, and meaning-focused coping mediated the relationship between meaning in life and psychological well-being resulting in a moderately high significant estimated total indirect effect on psychological well-being (beta = 0.47 (95% CL, 0.31–0.59). In other words, meaning in life (i.e., global meanings) was related to the use of problem-, emotion-, and meaning-related coping strategies which in turn enhanced psychological well-being. Replicating this study using longitudinal data would confirm the directionality of the path analytic relationships.

Conversely, situational meaning was associated with a negative indirect effect on psychological well-being via its negative direct effects on emotion-focused and meaning-focused coping efforts. The findings also showed that when emotion-focused and meaning-focused coping efforts were included in the path model, the direct effect of situational meaning on well-being was also insignificant, underscoring again the important mediating role of coping strategies in relation to psychological well-being (beta = 0.02, $p > 0.05$).

The finding that situational meaning was associated with poor psychological well-being in some cancer patients *due to an apparent lack of effective coping efforts* supports previous studies in which situational meanings (reflected by "violations" in global goals and beliefs) were associated with increased intrusive ideation, anxiety, and poor posttraumatic growth [3, 18, 27, 29].

Krok's study showed that situational meaning is associated with less emotion- and meaning-focused coping efforts and is unrelated to problem-focused coping efforts, highlighting a lack of effective coping efforts to restore order, purpose, and well-being. As Park has cautioned, some individuals may stop their search for meaning and, as implied by Krok's study, may accept their negative illness cognitions (situational meaning), preferring to accept their reintegrated self in a global meaning shift toward an unpredictable world with unattainable goals which together interfere with and even block the person's ability to reestablish order and purpose in life. These patients likely reinforce their negative situational meanings with negatively altered global assumptions. Consequently, they may embrace beliefs that cancer is uncontrollable and life-threatening with dire consequences regardless of medical facts and a clinical prognosis to the contrary. This ultimately works at cross purposes with the health-promoting goals of treatment due to their resultant emotional distress and stress-induced dysregulated neural physiological and immune structures and mediators [57, 58].

Cognitive Processing, Personal Resources (Optimism and Faith), Social Support, and Meaning-Focused Coping Strategies

In a review of 22 studies, the cancer threat, optimism and "being open," cognitive processing, problem-focused, meaning-making, spiritual/religion coping strategies, and social support were shown to be positively related to posttraumatic growth [49]. Of these variables, cognitive processing (such as deliberate rumination) and supportive relationships were identified as key cognitive processes that resulted in posttraumatic growth (see section "Facilitating Deliberate Rumination") [49]. This finding suggests that supportive relationships and cognitive ruminations were implicated in the search for meaning and that posttraumatic growth is an indicator of meaning found. Supportive relationships and sense of optimism were also shown to influence the selection of *meaning-making* coping *strategies*, such as reframing and cognitive reappraisals which led to posttraumatic growth (or meaning found) [49]; see Part II Chap. 5. A qualitative study has also provided strong support for the vital role of supportive relationships in promoting meaning making and meaning [59].

A path analysis using cross-sectional data from 201 cancer patients in China showed that positive reframing (as well as active coping and planning) were significant mediators between social support and posttraumatic growth among patients with diverse cancers [27]. High levels of perceived support had direct and positive effects on adaptive coping strategies including reframing which in turn positively increased posttraumatic growth. Longitudinal data are needed to confirm the directionality of the findings. Close personal relationships provide caring and support and are deeply meaningful in and of themselves within the context of a meaningful life [60]. It is not surprising therefore to also find that support has been strongly related to global meaning (meaning in life) in patients with cancer [61]. A sense of secure attachment within social relationship(s) was also significantly related to positive reframing and religion (as well as active coping efforts) which then were all predictive of posttraumatic growth [62].

Last faith is a personal resource imbued with personal meaning which has been associated with quality of life, suggesting that a sense of meaning is a mediator of the relationship between faith and quality of life [63]. A qualitative study of 29 patients with cancer in Malaysia also suggested that a Higher Being, cultural identity, and emotional affiliations with nature constituted existential, *spiritual and religious meaning-making coping strategies* [64]. Diverse beliefs, practices, and feelings associated with the sacred are meaning-making coping strategies that help individuals cope with distressing circumstances [65, 66]. Three meta-analyses based on individuals with cancer indicated that *R/S* strategies in terms of cognitive beliefs, affective feelings, and behavioral practices were significantly related to various patient-reported health outcomes (physical, mental, and social) [67–69]. Although directionality of effects needs further clarification, the relationship between faith or religion and meaning making/found is clearly evident.

In Park's overview of these meta-analyses, *affective R/S* (such as spiritual well-being, spiritual distress, and spiritual experiences) showed the largest effect sizes across mental, physical, and social health, but especially in relation to *mental health* (measures of well-being, depression, and anxiety) and *social health* (e.g., social roles, relationships, sense of connectedness to others) [68]. Affective *R/S* seems to establish a spiritual connectedness to something greater than the self that provides a sense of psychological well-being and comfort to those confronting the traumatizing experience of cancer. The relationship between affective *R/S* and social health underscores how *R/S* beliefs can shape and give meaning to an individual's relationships. The meaningfulness of social ties and a sense of connectedness to others may be strengthened through shared spiritual experiences.

The relationship of *cognitive R/S* (i.e., beliefs, perceptions, and causal attributions) with mental health suggests that cognitive beliefs assign meaning to the cancer-related experience which either improves or worsens the individual's psychological adjustment to cancer [66]. The significant relationship between *cognitive R/S* and social health (roles, relationships, and social responsibilities) similarly indicates how these *R/S* beliefs may shape and give meaning to an individual's relationships and social responsibilities. It is worth noting that these analyses did not include other coping strategies that may mediate the relationships between faith, religion, and health-related outcomes such as acceptance [49].

To summarize, when patients open themselves to the potential meaningful opportunities that adversity may unexpectedly offer, psychological healing, *the subjective state of feeling whole or a sense of personal growth*, may be realized through myriad meaning-making/meaning-made paths, for instance, through the cultivation of more meaningful personal relationships, the pursuit of beloved hobbies, a deeper appreciation of nature, a resonating philosophy of life, and for many, a belief in the spiritual and/or faith in a Higher Being.

10.6 Meaning-Making Clinical Interventions (Review Appendix in this Chapter and Appendix B)

Various meaning-making coping strategies facilitate meaning found in distressed individuals with cancer which may be utilized at the bedside or in the clinic (Table 10.2) (see Sect. 10.7). Manualized meaning-related interventions for distressed individuals with cancer have been developed for use on a one-on-one basis with patients or caregivers or in groups. In a meta-analysis of 29 RCTs ($n = 2305$), psychosocial interventions significantly improved meaning and purpose in adults with cancer [23]. Interventions that were specifically designed to increase meaning and purpose had significant effect size outcomes. These interventions included meaning-focused, cognitive existential, supportive expressive, and mindfulness-based stress reduction approaches.

Other meta-analyses have demonstrated that compared to controls, meaning-centered/making interventions exerted large positive effects on meaning in life with significant positive effects on quality of life, hope and optimism, self-efficacy, and social well-being, as well as negative effects on anxiety and depression in individuals with a history of cancer [53, 70, 71]. These findings were borne out across patients with early stage, advanced, and palliative cancer who received either an individualized or group meaning-based intervention to reduce existential distress [25, 72–74]. Significantly, a subanalysis of Breitbart's RCT indicated that the competence of the healthcare provider-led interventions was a significant factor in the clinical outcomes of the patients, with *the nurse displaying the largest effects*.

Nonetheless, meaning-centered interventions vary in terms of psychotherapeutic underpinnings, content, sequencing, topics, strategy, frequency, and duration of effects [73, 75, 76]. Overall, meaning-focused interventions were shown to benefit patients as well as family caregivers across illness stages [77, 78].

Two meaning-related interventions are closely aligned with nursing's philosophy of care and theoretical underpinnings: the life review derived from Erickson's stages of psychosocial development and the meaning-making intervention derived from stress-coping theory. These clinical interventions have distinct goals, objectives, and desired outcomes as a function of their respective perspectives. Selecting one or the other would depend on the individual's stated goals, concerns, and preferences.

Table 10.2 Meaning-focused resilient-promoting coping strategies

Nursing objectives	Content/strategies	Clinical outcomes	References
Promote meaning-focused coping strategies	*Manualized interventions* (a) Meaning-making intervention (b) Life review intervention *Individual strategies* (a) Reframing (b) Find clinical benefits in light of reality (c) Facilitate positive reappraisals (d) Propose alternative explanations, interpretations (e) Use of storytelling, narratives to integrate cancer into the person's life story to facilitate acceptance and a reintegrated self (f) Infuse ordinary daily events with positive meaning (g) Discuss changes in an individual's basic goals, values since diagnosis with the goal of reprioritizing patient goals, and reaffirming values intrinsic to the person *Indicators of meaning found given clinical reality* (a) Acceptance (b) Found benefits, new meaning, purpose (c) Reprioritized goals and values	↑QOL· ↑ Meaning in life ↑Hope ↑ Self-esteem, ¹optimism¹, self-efficacy ↓ Depression, ↓ Anxiety	[2, 7, 53, 73, 79, 85–88]

The Life Review (See Appendix B)

The life review refers to a personal review process led by a healthcare provider and based on Erikson's theory of psychological development in which the individual reviews his past highlighting both positive and negative experiences and their significance to himself [76, 79]. Unresolved issues are examined from the benefit of hindsight and then reintegrated into one's whole self resulting in a sense of overall well-being [76]. The life review has been shown to be an effective clinical intervention for alleviating emotional and existential distress in elderly persons and patients with palliative cancer.

In a meta-analysis of 15 studies of patients with cancer, a life review was significantly related to improved mental health and well-being as indicated by a decrease in depression and anxiety, and an increase in hope, self-esteem, and quality of life [76]. In a meta-analysis of 8 randomized controlled studies based on patients with terminal or advanced cancer, a life review was significantly related to the spiritual subscale of the meaning in life measure and quality of life as well as a reduction in general distress compared to usual care [80]. A life review may be of therapeutic benefit to individuals with advanced or terminal disease, and a full account of its goals, objectives, and clinical approach may be found in David Haber's article.

Meaning-Made Interventions (Appendix B)

A number of meaning-centered interventions exist in the literature [74, 78, 81, 82]. One meaning-making intervention was designed by a nurse scientist to address existential concerns that may arise in patients with cancer at any stage of the disease [83]. A clinical study randomly assigned 74 patients to receive a meaning-making intervention or usual care. Compared to usual care, those who received the meaning-making intervention during treatment for colorectal or breast cancer reported significant improvements in self-esteem, optimism, and self-efficacy, all essential determinants of resilience. The intervention consisted of up to four sessions, offered one on one and administered in the cancer clinic, a hospital unit or home setting.

A follow-up pilot study suggested that the meaning-making intervention was also effective in enhancing meaning in life in patients who were recently diagnosed with advanced ovarian cancer, as assessed at 1 and 3 months postintervention [25]. Three months postintervention, only 2/12 patients (17%) in the meaning-making group experienced clinical levels of depression and anxiety, whereas the control group had twice as many patients (5/12, 42%) based on the HADS (clinical cut off >16), suggesting that the intervention has clinical significance. The nonsignificant differences between the two groups on depression and anxiety when group means were used may be due to the small sample size [25]. The trends in the study data support the relevance of this meaning-making intervention for patients early in the diagnostic phase as well as during treatment, underscoring the need for a fully developed RCT to assess its clinical benefits.

In summary, meaning-making interventions have produced positive clinical outcomes in patients with cancer as well as in survivors, highlighting their importance for patients and loved ones, who are experiencing existential concerns or distress at any phase along the cancer continuum. The key to these interventions lies in their meaning-centered focus [84]. Vos and Vitali recommend a meaning-centered/meaning-making intervention particularly for individuals facing a life-threatening or chronic illness, as they are more likely to raise meaning-related issues.

10.7 Nursing Approaches

Nursing Assessment

Table 10.3 provides suggested components of meaning enhancing strategies. Existential concerns experienced at diagnosis may differ from those experienced prior to major surgery or toward the end of life. Regularly assess *patient meanings at identified stressful points* along their illness and recovery continuum so that relevant interventions may be implemented [16, 89].

Table 10.3 Components of a meaning-related nursing assessment

Clinical areas	Components
1. Screen for emotional distress	≥3 cutoff [10] (Review Part II Chap. 3)
a. Indicators of distress to look for:	Sadness, vulnerability, anxiety, fear, social isolation, depressed mood, recursive intrusive ideation [10]
b. Indicators of existential distress include	Death anxiety, fear of death, profound loneliness, grief, desire for hastened death [3, 10, 19]
c. Contributing factors	Poorly controlled symptoms, poor prognosis, progressive disease, fear of recurrence, stopped treatment, sense of hopelessness, loss of purpose and meaning in life [14, 90, 91]
2. Threats to global assumptions and global meanings (world and self)	a. World assumptions (1) orderly, predictability (controllability), (2) causality, (3) coherence, (4) ethics, and (5) justice b. Self global goals, values, and attitudes about family, self, future plans, for example, with respect to health, relationships, work, knowledge, achievement, and religion [24] c. Global meaning question: what makes your life meaningful [25]? Which global assumptions and global goals are most important to person before/after stressor event, for example, family, career, health, sense of personal control; see Sect. 10.2 d. Compare and contrast impact of threat on global meanings before and after cancer e. What has changed, stayed the same f. What do you attribute change to? [2, 7, 10, 14, 91]
3. Situational meanings (i.e., about the threat or stressor event)	(1) Meaning of threat, (2) impact on person's goals and beliefs, (3) impact on global assumptions and beliefs [3, 7]
4. Search for meaning	In terms of (1) length of time of search, (2) unwanted ideation and avoidant behaviors (how long, antecedent factors, impact on well-being) [2, 23]
5. Found meaning	(1) Acceptance, (2) made sense of what happened, (3) personal growth, (4) new meanings and purpose linked to current reality, and (5) contributing factors
6. Use of meaning-making strategies	(1) Reappraisal, reframing, existential, spiritual, religious, cultural, and nature-related strategies (rituals) [2, 7, 73] (2) What worked and what did not Compare with other stressor events
7. Resources that enhance sense of meaning	(1) Support of family, loved one, friends, (2) spiritual, religious, cultural, nature-based affiliations, and (3) use of storytelling with friends or supportive relationships [27, 73, 92]

Nursing Interventions: Global Assumptions, Situational Meanings, and Meaning Making

The nurse's goal is to facilitate meaning making and meaning found in emotionally distressed and existentially distressed individuals. Meaning-making nursing interventions have to do with facilitating the process of comparing and contrasting global goals, assumptions, and beliefs about the justness, controllability, and predictability of the world with situational meanings which challenge these world views [2]. The intent is for the individual to learn something about the world and the self by examining past and current experiences that may be used to reconcile the discrepancies between his or her global and situational beliefs, leading to a more compatible re alignment of these two meanings in keeping with the person's clinical reality. In the process, personal goals may be reprioritized, and acceptance or new meanings (order and purpose) become possible.

Many of the patient's global goals before cancer may still resonate (even more so) after the diagnosis : meaningful relationships, maintaining his health, stimulating his mind with various projects (work and knowledge may now be intensified in value or reordered in priority as a function of the patient's clinical reality). Whereas the patient once held global beliefs about the predictability and controllability of the world, his situational meanings may lead him to modify those assumptions, in light of the traumatizing cancer diagnosis, thereby causing emotional distress. Although the world may now be perceived as less controllable and more unpredictable, the nurse may help the patient realize that despite his altered global perspective, *he still maintains personal control* over most things in his life even with a chronic illness, and he can still promote his health and enjoy family and friends. This meaning-making process may be facilitated through narrative storytelling supported by strategies delineated in the next section [2, 14, 73, 83] (see Table 10.4 principles of meaning making).

Because the patient and the family caregiver influence one another's emotions, thoughts and well-being, consider offering a meaning-making intervention to the patient and his or her caregiver as parallel and separate interventions depending on their preferences [52, 93]. Meaning-making interventions should be individually tailored to specific concerns in order to facilitate desired outcomes of posttraumatic growth, enhanced meaning and purpose, acceptance, and well-being. Chapter 18 in section "More Cognitive Strategies" discusses strategies that may promote meaning in life through the relationship between meaning and spiritual and religious beliefs in individuals at the end of life.

Meaning-Making Strategies

A number of meaning-making strategies may be used to facilitate the person's ability to positively reappraise global and situational meanings so both are better aligned with the patient's current reality (Appendix in this chapter and Appendix B).

Encourage Cognitive Shift toward Neutral or Positive Reappraisals
(Review Part IV Chap. 9)
Encourage the Individual's More Neutral or Positive Reappraisals of His Circumstances Positive cognitive reappraisal is the positive interpretation an individual makes that can lead to meaning found; it can involve processes of reframing and reinterpreting emotionally distressing situations so that more constructive

Table 10.4 Principles of a meaning-making intervention [23, 79, 83, 84] (Review Sect. 10.5)

Steps	Content
(1) Explore situational meaning of cancer-related threat (section "Situational Meaning")	(1) Examine the patient's situational meanings and emotional reactions to the cancer experience in terms of Leventhal's five beliefs about the threatening situation: (a) threat to health (illness identity), (b) consequences, (c) timeline, and (d) causes (attributions), illness coherence (what patient understands about the disease and treatment), and perceived control (c) Identify what aspects of the situational meanings (beliefs) are most difficult to come to terms with (e.g., the unpredictability of the cancer causing uncertainty, given their assumptions about a predictable and controllable world)
(2) Global meaning assumptions (beliefs) about the world (section "Global Meaning-Orienting System")	(a) Explore how current situational meanings challenged global beliefs or assumptions about the world before cancer: assumptions the person held about *predictability, justness, controllability, causality, coherence*
(3) Explore global meaning goals with respect to self and relationships (section "Global Meaning-Orienting System")	(a) Explore patient's global meaning goals regarding relationships (family, friends, other), career, knowledge, achievement, religion. What priorities of life from these categories guided your life (b) Have these been altered by the cancer —if so, in what ways? (c) Have these global meaning goals been altered by stressful experiences in the past—if so, in what ways? What is similar/different? (d) Have these altered global meaning goals from the past informed the current cancer experience? Do some global assumptions about for eg family remain the same?
(4) Examine previous coping responses to similarly stressful experiences in the past and their applicability to current ways of managing cancer experience	(a) Ask patient to identify emotion-focused, meaning-focused, problem-focused strategies they have used to cope in relation to significant stressor events (situational meanings) in their past. Which strategies were effective? Not effective? What did they learn from these experiences? (b) Could these strategies and lessons from the past inform how to cognitively and emotionally manage the cancer experience, find positive meaning, purpose in the present? What adjustments in global meaning and goals could be made in light of a current realities (i.e., changes to life priorities, goals, and beliefs)
(5) Consolidation or embedding changes in a reintegrated self	(a) Reinforce the reintegration of altered priorities, values, and beliefs that establish a new meaning in life (b) Patient and nurse together (1) review the realigned global and situational (goals and beliefs) meanings giving rise to a new meaning in life (purpose) (2) review reordered priorities, goals, and purposes that are aligned with present demands and expectations of the cancer-related experience, and (3) review useful coping strategies

meanings and emotional responses may emerge [7, 94]. The process may include providing relevant information, reframing patient thoughts, use of cognitive restructuring, and breaking down catastrophic or exaggerated thoughts into manageable parts (Review Part IV Chap. 9). Positive reappraisal *not only guides the subsequent choice of coping strategies used in response* to a stressful situation that reduces emotional distress. It also may fuel personal growth via processes of self-reflection and comparative analysis; positive reappraisal may also potentially strengthen immune functioning [32, 95].

Decatastrophize Perceptions As the patient is encouraged to examine thoughts, feelings, and beliefs about the cancer experience, *de*catastrophize beliefs, myths, and cognitive distortions that may have warped the patient's ability to reconcile situational and global meanings [96]. Cancer- or treatment-related cognitive distortions feed emotional distress and debilitate the patient's ability to recognize new possibilities or meanings in their current life. Explore where these beliefs came from. Ask the individual for evidence that supports his distorted belief. Provide factual information and together compare it to the belief. Break generalizations into smaller more manageable parts and evaluate with the individual what can or cannot be changed (Chap. 9, section "Break Down Generalizations into Smaller Manageable Components").

Keeping a Diary Another strategy is to encourage the patient to write down his thoughts, feelings, and experiences as a reflection exercise that can facilitate a more pensive and objective examination of the threat and heighten his awareness of the behavioral and emotional responses that interfere with his ability to move toward adaptation [97].

Encourage the Meaning-Making Narrative

Meaning and purpose can materialize through narrative storytelling in which processes of reappraisal may lead to new meanings and priorities [47]. Therapeutic narratives are shaped by the goals of the narrative and organizing themes. Because cancer may challenge who we are to ourselves (i.e., our self-identity), encouraging the individual's narrative about the trauma event and its impact on the self offers the opportunity to revisit, retell, and reinterpret distressing aspects of the cancer experience within the healing context of the nurse–patient (caregiver) relationship [98]. A therapeutic narrative organized around topics/themes emanating from stress and meaning-making coping theory may include a reflection on the significance of supportive relationships, work/career, family and friends, meaningful personal activities/accomplishments, and health-oriented lifestyle behaviors before and after cancer. These reflections may promote a renewed sense of meaning and purpose in the individual's current life above and beyond the reality of cancer [2, 7, 14]. It may facilitate the process of reconciling the gap between global and situational meanings that has led to the emotional distress.

Through a process of examining meaningful aspects of the individual's previous assumptions about the world and the self in relation to perceived changes that characterize his situational meanings, the patient may come to realize that some elements of his global assumptions about the self and the world may have altered, but a lot of who he is remains. For instance, the desire for volunteering, creative expression (for instance, wanting to write a novel, poetry, or do carpentry), the importance of religion in family life, and a circle of supportive relationships constitute core values that can add up to a meaningful life in the present context, if the individual can recognize those values in part through a reordering of life priorities grounded in current reality.

In contrast to other psychotherapies that focus on negative affect and potentially pathologize existential distresses that are generally *normal* within the context of cancer-related experiences, storytelling narratives enable a healing-inducing context within which different meanings may evolve [99]. The life review narrative and the meaning-making intervention have been shown to be effective nurse-led approaches to help patients and caregivers find meaning in life while living with the uncertainty and sadness of cancer [79, 83].

Clinical Anecdote 10.4
It was Gary's 4th chemotherapy session. His depression seemed to deplete his energy despite psycho-pharmaco-therapeutic interventions. At 47 he had been at the top of his game as a well known financier with a loving wife and children. Though he had everything to live for, he seemed unable to mobilize any meaning-focussed strategies to help himself find meaning from a loving and concerned family. As far as he was concerned everything he valued, his work and family and friends were being taken from him. He was mourning the loss of the life he had known and a future he had made negative assumptions about, which blocked his ability to live fully in the present surrounded by all his blessings.

Facilitating Deliberate Rumination [100] (Chap. 9)

One clinical strategy that has achieved success in helping patients process a traumatic event is deliberate rumination [49]. Deliberate rumination targets the individual's intrusive ideation by *intentionally* facilitating cognitive processing via a more controlled and deliberate meaning-making process [50]. It involves the patient's active participation in examining aspects surrounding the intrusive ideation, relevant personal resources, and social support, generating reappraisals and identifying cognitive and behavioral coping responses within a supportive context that enable the person to arrive at new meanings which can facilitate the successful integration of the traumatic event [40, 50, 101]. Deliberate rumination may follow these general steps [100]:
1. Explain to the patient that the unwanted cognitive ideations are the brain's neurophysiological efforts to cognitively process or integrate distressing events

2. Provide the person with relevant information about the disease (cancer) and/or the treatment to serve as an informed clinical context within which deliberate rumination may be meaningfully discussed between nurse and patient/caregiver.
3. Invite the patient's narrative about the stressful ideation from different perspectives of the distressing experience: Identify perceived triggers, that is factors that triggered the unwanted thoughts; how frequently and how long do these intrusive episodes last; what coping strategies are used to stop these thoughts; what is the impact on daily life, personal relationships, him/herself; quality of sleep. Are there close personal relationships with whom the patient can share thoughts and feelings about the unwanted intrusions. Offer reframing, clarifications, and interpretations and manage distorted beliefs with facts. The goal is to facilitate the individual's ability to become "accustomed" to discussing these disturbing thoughts and, in so doing, experience greater habituation (ie reducing emotional reactivity) and greater personal control over them. The second and related goal is to encourage through the narratives the individual's ability to develop a cohesive meaningful narrative of the stressful experience, how it compares to previous stressors, and what benefits or opportunities may emerge from having cancer that altogether provides a meaningful context within which cognitive processing may be facilitated.
4. Concurrently, introduce the relaxation response technique or related mindfulness activities which can be helpful in enabling the person's awareness of disturbing thoughts without reacting emotionally [100, 102].
5. Last, the nurse's desired goal is to help the patient to realize through positive reappraisals that the patient or caregiver can still be the authors of their future by the choices they make regarding how to live their life going forward, for instance, recognizing their illness as an opportunity to deepen meaningful relationships, spiritual connections, and tap into different creative facets of the self.
6. There is some evidence that as a complementary modality, healing touch has been shown to have some success in reducing intrusive ideations [36].

A Word About Causal Attributions

With the desire to answer the question "why" or "why me," patients may develop beliefs about the causes for cancer which may or may not have a predicate in scientific knowledge and may or may not be modifiable [103]. Causal attributions are beliefs that tend to be part of the situational meanings associated with the perceived stressor event. Most causal attributions refer to lifestyle behaviors (I never exercised, that is the reason I got cancer) or biological. For instance, the patient who uses biological attributions such as "I was born with bad genes" may perceive cancer or a cancer recurrence to be *beyond his/her control*, which may induce further emotional distress and maladaptive behaviors that eventually lead to a greater health-related risk such as a cancer recurrence [103]. A study of survivors of glioblastoma (GBM) reported that many patients attributed their cancer to poor diet, previous head injury, smoking, and/or an increased workload and stress [104].

The significant issue, however, from a nursing perspective is to encourage patients to shift their cognitive thinking toward what they can do moving forward to promote their quality of life rather than perseverate on a possible cause over which they have no control and may make them feel potentially helpless. Nurses may help patients identify perceived causes they can and cannot "change" moving forward along a more empowered path toward health and possibly personal growth. For instance, share the fact that the individual is in a position to facilitate the downregulation of many cancer-producing genes by making health-promoting changes in lifestyle behaviors through physical exercise, a healthy diet, and/or mindful meditation practices, notwithstanding their causal beliefs [105]. In principle, human beings are more likely to change their behavior if they receive meaningful and factual explanations.

A Matter of Personal Choice

Ultimately, the ability to find meaning within a new personal reality may have to do with making a *fundamental choice*: whether to be emotionally defeated by a traumatizing event such as a cancer diagnosis or motivated to find something meaningful in the experience that enhances psychological healing and even acceptance of the disease [106]. Through the nurse's conversations with the patient, she may help the patient realize that personal benefits are possible, even if that choice falls within clinical constraints.

Clinical Anecdote 10.5
Jesse listened carefully to the doctor's feedback. The cancer had returned after 10 years. He weighed his good fortune against the bad: He was 74 years old, with a wonderful wife, family and 4 grandchildren. He had made the most of his retirement doing what he loved most-painting, skiing and travelling. He looked up at the oncologist—"You look worse than I am!" he laughed. "Don't feel so bad. You gave me 10 great years—and I have had a good life. Don't get me wrong—I plan to live well with whatever time I have left." Jesse chose the silver lining in the midst of another life-threatening situation which led him to a realistic acceptance that gave him emotional peace.

What is meaningful to the patient may be as simple as going on one last great family trip, attending a daughter's wedding or a much beloved sports game, or enjoying the company of loved ones. For some, there is a need to reach out to those in need, to share lessons learned with others who have cancer, it is about extending beyond the self toward some common good. And for others, the goal may simply be to have a dignified death surrounded by loved ones. Thus, personal growth may be realized through the patient's positive changes in life goals and priorities that are grounded in their clinical circumstances and may vary with disease progression and survivorship [31, 32].

In contrast, suffering without meaning is meaningless according to Frankl, who suffered greatly during World War II, incarcerated as a young Jewish man first in Theresienstadt and then at Dachau concentration camp. He argued that suffering without meaning precluded the possibility of healing. And yet many people find little that is meaningful in living with cancer. Although a cure may lie beyond medical control, how the individual responds to cancer or interprets it does lie within the patient's purview and is *in itself* a meaningful response to suffering [1, 106]. Knowing that this fundamental *choice of how to live* lies within oneself even when there is no cure can provide the impetus for *personal growth* [107]. According to Cordova, the greater the threat, the greater the opportunity to grow [108]. But this requires *an ability to let go of the past and even future expectations in order to find personal meaning in the present moment.*

Clinical Anecdote 10.6
Meaning through nature buoyed the spirit of a young patient in the last terminal phase of her life. E, a young and single mother would ask to have her bed turned toward the east-facing window in order to intently follow the arc of the early rising sun; and then later to have her bed re-positioned toward the west-facing window to watch the sun sink below the horizon leaving in its wake a kaleidoscopic display of color that shouted out the dying of the day. E's sense of meaning was anchored in nature all around her, and in the belief that her whole being was an integral part of an encompassing universe, and so she stood fearlessly at the precipice of her corporeal demise, knowing that somehow, her spirit would live everywhere.

10.8 Final Thoughts

What resonates as meaningful to one person will vary in others, depending on the perceived threat as much as the quality of personal and social resources and meaning-focused strategies in the patient's life. But finding something meaningful in an insufferable experience can allow for positive "life changes" such as hope and a reason to live in the potential of the moment [8, 40]. Feelings of overall well-being or a sense of wholeness can occur when personal desires and aspirations are successfully realigned with clinical realities so that new meanings and purposes can take hold in one's present life (Mount 2007). The nurse is in an optimal position to facilitate this process, which becomes especially relevant in the advanced stages of the disease. It is a critical intervention that depends on clinical competence in managing the key concepts inherent in meaning making. For that to occur, consider inviting clinical experts, such as Dr Virginia Lee, who have developed and tested their own meaning-making interventions to give clinical courses so that both university nursing students and oncology nurses may acquire the necessary scientific knowledge and clinical skillfulness.

Appendix: Psychosocial Interventions—Meaning-Related Studies

Author	Purpose/interventions	Study design	Sample phase	Outcomes
Park et al. [23]	To evaluate effects of psychosocial interventions on meaning/purpose in adults with cancer *Interventions* Included (a) meaning focused (b) meditation (c) coping skills strategies (d) creative arts (e) health education (f) yoga	Systematic review and meta-analysis of 29 RCTs	2305 adults with cancer	(1) Psychosocial interventions were associated with significant improvements in meaning/purpose ($g = 0.37$, 95% CI, 0.22–0.52, $p < 0.0001$ (2) Interventions specifically designed to increase meaning/purpose ($g = 0.42$, 95% CI, 0.24–0.60) showed significantly higher effect sizes compared to those aimed at other primary outcomes ($g = 0.18$, 95% CI, 0.09–0.27); $p = 0.009$ *Conclusion*: Psychosocial interventions showed small to medium effect size on increased meaning/purpose Methodological issues around small samples and issues around concealment

| Lee et al. [73] | To examine the efficacy of a meaning-making coping intervention on psychological adjustment to cancer

Intervention (4 sessions)
To address existential issues based on stress-coping theory [3] Used narrative story to explore
(a) meaning of cancer-related events and emotions since diagnosis
(b) within broader context of past life events and coping strategies that may inform current cancer experience
(c) the development of realistic goals in the context of one's mortality | RCT
(a) meaning-making intervention
(b) usual care
Measures
(a) the Rosenberg Self-Esteem Scale (RSES)
(b) Life Orientation Test-revised (LOT) assessed optimism
(c) Generalized self-efficacy scale (GSES) | 82 breast or colorectal patients diagnosed in last 6 months and during treatment | (1) *Compared to usual care, and controlling for baseline data, the meaning-making intervention demonstrated significantly higher levels of*
(a) self-esteem ($F = 8.01, p = 0.006$)
(b) optimism ($F = 5.78, p = 0.019$)
(c) self-efficacy ($F = 10.76, p = 0.002$)
(2) A posttest *mean difference* between the two groups based on
(a) the self-esteem measure (RSES) of 1.66 points corresponded to an estimated change of 5.4% on the 31-point scale or a small effect size of 0.26
(b) the optimism measure (LOT) of 3.08 points revealed a 9.3% change on the 33-point optimism scale or an effect size of 0.24
(c) the self-efficacy measure (GSES) of 2.41 points showed a 7.7% change on the 31-point self-efficacy scale or an effect size of 0.22.

Conclusion: A theoretically grounded meaning-making intervention developed by a nurse with clinical benefits for patients with existential distress that needs to be replicated across illness stages *in rigorously designed trials* |

(continued)

(continued)

Author	Purpose/interventions	Study design	Sample phase	Outcomes
Life review				
Wang et al. [80]	To evaluate therapeutic life review on spiritual well-being, psychological distress, and quality of life in patients with terminal or advanced cancer *Interventions* Process aimed at reconciling past conflicts into reintegrated self resulting in peace, based on three different pathways (a) *Life completion*—by reviewing life history, family, achievements, social roles that lead to personally meaningful goals, confirmation of self-identity which results in sense of life completion or peace and increased well-being (b) *Burden relief*—a review of memories of raising children, taking care of family in order to reduce patient feelings of being a burden, thereby reducing psychological distress (c) *Hope promotion*—review of life history to improve patient's feelings about family relationships including their progeny's growth resulting in greater feelings of hope	Systematic review and meta-analysis of 8 RCTs	People with advanced, terminal cancer	Pooled results showed significant effect of life review compared to usual care on (1) Meaning of life (SMD = 0.33; 95% CI, 0.12–0.53) (2) General distress (SMD = −0.32, 95% CI, −0.55 to −0.09) (3) Overall quality of life (SMD = 0.35; 95% CI, 0.15–0.56) (4) Findings remained significant at 3-month follow-up *Conclusion*: Potentially beneficial for individuals toward end of life; small number of RCTs and methodological problems necessitate more rigorous RCTs

Campo et al. [109]	Assessed relationship of resilient personal resources on psychological outcomes every 4 months Whether this relationship was mediated by reductions in depressive symptoms and/or four meaning-making processes (search for meaning and finding reasons for one's illness; search for and finding benefit from the illness)	Longitudinal study subjected to hierarchical regression analyses	254 posttransplant cancer survivors, 9 months to 3 years post-stem cell transplant	(1) A composite measure of personal resilience resources (self-esteem, mastery, optimism) predicted significant decrease in PTSD stress symptoms ($b = -0.07$, $p = 0.005$) mediated by significant reductions in depressive symptoms ($b = -0.011$, 95% CI, -0.034 to -0.003) and significant reductions in the search for the reason for the illness ($b = -0.012$, 95% CI -0.027 to -0.003) (2) Greater personal resilience resources were also predictive of significant increases in purpose in life ($b = 0.10$, $p < 0.001$), mediated by reductions in depressive symptoms ($b = 0.015$, 95% CI 0.003–0.033) Conclusion: Finding meaning was not an important factor in this study, suggesting that individuals with greater personal resources may not need to find meaning in order to psychologically adjust to cancer Alternatively many of the survivors in this study had already found meaning, closer to the diagnosis and treatment

(continued)

(continued)

Author	Purpose/interventions	Study design	Sample phase	Outcomes
Krok and Telka [28]	To assess mediating effects of coping strategies in relationships between global and situational meaning and psychological well-being	Cross sectional using structural equation modeling	187 patients with gastric cancer	(1) Path model showed that the direct effect of meaning in life (MIL) on psychological well-being (PWB) was not significant ($b = 0.09, p > 0.05$) (2) The direct effect of changes of beliefs and goals (situational meaning) on PWB was also NS ($b = 0.02, p > 0.05$) (3) Standardized indirect effects with 95% CI for final mediation model showed that (a) MIL → Problem-, emotional-, and meaning-focused coping → PWB had a significant estimated total indirect effect of 0.47 (95% CI, 0.31–0.59) (b) Changes of beliefs/goals → emotional coping → PWB had a significant estimated total indirect negative effect of -0.17 (95% CI, -0.33 to -0.01) on psychological well-being Main finding is that coping strategies serve as important mediators in the relationship between MIL and PWB, and between changes in beliefs and goals and PWB The cross-sectional data indicates the need to replicate the path results using longitudinal data, as there is no cause and effect in the actual data as opposed to the assumptions inherent on the path analysis

Life review

Zhang et al. [76]	To assess evidence on the effect of a life review on well-being and mental health in patients with cancer	Systematic review of RCTs and clinical controlled trials	15 studies ($n = 899$) participants	(1) 9/15 studies rated as providing "strong quality evidence"; 6 were of "moderate quality" (2) Studies guided by structured interviews, and use of memory prompts, and proposing a legacy gift (3) Majority of studies reported that a life review helped patients with cancer by reducing anxiety and depression; and also by increasing hope, self-esteem, and quality of life Conclusion: Life review can improve the psychological health and well-being of patients with cancer More research based on more rigorous research designs and methods required to fully investigate the potential clinical outcomes of life reviews

(continued)

(continued)

Author	Purpose/interventions	Study design	Sample phase	Outcomes
Park et al. [110]	Assess effects of a brief supportive expressive group therapy combined with mindfulness intervention *Intervention* (1) SEGT—develop strategies to express emotions, enhance SS, individual resources, opportunities to review life, increase sense of control, address meaning of cancer (2) Mindfulness meditation component	Open-label, single arm, pre-/postdesign Feasibility study 4 weeks, 3-h sessions (1) HRV—The normalized spectral heart rate variability (HRV) measures relationship between (a) *low frequency (LF)* nu (e.g., 0.04–0.15 Hz) and (b) *high frequency (HF)* nu (e.g., 0.15–0.40 Hz) To measure modulation of the sympathetic and parasympathetic branches of the ANS (2) LF (measure of SNS) (3) HF measure of PNS (4) People with SDNN values <50 ms → unhealthy (5) 50–100 m → compromised (6) >100 m → healthy	28 distressed women with nonmetastatic breast cancer who had completed coadjuvant chemotherapy	(1) HRV (i.e., LF/HF ratio) and psychological stress at BASELINE Re SNS: LFnu associated with (a) anxiety ($r = 0.471, p = 0.017$) (b) depression ($r = 0.543, p = 0.005$) (c) perceived support (PSS) ($r = 0.40, p = 0.048$) (d) state anxiety ($r = 0.554, p = 0.004$) (e) well-being ($r = -0.658, p < 0.001$) Re: PNS: HFnu associated with (a) distress ($r = -0.471, p = 0.017$) (b) depression ($r = -0.543, p = 0.005$) (c) PSS ($r = -0.400, p = 0.048$) (d) state anxiety ($r = -0.554, p = 0.004$) (e) wbg ($r = 0.658, p < 0.001$) Re LF/HV (i.e., ↑ed HRV) associated with (a) anxiety ($r = 0.474, p = 0.017$) (b) depression ($r = 0.565, p = 0.003$) (c) PSS ($r = 0.548, p = 0.005$) (d) state anxiety ($r = 0.447, p = 0.025$) (v) wbg ($r = -0.657, p < 0.001$) (2) A significantly increased SDNN (i.e., mean of the standard deviation of all normal node to node intervals of the QRS) in a 5-min segment and a normalized high frequency (HF 0.15 to 0.4 Hz) posttreatment signified slower HRV (which is healthier) (3) Low HF (i.e., low PNS) was associated with greater depression, anxiety, perceived stress and anger at baseline (4) An increase in HP power posttreatment was related to reduced anger over baseline scores

References

1. Mount BM, Boston PH, Cohen SR. Healing connections: on moving from suffering to a sense of well-being. J Pain Symptom Manag. 2007;33(4):372–88. PubMed PMID: 17397699. Epub 2007/04/03. eng.
2. Park CL. Making sense of the meaning literature: an integrative review of meaning making and its effects on adjustment to stressful life events. Psychol Bull. 2010;136(2):257–301. PubMed PMID: 20192563. Epub 2010/03/03. eng.
3. Park CL, Edmondson D, Fenster JR, Blank TO. Meaning making and psychological adjustment following cancer: the mediating roles of growth, life meaning, and restored just-world beliefs. J Consult Clin Psychol. 2008;76(5):863–75. PubMed PMID: 18837603. Epub 2008/10/08. eng.
4. Janoff-Bulman R. Assumptive worlds and the stress of traumatic events: applications of the scheme construct. Soc Cogn. 1989;7:113–36.
5. Folkman S, Greer S. Promoting psychological well-being in the face of serious illness: when theory, research and practice inform each other. Psycho-Oncology. 2000;9(1):11–9. PubMed PMID: 10668055. Epub 2000/02/11. eng.
6. Seiler A, Jenewein J. Resilience in cancer patients. Front Psych. 2019;10:208. PubMed PMID: 31024362. Pubmed Central PMCID: PMC6460045. Epub 2019/04/27. eng.
7. Park C, Folkman S. Meaning in the context of stress and coping. Rev Gen Psychol. 1997;1:115–44.
8. Folkman S, Moskowitz J. Positive affect and meaning-focused coping during significant psychological stress. In: Hewstone M, de Wit JB, van den Bos K, Stroebe MS, editors. The scope of social psychology: theory and applications. New York: Psychology Press; 2007. p. 193–208.
9. Folkman S. Positive psychological states and coping with severe stress. Soc Sci Med. 1997;45(8):1207–21. PubMed PMID: 9381234. Epub 1997/09/25. eng.
10. Riba MB, Donovan KA, Andersen B, Braun I, Breitbart WS, Brewer BW, et al. Distress management, version 3.2019, NCCN clinical practice guidelines in oncology. JNCCN. 2019;17(10):1229–49. PubMed PMID: 31590149. Pubmed Central PMCID: PMC6907687. Epub 2019/10/08. eng.
11. McEwen BS. In pursuit of resilience: stress, epigenetics, and brain plasticity. Ann N Y Acad Sci. 2016;1373(1):56–64. PubMed PMID: 26919273. Epub 2016/02/27. eng.
12. McEwen BS, Gray J, Nasca C. Recognizing resilience: learning from the effects of stress on the brain. Neurobiol Stress. 2015;1:1–11. PubMed PMID: 25506601. Pubmed Central PMCID: PMC4260341. Epub 2014/12/17. Eng.
13. Lee V. The existential plight of cancer: meaning making as a concrete approach to the intangible search for meaning. Support Care Cancer. 2008;16(7):779–85. PubMed PMID: 18197427. Epub 2008/01/17. eng.
14. Park CL. Meaning making in the context of disasters. J Clin Psychol. 2016;72(12):1234–46. PubMed PMID: 26900868. Epub 2016/02/24. eng.
15. Vehling S, Kissane DW. Existential distress in cancer: alleviating suffering from fundamental loss and change. Psycho-Oncology. 2018;27(11):2525–30. PubMed PMID: 30307088. Epub 2018/10/12. eng.
16. Vehling S, Philipp R. Existential distress and meaning-focused interventions in cancer survivorship. Curr Opin Support Palliat Care. 2018;12(1):46–51. PubMed PMID: 29251694. Epub 2017/12/19. eng.
17. Dekker J, Braamse A, Schuurhuizen C, Beekman ATF, van Linde M, Sprangers MAG, et al. Distress in patients with cancer - on the need to distinguish between adaptive and maladaptive emotional responses. Acta Oncol. 2017;56(7):1026–9. PubMed PMID: 28145789. Epub 2017/02/02. eng.
18. Vehling S, Lehmann C, Oechsle K, Bokemeyer C, Krull A, Koch U, et al. Global meaning and meaning-related life attitudes: exploring their role in predicting depression, anxiety, and

demoralization in cancer patients. Support Care Cancer. 2011;19(4):513–20. PubMed PMID: 20306275. Epub 2010/03/23. eng.
19. Kissane DW. The relief of existential suffering. Arch Intern Med. 2012;172(19):1501–5. PubMed PMID: 22945389. Epub 2012/09/05. eng.
20. Kissane DW. Psychospiritual and existential distress. The challenge for palliative care. Aust Fam Physician. 2000;29(11):1022–5. PubMed PMID: 11127057. Epub 2000/12/29. eng.
21. Robinson S, Kissane DW, Brooker J, Burney S. A systematic review of the demoralization syndrome in individuals with progressive disease and cancer: a decade of research. J Pain Symptom Manag. 2015;49(3):595–610. PubMed PMID: 25131888. Epub 2014/08/19. eng.
22. Vehling S, Lehmann C, Oechsle K, Bokemeyer C, Krüll A, Koch U, et al. Is advanced cancer associated with demoralization and lower global meaning? The role of tumor stage and physical problems in explaining existential distress in cancer patients. Psycho-Oncology. 2012;21(1):54–63. PubMed PMID: 21061407. Epub 2010/11/10. eng.
23. Park CL, Pustejovsky JE, Trevino K, Sherman AC, Esposito C, Berendsen M, et al. Effects of psychosocial interventions on meaning and purpose in adults with cancer: a systematic review and meta-analysis. Cancer. 2019;125(14):2383–93. PubMed PMID: 31034600. Pubmed Central PMCID: PMC6602826. Epub 2019/04/30. eng.
24. Emmons RA. Personal goals, life meaning, and virtue: well springs of a positive life. Washington: American Psychological Association; 2003.
25. Henry M, Cohen SR, Lee V, Sauthier P, Provencher D, Drouin P, et al. The meaning-making intervention (MMi) appears to increase meaning in life in advanced ovarian cancer: a randomized controlled pilot study. Psycho-Oncology. 2010;19(12):1340–7. PubMed PMID: 20878857. Epub 2010/09/30. eng.
26. Leventhal H, Phillips LA, Burns E. The common-sense model of self-regulation (CSM): a dynamic framework for understanding illness self-management. J Behav Med. 2016;39(6):935–46. PubMed PMID: 27515801. Epub 2016/08/16. eng.
27. Cao W, Qi X, Cai DA, Han X. Modeling posttraumatic growth among cancer patients: the roles of social support, appraisals, and adaptive coping. Psycho-Oncology. 2018;27(1):208–15. PubMed PMID: 28171681. Epub 2017/02/09. eng.
28. Krok D, Telka E. The role of meaning in gastric cancer patients: relationships among meaning structures, coping, and psychological well-being. Anxiety Stress Coping. 2019;32(5):522–33. PubMed PMID: 31234657. Epub 2019/06/27. eng.
29. Scharloo M, Baatenburg de Jong RJ, Langeveld TP, van Velzen-Verkaik E, Doorn-Op den Akker MM, Kaptein AA. Illness cognitions in head and neck squamous cell carcinoma: predicting quality of life outcome. Support Care Cancer. 2010;18(9):1137–45. PubMed PMID: 19718524. Pubmed Central PMCID: PMC2910308. Epub 2009/09/01. eng.
30. Tomich PL, Helgeson VS. Five years later: a cross-sectional comparison of breast cancer survivors with healthy women. Psycho-Oncology. 2002;11(2):154–69. PubMed PMID: 11921331. Epub 2002/03/29. eng.
31. Bower JE, Meyerowitz BE, Desmond KA, Bernaards CA, Rowland JH, Ganz PA. Perceptions of positive meaning and vulnerability following breast cancer: predictors and outcomes among long-term breast cancer survivors. Ann Behav Med. 2005;29(3):236–45. PubMed PMID: 15946118. Epub 2005/06/11. eng.
32. Bower JE, Kemeny ME, Taylor SE, Fahey JL. Finding positive meaning and its association with natural killer cell cytotoxicity among participants in a bereavement-related disclosure intervention. Ann Behav Med. 2003;25(2):146–55. PubMed PMID: 12704017. Epub 2003/04/22. eng.
33. Lutgendorf SK, Andersen BL. Biobehavioral approaches to cancer progression and survival: mechanisms and interventions. Am Psychol. 2015;70(2):186–97. PubMed PMID: 25730724. Pubmed Central PMCID: PMC4347942. Epub 2015/03/03. eng.
34. Schroevers MJ, Kraaij V, Garnefski N. Cancer patients' experience of positive and negative changes due to the illness: relationships with psychological well-being, coping, and goal reengagement. Psycho-Oncology. 2011;20(2):165–72. PubMed PMID: 20217657. Epub 2010/03/11. eng.

35. Creamer M, Burgess P, Pattison P. Reaction to trauma: a cognitive processing model. J Abnorm Psychol. 1992;101(3):452–9. PubMed PMID: 1500602. Epub 1992/08/01. eng.
36. Reeve K, Black PA, Huang J. Examining the impact of a healing touch intervention to reduce posttraumatic stress disorder symptoms in combat veterans. Psychol Trauma. 2020;12(8):897–903. PubMed PMID: 33346680. Epub 2020/12/22. eng.
37. Kernan WD, Lepore SJ. Searching for and making meaning after breast cancer: prevalence, patterns, and negative affect. Soc Sci Med. 2009;68(6):1176–82. PubMed PMID: 19157667. Epub 2009/01/23. eng.
38. Vickberg SM, Bovbjerg DH, DuHamel KN, Currie V, Redd WH. Intrusive thoughts and psychological distress among breast cancer survivors: global meaning as a possible protective factor. Behav Med. 2000;25(4):152–60. PubMed PMID: 10789021. Epub 2000/05/02. eng.
39. Helgeson VS, Reynolds KA, Tomich PL. A meta-analytic review of benefit finding and growth. J Consult Clin Psychol. 2006;74(5):797–816. PubMed PMID: 17032085. Epub 2006/10/13. eng.
40. Folkman S. The case for positive emotions in the stress process. Anxiety Stress Coping. 2008;21(1):3–14. PubMed PMID: 18027121. Epub 2007/11/21. eng.
41. Winger JG, Adams RN, Mosher CE. Relations of meaning in life and sense of coherence to distress in cancer patients: a meta-analysis. Psycho-Oncology. 2016;25(1):2–10. PubMed PMID: 25787699. Pubmed Central PMCID: PMC4575247. Epub 2015/03/20. eng.
42. Bower JE, Kemeny ME, Taylor SE, Fahey JL. Cognitive processing, discovery of meaning, CD4 decline, and AIDS-related mortality among bereaved HIV-seropositive men. J Consult Clin Psychol. 1998;66(6):979–86. PubMed PMID: 9874911. Epub 1999/01/06. eng.
43. Karatsoreos IN, McEwen BS. Annual research review: the neurobiology and physiology of resilience and adaptation across the life course. J Child Psychol Psychiatry. 2013;54(4):337–47. PubMed PMID: 23517425. Epub 2013/03/23. eng.
44. McEwen BS, Gianaros PJ. Stress- and allostasis-induced brain plasticity. Annu Rev Med. 2011;62:431–45. PubMed PMID: 20707675. Epub 2010/08/17. eng.
45. Avdi E, Evans C. Exploring conversational and physiological aspects of psychotherapy talk. Front Psychol. 2020;11:591124. PubMed PMID: 33250829. Pubmed Central PMCID: PMC7676902. Epub 2020/12/01. eng.
46. Park CL, Helgeson VS. Introduction to the special section: growth following highly stressful life events–current status and future directions. J Consult Clin Psychol. 2006;74(5):791–6. PubMed PMID: 17032084. Epub 2006/10/13. eng.
47. Tedeschi RG, Calhoun LG. Posttraumatic growth: conceptual foundations and empirical evidence. Psychol Inq. 2004;15:1–18.
48. Tedeschi RG, Calhoun LG. Beyond the concept of recovery: growth and the experience of loss. Death Stud. 2008;32(1):27–39. PubMed PMID: 18652064. Epub 2008/07/26. eng.
49. Kolokotroni P, Anagnostopoulos F, Tsikkinis A. Psychosocial factors related to posttraumatic growth in breast cancer survivors: a review. Women Health. 2014;54(6):569–92. PubMed PMID: 24911117. Epub 2014/06/10. eng.
50. Taku K, Calhoun LG, Cann A, Tedeschi RG. The role of rumination in the coexistence of distress and posttraumatic growth among bereaved Japanese university students. Death Stud. 2008;32(5):428–44. PubMed PMID: 18767236. Epub 2008/09/05. eng.
51. Kamijo N, Yukawa S. The role of rumination and negative affect in meaning making following stressful experiences in a Japanese sample. Front Psychol. 2018;9:2404. PubMed PMID: 30546340. Pubmed Central PMCID: PMC6279863. Epub 2018/12/14. eng.
52. Ellis EM, Orehek E, Ferrer RA. Patient-provider care goal concordance: implications for palliative care decisions. Psychol Health. 2019;34(8):983–98. PubMed PMID: 30905185. Epub 2019/03/25. eng.
53. Vos J, Vitali D. The effects of psychological meaning-centered therapies on quality of life and psychological stress: a metaanalysis. Palliat Support Care. 2018;16(5):608–32. PubMed PMID: 30246682. Epub 2018/09/25. eng.
54. Aerts H, Van Vrekhem T, Stas L, Marinazzo D. The interplay between emotion regulation, emotional well-being, and cognitive functioning in brain tumor patients and their caregivers:

an exploratory study. Psycho-Oncology. 2019;28(10):2068–75. PubMed PMID: 31385377. Epub 2019/08/07. eng.
55. Bernard M, Strasser F, Gamondi C, Braunschweig G, Forster M, Kaspers-Elekes K, et al. Relationship between spirituality, meaning in life, psychological distress, wish for hastened death, and their influence on quality of life in palliative care patients. J Pain Symptom Manag. 2017;54(4):514–22. PubMed PMID: 28716616. Epub 2017/07/19. eng.
56. Wise M, Marchand LR, Roberts LJ, Chih MY. Suffering in advanced cancer: a randomized control trial of a narrative intervention. J Palliat Med. 2018;21(2):200–7. PubMed PMID: 29135330. Pubmed Central PMCID: PMC5797325. Epub 2017/11/15. eng.
57. Mathew A, Doorenbos AZ, Li H, Jang MK, Park CG, Bronas UG. Allostatic load in cancer: a systematic review and mini meta-analysis. Biol Res Nurs. 2021;23(3):341–61. PubMed PMID: 33138637. Epub 2020/11/04. eng.
58. Mathews HL, Konley T, Kosik KL, Krukowski K, Eddy J, Albuquerque K, et al. Epigenetic patterns associated with the immune dysregulation that accompanies psychosocial distress. Brain Behav Immun. 2011;25(5):830–9. PubMed PMID: 21146603. Pubmed Central PMCID: PMC3079772. Epub 2010/12/15. eng.
59. Sloan DH, BrintzenhofeSzoc K, Mistretta E, Cheng MJ, Berger A. The influence of relationships on the meaning making process: patients' perspectives. Ann Palliat Med. 2017;6(3):220–6. PubMed PMID: 28724296. Epub 2017/07/21. eng.
60. Sjolander C, Ahlstrom G. The meaning and validation of social support networks for close family of persons with advanced cancer. BMC Nurs. 2012;11:17. Pubmed Central PMCID: PMC3488574. Epub 2012/09/18. eng.
61. Lethborg C, Aranda S, Cox S, Kissane D. To what extent does meaning mediate adaptation to cancer? The relationship between physical suffering, meaning in life, and connection to others in adjustment to cancer. Palliat Support Care. 2007;5(4):377–88. PubMed PMID: 18044415. Epub 2007/11/30. eng.
62. Schmidt SD, Blank TO, Bellizzi KM, Park CL. The relationship of coping strategies, social support, and attachment style with posttraumatic growth in cancer survivors. J Health Psychol. 2012;17(7):1033–40. PubMed PMID: 22253327. Epub 2012/01/19. eng.
63. Canada AL, Murphy PE, Fitchett G, Stein K. Re-examining the contributions of faith, meaning, and peace to quality of life: a report from the American Cancer Society's Studies of Cancer Survivors-II (SCS-II). Ann Behav Med. 2016;50(1):79–86. PubMed PMID: 26384498. Epub 2015/09/20. eng.
64. Ahmadi F, Mohamed Hussin NA, Mohammad MT. Religion, culture and meaning-making coping: a study among cancer patients in Malaysia. J Relig Health. 2019;58(6):1909–24. PubMed PMID: 29948793. Pubmed Central PMCID: PMC6842329. Epub 2018/06/28. eng.
65. Tarakeshwar N, Vanderwerker LC, Paulk E, Pearce MJ, Kasl SV, Prigerson HG. Religious coping is associated with the quality of life of patients with advanced cancer. J Palliat Med. 2006;9(3):646–57. PubMed PMID: 16752970. Pubmed Central PMCID: PMC2504357. Epub 2006/06/07. eng.
66. Park CL, Sherman AC, Jim HS, Salsman JM. Religion/spirituality and health in the context of cancer: cross-domain integration, unresolved issues, and future directions. Cancer. 2015;121(21):3789–94. PubMed PMID: 26258608. Pubmed Central PMCID: PMC4618033. Epub 2015/08/11. eng.
67. Sherman AC, Merluzzi TV, Pustejovsky JE, Park CL, George L, Fitchett G, et al. A meta-analytic review of religious or spiritual involvement and social health among cancer patients. Cancer. 2015;121(21):3779–88. PubMed PMID: 26258730. Pubmed Central PMCID: PMC4618183. Epub 2015/08/11. eng.
68. Salsman JM, Fitchett G, Merluzzi TV, Sherman AC, Park CL. Religion, spirituality, and health outcomes in cancer: a case for a meta-analytic investigation. Cancer. 2015;121(21):3754–9. PubMed PMID: 26258400. Epub 2015/08/11. Eng.
69. Jim HS, Pustejovsky JE, Park CL, Danhauer SC, Sherman AC, Fitchett G, et al. Religion, spirituality, and physical health in cancer patients: a meta-analysis. Cancer. 2015;121(21):3760–8. PubMed PMID: 26258868. Epub 2015/08/11. Eng.

70. Bauereiß N, Obermaier S, Özünal SE, Baumeister H. Effects of existential interventions on spiritual, psychological, and physical well-being in adult patients with cancer: systematic review and meta-analysis of randomized controlled trials. Psycho-Oncology. 2018;27(11):2531–45. PubMed PMID: 29958339. Epub 2018/06/30. eng.
71. Vos J, Craig M, Cooper M. Existential therapies: a meta-analysis of their effects on psychological outcomes. J Consult Clin Psychol. 2015;83(1):115–28. PubMed PMID: 25045907. Epub 2014/07/22. eng.
72. Breitbart W, Pessin H, Rosenfeld B, Applebaum AJ, Lichtenthal WG, Li Y, et al. Individual meaning-centered psychotherapy for the treatment of psychological and existential distress: a randomized controlled trial in patients with advanced cancer. Cancer. 2018;124(15):3231–9. PubMed PMID: 29757459. Pubmed Central PMCID: PMC6097940. Epub 2018/05/15. eng.
73. Lee V, Cohen SR, Edgar L, Laizner AM, Gagnon AJ. Meaning-making and psychological adjustment to cancer: development of an intervention and pilot results. Oncol Nurs Forum. 2006;33(2):291–302. PubMed PMID: 16518445. Epub 2006/03/07. eng.
74. Breitbart W, Rosenfeld B, Pessin H, Applebaum A, Kulikowski J, Lichtenthal WG. Meaning-centered group psychotherapy: an effective intervention for improving psychological well-being in patients with advanced cancer. J Clin Oncol. 2015;33(7):749–54. PubMed PMID: 25646186. Pubmed Central PMCID: PMC4334778 online at www.jco.org. Author contributions are found at the end of this article. Epub 2015/02/04. eng.
75. van der Spek N, Vos J, van Uden-Kraan CF, Breitbart W, Cuijpers P, Holtmaat K, et al. Efficacy of meaning-centered group psychotherapy for cancer survivors: a randomized controlled trial. Psychol Med. 2017;47(11):1990–2001. PubMed PMID: 28374663. Pubmed Central PMCID: PMC5501751. Epub 2017/04/05. eng.
76. Zhang X, Xiao H, Chen Y. Effects of life review on mental health and well-being among cancer patients: a systematic review. Int J Nurs Stud. 2017;74:138–48. PubMed PMID: 28692880. Epub 2017/07/12. eng.
77. Applebaum AJ, Buda KL, Schofield E, Farberov M, Teitelbaum ND, Evans K, et al. Exploring the cancer caregiver's journey through web-based meaning-centered psychotherapy. Psycho-Oncology. 2018;27(3):847–56. PubMed PMID: 29136682. Epub 2017/11/15. eng.
78. Applebaum AJ, Kulikowski JR, Breitbart W. Meaning-centered psychotherapy for cancer caregivers (MCP-C): rationale and overview. Palliat Support Care. 2015;13(6):1631–41. PubMed PMID: 26000705. Pubmed Central PMCID: PMC5084443. Epub 2015/05/23. eng.
79. Haber D. Life review: implementation, theory, research, and therapy. Int J Aging Hum Dev. 2006;63(2):153–71. PubMed PMID: 17137032. Epub 2006/12/02. eng.
80. Wang CW, Chow AY, Chan CL. The effects of life review interventions on spiritual well-being, psychological distress, and quality of life in patients with terminal or advanced cancer: a systematic review and meta-analysis of randomized controlled trials. Palliat Med. 2017;31(10):883–94. PubMed PMID: 28488923. Epub 2017/05/11. eng.
81. Gagnon P, Fillion L, Robitaille MA, Girard M, Tardif F, Cochrane JP, et al. A cognitive-existential intervention to improve existential and global quality of life in cancer patients: a pilot study. Palliat Support Care. 2015;13(4):981–90. PubMed PMID: 25050872. Pubmed Central PMCID: PMC5485259. Epub 2014/07/23. eng.
82. Breitbart W, Poppito S, Rosenfeld B, Vickers AJ, Li Y, Abbey J, et al. Pilot randomized controlled trial of individual meaning-centered psychotherapy for patients with advanced cancer. J Clin Oncol. 2012;30(12):1304–9. PubMed PMID: 22370330. Pubmed Central PMCID: PMC3646315 found at the end of this article. Epub 2012/03/01. eng.
83. Lee V, Robin Cohen S, Edgar L, Laizner AM, Gagnon AJ. Meaning-making intervention during breast or colorectal cancer treatment improves self-esteem, optimism, and self-efficacy. Soc Sci Med. 2006;62(12):3133–45. PubMed PMID: 16413644. Epub 2006/01/18. eng.
84. Kissane DW, Lethborg C, Brooker J, Hempton C, Burney S, Michael N, et al. Meaning and purpose (MaP) therapy II: feasibility and acceptability from a pilot study in advanced cancer. Palliat Support Care. 2019;17(1):21–8. PubMed PMID: 30600794. Epub 2019/01/03. eng.

85. Zhang H, Zhao Q, Cao P, Ren G. Resilience and quality of life: exploring the mediator role of social support in patients with breast cancer. Med Sci Monit. 2017;23:5969–79. PubMed PMID: 29248937. Pubmed Central PMCID: PMC5744469. Epub 2017/12/19. eng.
86. Zhang J, Yin Y, Wang A, Li H, Li J, Yang S, et al. Resilience in patients with lung cancer: structural equation modeling. Cancer Nurs. 2020;44(6):465–72. PubMed PMID: 32618622. Epub 2020/07/04. eng.
87. Teo I, Baid D, Ozdemir S, Malhotra C, Singh R, Harding R, et al. Family caregivers of advanced cancer patients: self-perceived competency and meaning-making. BMJ Support Palliat Care. 2019;10(4):435–42. PubMed PMID: 31806656. Epub 2019/12/07. eng.
88. Beesley VL, Smith DD, Nagle CM, Friedlander M, Grant P, DeFazio A, et al. Coping strategies, trajectories, and their associations with patient-reported outcomes among women with ovarian cancer. Support Care Cancer. 2018;26(12):4133–42. PubMed PMID: 29948398. Epub 2018/06/28. eng.
89. Sherman AC, Simonton S, Latif U, Bracy L. Effects of global meaning and illness-specific meaning on health outcomes among breast cancer patients. J Behav Med. 2010;33(5):364–77. PubMed PMID: 20502953. Epub 2010/05/27. eng.
90. Kissane DW, Clarke DM, Street AF. Demoralization syndrome–a relevant psychiatric diagnosis for palliative care. J Palliat Care. 2001;17(1):12–21. PubMed PMID: 11324179. Epub 2001/04/28. eng.
91. Park CL, Cho D, Blank TO, Wortmann JH. Cognitive and emotional aspects of fear of recurrence: predictors and relations with adjustment in young to middle-aged cancer survivors. Psycho-Oncology. 2013;22(7):1630–8. PubMed PMID: 23060271. Epub 2012/10/13. eng.
92. Park CL, Edmondson D, Hale-Smith A, Blank TO. Religiousness/spirituality and health behaviors in younger adult cancer survivors: does faith promote a healthier lifestyle? J Behav Med. 2009;32(6):582–91. PubMed PMID: 19639404. Epub 2009/07/30. eng.
93. Ellis KR, Janevic MR, Kershaw T, Caldwell CH, Janz NK, Northouse L. Meaning-based coping, chronic conditions and quality of life in advanced cancer & caregiving. Psycho-Oncology. 2017;26(9):1316–23. PubMed PMID: 27147405. Pubmed Central PMCID: PMC5097695. Epub 2016/05/06. eng.
94. Gross JJ, John OP. Individual differences in two emotion regulation processes: implications for affect, relationships, and well-being. J Pers Soc Psychol. 2003;85(2):348–62. PubMed PMID: 12916575. Epub 2003/08/15. eng.
95. Cordova MG-FJ, Golant M, Kronenwetter C, Chang V, Spiegel D. Breast cancer as trauma: posttraumatic stress and posttraumatic growth. J Clin Psychol Med Settings. 2007;14:308–19.
96. Karademas EC, Paschali A, Hadjulis M, Papadimitriou A. Maladaptive health beliefs, illness-related self-regulation and the role of the information provided by physicians. J Health Psychol. 2016;21(6):994–1003. PubMed PMID: 25104783. Epub 2014/08/12. eng.
97. Benson H, Stuart E. The wellness book: the comprehensive guide to maintaining health and treating stress-related illness. New York: Simon and Schuster; 1992.
98. Atkinson S, Rubinelli S. Narrative in cancer research and policy: voice, knowledge and context. Crit Rev Oncol. 2012;84:11–6. PubMed PMID: 23347413. Pubmed Central PMCID: PMC4241714. Epub 2013/02/01. eng.
99. Chippendale T, Boltz M. Living legends: effectiveness of a program to enhance sense of purpose and meaning in life among community-dwelling older adults. Am J Occup Ther. 2015;69(4):1–11. PubMed PMID: 26114464. Epub 2015/06/27. eng.
100. Tedeschi RG, Taku K, Calhoun LG. Post traumatic growth: theory, research, and applications. New York: Routledge; 2018.
101. Morris BA, Shakespeare-Finch J. Rumination, post-traumatic growth, and distress: structural equation modelling with cancer survivors. Psycho-Oncology. 2011;20(11):1176–83. PubMed PMID: 20731009. Epub 2010/08/24. eng.
102. Kabat ZJ. Full catastrophe living: using the wisdom of your body and mind to face stress, pain and illness. New York: Delacourt; 1990.
103. Ferrucci LM, Cartmel B, Turkman YE, Murphy ME, Smith T, Stein KD, et al. Causal attribution among cancer survivors of the 10 most common cancers. J Psychosoc Oncol.

2011;29(2):121–40. PubMed PMID: 21391066. Pubmed Central PMCID: PMC3074193. Epub 2011/03/11. eng.
104. Birudu R, Reddy K. Illness perceptions and perceived social support among glioblastoma survivors during hospitalization. J Cancer Res Ther. 2020;16(6):1449–53. PubMed PMID: 33342811. Epub 2020/12/22. eng.
105. Bhasin MK, Dusek JA, Chang BH, Joseph MG, Denninger JW, Fricchione GL, et al. Relaxation response induces temporal transcriptome changes in energy metabolism, insulin secretion and inflammatory pathways. PLoS One. 2013;8(5):e62817. PubMed PMID: 23650531. Pubmed Central PMCID: PMC3641112. Epub 2013/05/08. eng.
106. Frankl V. Man's search for meaning. Boston: Beacon Press; 2006.
107. Remen RN. Kitchen table wisdom: stories that heal. New York: Riverhead Books; 2006.
108. Cordova MJ, Cunningham LL, Carlson CR, Andrykowski MA. Posttraumatic growth following breast cancer: a controlled comparison study. Health Psychol. 2001;20(3):176–85. PubMed PMID: 11403215. Epub 2001/06/14. eng.
109. Campo RA, Wu LM, Austin J, Valdimarsdottir H, Rini C. Personal resilience resources predict post-stem cell transplant cancer survivors' psychological outcomes through reductions in depressive symptoms and meaning-making. J Psychosoc Oncol. 2017;35(6):666–87. PubMed PMID: 28613996. Pubmed Central PMCID: PMC5844182. Epub 2017/06/15. eng.
110. Park H, Oh S, Noh Y, Kim JY, Kim JH. Heart rate variability as a marker of distress and recovery: the effect of brief supportive expressive group therapy with mindfulness in cancer patients. Integr Cancer Ther. 2018;17(3):825–31. PubMed PMID: 29417836. Pubmed Central PMCID: PMC6142099. Epub 2018/02/09. eng.

Strengthening Supportive Relationships 11

11.1 Introduction

A family member with cancer is a distressing experience for the whole family. When cancer strikes, it disrupts the family's assumptive world and the nature of their relationships with one other, including the patient [1]. It may lead family members to question their own values and beliefs about life and death. Although society expects family members to nurture and care for their ill family member, the health risks posed by the progressive burden of caregiving and the family caregiver's own need for support are related with consequential health-related outcomes for both the caregiver and patient [2].

Social support is widely shown to exert a protective function against disease onset, progression, and mortality in western countries [3–7]. It is a significant predictor of health-related outcomes, such as psychological resilience, post-traumatic personal growth, and longer survival rates, as evidenced mainly in overrepresented studies of breast cancer patients [6–10].

The purpose of this chapter is to examine the concept of support within the context of the patient with cancer and his or her informal caregiver (i.e., an intimate member of the patient's inner circle of loved ones) and strategies nurses may consider to strengthen their supportive relationships.

11.2 Objectives

At the end of this chapter you will be able to:

1. Draw on scientific theory and evidence of the therapeutic effects of support to guide clinical interventions that can enhance support.
2. Identify empirically known resilient-promoting supportive behaviors.
3. Understand the clinical context in which support may or may not be perceived to be therapeutic by the patient or family caregiver.

Clinical Anecdote 11.1

One blessing of having cancer was the coordinated and continuous acts of loving support from family and friends. Each morning I would rise early to meet a good friend for a walk before she went off to work, and I collapsed at home for a sound sleep. This continued even through chemotherapy. It was an essential component of my healing because it not only promoted my physical health but critically, it provided a daily opportunity to normalize my life, to talk about anything on my mind. Sometimes we talked about cancer but only at my initiative. We discussed all the things that had knitted us together in friendship throughout the years- family, travels, books, bird watching and imagined other sundry things we still wanted to do. It carved out a sacred time from the reality of illness that enabled lots of laughs so that I could temporarily forget that I was still very ill. It buoyed my spirits, and was an invaluable part of my healing throughout treatment and the transition into survivorship, and this walking and talking continue to this day.

Other good friends biked with me, prepared meals that could be frozen so I did not need to cook- and even created fun nights 'in' to eat- at home. One of my most wonderful clinic nurses occasionally gave me frozen homemade meals (she did this for other patients, as well) that made me feel deeply cared for and validated as a person.

Above all, my family was always there- my husband to take walks in the evening when I wasn't too tired, or to go away for a weekend, or during the third 'restorative' week of the chemotherapy cycle. Husband and daughter took turns driving me to our favorite summer retreat for week-long visits. All of this caring attention lightened my emotional burden, validated the myriad blessings to be experienced in the present, and gave me hope.

There are patients who for various reasons are unable to access the support that buffered me from too much anxiety or even the potential loneliness that could have been triggered by knowing that I could be travelling along a different pathway with a shortened lifespan compared to everyone I cared about. These patients deserve our special attention. Patients who are not getting the support they need must be identified and assessed. As feasible, their supportive relationships with family and friends or other resources need to be strengthened. At the very least these patients need greater support from the nurse, and the healthcare team so that feelings of loneliness and possible despair may be attenuated.

11.3 Definitions (Review Appendix in this Chapter and Appendix B)

Social support is defined in various ways, but essentially refers to the individual's perception that he or she is loved, cared for, and esteemed and belongs to a reciprocal and meaningful network of individuals with mutual obligations, who give and receive emotional, informational, and instrumental (tangible aid, materials, services) support (Table 11.1) [13, 14]. Emotional support has to do with caring, love, trust, and empathy [5, 11]. House's conceptualization includes appraisal support, that is, providing affirmation and feedback. Support also refers to the structure and

Table 11.1 Four classes of support [5, 11, 12]

Classes	Description
1. Emotional support	Provides/receives empathy, caring, love, esteem, active listening, comfort, and reassurance
2. Instrumental support	Gives help, material assistance, services such as taking care of the patient, doing the grocery shopping
3. Informational support	Provides advice, suggestions, relevant information to use in coping with challenges/stressors
4. Appraisal support	Provides affirmation, feedback, alternative explanations, facilitates social comparison, and self-evaluation

extent of connectedness one experiences with one's social relationships as well as the quality and quantity of social interactions [12].

Other conceptualizations of support make distinctions between the actual receipt of support, perceived availability of support, and, significantly, the fit between the type of support being offered and the person's need for support under various conditions [10]. The therapeutic impact of support tends to vary according to the type of support offered, how it is perceived by the intended recipient, the phase of illness and treatment, as well as the source of support.

Family Support

One of the most important sources of potential support for most patients with cancer is the family, conceptualized in this book mainly in terms of informal caregivers such as spouses, partners, and/or significant others [15–18]. Family support has to do with the extent to which family members or the patient's network of significant others relate to and communicate with each other in the pursuit of shared goals and various activities, such as caring for or providing needed support to one another, including their ill loved one [4, 19]. Family support is reflected by the sense of cohesiveness and connectedness among its members, the extent of open communication, and lack of conflict. Family support is associated with less anxiety and fewer chemotherapy-related symptoms in patients and less depression and higher quality of life in caregivers [18, 20, 21].

Partner and Spousal Support

A close personal relationship, such as a spouse, partner, or confidant, often serves as the patient's informal caregiver [1, 22]. The supportive nature of these relationships is conveyed through social and emotional support, meaningful communication, interdependent dyadic coping, and mutual satisfaction with the relationship [1, 23].

Affectionate displays of support, such as expressions of love and fondness, validate a patient's sense of worthiness, connectedness, belonging, and emotional security which buffers him from the ill effects of various stressors [24]. Compassionate understanding, encouraging the patient's expression of feelings, and offering relevant suggestions, interpretations, information, feedback, and guidance are supportive behaviors that foster effective patient reappraisals and coping responses to major stressors [25, 26].

Spousal and partner supports also provide tangible support, such as material and behavioral assistance, accompanying the patient to clinic appointments and treatments, doing the weekly grocery shopping, cooking, and providing financial assistance. A secure attachment style between patients and family caregivers is associated with the ability to *receive* support and, in caregivers, the added ability to find meaning in caregiving [27, 28]. Although spouses and partners are important sources of support for patients, they also are most likely to suffer as a result of their loved one's illness, which may compromise their own coping capabilities, health, and ability to provide meaningful support to their ill loved one.

11.4 Models of Support and Clinical Findings

The role of social support in promoting resilience, quality of life, and survivability has been explained by at least two important models: the direct or main effects model and the protective or buffering model of support [7, 13, 14, 29–31]. The third way in which support may foster resilience and health-related quality of life is via indirect or mediating coping pathways [32].

Stress-Buffering Model

Social support has been widely shown to protect the patient by moderating the toxic effects of stress on health outcomes. The buffering mechanism occurs in highly stressed contexts in which high levels of support reduce the toxic physiological and behavioral effects of a stressor, thereby protecting an individual's resilience and health-related outcomes [13, 31]. When the patient perceives support as high and relevant to his needs, the impact of stress on health outcomes is reduced or attenuated [13].

In a study of the buffering (and direct) effects of support in women who had survived gynecological cancer, different types and amounts of support were examined [33]. A summary measure of functional or perceived availability of support was based on the following subscales: (1) *appraisal* support which referred to a confidant with whom problems might be discussed, (2) *companionship* support which provided a sense of belonging, as well as (3) subscales of self-esteem and material assistance (all based on the Interpersonal Support Evaluation measure). Structural support referred to the number of social ties and frequency of contacts, based on the Social Network Index. The findings indicated that the positive relationship between physical symptoms (i.e., the stressor) and cancer-related perceived stress (psychological adjustment) was buffered by high levels of perceived support in that levels of perceived stress were significantly lower than among women with low levels of perceived support. Similar buffering effects were noted with the measure of structural support.

Post hoc tests further revealed that the perceived availability of a confidant or companionship was also a buffer of cancer-related perceived stress [33]. Other studies of people with cancer have shown significant buffering effects of perceived support in survivors of breast cancer and other cancers [22, 34]. Supportive "secondary" caregivers of children with cancer buffered stress effects on family functioning associated with caring for their children with cancer [35]. Other studies showed that attachment security was an effective stress-related buffer in patients with metastatic cancer [36], and perceived support effectively buffered emotional distress in survivors of hematopoietic cell transplantation [37]. When perceived stress associated with disease- or treatment-related symptoms is high (i.e., the stressor), the greater the perceived support, the greater the improvement in psychological outcomes compared to those with less support available [33], depending on the clinical condition and contextual factors involved.

In contrast, neither perceived support nor structural support demonstrated buffering effects on the relationship between physical symptoms (the stressor) and depressive symptoms (psychological adjustment) in Carpenter's study of survivors of gynecological cancers. Finding non-buffering effects is consistent with other findings in which, for instance, perceived support was not shown to buffer the deleterious relationship of perceived stressful life events on psychological distress in women with breast cancer [38]. One possible explanation is that the *perceived availability of support was not sufficiently high* to exert a therapeutic reduction in psychological distress (psychological adjustment) via its buffering interactional effects on perceived stressful life events. The buffering effects of support appear to depend on the type, amount, and source of support, the level of perceived stress (the stressor), and the type of psychological adjustment [33]. Findings may also be influenced by the measures used to assess support.

Main Effects Model

The second essential function of support lies in its direct, main effects on health-related outcomes independent of the presence of other independent variables, specifically perceived stress [39]. It is important to underscore that although perceived support was not found to buffer the deleterious relationship between physical symptomatology (the stressor) and depressive symptoms (psychological adjustment) in survivors of gynecological cancer (discussed above), analyses revealed a direct or main effect on psychological adjustment independent of the presence of physical symptoms (stressor) [33].

Converging evidence confirms the positive direct effects of social support on various health outcomes such as quality of life, psychological resilience, a sense of well-being, and survival and reduction of emotional distress and biological indicators of allostatic load in mainly cancer patients [1, 23, 40–42]. Patients with high levels of support and who feel socially integrated have less stress-related reactions to a diagnosis of breast cancer.

Conversely, other studies demonstrate that a lack or decrease of social support in survivors of breast cancer is associated with greater depression, negative affect, and stress as well as a key determinant of the stage of cancer at diagnosis [43, 44]. Moreover, socially isolated women survivors of breast cancer as well as women with low support and small social networks have a *significantly higher risk of mortality* than women with high levels of support and larger social networks or women with high levels of support [44, 45]. Whereas large networks were associated with better psychological adjustment in patients after the cancer diagnosis, this also depended significantly on the quality and "burden" that distinguished family relationships. In other words, not all family networks are supportive.

In another study, low social support and measures of structural indices of support were associated with cancer progression in patients with breast cancer, although these same associations did not bear out for other cancers, and further research is needed [6]. Higher levels of spousal or family negativity were significantly related to higher levels of allostatic load in a national study of adults [42].

Last, there is some evidence that received support or the support offered must fit the individual's need for support in order for the support to be positively associated with psychological adjustment in patients with cancer as well as the general population [22, 46]. For instance, the type of support a patient with cancer may need at the time of a new diagnosis may differ during treatment and as a survivor. Too much support may convey a lack of confidence in the patient's ability to recover, or it may make the patient feel guilty that the support cannot be adequately reciprocated, or worse, the support provided or offered does not match the needs of the patient.

Mediating Effects

Support also has an essential role to play in encouraging relevant coping behaviors that enhance the individual's resilient capabilities (see Fig. 11.1). In studies of support and coping based on path analytic techniques, the direct effects of support on health-related outcomes and post-traumatic growth (PTG) in particular were observed to dissipate when the mediating effects of active coping behaviors or personal resources, such as optimism or resilience, were added to regression path analytic models [9, 48]. The mediating effects of coping behaviors on the direct relationship between support and PTG suggest that support directly promotes active coping responses that subsequently enhance health outcomes. Individuals who are secure in their supportive relationships are more amenable to learning ways to reframe the stressor event, enabling the possibility for personal growth as well as positive health-related outcomes.

The fact that support has been shown to exert buffering, mediating, and direct effects on resilience and psychosocial adjustment in stressful and non-stressful environments testifies to its important diverse and positive influences on the

11.5 Support and Personal Resources

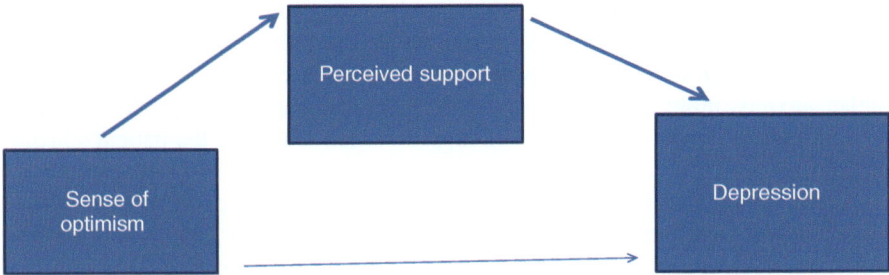

Fig. 11.1 Perceived support as mediator of a sense of optimism and depression [47]

individual's health potential. Researchers continue to study the conditions and reasons for these differential models to be evidenced across the cancer trajectory in patients with breast cancer, but significantly in other forms of cancer as well.

11.5 Support and Personal Resources

Personal resources play an essential role in a person's ability to accept and seek support and include the quality of attachments, self-efficacy beliefs, optimism, and resilience.

Support and Attachment

Attachment lies at the core of meaningful human relationships and is closely linked to the quality of support patients need and experience from others [28, 49]. Typically, individuals derive their greatest emotional support from close personal relationships such as family and friends with whom they are closely bonded [50].

Attachment theory posits that we are born with a psychobiological system that drives us to seek closeness to significant others at stressful times when we need to feel secure and to better regulate our emotions [51, 52]. Studies of mother-infant attachment show that a nurturing, encouraging, protective, and loving relationship provides feelings of security, alleviates infant distress (emotion regulation), and is a source of comfort and reassurance to the growing child [53]. Studies have also shown a relationship between adult attachment caregiving behaviors and activity in the limbic, prefrontal, basal ganglia, and HPA regions of the brain [53]. Securely attached individuals from infancy tend to replicate the same sense of emotional connectedness within adult supportive relationships.

A sense of connectedness with significant others deepens the quality of adult relationships. The need for secure attachment, proximity to loved ones, and a safe emotional haven lies at the core of quality adult relationships. Attachment security and socioemotional support are interrelated conceptually, psychologically, and biologically [54]. For instance, social support has been shown to reduce stress levels in securely attached individuals. Individuals who received support but did not feel securely attached had fewer social resources and poorer health-related outcomes [28, 49, 55]. Insecurely attached cancer patients and caregivers were found to have higher anxiety, more depression, and poor *perceived* support [50]. Secure attachment appears to enable the receipt of support which enhances the patient's health outcomes.

An interesting experimental study showed that perceived support without a sense of attachment significantly reduced cortisol levels in volunteers exposed to a stress test. Conversely, attached individuals who did not receive support did not improve cortisol levels [54]. It seems that during stress, support reduces biological stress (as assessed by cortisol levels) even in the absence of perceived attachment. A sense of attachment without commensurate support suggests emotional dependence rather than the basis of an authentic supportive relationship. Ditzen's findings also suggest by extension that patients who are in the stressful anticipation phase such as waiting for a diagnosis, frightening procedure, surgery, radiation, or chemotherapy would likely benefit from a nurse's supportive presence, reassurances, and explanations.

Support and Self-Efficacy (See Part II, Chap. 5)

Self-efficacy is the belief in one's own capability to draw on behaviors that can achieve desired goals even in the face of apparent obstacles [56, 57]. Self-efficacy and support in the context of cancer-related stress are important components of patient coping [58]. For instance, received support was shown to enhance self-efficacy in a repeated measures study that replicated findings from earlier cross-sectional studies [32, 59]. These results are consistent with social cognitive theory and the enabling hypothesis in which the *receipt of* needed support (emotional, informational, and material) can strengthen an individual's sense of self-efficacy which (according to these findings) subsequently can improve adherence to treatment and physical functioning [59, 60]. A longitudinal study based on partner perceptions also showed that the self-efficacy of one partner appeared to elicit the support provided by the other [61]. That is, the patient's own self-efficacy beliefs appear to be instrumental in seeking and obtaining needed support from another person, in this case one's spouse. Self-efficacy and support generally *interact* and, based on these and other findings, suggest the importance of the nurse in promoting a patient's ability to seek and maintain needed support [58].

Support and Optimism

Optimism refers to the generalized expectation of positive outcomes [62]. Perceived support has been found to mediate the relationship between optimism and depression in at-risk women for breast cancer [47] (see Fig. 11.2). Optimism has also been found to moderate the relationship between perceived support and anxiety: Patients with advanced cancer and low optimism were shown to have fewer symptoms of anxiety if their level of support was perceived to be high. Conversely, support did

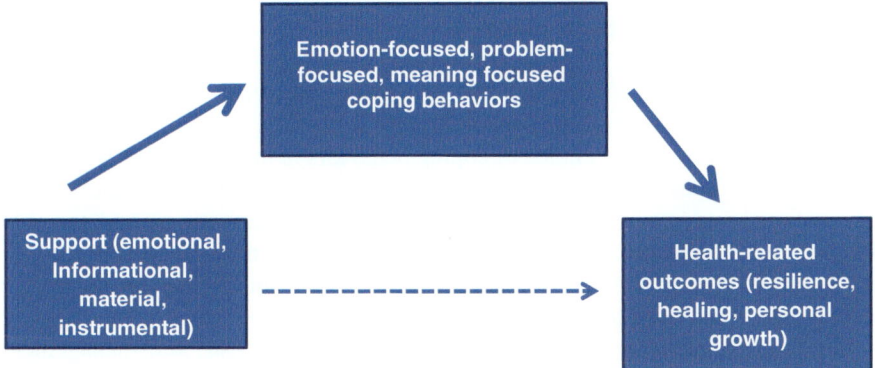

Fig. 11.2 Mediating effects of coping behaviors

not appear to reduce anxiety in patients with high levels of optimism [63]. Because optimistic individuals tend to attract support, it is possible that in these individuals, a further increase in support may be interpreted as an indicator of declining health status, thereby accounting for their anxiety. Other analyses suggest that perceived support is a mediator of the relationship between optimism and depression, suggesting that optimistic individuals may also elicit greater support which subsequently has an impact on depression [47]. These findings have clinical implications in caring for patients with cancer (Fig. 11.1).

Support and Resilience

Resilience is the desired overall outcome of biological and psychological processes of stress-coping adaptation assessed at one moment in time [64]. An individual's overall resilience serves as a personal resource within stressful circumstances (review Part II, Chaps. 4 and 5). In other words, one's overall resilience based on a cross-sectional measure may be said to reflect an individual's accrued, resilient-promoting capabilities at that moment in time. Support and resilience have reciprocating effects.

A recent finding suggested that the resilience of survivors of colorectal cancer mediated the relationship between support and post-traumatic growth based on path analytic models using cross-sectional data [9]. Support appears to *strengthen* resilient capabilities which in turn enhance clinical outcomes such as post-traumatic growth in survivorship. Thus, support has a critical indirect role in promoting post-traumatic growth via its direct positive effects on overall resilience (i.e., fostering relevant coping strategies) in survivors of colorectal cancer. Conversely, social support was found to mediate the relationship between resilience and quality of life [65]. That is, resilient patients with breast cancer were better able to obtain the support they needed in order to enhance their quality of life. Although these studies testify to the reciprocal effects between support and resilience, a study based on a longitudinal design is required to confirm the direction of effects.

Support and Coping Behaviors

Coping behaviors tend to mediate the relationship between support and health-related outcomes (Fig. 11.2). Support directly influences the patient's cognitive appraisals/reappraisals and choice of coping behaviors in the face of stressful situations [25, 48]. Types of support influencing coping behaviors included emotion and informational support, affectionate behaviors, positive interactions, and tangible support. These supportive behaviors have not always been observed across studies, which may have to do with the phase of illness and treatment and the type of support desired by and provided to patients [22].

Informal sources of support have been shown to directly foster self-management capabilities (communication, information seeking, and exercise) and indirectly by influencing coping style in Chinese survivors of cancer [66]. Informational support may help to modify distorted appraisals by cancer patients, which have important clinical implications throughout the disease trajectory, including the survival phase. Support indirectly promotes personal growth via its direct positive effects on active coping, planning, and positive reframing which subsequently have been shown to enhance a sense of personal growth in cancer patients [25].

Not All Support Is Supportive

The support patients derive from their interactions with family and friends is a critical resource, as clinical findings above illustrate. Yet not all support has been shown to result in positive health-related outcomes for a number of reasons [22, 67, 68]. The type of support offered by the family, caregiver, or close friend may not be *sufficient* or what the patient feels *she or he needs* as a function of the clinical situation. A patient may perceive him- or herself as a burden rather than a loved one to whom support has been freely given [69]. The husband who visits his wife in the palliative care unit each evening may appear to staff as being supportive to his wife. But staff may not have been privy to his constant daily deflating comments to his wife, such as "I still have lots to do, I haven't eaten yet, I am so tired or I cannot stay long." This would undoubtedly negatively affect the quality and quantity of the patient's support, by making her feel that she is a burden rather than a beloved spouse.

Many studies report that neither perceived availability of support nor received emotional support *during the early post-diagnostic phase was* supportive according to long-term survivors of various cancer types [10]. Conveying to a patient that support was available "on request" fell short for most patients with cancer during the extremely stressful diagnostic phase. However, patient perceptions changed as they got better, so that the perceived *availability* of support from family and friends was more appreciated in survivorship. In a crisis, support from loved ones was about showing up and being fully present without being asked.

A study of patients with head and neck cancer found that support had differential effects on psychological well-being depending on how support was assessed by the patient ("available" versus "received"), the medical diagnosis, and the number of physical health problems at diagnosis and 6 months later [70]. Interestingly, especially in patients with *few health* complaints, received support at baseline was significantly related to depressed symptoms in head and neck cancer patients before rather than after treatment. Patients who received more support showed more depressive sympotmatology that those who received less support. The researchers hypothesized that the patients who reported *receiving* more emotional and instrumental support at diagnosis may have *received support* because of their greater depressive symptoms. Alternatively, patients who received support may have experienced more depressive symptoms because the received support elicited feelings of low esteem or feelings that their autonomy had been infringed upon. In contrast, patients also with few health complaints who reported *perceived support availability* at diagnosis and 6 months later were shown to have significantly fewer depressed symptoms [70]. The availability of support had a significant direct main effect on health-related outcomes independent of stress and suggests that available support was sufficient to meet the patient's needs before and after treatment given the paucity of health complaints. These findings are consistent with those from a study of patients with colorectal cancer with high perceived support (perceived confidant and affective support) who manifested higher quality of life *in the absence of* psychological or physical symptoms [71]. These findings suggest that received support versus available support can be complicated and underscore the importance of assessing the patient's and caregiver's support needs.

Other findings have shown that emotional support from family and friends was important but still *required* an active clinical intervention *by a healthcare provider* particularly when the clinical context became more critical [28]. The significance of these findings is that *healthcare provider support* serves a specific function, offering health-related support that cannot be provided by family and friends.

When Patients Lack Support

Some patients are lonely due to a lack of support. This loneliness, defined as the discrepancy between one's desired and actual relationships, causes social distress but also may be attributed to cognitive decline [72]. Patients lacking support or experiencing significant burdens in their relationships were found to have poorer health outcomes [45, 73]. Loneliness and inadequate support have been associated with increased stress, anxiety, depression, impaired mood effects, and an increased risk of mortality and morbidity [40, 43, 45].

Support and Neurobiological Effects (Part III Chap. 7)

The protective function of support on an individual's biology involves triggering the downregulation of the stress-induced HPA axis, the sympathetic nervous system (SNS), and their corresponding stress mediators to normalizing levels, enabling the reactivation of the parasympathetic nervous system (PNS) and immune system functions [74, 75].

Immune cells such as natural killer cell functions and numbers, cytotoxic T-cells, and various cytokines that play a central role in hunting and eliminating cancer cells were shown to be reactivated when patients experienced high levels of perceived support [7, 76]. Patients with ovarian cancer, for example, who reported high levels of support were found to have significantly lower levels of pro-inflammatory factors, such as VEGF, IL-6, and MMP-9 *within the tumor microenvironment*. Cancer cells depend on these markers *to promote the growth and proliferation* of the tumor [7, 40, 77]. Natural killer cell activity in tumor-invading lymphocytes was also higher in patients with perceived support compared to distressed patients [77]. The positive relationship between perceived support and cell-mediated immunity may be a causative factor in the longer survival of supported patients with cancer [7, 78].

The extent to which one feels loved and cared for, that is, emotionally connected with another, appears to activate reward-related neural circuits that may embed or reinforce the therapeutic physiological experience of being supported [31]. There are probably myriad interrelated neuroendocrine pathways activated by perceived support, but two important neural circuits that likely mediate the process of social buffering include the inhibitory activities of the ventromedial prefrontal cortical neural endocrine circuits that suppress amygdala activity and the oxytocinergic systems [75, 79]. Oxytocin is involved in promoting social bonds directly and also suppressing the stress-induced activity of the HPA axis and SNS, as measured by anxiety levels [74, 80]. Oxytocin may inhibit the release of stress-induced neurohormones and other neurotransmitters. Once basal levels of physiological activity have been restored, PNS (healing) processes re-emerge to foster the resilience-promoting capabilities of human beings.

A Lack of Support A DNA microarray analysis of the leukocytes of individuals who were lonely versus not lonely showed differential expression among 209 genes [81]. Lonely individuals expressed significantly fewer leukocyte genes associated with *anti-inflammatory glucocorticoid elements* compared to non-lonely persons. Moreover, lonely people overexpressed the genes associated with triggering pro-inflammatory NFkB/Rel transcription factors that have been implicated in inflammatory diseases including cancer [81]. Similarly, pro-inflammatory transcription factors such as NFkB and STAT3 were significantly *increased* within the tumors of lonely and depressed patients with ovarian cancer compared to the tumors of non-depressed and supported persons [82]. The poor support of depressed patients with ovarian cancer was also associated with increased *intra-tumor norepinephrine* suggesting that an activated sympathetic nervous system serves as one mechanism by which pro-inflammatory biobehavioral factors *continue to modulate corresponding gene expression* in solid tumors [73, 82]. These findings provide invaluable insights into the neuroendocrinal pathways that are triggered in lonely or unsupported patients with cancer which put them at significant risk for disease progression and a shortened life. This biological knowledge supports the need for clinical interventions that downregulate stress and enhance the supportive relationships of patients and their caregivers.

11.6 The Importance of a Patient-Family Caregiver Dyad as the Focus of a Supportive Intervention

Informal sources of support, such as close family members, spouses, and significant others, are the greatest predictors of adaptive resilience and survivability in cancer patients [76]. Spouses and cancer patients with low perceived personal control but high levels of perceived spousal support were shown to experience significantly less distress than dyads with low support [83, 84]. Dagan and colleagues' longitudinal study showed that the partner's emotional responsiveness to the patient's high need for emotional expression predicted low levels of depression in patients with cancer. Emotional support, in the form of *validating and understanding* the patient's emotional expressions, was more important in accounting for the patient's low level of depressed symptoms than the partner's caring *expressions* of love [83]. The relational context between caregiver and patient is essential to consider in caring for patients.

Furthermore, unsupportive compared to supportive spousal behaviors were shown to have a bigger impact on the partner's distress whether or not the latter had cancer [84]. Findings from a study of couple intimacy suggested that an inability to discuss concerns about prostate cancer, for instance, was associated with couple distress, relationship dissatisfaction, and lack of intimacy [85]. A meta-analysis of distress within dyads' coping with cancer found a significant low-to-moderate relationship between the patient and the caregiver's distress, suggesting that couples function as a mutually reciprocating and interactive emotional system [86]. The findings highlight the clinical importance of assessing the nature of the dyad's support toward one another, and feelings of dissatisfaction or resentment toward one another, given the respective impact of one another's moods and health on each other's resilient capabilities and health.

Both theory and research findings strongly highlight the importance of strengthening supportive behaviors between family members and patients due in part to the key caregiver role in promoting resilience and post-traumatic growth in patients [22, 23]. The support data also suggest that the nature of this informal support must be sensitively *tailored* to the patient's changing needs and be capable of adapting to the patient as a function of the nature of the disease, its progression, treatment, and overall psychological well-being. This also may be said of the caregiver and his or her need for different types of support from professionals, family members, or close friends [87, 88]. A supportive intervention should include both patients and family caregivers, whenever possible with opportunities to intervene with each separately as needed [87, 89].

The receipt of emotional support, a sense of emotional closeness, and connectedness have been shown to promote post-traumatic growth and resilience, as well as prolong survival (Table 11.2) [40, 76]. Schroever's study indicated that emotional support and specifically comforting, reassuring, and problem-solving behaviors received by patients reported 3 months post-diagnosis were associated with finding meaning in the cancer experience 8 years later. In a recent study, patients with cancer identified the types of support they wanted from caregivers. These included

Table 11.2 Examples of support valued by patients and family caregivers

Support behaviors
Emotional support, providing reassurance, comfort, promoting problem-solving behaviors, validating thoughts and feelings [10, 83, 84]
Companionship, empathy, information, instrumental support (help to/from appointments) [90]
Emotional closeness, sense of connectedness [40, 90]
Providing education and relevant information, counseling, and enhancing supportive relationships with family, friends [91]

companionship, empathy, information, and help getting to and from appointments [90]. Patients and caregivers are both affected by the disease and treatment [86]. Their respective distress and the nature of the support perceived received from one another have been shown to influence one another with either beneficial or detrimental psychological outcomes.

11.7 Controlled Trials: Supportive Expressive Intervention Studies (Review Appendix in this Chapter and Appendix B)

Most supportive interventions occur as an integral part of nursing patients and the family caregiver, either individually or together. However, randomized controlled studies have evaluated the effectiveness of a supportive expressive group intervention (SEGT) mainly in women with breast cancer at different phases of the disease on a variety of biobehavioral outcomes [92–94]. The findings generally supported the effectiveness of the SEGT in reducing total mood disturbances, depression, anxiety, anger, confusion, intrusive ideation, and avoidant behaviors as well as a sense of hopelessness and helplessness particularly in those with metastatic breast cancer or a breast cancer recurrence. One RCT also showed a significant improvement in social functioning [93]. Women with high distress at baseline benefited more from the intervention compared to women with no or low levels of distress.

Conversely, two systematic reviews and meta-analyses reported mixed results. A meta-analysis of four RCTs showed that SEGT was related to a *reduction* in quality of life, a slight *increase* in anxiety, and a slight reduction in depression in women with breast cancer [95]. The other meta-analysis indicated that 4/5 RCTs demonstrated inconclusive results, and only one study ($n = 50$) reported significant improvements in mood disturbances [67]. Both meta-analyses were hindered by poor-quality evidence based on high heterogeneity among the studies.

One hypothesis however is that SEGT may be effective in improving the symptoms and side effects experienced by patients with breast cancer when provided earlier in the course of the disease and treatment, enabling the patient to benefit from the therapeutic effects of the intervention over time [93, 94]. A qualitative study of women in the early phase of their breast cancer who participated in a SEGT intervention revealed a number of benefits including the receipt of support from the group, learning from the experiences of the other women, and feeling empowered by their increased ability to be more open and to share their feelings and thoughts with others [96]. The supportive group intervention was also credited for helping some participants to reorder priorities in their life, improve the quality of personal relationships, and experience a greater sense of optimism. Whereas a few participants felt uncomfortable discussing intimate aspects of their couple relationship or dealing with the needs of others within the group, the majority derived a number of clear benefits.

Although SEGT studies based on patients in the advanced stages of their illness showed that participants improved quality of life, the supportive intervention attracted less than half the eligible patients as reported by one study, suggesting that a group intervention may not be optimal for patients in the advanced stages of cancer [93]. Rather, the SEGT intervention appears to be more relevant for patients evidencing high levels of distress in the earlier phases of the disease continuum in order to relieve anxiety and other symptoms. The SEGT intervention also may not be appropriate for individuals in transition to survival. Classen's 12-week, supportive expressive group intervention was designed to strengthen patient support, encourage emotional expression, and explore existential issues in patients with primary, non metastatic breast cancer. Individuals had successfully completed cancer-related treatments and were disease-free. The nonsignificant findings suggest that (1) given their clinical status at the time of the SEGT intervention, these patients were unlikely to have experienced high levels of distress at baseline (which was not measured). Moreover, they were unlikely to clinically benefit from an SEGT program that typically included a discussion on existential issues such as death and dying, particularly when their personal expectations were oriented toward finding a healthy life after cancer [97]. The SEGT, like many other psychosocial interventions, must be tailored in content and delivery format to the needs of the participants.

SEGT and Survivability

The question of whether supportive expressive group interventions (SEGT) lengthen survival in patients with cancer has also been examined with mixed results. For instance, a RCT of patients with a primary diagnosis of stomach, pancreatic, primary liver, or colorectal cancer, who were randomly assigned to receive a therapeutic supportive intervention compared to usual care, showed significantly longer survival based on Kaplan-Meier survival curves 10 years later [91]. The support intervention consisted of education and information, counseling, encouraging support from family and friends, exploring the patient's thoughts and feelings about the surgery, providing assertiveness training to more effectively interact with healthcare providers, and helping patients plan for the future at discharge.

In contrast, other survival analyses have shown that the SEGT intervention failed to lengthen survivorship in patients with metastatic breast cancer (e.g., [94, 98]) or had recently experienced a cancer recurrence [93].

Andersen and her colleagues reported significant biobehavioral improvements and a longer survival over a median of 11 years in women who participated in a multimodal psychosocial supportive intervention following surgery for regional breast cancer [76, 78, 99]. Interventions included a supportive component as an integral part of a more comprehensive clinical intervention which consisted of many of the following key components: psychoeducation about the disease and treatment, promoting cognitive and behavioral coping strategies, goal setting and problem-solving approaches to practical problems, communication skills for obtaining and maintaining support and for strengthening personal relationships, and information about diet and exercise.

The intervention showed significant improvements in mood disturbances, anxiety, fatigue, *the ability to find and retain support*, family relationships, dietary habits, and exercise over time [76]. Although disease recurred in both the supportive arm and assessment-only arm, the intent-to-treat analysis showed that the intervention group had a significantly lower risk of death after the cancer recurrence compared to the control group and had a 56% reduction in the risk of death from breast cancer or all death-related causes. The researchers hypothesized that the stable and improved supportive relationships during stressful periods may have enhanced natural killer cell cytotoxicity which is essential in controlling the spread of cancer after surgery and other cancer-related treatments including chemotherapy or radiotherapy. This hypothesis has gained consistent scientific support from other subsequent research findings [7]. The patients' perceived support was deemed to be an essential contributing factor in prolonging survival of patients, but it was the quality of informal support starting at baseline that was thought to be the determining factor [40].

11.8 Nursing Approaches

Nursing goals are to (1) strengthen overall support within the patient-caregiver relationship and (2) address the individual supportive needs of the patient and caregiver. Family-focused interventions to enhance the quality and frequency of support across family members may also be important but exceed the goals of this book.

Nursing Assessment of Patients and Family Caregivers

Regular nursing assessments of the patient's quality of support from family and friends start at diagnosis and continue throughout the cancer experience and into survivorship. These assessments enable supportive interventions to be tailored according to the changing support needs of patient and caregiver and the quality of their relationship(s). Patients lacking support as well as those experiencing toxic social relationships need to be identified, and a plan put in place to counter those deleterious effects on the individual's potential capabilities for psychosocial resilience. Negative or inadequate social relationships can jeopardize treatment efficacy and the patient's ability to tolerate or continue the treatment to completion [100].

Social Resources
Social resources may be assessed with the patient and caregiver present and/or individually. Ascertain the individuals who constitute the family and/or close friends from both patient and caregiver perspectives (they may differ). Identify the normal roles and functions within the family. Identify the important supportive relation-

ships of the patient and the family caregiver within the family and from close friends (support functions, quality, quantity, connectedness, availability, accessibility, and perceived/receipt of support). What is the quality of communication among family members (e.g., angry, caring, patient, impatient, respectful, interrupting, and so on)? Consider the impact of the cancer-related threat on the availability and stability of supportive relationships, particularly if family members themselves are fragile to begin with [101, 102].

Support Functions
Assess emotional, informational, material, and instrumental functions. Ask the patient and caregiver, respectively, to rate their satisfaction with support on a visual analogue 10-point scale. Ask the patient or caregiver to explain their response, and in addition to identify the source, type, and quantity of support they have received versus support they need, and whether *their need* is of short, frequent, or indefinite duration. Assess the nature of the support in relation to cancer- and treatment-related challenges they must confront over the continuum [9, 59]. Explore whether specific sources of support have facilitated positive reappraisals and more effective coping responses to stress [25]. If so, what types of support were most effective? What other types of support would be appreciated by the patient *and* the caregiver? It is equally essential that the caregiver feel supported by family and/or significant others in order to minimize the chances of caregiver burden and its potential damaging effects on the quality of the patient and caregiver relationship [103].

The Quality of the Patient-Family Caregiver Relationship
The quality of the patient-caregiver relationship has to do with the affective state, shared understanding, mutual affinity, sense of connectedness, and informational and instrumental components of support that characterize the relationship.

Patterns of Support May Change Over Time Explore the quality and frequency of giving and receiving emotional, informational, and instrumental support within the patient-caregiver relationship over the course of the illness, treatment, survival, and/or end-of-life phases [43]. You might start with a patient's or caregiver's main concern and invite each individual to share their thoughts and feelings about the types of support they have experienced in response to that concern or other stressors, identifying those supportive behaviors that have been most meaningful and why [103]. Explore the types of well-intentioned supports that were less valued and why.

Sense of Connectedness Between Patient and Caregiver (See Part IV Chap. 8) A sense of connectedness between two individuals is characterized by shared beliefs and a mutual understanding, trust, and regard. People generally desire deep human and/or spiritual connections to feel secure and less lonely and to help make sense of a situation [104, 105]. Assessing the quality of affective bonds within a supportive relationship gets at the therapeutic core of human relationships [28]. However, emotional attachment in the absence of support is not therapeutic and bears a greater resemblance to dependency [54]. Invite the patient and family caregiver to share their perceptions about their relationship. You might ask the patient and caregiver to describe their relationship before cancer and currently. What if anything has changed since cancer, the reasons, and the possible solutions. Explore their current relationship in terms of what works and descriptors or characteristics that exemplify it. Explore their relationship in terms of shared values, sense of connectedness, and normal participation in one another's lives and its impact on one another's sense of well-being. Explore what they value most and least about their relationship, whether it is a particularly close relationship, emotionally, and how it fits within the relational context of their family. For instance:

Clinical Anecdote 11.2
In an interview with the patient, Jeff and his wife Anne described their relationship as "solid" although marked by few outward expressions of love and affection. "Anne arrives everyday with something good for me to eat since I have been hospitalized. After the meal, she leaves to take care of the family. We do things for one another- that's how we show up for each other." This relationship might be described in terms of mostly instrumental displays of support in this vignette.

Invite respective descriptions of being close or connected, sources of comfort, and physical displays of affection (such as warm touches, hand holding, and hugs) toward one another. Listen for statements such as "We know what one another is thinking before it is said" and "She/he immediately understands how I feel, think about things."

Explore the effects of stress on the relationship. Ask how each handles adversity, whether they find themselves disagreeing more than they would like to, and what actions they take in those instances to restore a sense of mutual harmony. Are there topics in which there appears to be disagreement, and how are these managed (avoided, discussed rationally or in anger)? *Often these assessments are an intervention in themselves* by providing an opportunity to share and examine thoughts, feelings, and behaviors through a discussion that can lead to heightened insights that trigger positive changes.

Observe for signs of shared understanding and emotional and behavioral connectivity within the dyad. For instance, are both members engaged, distracted, or uninterested in what the other is saying? When one person is distressed, does the other person share their concern verbally, behaviorally (e.g., reaching out to physically console the person with a touch or hug? Do they finish one another's sentences or anticipate what the other is feeling, thinking? Are they one another's greatest advocate or cheerleader?

Fit Between Need for and Receipt of Support Assess potential gaps between the individual's need for and perceived receipt of support from the family caregiver, and relevant sources [68]. For instance, emotional support, which is an essential component of feeling validated, loved, and cared for, may be perceived by patients as *inadequate* at times, depending on the nature of the stressor and the source and type of support [32]. Patients may appreciate offers of support availability during survivorship when things are going well. But offers of "I am available if you need me" just before a major surgical procedure may not be regarded as sincere or reassuring. A lack of fit between the emotional support provided by the caregiver and the patient's need for a different type of support in a clinical situation may fray at their essentially loving relationship [22]. Because the type and amount of support may not meet individual needs, ask the dyad to estimate the frequency and type of support each experiences in a typical week and whether the support is "generally enough," "more than enough," or "not enough" and why. This is important because perceived support is affected by whether the individual sought and received *the needed type of* support.

The type and sources of support they need (or lack) versus what they perceive receiving can be a function of the phase of treatment, clinical status, symptoms and side effects, self-efficacy beliefs, problem-solving skills, emotional distress, and clinical state of health of either the patient or caregiver. For instance, a lack of fit between *unsolicited received support* and the level of stress currently being experienced (which may be manageable) was shown to result in depressed symptoms in patients with head and neck cancer who were assessed before treatment and 6 months later [70]. Conversely receipt of needed support has been associated with increased self-efficacy beliefs, adherence to treatment, and improved physical functioning [59]. The findings underscore the importance of the caregiver clarifying with the patient the kind of support that the patient would prefer as opposed to providing support based on untested assumptions that were made.

Quality of Communication (Review Part IV Chap. 8)

Communication skills are essential in successfully eliciting and maintaining needed support. It is a critical predicate for giving and receiving support and for providing supportive care [106]. This should be assessed within two important domains: (1) the quality, types, and frequency of communications within the dyad and also (2) the quality of communication between the dyad and the nurse as well as with the oncologist (other healthcare providers).

Dyadic Communication Explore the dyad's facility for shared emotional expression, that is, their propensity to share thoughts and feelings with one another in an open and timely manner and to accurately read one another's behaviors such as facial expressions. Explore different patterns of communication: who generally starts conversations; are conversations in synch with one another, mutually reciprocal and convey understanding; how responsive is each party to one another's comments, fears, and anxieties? Can the caregiver and patient read behavioral cues? What behavioral gestures or grimaces appear to shut down communication or encourage it? Do they maintain eye contact when they are conversing with one another? Where does the caregiver sit in relation to the patient? Are both positioned within reach of a comforting touch or hug? Does the caregiver lean toward the patient when they are talking? Or vice versa.

Describe the tone of their voices when they speak to one another. Warm, diffident, hostile, or adversarial? Is the caregiver, in particular patient centered, fully present and responsive to the needs of the patient? Does the patient convey concerns for the health or well-being of the caregiver? Ask each person to describe the frequency, quality, and substance of their communications with one another. How do they make decisions about the patient's care, and other related matters, such as medical appointments or end-of-life care. Ask them what they desire to modify in one another's mode of communications, if possible. This assessment may lead the nurse to determine that the nature of the dyadic communication requires a clinical referral to psychology.

A lack of communication skills or a history of loneliness and few supportive resources are clear obstacles to deriving the therapeutic benefits of being supported [49]. Lack of support is associated with increased stress, anxiety, depression, impaired mood effects, and an increased risk of mortality and morbidity [45, 107]. Patients and caregivers whose behavioral patterns of interacting with one another appear dysfunctional must be addressed and/or referred to psychologist. Examples might include a patient who is in the process of sharing a lack of needed support as the caregiver appears disinterested or lacks empathy, based on the caregiver's verbal and nonverbal behaviors and lack of emotional and behavioral connection with the patient.

To summarize, an in-depth support-related clinical assessment may serve as a therapeutic intervention in its own right. Below are other strategies that can promote feelings of support in patients and caregivers and within the patient-caregiver dyad.

Nursing Interventions (Review Appendix in this Chapter and Appendix B)

The goals and content of supportive interventions must be congruent with the clinical context and supportive needs of the patient and/or family caregiver (Table 11.3). Nurse-led discussions between the patient and family caregiver might be organized around one or more relevant topics identified through the support assessment: (1) enhancing the patients' supportive relationships with family and friends, (2) promoting strategies to help patients elicit and maintain needed support, (3) identifying ways that the family caregiver and significant others may be supportive to one another in order to more effectively support the patient, (4) addressing relational difficulties impeding the possibility of giving or receiving needed support, and (5) exploring strategies of support within the patient-caregiver relationship. Generating supportive behaviors is more likely to be effective when these behaviors are proposed by the patient and caregiver (and family members as needed), working together to find meaningful solutions [112]. Growing evidence supports the clinical imperative of nurses and other healthcare providers improving their ability to be supportive by strengthening *their* communication skills through formal workshops [106, 113, 114].

Table 11.3 Suggested interventions to promote support (review Appendix in this Chapter and Appendix B) [22, 23, 25, 88, 97, 108–111]

Suggested support specific strategies
(1) Promote a supportive environment in which patient and caregiver may share feelings and thoughts and support one another (e.g., quiet space, regular meaningful interactions, active listening, and being fully present with one another)
(2) Enhance patient and family caregiver communication skills (as needed): such as the importance of conversing without anger, judgment, criticism; suggest starting a sentence with "I *feel*"… rather than "*You always do*"…, and promote the discussion of difficult issues without hurting one another's feelings
(3) Promote dyadic emotional expressions of empathy, understanding, encouragement, comfort
(4) Elicit the dyad's feelings and thoughts regarding behaviors that enhance a sense of connectedness between them (for instance, use of physical touch, active listening without judgment, maintaining eye contact, leaning into the conversation, nodding in agreement)
(5) Discuss and invite dyad to share meaningful examples of functional, emotional, informational support
(6) Invite dyad to share examples of well-intentioned support that was not supportive, possible reasons why, and their preferred support in various clinical contexts
(7) Encourage caregivers to share and promote relevant coping strategies and information with the patient (review Chap. 9)
(8) Use an unstructured, nondidactic approach: open-ended questions, invite patient and family to identify topics of importance to them

Encourage Open Communication and Emotional Expression [97, 110, 98]

Generate mutually agreed ways of communication between the patient and caregiver during each meeting (as relevant): Set the tone by reviewing/generating together supportive ways to communicate (e.g., listening to one another without judgment, without interruptions, leaning in toward one another during discussions, maintaining eye contact, employing behavioral gestures such as nodding in agreement to convey understanding or support, seeking clarification, paraphrasing what has been said to validate the concern and to acknowledge one another's thoughts and feelings).

Encourage open expression of thoughts and feelings between the patient and caregiver. Invite the dyad to describe the nature of their relationship, comparing and contrasting their relationship before and after the patient was diagnosed, as well as over time since diagnosis. Ask each to describe positive, meaningful aspects of their relationship, what each person means to the other, and to share examples of what binds them as a dyad. Invite them to also share what may interfere with their ability to be open with one another, family or loved ones, such as having concerns about hurting one another's feelings.

Offer relevant contextual information and guided mentorship. Encourage dyadic problem-solving. Consider using vignettes of relationships between hypothetical patients and informal caregivers, which illustrate supportive/nonsupportive interactions that have an impact on open communication and the ability to honestly share feelings and thoughts with one another. The vignettes are intended to generate caregiver-patient discussion through sharing their thoughts, feelings, and behaviors in response to each vignette. These vignettes are meant to lead to solutions and highlight connections between behaviors, feelings, and thoughts of one another through discussions within a more objective (safe) context (i.e., the vignette).

Strengthen the Patient's and Family Caregiver's Sense of Connectedness with One Another (as well as More Broadly with Their Family/Significant Others)

The conversation might begin with inviting one another to share perceptions of what being "emotionally connected" to a significant other means and feels like and the ways it may be conveyed through various words and behaviors. Invite the patients and partners to share their understanding of the meaning of support with one another, and invite them to provide examples of support behaviors they appreciate from one another. Identify other possible supportive behaviors that patient and caregiver may welcome in order to strengthen their relationship.

Mutual feelings of connectedness may be strengthened by fostering open communication without judgment, encouraging stated recognitions of one another's strengths, providing regular expressions of mutual appreciation and love, engaging in collaborative problem-solving, respecting differences of opinion, and encouraging emotionally supportive behaviors with one another [115].

Heighten Awareness of the Unspoken Meanings Conveyed by Patient-Caregiver's Respective Behaviors

Often people are unaware of the impact that their behaviors have on loved ones. Because not all behaviors convey support, such as a raised quizzical eyebrow when the patient is talking, an exploration of the potential negative effects of unintentional behavioral displays is an important exercise within a dyadic intervention that also highlights how the quality of support may be consequentially affected. Highlight the importance of both patient and caregiver *checking in with one another regularly* to ensure mutual understanding and also that needed support is being given and received [22, 23].

Closing the Gap

The patient's and caregiver's expressed needs for support, and what actually is provided by *other family members and healthcare providers* is an essential part of nursing the patient-caregiver dyad [22]. Support is context-dependent, increasing during a crisis and abating over time. This is a topic for discussion with both patient and caregiver sharing their thoughts and feelings. Thus the type and quantity of support should be revisited especially at potential moments of uncertainty and vulnerability, that is, the diagnosis, before major surgery, chemotherapy, radiation therapy, a cancer recurrence, and transition to survivorship or end of life when emotional distress may skyrocket.

Discussion may be expanded, as needed, to include close members of the social network for the purpose of working together to find solutions to various tasks or activities (instrumental support) such as accompanying the patient to clinic appointments or buying the groceries or keeping the patient company so that the caregiver has some time off to regenerate and care for her or his own health.

Supportive Needs of Family Caregivers (Review Appendix B)
Informal caregivers tend to be the spouse, partner, or close friend with whom the patient may share a sense of shared intimacy, attachment, affection, self-disclosure, and mutual understanding, leading both partners to feel understood, validated, and cared for [116, 117]. The caregiving role is widely known to cause emotional distress as they observe the disease progression of their loved one. At the same time, they are expected to assume multiple and unfamiliar and often time-consuming caregiving duties that challenge their caregiver skill set and clinical knowledge needed to care for the patient [88]; see Part V Chap. 18 on supportive care.

A systematic review and meta-analysis investigated supportive interventions for caregivers of patients with cancer [88]. Three support categories were identified: (1) providing psychoeducation to the caregiver concerning the patient's cancer, (2) enhancing coping efforts and skill development in communication and problem-solving, and (3) counseling caregivers in response to their emotional reactions in caring for their loved one. (These categories are also applicable in supporting patients as well.) Caregivers require regular emotional, informational, and instrumental support from the nurse starting from diagnosis throughout the disease trajectory. This becomes even more imperative with disease progression at end of life [108, 118–120].

Accordingly, help caregivers, as needed, to interpret patient cues in a way that enhances their own compassionate understanding and emotional responsiveness to the patient. Suggest sensitive responses to a patient's bad test result or prognosis, such as "Whatever it is, we will do this together." Encourage the caregiver to reminisce with the patient about happy times in the past or just the previous week as a form of shared therapeutic distraction that offers temporary relief from the cancer-related reality.

Caregivers may require help in developing support seeking strategies to obtain the support they need, particularly when it involves getting family or friends to share some caregiving activities. Brainstorming with the nurse may help the caregiver identify interfering factors that account for the lack of family support. These factors can then serve as the basis for the caregiver's preferred solution.

Controlled studies have shown that the beneficial effects of psychosocial interventions on caregiver health-related outcomes are inconsistent and require further investigation [121, 122]. It is possible that health outcomes may be enhanced by regular clinic visits with the nurse or by supportive booster sessions via telephone or skype or even home visits in order to enable a closer fit between the changing supportive needs of caregivers based on the patient's clinical status and the support offered by the nurse.

Obtaining Needed Support from the Nurse and Physician

Each time the nurse is *present* for the patient and caregiver, actively listens, engages in interventions that promote the patient's or caregiver's coping skills including strategies to downregulate stress, provides relevant information, advocates for the patient or caregiver, and clarifies and *regularly meets* with the patient and family caregiver to address concerns and worries and to monitor changing supportive needs and well-being, the nurse is being supportive. The Appendix below summarizes numerous strategies that at their core are intended to provide the emotional, informational, and instrumental support needed by most patients and caregivers.

It is a clinical imperative that the nurse regularly examines whether the patient and caregiver are receiving the support they need from the nurse and oncologist or other healthcare providers, and then engages with both to generate the solutions that address their concerns. Patients and caregivers may seek the nurse's assistance in discussing a clinical issue with the physician. Simple recommendations may range from helping them to write down their concerns on paper for their meeting with the doctor, offering clinical information to clarify certain medically related concerns, role-playing various scenarios, and/or accompanying the patient and caregiver to a medical appointment in the role of patient advocate. Last, provide email addresses and/or texting numbers so patients and caregivers may reach out to the nurse or oncologist as needed.

11.9 Final Thoughts

One clinical concern in the literature is why an estimated third of distressed cancer patients tend to decline supportive "services" [123]. Is it possible that for some, the support being offered as a "service" lacks the depth of emotional support which is normally associated with feeling known and cared for [105]? Another potential reason is that the support being offered is embedded in cultural interpretations with differential effects on people from different cultures [74].

Certainly conceptual and methodological issues have contributed to the variable results in clinical intervention studies to date [124]. Early-phase clinical intervention studies to investigate the effectiveness of nursing interventions aimed at strengthening patient-caregiver support, on resilience and long-term survival across people with different cancers, would inform the field of supportive relationships and cancer care. Future RCT studies that target the primary supportive relationship(s) of the patient and his or her partner might offer tailored dyadic as well as individual parallel supportive interventions to meet the individual as well as dyadic needs of the patient and caregiver [89].

Appendix: Psychosocial Support-Related Interventions

Author	Purpose/intervention	Study design	Sample/phase of disease	Outcomes
Kissane [93]	To evaluate a supportive expressive group intervention (SEGT) on survival, i.e., primary outcomes and psychological well-being *Intervention* (a) Enhance relationships with family, friends, hcps (b) develop a network of support within group (c) fostered expression of feelings and thoughts related to existential distress	RA within 10 months after recurrence (a) SEGT plus 3 relaxation classes for weekly sessions/12 months ($n = 147$) (b) 3 relaxation classes ($n = 80$)	227 women with breast cancer recurrence	(1) *SEGT did not prolong survival* (median survival: 24 months versus 18.3 months) (2) Significant predictors of survival: treatment with chemotherapy, hormone therapy, visceral metastases, advanced cancer at diagnosis (3) SEGT improved and prevented depression ($p = 0.002$), reduced hopelessness and helplessness ($p = 0.004$), improved social functioning ($p = 0.03$) (4) Lacked a distress assessment as part of inclusion criteria to target those with high distress *Conclusion* improved QOL Findings consistent with earlier supportive expressive RCT [94]

(continued)

Appendix (continued)

Author	Purpose/intervention	Study design	Sample/phase of disease	Outcomes
Andersen et al. [78]	To assess the effectiveness of a psychosocial intervention to reduce emotional distress, improve health behaviors and immune responses Multimodal support Intervention—met weekly × 1.5 h × 18 sessions over 4 months (1) Understand stress responses, progressive muscle relaxation techniques (2) Promote positive coping, problem solving for common symptoms, and tx side effects (3) Identify social network, support needed, specific support contact (4) Communication training (5) Healthy diet, energy balance information, smoking cessation, treatment adherence (6) Stretch and walk protocol (20 min/day, 3 times a week) referral information (7) Disease/treatment information, assertive communication skills, monitoring of treatment/ follow-up appointments, goal setting	RCT with women postsurgery and before adjuvant therapy started RA to (1) intervention group (2) assessment group (asst) Small group sessions, weekly × 4 months, then monthly for 8 month (26 sessions/year) Hypotheses (1) Psychosocial interventions improve survival due to social support (2) A multicomponent biobehavioral intervention would impact the incidence of and time of recurrence for women with localized breast cancer (3) Reducing stress may lead to healthier behaviors (i.e., healthier diet, increased physical activity, and/or increased treatment adherence)	227 women post-surgery for regional breast cancer	(1) Emotional distress (a) Mood disturbance Intervention group showed 36% reduction in total mood disturbance compared to asst group which decreased 12% (b) Significant difference in the reduction of mood disturbance associated with the intervention compared to controls ($F = 1.93 = 4.13$, $P = 0.04$) for patients with the highest baseline stress (c) Anxiety Intervention showed a greater reduction in anxiety compared to controls ($F1, 193 = 4.15$, $P = 0.04$) The intervention was equally effective for patients with low or high cancer-related stress (d) Fatigue Intervention decreased fatigue in patients with high stress but not low stress based on 3-way interaction ($F1, 193 = 5.14$, $P = 0.02$) (2) Social adjustment (a) Intervention showed a significant 2-way interaction for social adjustment ($F4, 140 = 2.41$, $P = 0.048$) (b) Follow-up analysis showed a significant 2-way interaction for PSS family ($F1, 143 = 5.36$, $P = 0.02$), that is perceived support from family significantly improved in the intervention group but decreased among controls (3) Dietary habits (a) A significant 2-way interaction ($F1, 194 = 5.01$, $P = 0.03$) showed intervention increased healthy food habits at 4 months (4) Exercise Increase in physical exercise that approached significance in the intervention group ($p = 0.08$) (5) Immune functions (a) NS differences in CD3, CD4, CD8 counts (b) T cell blastogenesis; mancova showed significant effect for the Con-A-induced T cell blastogenesis ($F3, 154 = 6.37$, $p = 0.0004$) (c) NK cell count and lysis were nonsignificant Conclusion (1) Strength of intervention is that it purposefully designed strategies to improve specific survival promoting biological and behavioral indicators of healthy adjustment (2) The intervention appeared to have limited effects on cell-mediated immune functions but needs further investigation and analysis given the significant effects based on the Con-A-induced T cell blastogenesis

Andersen et al. [99]	To evaluate a psychological intervention designed to reduce the risk of cancer recurrence and improve survival before start of adjuvant tx Intervention See Andersen et al. [78]	Follow-up of a RCT after a median of 11 years	(1) Disease recurrence known in 93% of patients (212/227) (a) Disease recurred in 62/212 patients (29%), i.e., 29 in intervention group versus 33 in controls (b) Intervention compared to controls significantly reduced risk of breast cancer recurrence (HR: 0.55; $P = 0.034$) (c) Intervention had a 45% reduction in risk of cancer recurrence (d) Recurrence: Intervention group (Median 2.8 years; Range = 0.9–11 years); controls (Median 2.2 years; Range = 0.2–12 years) (2) Death occurred in 54/227 (24%) (Intervention grp: 24; Controls: 30) (a) Intervention also had a reduced risk of death from breast cancer (HR: 0.44, $P = 0.016$) compared to controls (b) Intervention group also had a reduced risk of death from all causes compared to controls (HR: 0.51; $P = 0.028$) (c) For those who died, median survival time for intervention group: (Median 6 years (range = 0.3–11.1 years); for controls: 5 years (range = 0.4–12.4 years) Conclusion The intervention may have boosted or enhanced immune cells to eliminate cancer cells providing an edge on later survivorship. Patients in intervention group had the greatest decrease in distress

(continued)

Appendix (continued)

Author	Purpose/intervention	Study design	Sample/phase of disease	Outcomes

Andersen et al. [76]	To evaluate hypothesis that intervention group would show longer survival after cancer recurrence	Follow-up (see start of study: Andersen et al. [78]) Tested at time of recurrence, 4, 8, 12 months later	All patients were followed N=62 patients recurred in intervention and control groups	(1) Survival analysis: 62 patients had a recurrence
				  (a) at recurrence median disease-free interval was 30 months; 90% received treatment
				  (b) 41/62 patients consented to be followed (Intervention group: 29; Assessment control group: 33
				  (c) 44/62 (71%) later died: intervention arm: 19; and controls 25
				  (d) All patients showed high levels of psychological distress at recurrence
				  (e) Intent to treat analysis showed a reduced risk of death after recurrence for the intervention compared to control group (HR, 0.41; 95% CI, 0.20–0.83, $P = 0.014$)
				  (f) After the distress of recurrence the intervention group compared to controls showed a significant reduction in distress that improved over 12 months with a significant difference between the two groups ($P = 0.008$)
				  (g) After recurrence there was a 59% decrease in risk of dying of breast cancer in intervention group
				(2) Social support
				  (a) Intervention group showed a significantly higher level of social support at baseline compared to controls ($P = 0.001$) which was maintained across the 12 months, whereas the control assessment group level of support declined ($P = 0.002$)
				  (b) The intervention group also perceived more support at the recurrence from family ($P = 0.007$) than the assessment group
				  (c) Support was similarly higher albeit only trending toward significance ($P = 0.086$)
				(3) Immune functions
				  (a) The intervention group showed no significant decline in Natural killer cell cytotoxicity NKCC (P)
				  (b) The time effect showed a significant decline in Natural killer cell cytotoxicity NKCC for the assessment group ($P < 0.001$)
				  (c) The study arm × time showed the intervention with a significantly slower decline in NKCC

			(4) Differential immune levels at 12 months
			   (a) Results showed significantly higher NKCC ($P = 0.001$), Con A blastogenesis ($P = 0.021$), and PHA blastogenesis ($P = 0.007$) at 12 months in the intervention compared to assessment group
			(5) Conclusion
			   (a) Individuals in the intervention group appeared to be more capable at finding and retaining needed support
			   (b) As observed in the Andersen 2004 earlier phase of this study, support from family appeared to improve in the intervention group compared to controls during the intervention phase of the study
			   (c) This may have resulted in stable and supportive relationships during periods of stress afterward—this is critical due to relationship between support and NKCC which is needed to maintain immune surveillance and cancer suppression after surgery and adjuvant cancer treatments according to current research models and empirical findings [125]

Andersen et al. [126]	To test whether a psychosocial intervention contributes to increased health
	Intervention
	See Andersen et al. [78]
		Postsurgery 227 patients with breast cancer RA to
		(1) Intervention
		(2) Control group
			An estimated 1 year after baseline measures take post-surgery	(1) Path analysis
				   (a) Showed that intervention directly improved health (beta = $0.18\ P < 0.05$) at 12 months also after controlling for baseline variables of distress, immunity, and health
				   (b) The path analysis showed that the support intervention directly reduced distress at 4 months (beta = -0.17) which then improved health by 12 months (beta = -0.32) and was overall significant ($z = 2.11, P < 0.04$)
				   (c) The intervention also improved T cell blastogenesis ($b = 0.26, p < 0.05$) (in response to the lab-induced phytohemagglutinin) which was unrelated to measures of improved health (functional health, medical symptoms/side effects)
				(2) Symptom toxicities increased by 29% in assessment control group compared to 14% in intervention group at 12 months
				Conclusion
				Supportive intervention appeared to improve health outcomes at 12 months by reducing distress 4 months after baseline

(continued)

Appendix (continued)

Author	Purpose/intervention	Study design	Sample/phase of disease	Outcomes
Classen et al. [92]	To assess the effectiveness of supportive expressive group interventions on the psychological adjustment of women with metastatic breast cancer Intervention 12 month weekly Aim: To help patients with cancer adjust to existential concerns (1) encouraged to express and manage disease-related emotions, increase social support, increase relationships with family and MDs, improve symptom control (2) unstructured and non-didactic	RCT RA to: (1) SET $n = 64$ (2) Controls $n = 61$ Data at baseline and every 4 months for 1 year	125 women with metastatic breast cancer	(1) Intervention group had significantly greater decrease in mean IES (intrusiveness and avoidance behavior) compared to controls ($F1,90 = 4.63, p = 0.03$) with an effect size = 0.25 (small-medium) (2) Significant difference in slope of IES total scores across various recruitment sites ($F2,90 = 4.39, P = 0.02$), but there were no site by treatment interactions ($F2,90 = 0.57, P = 0.57$) (3) Baseline IES total scores were significantly related to the slope of change on the IES ($F1,90 = 34.79, p < 0.001$) with the women at baseline with the highest distress showing the greatest decrease in symptoms over time (4) There was an effect size difference favoring the intervention for mood (effect size = 0.25) and for traumatic stress symptoms (effect size = 0.33) Conclusion Study indicates that SET may have a therapeutic effect on cancer-related stress in women with advanced metastatic breast cancer

Goodwin et al. [94]	Evaluating whether SET prolonged survival in patients with metastatic cancer	RCT multicentered trial
		RA to
		(1) SET (n = 158)
		(2) Controls (n = 77)
			235 patients with metastatic cancer expected to survive at least 3 months	(1) Symptoms
				  (a) Change scores for the intervention group compared to the controls were significant in favor of a significant reduction in total mood disturbance ($P = 0.02$), depression-dejection ($P = 0.002$), tension-anxiety ($P = 0.002$), anger hostility ($P = 0.007$), and confusion ($P = 0.02$)
				  (b) Adjustments for baseline scores decreased the differences between the two groups but revealed a significant interaction between baseline score and effect of treatment
				    • That is, distressed women at baseline benefited from the intervention, whereas women who were not as distressed did not benefit
				    • The magnitude of the benefit for the distressed women was 13.5% of the possible range of the scale
				  (c) NS differences for fatigue or vigor
				(2) Pain and suffering
				  (a) Women in the intervention reported less worsening pain over the year than controls ($P = 0.04$)
				  (b) A significant interaction between treatment and baseline showed that the intervention group benefited only if their scores were high with a magnitude of 15% of the scale range
				(3) Survival
				  (a) Kaplan-Meier survival analysis indicated that median survival was 17.9 months in the intervention group and 17.6 months in the control group
				  (b) Univariate Cox model showed the hazard ratio for death in the intervention compared to control group was NS (HR =1.06, 95% CI 0.78 to 1.45; $P = 0.72$).
				  (c) A multivariate Cox model showed NS effect of the intervention for survival (HR: 1.23, 95% CI, 0.88–1.72, $P = 0.22$) and effects remained the same after accounting for other potential variables
				Conclusion
				SET does not prolong life in women with metastatic breast
				It improves pain and mood in women who were initially highly distressed

(continued)

Appendix (continued)

Author	Purpose/intervention	Study design	Sample/phase of disease	Outcomes

Guarino et al. [95]	To assess efficacy of CBT, supportive expressive therapy (SET) and psychoeducational therapy (PET) for women with breast cancer
	(1) CBT ($K = 17$)
	  (a) Focus on ↑affective state and coping with cancer by modifying maladaptive mental schema and ↓ distress, ↓intrusive ideation
	(2) SET ($K = 4$)
	  (a) Cognitive-emotional focused therapy aimed at ↑ development of social support (SS) and emotional expression and examines existential concerns
	(3) Psychoeducation (PET) ($K = 4$) interdisciplinary approach includes
	  (a) Education—knowledge regarding disease, treatments
	  (b) Psychological—provides affective, cognitive skills related to coping with experience of illness
		Systematic review/meta-analysis of 25 studies	7834 out of 8472 women with breast cancer who completed pre-/postassessments	(1) QOL
				  (a) Meta-analysis based on all 3 interventions ($k = 13$) showed a nonsignificant improvement in QOL based on a medium effect size (0.38, 95% CI, −0.07 to 0.84) $I^2 = 98\%$
				Subanalyses
				  (b) CBT ($k = 8$) improved QOL life based on the highest effect size although not significant ($d = 0.55$ (−0.25 to 1.35) $I^2 = 0.99\%$)
				  (c) SET ($k = 1$) decreased quality of life with a small nonsignificant effect size ($d = 0.11$ (−0.15 to −0.07))
				(2) Anxiety
				  (a) Meta-analysis with 10 studies showed anxiety was reduced posttreatment with a medium effect size that was nonsignificant ($d = −0.39$ (−0.91 to 0.14) $I^2 = 98\%$
				  (b) PET ($K = 1$) showed medium posttreatment reduction in anxiety that was significant ($d = −0.45$ (−0.49 to −0.40))
				  (c) SET ($K = 1$) showed a small increased effect posttreatment in anxiety that was significant ($d = 0.10$ (0.02–0.18))
				(3) Depression
				  (a) Meta-analysis with 12 studies showed a significant medium posttreatment effect that reduced depression ($d = −0.35$ (−0.79 to −0.10) $I^2 = 98\%$)
				  (b) CBT ($k = 10$) showed a medium effect size reduction in depression that was not significant ($d = −0.42$ (−0.06 to 0.12))
				  (c) SET ($k = 2$) showed a nonsignificant small effect size decrease in depression ($d = −0.10$ (−2.18 to 2.16) $I^2 = 0.98\%$)
				(4) Mood ($K = 10$)
				  (a) Meta-analysis with 10 studies produced a nonsignificant small effect reduction in mood (i.e., improved mood) ($d = −0.17$ (−0.41 to 0.06))
				  (b) PET ($K = 3$) showed a nonsignificant medium effect reduction for mood ($d = −0.34$ (−1.05 to 0.36) $I^2 = 97\%$)
				  (c) SET ($K = 2$) showed a nonsignificant minimal effect size reduction for mood ($d = −0.07$ (−1.70 to 1.56), $I^2 = 99\%$)
				Conclusion
				Poor quality evidence with high heterogeneity across studies

Study	Intervention	Sample	Results

Spiegel et al. [98] Follow-up of earlier study See Classen et al. [92]	To assess whether supportive expressive group therapy (SEGT) prolonged survival of women with metastatic breast cancer Intervention 90 min weekly for 12 months though some participants continued for 12.5 years
	(1) participants encouraged to confront problems
	(2) strengthen relationships
	(3) find greater meaning in their lives
	(4) semistructured, nondidactic
	Themes included
	(1) building strengthening supportive bonds
	(2) facilitating expression of emotion
	(3) confronting fears of dying including death of group members
	(4) reordering life priorities
	(5) improving support from/communication with family and friends
	(6) improving MD communications
	(7) learning self-hypnosis for anxiety and pain control
		125 women RA to
		(1) SEGT with 64 women
		(2) 61 women received educational materials
		122 women with advanced metastatic breast cancer and 3 with locally recurrent breast cancer
			(1) Mortality
			  (a) Overall mortality 14 years after baseline was 86% and median survival time was 32.8 months
			  (b) NS effect of intervention on survival (treatment median = 30.7 m) compared to controls (median 33.3 months)
			  (c) Moderator analysis showed a significant overall interaction between estrogen receptor (ER) status and treatment condition ($P = 0.002$) that is among the 25 ER-negative women, those RA to the treatment survived longer (median = 29.8 months) compared to those assigned to controls (median = 9.3 months)
			  (d) The ER positive women showed no treatment effect
			Conclusion
			(1) NS for longer survival which also did not replicate the earlier study
			(2) Findings suggest that more work needs to be done to identify which individuals are more likely to benefit from the SET intervention based on disease but possibly other factors such as baseline levels of distress or perceived support from loved ones
			(3) No blinding; large differential findings in both groups depending on the hospital accrual site

(continued)

Appendix (continued)

Author	Purpose/intervention	Study design	Sample/phase of disease	Outcomes
Brandao et al. [96]	Aim: explore perceptions and experiences of patients with breast cancer who attended supportive expressive group interventions (SEGT) 16 sessions Intervention Aimed to improve (1) SS (2) Coping strategies (3) Healthy emotional processing	Qualitative	12 women facing breast cancer during initial phase of illness, after completing SET	Content analysis produced four main themes (1) Expectations/motivations to participate in SEGT, i.e., (a) learn at other experiences of women (b) looking for support (SS) (c) the group context (d) altruism: found meaning by helping others (2) Group processes/experiences (a) helpful aspects—learning/sharing experiences, increase in SS, realizing they were not alone which normalized feelings, sense of empowerment, catharsis, emotional expression, improved interpersonal relationships, increased hope, openness (b) unhelpful aspects—difficulty discussing intimate couple issues, or dealing with others' opinions/needs, or leaving children home to attend the meeting, size of group, frequency and duration of sessions also varied in preference (3) Perceived changes promoted/triggered by SEGT, i.e.. (a) greater capacity to express emotions, in the group and with family (b) ↑ed ease with own thoughts and emotions (c) reordering of life priorities (d) ↑optimism, coping with practical issues, self-esteem, security, SS, improved interpersonal relationships (4) Perceptions about the therapeutic relationship: (a) characteristics of therapist: most important are empathy, active listening (b) leadership: allowing patients to discuss issues important to them; ensure a balance across members regarding who talks the most (c) promoting personal skills—helped refine personal skills of emotional expression and coping strategies (5) Most helpful aspects of SEGT (a) normalization/expression of feelings, thoughts, reactions (b) improvement of social support (c) learning about cancer and what occurred via sharing experiences among attendees (d) SEGT also helped to improve personal and social skills, for instance, express emotions and establish satisfying interpersonal relationships Conclusion (1) Findings helped link how the intervention might be connected to patient outcomes, i.e., ↑ed QOL, ↓ed psychological distress in intervention studies (2) The clinical therapist was trained in SEGT and Dr Spiegel served as consultant

Study	Aim/Intervention	Design/Sample	Measures	Results
Park et al. [127]	Assess effects of a brief supportive expressive group therapy combined with mindfulness intervention Intervention (1) SEGT—develop strategies to express emotions, enhance SS, individual resources, opportunities to review life, increase sense of control, address meaning of cancer (2) mindfulness meditation component	Open-label, single arm, pre-/postdesign Feasibility study 4 weeks, 3-hour sessions 28 distressed women with non-metastatic breast cancer who had completed coadjuvant chemotherapy	(1) HRV—the normalized spectral heart rate variability (HRV) measures relationship between (a) low frequency (LF) nu (e.g., 0.04–0.15 Hz) and (b) high frequency (HF) nu (e.g., 0.15 to 0.40 Hz) to measure modulation of the sympathetic and parasympathetic branches of the ANS (2) LF (measure of SNS) (3) HF measure of PNS (4) People with SDNN values <50 ms → unhealthy (5) 50–100 m → compromised (6) >100 m → healthy	(1) HRV (i.e., LF/HF ratio) and psychological stress at baseline Re SNS: LFnu associated with (a) anxiety ($r = 0.471$, $p = 0.017$) (b) depression ($r = 0.543$, $p = 0.005$) (c) perceived support (PSS) ($r = 0.40$, $p = 0.048$) (d) state anxiety ($r = 0.554$, $p = 0.004$) (e) well-being (wbg) ($r = -0.658$, $p < 0.001$) Re: PNS: HFnu associated with (a) distress ($r = -0.471$, $p = 0.017$) (b) depression ($r = -0.543$, $p = 0.005$) (c) PSS ($r = -0.400$, $p = 0.048$) (d) state anxiety ($r = -0.554$, $p = 0.004$) (e) wbg ($r = 0.658$, $p < 0.001$) Re LF/HV (i.e., ↑ed HRV) associated with (a) anxiety ($r = 0.474$, $p = 0.017$) (b) depression ($r = 0.565$, $p = 0.003$) (c) PSS ($r = 0.548$, $p = 0.005$) (d) state anxiety ($r = 0.447$, $p = 0.025$) (e) wbg ($r = -0.0657$, $p < 0.001$) (2) A significantly increased SDNN (i.e., mean of the standard deviation of all normal node to node intervals of the QRS) in a 5-min segment and a normalized high frequency (HF 0.15 to 0.4 Hz) posttreatment which signifies slower HRV (which is healthier) (3) Low HF (i.e., low PNS) was associated with greater depression, anxiety, perceived stress and anger at baseline Conclusion (1) Results provide preliminary evidence for the effectiveness of the combined (MM and SET) approach to reducing distress (2) Also preliminary evidence for using HRV as a biomarker of distress and recovery

(continued)

Appendix (continued)

Author	Purpose/intervention	Study design	Sample/phase of disease	Outcomes
Carlson et al. [128]	To compare effectiveness of mindfulness-based cancer recovery (MBCR) interventions with supportive expressive group therapy (SEGT) *Interventions* See Carlson et al. [129]	Follow-up analysis from a 3-arm RCT Comparative study in which survivors were RA to (a) MBCR (b) SEGT	Distressed 165/252 survivors of stage 1–111 breast cancer	Posttreatment, compared to SEGT (1) MBCR showed greater reduction in mood disturbance (fatigue, anxiety, confusion), stress symptoms (tension, sympathetic arousal, cognitive symptoms) (2) MBCR showed significant increase in emotional/functional quality of life, emotional, affective and positive social support, spirituality (feelings of peace, meaning in life) and posttraumatic growth (appreciating life, identifying new possibilities) RE SEGT (1) also improved albeit to a lesser extent Re effect sizes (1) over time ranged from small to medium, and most sustained for 12 months Conclusion (1) Study demonstrates importance in identifying *distressed* individuals who can benefit most from these interventions (2) MBCR showed sustained benefits of MBCR in enhancing well-being suggesting that the women learned important coping strategies

| Carlson et al. [129] | Assessing effects of MBCR and SEGT in distressed survivors of breast cancer Intervention (1) MBCR Derived from spiritual traditions and practices captured by Kabat Zinn and tailored to persons with cancer experience; centered on mindfulness practices, i.e., conscious awareness in the present, open and nonjudgmental manner, cultivated by practices in mindful meditation and gentle yoga-helps ↑ emotion regulation via gradual exposure to feared thoughts/feelings, ruminations, experiential avoidance within nonjudgmental inner context so stimuli lose their power—result—↑ed control, calm, peace, in face of uncontrollable aspects of cancer (2) SET Goals are to facilitate mutual support, family support; emotional expressiveness and openness; increase coping skills; doctor-patient relations; alleviate distress surrounding death and dying | 3-arm multisite RCT RA to (1) MBCR (2) SET (3) control | 271 Stage 1-111 distressed survivors of breast cancer | Based on linear mixed effects models, intent to treat analyses (1) RE diurnal cortisol slopes: Normal downward cortisol slopes for both SET and MBSR maintained whereas controls sloped gently upward between baseline and posttreatment with small effect size differences between SET and controls ($P = 0.002$) and between MBCR and controls ($P = 0.011$) (2) MBCR > SET ($p = 0.009$) or controls ($p = 0.024$) significantly reduced stress symptoms (3) MBCR compared to controls showed significant increase in quality of life (QOL) ($p = 0.005$) (4) MBCR showed significant improvement in social support compared with the SET group ($p = 0.012$) Conclusion (1) MBCR showed greater improvements for stress levels, quality of life, and social support than SET or controls (2) Both SET and MBCR showed greater normative cortisol slopes than controls for diurnal cortisol (3) Appears that SET and MBCR served to protect individuals from deleterious effects of dysregulated cortisol levels |

(continued)

Appendix (continued)

Author	Purpose/intervention	Study design	Sample/phase of disease	Outcomes
Bjorneklett et al. [130]	Follow-up (i.e., mean 6.5 years after randomization) of a RCT to assess a support group intervention for women after primary treatment for breast cancer Intervention (1) 1 week intervention (2) 4 days of follow-up 2 months later (3) combined approach based on a support group intervention (4) received information about cancer, risk factors, physical and psychological effects, coping strategies, physical exercise, relaxation, imagery, and nonverbal communication [110]	RCT with RA to: (1) 181 women in support group (2) 181 women in control group	382 women with primary breast cancer posttreatment	(1) Significant improvement in physical, mental and total fatigue, cognitive function, body image, and future perspective compared to controls after adjusting for chemotherapy tx, marriage, education, children at home, age (2) The proportion of women experiencing anxiety and depression did not differ between the two groups Conclusion (1) Support intervention improved several parameters of well-being but not anxiety or depression

Author	Aim / Intervention	Design	Sample	Results
Kuchler et al. [91]	To evaluate effectiveness of a psychotherapeutic support intervention on survival in patients with GI cancer and undergoing surgery: a 10-year follow-up Intervention (1) Patients received educational information, counseling, a supportive relationship to patients at the bedside (2) provided on going emotional and cognitive support to enhance fighting spirit and hope and to counter hopelessness (3) Assisted the patient in forming questions for other caregivers (4) also encouraged family and social support (5) relaxation therapy (6) before discharge therapist explored patient understanding and feelings about the surgery, and helped patient in planning for the future-targeting emotional integration of experience including aspects of cognitive-existential therapy (similar to [93, 98])	RCT	217 patients with a preliminary diagnosis of local, regional, or metastatic cancer of the esophagus, stomach, liver/gall bladder, pancreas, or colon/rectum	(1) Kaplan-Meier survival curves showed significantly better survival for the experimental than control group (unadjusted significance level for group differences was $P = 0.0006$ for survival at 10 years) (Log rank $X^2 = 11.73$; $p = 0.006$) (a) In adjusted analyses: Cox regression models that took TNM staging of the residual tumor classification and tumor site into account showed significant differences at 10 years (b) Secondary analyses showed greater longer-term survival for patients with stomach, pancreatic, primary liver, or colorectal cancer (c) 29/136 intervention patients versus 13/135 controls, survived (d) Among patients with metastases only 3 in each group remained Conclusion (1) Patients with GI cancers appear to benefit from a presurgical supportive intervention during the inpatient hospital stay in terms of lengthened survival (a) This intervention focused on active coping but also information about the surgery and cancer treatment (b) Researchers hypothesized that 1 reason why expecting positive outcomes does not occur may be due to the fact the intervention started too late in patients with advanced disease

References

1. Kayser K, Acquati C, Reese JB, Mark K, Wittmann D, Karam E. A systematic review of dyadic studies examining relationship quality in couples facing colorectal cancer together. Psycho-Oncology. 2018;27(1):13–21. PubMed PMID: 27943551. Epub 2016/12/13. eng.
2. Kim Y, Shaffer KM, Carver CS, Cannady RS. Quality of life of family caregivers 8 years after a relative's cancer diagnosis: follow-up of the National Quality of Life Survey for Caregivers. Psycho-Oncology. 2016;25(3):266–74. PubMed PMID: 25976620. Epub 2015/05/16. eng.
3. Chou AF, Stewart SL, Wild RC, Bloom JR. Social support and survival in young women with breast carcinoma. Psycho-Oncology. 2012;21(2):125–33. PubMed PMID: 20967848. Pubmed Central PMCID: PMC3036767. Epub 2010/10/23. eng.
4. Holt-Lunstad J, Smith TB, Layton JB. Social relationships and mortality risk: a meta-analytic review. PLoS Med. 2010;7(7):e1000316. PubMed PMID: 20668659. Pubmed Central PMCID: PMC2910600. Epub 2010/07/30. eng.
5. House JS, Landis KR, Umberson D. Social relationships and health. Science. 1988;241(4865):540–5. PubMed PMID: 3399889. Epub 1988/07/29. eng.
6. Nausheen B, Gidron Y, Peveler R, Moss-Morris R. Social support and cancer progression: a systematic review. J Psychosom Res. 2009;67(5):403–15. PubMed PMID: 19837203. Epub 2009/10/20. eng.
7. Lutgendorf SK, Andersen BL. Biobehavioral approaches to cancer progression and survival: mechanisms and interventions. Am Psychol. 2015;70(2):186–97. PubMed PMID: 25730724. Pubmed Central PMCID: PMC4347942. Epub 2015/03/03. eng.
8. Nenova M, DuHamel K, Zemon V, Rini C, Redd WH. Posttraumatic growth, social support, and social constraint in hematopoietic stem cell transplant survivors. Psycho-Oncology. 2013;22(1):195–202. PubMed PMID: 21972000. Pubmed Central PMCID: PMC3760719. Epub 2011/10/06. eng.
9. Dong X, Li G, Liu C, Kong L, Fang Y, Kang X, et al. The mediating role of resilience in the relationship between social support and posttraumatic growth among colorectal cancer survivors with permanent intestinal ostomies: a structural equation model analysis. Eur J Oncol Nurs. 2017;29:47–52. PubMed PMID: 28720265. Epub 2017/07/20. eng.
10. Schroevers MJ, Helgeson VS, Sanderman R, Ranchor AV. Type of social support matters for prediction of posttraumatic growth among cancer survivors. Psycho-Oncology. 2010;19(1):46–53. PubMed PMID: 19253269. Epub 2009/03/03. eng.
11. House J. Work, stress and social support. Reading: Addison-Wesley; 1981.
12. House J. Measures and concepts of social support. New York: Academic Press; 1985.
13. Cohen S, Wills TA. Stress, social support, and the buffering hypothesis. Psychol Bull. 1985;98(2):310–57.
14. Cobb S. Social support as a moderator of life stress. Psychosom Med. 1976;38(5):300–14.
15. Sarma EA, Kawachi I, Poole EM, Tworoger SS, Giovannucci EL, Fuchs CS, et al. Social integration and survival after diagnosis of colorectal cancer. Cancer. 2018;124(4):833–40. PubMed PMID: 29160897. Pubmed Central PMCID: PMC5800969. Epub 2017/11/22. eng.
16. Koffman J, Morgan M, Edmonds P, Speck P, Higginson IJ. 'The greatest thing in the world is the family': the meaning of social support among black Caribbean and white British patients living with advanced cancer. Psycho-Oncology. 2012;21(4):400–8. PubMed PMID: 21259379. Epub 2011/01/25. eng.
17. Kim Y, Given BA. Quality of life of family caregivers of cancer survivors: across the trajectory of the illness. Cancer. 2008;112(11):2556–68. PubMed PMID: 18428199. Epub 2008/04/23. eng.
18. Kim Y, Morrow GR. The effects of family support, anxiety, and post-treatment nausea on the development of anticipatory nausea: a latent growth model. J Pain Symptom Manag. 2007;34(3):265–76. PubMed PMID: 17604591. Epub 2007/07/03. eng.
19. Sjolander C, Ahlstrom G. The meaning and validation of social support networks for close family of persons with advanced cancer. BMC Nurs. 2012;11:17. PubMed PMID: 22978508. Pubmed Central PMCID: PMC3488574. Epub 2012/09/18. eng.

20. Hebdon M, Badger TA, Segrin C, Pasvogel A. Social support and healthcare utilization of caregivers of Latinas with breast cancer. Support Care Cancer. 2021;29(8):4395–404. Pubmed Central PMCID: PMC8475626. Epub 2021/03/20. eng.
21. Molassiotis A, van den Akker OB, Boughton BJ. Perceived social support, family environment and psychosocial recovery in bone marrow transplant long-term survivors. Soc Sci Med. 1997;44(3):317–25. PubMed PMID: 9004367. Epub 1997/02/01. eng.
22. Merluzzi TV, Philip EJ, Yang M, Heitzmann CA. Matching of received social support with need for support in adjusting to cancer and cancer survivorship. Psycho-Oncology. 2016;25(6):684–90. PubMed PMID: 26126444. Pubmed Central PMCID: PMC4960824. Epub 2015/07/02. eng.
23. Merluzzi TV, Serpentini S, Philip EJ, Yang M, Salamanca-Balen N, Heitzmann Ruhf CA, et al. Social relationship coping efficacy: a new construct in understanding social support and close personal relationships in persons with cancer. Psycho-Oncology. 2019;28(1):85–91. PubMed PMID: 30303251. Epub 2018/10/12. eng.
24. Sherbourne CD, Stewart AL. The MOS social support survey. Soc Sci Med. 1991;32(6):705–14. PubMed PMID: 2035047. Epub 1991/01/01. eng.
25. Cao W, Qi X, Cai DA, Han X. Modeling posttraumatic growth among cancer patients: the roles of social support, appraisals, and adaptive coping. Psycho-Oncology. 2018;27(1):208–15. PubMed PMID: 28171681. Epub 2017/02/09. eng.
26. Kalbfleisch M, Cyr A, Gregorio N, Nyhof-Young J. Investigating coping strategies and social support among Canadian melanoma patients: a survey approach. Can Oncol Nurs J. 2015;25(1):60–72. PubMed PMID: 26642495. Epub 2015/12/09. eng
27. Hasson-Ohayon I, Goldzweig G, Sela-Oren T, Pizem N, Bar-Sela G, Wolf I. Attachment style, social support and finding meaning among spouses of colorectal cancer patients: gender differences. Palliat Support Care. 2015;13(3):527–35. PubMed PMID: 23928072. Epub 2013/08/10. eng.
28. Kammrath LK, Armstrong BF, Lane SP, Francis MK, Clifton M, McNab KM, et al. What predicts who we approach for social support? Tests of the attachment figure and strong ties hypotheses. J Pers Soc Psychol. 2019;118(3):481–500. PubMed PMID: 27162423. Pubmed Central PMCID: PMC4843551. Epub 2016/05/11. eng.
29. Somasundaram RO, Devamani KA. A comparative study on resilience, perceived social support and hopelessness among cancer patients treated with curative and palliative care. Indian J Palliat Care. 2016;22(2):135–40. PubMed PMID: 27162423. Pubmed Central PMCID: PMC4843551. Epub 2016/05/11. eng.
30. Kim J, Han JY, Shaw B, McTavish F, Gustafson D. The roles of social support and coping strategies in predicting breast cancer patients' emotional well-being: testing mediation and moderation models. J Health Psychol. 2010;15(4):543–52. PubMed PMID: 20460411. Pubmed Central PMCID: PMC3145334. Epub 2010/05/13. eng.
31. Eisenberger NI, Cole SW. Social neuroscience and health: neurophysiological mechanisms linking social ties with physical health. Nat Neurosci. 2012;15(5):669–74. PubMed PMID: 22504347. Epub 2012/04/17. eng.
32. Deno M, Tashiro M, Miyashita M, Asakage T, Takahashi K, Saito K, et al. The mediating effects of social support and self-efficacy on the relationship between social distress and emotional distress in head and neck cancer outpatients with facial disfigurement. Psycho-Oncology. 2012;21(2):144–52. PubMed PMID: 22271534. Epub 2012/01/25. eng.
33. Carpenter KM, Fowler JM, Maxwell GL, Andersen BL. Direct and buffering effects of social support among gynecologic cancer survivors. Ann Behav Med. 2010;39(1):79–90. PubMed PMID: 20151235. Pubmed Central PMCID: PMC3645934. Epub 2010/02/13. eng.
34. Huang CY, Hsu MC. Social support as a moderator between depressive symptoms and quality of life outcomes of breast cancer survivors. Eur J Oncol Nurs. 2013;17(6):767–74. PubMed PMID: 23623178. Epub 2013/04/30. eng.
35. Keim MC, Fladeboe K, Galtieri LR, Kawamura J, King K, Friedman D, et al. Primary and secondary caregiver depressive symptoms and family functioning following a pediatric cancer diagnosis: an exploration of the buffering hypothesis. Psycho-Oncology. 2021;30(6):928–35. PubMed PMID: 33724595. Epub 2021/03/17. eng.

36. Rodin G, Walsh A, Zimmermann C, Gagliese L, Jones J, Shepherd FA, et al. The contribution of attachment security and social support to depressive symptoms in patients with metastatic cancer. Psycho-Oncology. 2007;16(12):1080–91. PubMed PMID: 17464942. Epub 2007/04/28. eng.
37. Nørskov KH, Yi JC, Crouch ML, Fiscalini AS, Flowers MED, Syrjala KL. Social support as a moderator of healthcare adherence and distress in long-term hematopoietic cell transplantation survivors. J Cancer Surviv. 2021;15(6):866–75. PubMed PMID: 33420905. Pubmed Central PMCID: PMC8267051. Epub 2021/01/10. eng.
38. Kornblith AB, Herndon JE 2nd, Zuckerman E, Viscoli CM, Horwitz RI, Cooper MR, et al. Social support as a buffer to the psychological impact of stressful life events in women with breast cancer. Cancer. 2001;91(2):443–54. PubMed PMID: 11180093. Epub 2001/02/17. eng.
39. Cohen S. Social relationships and health. Am Psychol. 2004;59(8):676–84. PubMed PMID: 15554821. Epub 2004/11/24. eng.
40. Lutgendorf S, De Geest K, Bender D, Ahmed A, Goodheart M, Dahmoush L, Zimmerman M, et al. Social influences on clinical outcomes of patients with ovarian cancer. J Clin Oncol. 2012;30(23):2885–90.
41. Gonzalez-Saenz de Tejada M, Bilbao A, Bare M, Briones E, Sarasqueta C, Quintana JM, et al. Association of social support, functional status, and psychological variables with changes in health-related quality of life outcomes in patients with colorectal cancer. Psycho-Oncology. 2016;25(8):891–7. PubMed PMID: 26582649. Epub 2015/11/20. eng.
42. Brooks KP, Gruenewald T, Karlamangla A, Hu P, Koretz B, Seeman TE. Social relationships and allostatic load in the MIDUS study. Health Psychol. 2014;33(11):1373–81. PubMed PMID: 24447186. Pubmed Central PMCID: PMC4104264. Epub 2014/01/23. eng.
43. Fong AJ, Scarapicchia TMF, McDonough MH, Wrosch C, Sabiston CM. Changes in social support predict emotional well-being in breast cancer survivors. Psycho-Oncology. 2017;26(5):664–71. PubMed PMID: 26818101. Epub 2016/01/29. eng.
44. Coughlin SS. Social determinants of breast cancer risk, stage, and survival. Breast Cancer Res Treat. 2019;177(3):537–48. PubMed PMID: 31270761. Epub 2019/07/05. eng.
45. Kroenke CH, Quesenberry C, Kwan ML, Sweeney C, Castillo A, Caan BJ. Social networks, social support, and burden in relationships, and mortality after breast cancer diagnosis in the life after breast cancer epidemiology (LACE) study. Breast Cancer Res Treat. 2013;137(1):261–71. PubMed PMID: 23143212. Pubmed Central PMCID: PMC4019377. Epub 2012/11/13. eng.
46. Chen E, Lam PH, Finegood ED, Turiano NA, Mroczek DK, Miller GE. The balance of giving versus receiving social support and all-cause mortality in a US national sample. Proc Natl Acad Sci U S A. 2021;118:24. PubMed PMID: 34099550. Pubmed Central PMCID: PMC8214686. Epub 2021/06/09. eng.
47. Garner MJ, McGregor BA, Murphy KM, Koenig AL, Dolan ED, Albano D. Optimism and depression: a new look at social support as a mediator among women at risk for breast cancer. Psycho-Oncology. 2015;24(12):1708–13. PubMed PMID: 25782608. Pubmed Central PMCID: PMC6598678. Epub 2015/03/19. eng.
48. Schmidt SD, Blank TO, Bellizzi KM, Park CL. The relationship of coping strategies, social support, and attachment style with posttraumatic growth in cancer survivors. J Health Psychol. 2011;17(7):1033–40. PubMed PMID: 22253327. Epub 2012/01/19. eng.
49. Kizuki M, Fujiwara T. Adult attachment patterns modify the association between social support and psychological distress. Front Public Health. 2018;6:249. PubMed PMID: 30255007. Pubmed Central PMCID: PMC6141781. Epub 2018/09/27. eng.
50. Nissen KG. Correlates of self-rated attachment in patients with cancer and their caregivers: a systematic review and meta-analysis. Psycho-Oncology. 2016;25(9):1017–27. PubMed PMID: 26763738. Epub 2016/01/15. eng.
51. Ainsworth M. Attachment across the lifespan. Bull N Y Acad Med. 1985;61:792–812.
52. Bowlby J. Developmental psychiatry comes of age. Am J Psychiatry. 1988;145(1):1–10. PubMed PMID: 3276225. Epub 1988/01/01. eng.

53. Lenzi D, Trentini C, Tambelli R, Pantano P. Neural basis of attachment-caregiving systems interaction: insights from neuroimaging studies. Front Psychol. 2015;6:1241. PubMed PMID: 26379578. Pubmed Central PMCID: PMC4547017. Epub 2015/09/18. eng.
54. Ditzen B, Schmidt S, Strauss B, Nater UM, Ehlert U, Heinrichs M. Adult attachment and social support interact to reduce psychological but not cortisol responses to stress. J Psychosom Res. 2008;64(5):479–86. PubMed PMID: 18440400. Epub 2008/04/29. eng.
55. Shallcross SL, Frazier PA, Anders SL. Social resources mediate the relations between attachment dimensions and distress following potentially traumatic events. J Couns Psychol. 2014;61(3):352–62. PubMed PMID: 25019539. Epub 2014/07/16. eng.
56. Bandura A. The assessment and predictive generality of self-percepts of efficacy. J Behav Ther Exp Psychiatry. 1982;13(3):195–9. PubMed PMID: 7142408. Epub 1982/09/01. eng.
57. Bandura A. Self-efficacy: toward a unifying theory of behavioral change. Psychol Rev. 1977;84(2):191–215. PubMed PMID: 847061. Epub 1977/03/01. eng.
58. Haugland T, Wahl AK, Hofoss D, DeVon HA. Association between general self-efficacy, social support, cancer-related stress and physical health-related quality of life: a path model study in patients with neuroendocrine tumors. Health Qual Life Outcomes. 2016;14:11. PubMed PMID: 26787226. Pubmed Central PMCID: PMC4717553. Epub 2016/01/21. eng.
59. Banik A, Luszczynska A, Pawlowska I, Cieslak R, Knoll N, Scholz U. Enabling, not cultivating: received social support and self-efficacy explain quality of life after lung cancer surgery. Ann Behav Med. 2017;51(1):1–12. PubMed PMID: 27418357. Epub 2016/07/16. eng.
60. Luszczynska A, Sarkar Y, Knoll N. Received social support, self-efficacy, and finding benefits in disease as predictors of physical functioning and adherence to antiretroviral therapy. Patient Educ Couns. 2007;66(1):37–42. PubMed PMID: 17097259. Epub 2006/11/14. eng.
61. Hohl DH, Schultze M, Keller J, Heuse S, Luszczynska A, Knoll N. Inter-relations between partner-provided support and self-efficacy: a dyadic longitudinal analysis. Appl Psychol Health Well Being. 2019;11(3):522–42. PubMed PMID: 31231970. Epub 2019/06/25. eng.
62. Carver CS, Scheier MF. Dispositional optimism. Trends Cogn Sci. 2014;18(6):293–9. PubMed PMID: 24630971. Pubmed Central PMCID: PMC4061570. Epub 2014/03/19. eng.
63. Applebaum AJ, Stein EM, Lord-Bessen J, Pessin H, Rosenfeld B, Breitbart W. Optimism, social support, and mental health outcomes in patients with advanced cancer. Psycho-Oncology. 2014;23(3):299–306. PubMed PMID: 24123339. Pubmed Central PMCID: PMC4001848. Epub 2013/10/15. eng.
64. McEwen BS. Physiology and neurobiology of stress and adaptation: central role of the brain. Physiol Rev. 2007;87(3):873–904. PubMed PMID: 17615391. Epub 2007/07/07. eng.
65. Zhang H, Zhao Q, Cao P, Ren G. Resilience and quality of life: exploring the mediator role of social support in patients with breast cancer. Med Sci Monit. 2017;23:5969–79. PubMed PMID: 29248937. Pubmed Central PMCID: PMC5744469. Epub 2017/12/19. eng.
66. Geng Z, Ogbolu Y, Wang J, Hinds PS, Qian H, Yuan C. Gauging the effects of self-efficacy, social support, and coping style on self-management behaviors in Chinese cancer survivors. Cancer Nurs. 2018;41(5):1–10. PubMed PMID: 29461285. Epub 2018/02/21. eng.
67. Fors EA, Bertheussen GF, Thune I, Juvet LK, Elvsaas IK, Oldervoll L, et al. Psychosocial interventions as part of breast cancer rehabilitation programs? Results from a systematic review. Psycho-Oncology. 2011;20(9):909–18. PubMed PMID: 20821803. Epub 2010/09/08. eng.
68. Cutrona C. Stress and social support: in search of optimal matching. J Soc Clin Psychol. 1990;9:3–14.
69. Kroenke CH, Kwan ML, Neugut AI, Ergas IJ, Wright JD, Caan BJ, et al. Social networks, social support mechanisms, and quality of life after breast cancer diagnosis. Breast Cancer Res Treat. 2013;139(2):515–27. PubMed PMID: 23657404. Pubmed Central PMCID: PMC3906043. Epub 2013/05/10. eng.
70. De Leeuw JR, De Graeff A, Ros WJ, Hordijk GJ, Blijham GH, Winnubst JA. Negative and positive influences of social support on depression in patients with head and neck cancer: a prospective study. Psycho-Oncology. 2000;9(1):20–8. PubMed PMID: 10668056. Epub 2000/02/11. eng.

71. Gonzalez-Saenz de Tejada M, Bilbao A, Baré M, Briones E, Sarasqueta C, Quintana JM, et al. Association between social support, functional status, and change in health-related quality of life and changes in anxiety and depression in colorectal cancer patients. Psycho-Oncology. 2017;26(9):1263–9. PubMed PMID: 28872742. Epub 2017/09/06. eng.
72. Cacioppo JT, Hawkley LC. Perceived social isolation and cognition. Trends Cogn Sci. 2009;13(10):447–54. PubMed PMID: 19726219. Pubmed Central PMCID: PMC2752489. Epub 2009/09/04. eng.
73. Lutgendorf SK, DeGeest K, Dahmoush L, Farley D, Penedo F, Bender D, et al. Social isolation is associated with elevated tumor norepinephrine in ovarian carcinoma patients. Brain Behav Immun. 2011;25(2):250–5. PubMed PMID: 20955777. Pubmed Central PMCID: PMC3103818. Epub 2010/10/20. eng.
74. Hostinar CE. Recent developments in the study of social relationships, stress responses, and physical health. Curr Opin Psychol. 2015;5:90–5. PubMed PMID: 26366429. Pubmed Central PMCID: PMC4562328. Epub 2015/09/15. Eng.
75. Hostinar CE, Sullivan RM, Gunnar MR. Psychobiological mechanisms underlying the social buffering of the hypothalamic-pituitary-adrenocortical axis: a review of animal models and human studies across development. Psychol Bull. 2014;140(1):256–82, PubMed PMID: 23607429. Pubmed Central PMCID: PMC3844011. Epub 2013/04/24. eng.
76. Andersen BL, Thornton LM, Shapiro CL, Farrar WB, Mundy BL, Yang HC, et al. Biobehavioral, immune, and health benefits following recurrence for psychological intervention participants. Clin Cancer Res. 2010;16(12):3270–8. PubMed PMID: 20530702. Pubmed Central PMCID: PMC2910547. Epub 2010/06/10. eng.
77. Lutgendorf SK, Sood AK, Anderson B, McGinn S, Maiseri H, Dao M, et al. Social support, psychological distress, and natural killer cell activity in ovarian cancer. J Clin Oncol. 2005;23(28):7105–13. PubMed PMID: 16192594. Epub 2005/09/30. eng.
78. Andersen BL, Farrar WB, Golden-Kreutz DM, Glaser R, Emery CF, Crespin TR, et al. Psychological, behavioral, and immune changes after a psychological intervention: a clinical trial. J Clin Oncol. 2004;22(17):3570–80. PubMed PMID: 15337807. Pubmed Central PMCID: PMC2168591. Epub 2004/09/01. eng.
79. Hostinar CE, Gunnar MR. Future directions in the study of social relationships as regulators of the HPA axis across development. J Clin Child Adolesc Psychol. 2013;42(4):564–75. PubMed PMID: 23746193. Epub 2013/06/12. eng.
80. Heinrichs M, Baumgartner T, Kirschbaum C, Ehlert U. Social support and oxytocin interact to suppress cortisol and subjective responses to psychosocial stress. Biol Psychiatry. 2003;54(12):1389–98. PubMed PMID: 14675803. Epub 2003/12/17. eng.
81. Cole SW, Hawkley LC, Arevalo JM, Sung CY, Rose RM, Cacioppo JT. Social regulation of gene expression in human leukocytes. Genome Biol. 2007;8(9):R189. PubMed PMID: 17854483. Pubmed Central PMCID: PMC2375027. Epub 2007/09/15. eng.
82. Lutgendorf SK, DeGeest K, Sung CY, Arevalo JM, Penedo F, Lucci J, et al. Depression, social support, and beta-adrenergic transcription control in human ovarian cancer. Brain Behav Immun. 2009;23(2):176–83. PubMed PMID: 18550328. Pubmed Central PMCID: PMC2677379. Epub 2008/06/14. eng.
83. Dagan M, Sanderman R, Hoff C, Meijerink WJ, Baas PC, van Haastert M, et al. The interplay between partners' responsiveness and patients' need for emotional expression in couples coping with cancer. J Behav Med. 2014;37(5):828–38. PubMed PMID: 24113912. Epub 2013/10/12. eng.
84. Dagan M, Sanderman R, Schokker MC, Wiggers T, Baas PC, van Haastert M, et al. Spousal support and changes in distress over time in couples coping with cancer: the role of personal control. J Fam Psychol. 2011;25(2):310–8. PubMed PMID: 21480710. Epub 2011/04/13. eng.
85. Manne SL, Kissane D, Zaider T, Kashy D, Lee D, Heckman C, et al. Holding back, intimacy, and psychological and relationship outcomes among couples coping with prostate cancer. J Fam Psychol. 2015;29(5):708–19. PubMed PMID: 26192132. Pubmed Central PMCID: PMC5225663. Epub 2015/07/21. eng.

86. Hagedoorn M, Sanderman R, Bolks HN, Tuinstra J, Coyne JC. Distress in couples coping with cancer: a meta-analysis and critical review of role and gender effects. Psychol Bull. 2008;134(1):1–30. PubMed PMID: 18193993. Epub 2008/01/16. eng.
87. Northouse LL, Katapodi MC, Schafenacker AM, Weiss D. The impact of caregiving on the psychological well-being of family caregivers and cancer patients. Semin Oncol Nurs. 2012;28(4):236–45. PubMed PMID: 23107181. Epub 2012/10/31. eng.
88. Frambes D, Given B, Lehto R, Sikorskii A, Wyatt G. Informal caregivers of cancer patients: review of interventions, care activities, and outcomes. West J Nurs Res. 2018;40(7):1069–97. PubMed PMID: 28381113. Epub 2017/04/07. eng.
89. Dionne-Odom JN, Azuero A, Lyons KD, Hull JG, Tosteson T, Li Z, et al. Benefits of early versus delayed palliative care to informal family caregivers of patients with advanced cancer: outcomes from the ENABLE III randomized controlled trial. J Clin Oncol. 2015;33(13):1446–52. PubMed PMID: 25800762. Pubmed Central PMCID: PMC4404423 online at www.jco.org. Author contributions are found at the end of this article. Epub 2015/03/25. eng.
90. Korotkin BD, Hoerger M, Voorhees S, Allen CO, Robinson WR, Duberstein PR. Social support in cancer: how do patients want us to help? J Psychosoc Oncol. 2019;2019:1–14. PubMed PMID: 30929593. Epub 2019/04/02. eng.
91. Kuchler T, Bestmann B, Rappat S, Henne-Bruns D, Wood-Dauphinee S. Impact of psychotherapeutic support for patients with gastrointestinal cancer undergoing surgery: 10-year survival results of a randomized trial. J Clin Oncol. 2007;25(19):2702–8. PubMed PMID: 17602075. Epub 2007/07/03. eng.
92. Classen C, Butler LD, Koopman C, Miller E, DiMiceli S, Giese-Davis J, et al. Supportive-expressive group therapy and distress in patients with metastatic breast cancer: a randomized clinical intervention trial. Arch Gen Psychiatry. 2001;58(5):494–501. PubMed PMID: 11343530. Epub 2001/05/16. eng.
93. Kissane DW, Grabsch B, Clarke DM, Smith GC, Love AW, Bloch S, et al. Supportive-expressive group therapy for women with metastatic breast cancer: survival and psychosocial outcome from a randomized controlled trial. Psycho-Oncology. 2007;16(4):277–86. PubMed PMID: 17385190. Epub 2007/03/27. eng.
94. Goodwin PJ, Leszcz M, Ennis M, Koopmans J, Vincent L, Guther H, et al. The effect of group psychosocial support on survival in metastatic breast cancer. N Engl J Med. 2001;345(24):1719–26. PubMed PMID: 11742045. Epub 2001/12/14. eng.
95. Guarino A, Polini C, Forte G, Favieri F, Boncompagni I, Casagrande M. The effectiveness of psychological treatments in women with breast cancer: a systematic review and meta-analysis. J Clin Med. 2020;9:1. PubMed PMID: 31940942. Pubmed Central PMCID: PMC7019270. Epub 2020/01/17. eng.
96. Brandão T, Tavares R, Schulz MS, Matos PM. Experiences of breast cancer patients and helpful aspects of supportive-expressive group therapy: a qualitative study. Eur J Cancer Care. 2019;28(5):e13078. PubMed PMID: 31038245. Epub 2019/05/01. eng.
97. Classen CC, Kraemer HC, Blasey C, Giese-Davis J, Koopman C, Palesh OG, et al. Supportive-expressive group therapy for primary breast cancer patients: a randomized prospective multicenter trial. Psycho-Oncology. 2008;17(5):438–47. PubMed PMID: 17935144. Pubmed Central PMCID: PMC3037799. Epub 2007/10/16. eng.
98. Spiegel D, Butler LD, Giese-Davis J, Koopman C, Miller E, DiMiceli S, et al. Effects of supportive-expressive group therapy on survival of patients with metastatic breast cancer: a randomized prospective trial. Cancer. 2007;110(5):1130–8. PubMed PMID: 17647221. Epub 2007/07/25. eng.
99. Andersen BL, Yang HC, Farrar WB, Golden-Kreutz DM, Emery CF, Thornton LM, et al. Psychologic intervention improves survival for breast cancer patients: a randomized clinical trial. Cancer. 2008;113(12):3450–8. PubMed PMID: 19016270. Pubmed Central PMCID: PMC2661422. Epub 2008/11/19. eng.
100. Litzelman K, Reblin M, McDowell HE, DuBenske LL. Trajectories of social resource use among informal lung cancer caregivers. Cancer. 2020;126(2):425–31. PubMed PMID: 31626343. Pubmed Central PMCID: PMC6952577. Epub 2019/10/19. eng.

101. Ferrell B, Wittenberg E. A review of family caregiving intervention trials in oncology. CA Cancer J Clin. 2017;67(4):318–25. PubMed PMID: 28319263. Epub 2017/03/21. eng.
102. Ferrell BR, Temel JS, Temin S, Alesi ER, Balboni TA, Basch EM, et al. Integration of palliative care into standard oncology care: American Society of Clinical Oncology clinical practice guideline update. J Clin Oncol. 2017;35(1):96–112. PubMed PMID: 28034065. Epub 2016/12/31. eng.
103. Shiba K, Kondo N, Kondo K. Informal and formal social support and caregiver burden: the AGES caregiver survey. J Epidemiol. 2016;26(12):622–8. PubMed PMID: 27180934. Pubmed Central PMCID: PMC5121430. Epub 2016/05/18. eng.
104. Mount BM, Boston PH, Cohen SR. Healing connections: on moving from suffering to a sense of well-being. J Pain Symptom Manag. 2007;33(4):372–88. PubMed PMID: 17397699. Epub 2007/04/03. eng.
105. Thorne SE, Kuo M, Armstrong EA, McPherson G, Harris SR, Hislop TG. 'Being known': patients' perspectives of the dynamics of human connection in cancer care. Psycho-Oncology. 2000;14(10):887–98. PubMed PMID: 16200520. Epub 2005/10/04. eng.
106. Kissane DW, Bylund CL, Banerjee SC, Bialer PA, Levin TT, Maloney EK, et al. Communication skills training for oncology professionals. J Clin Oncol. 2012;30(11):1242–7. PubMed PMID: 22412145. Pubmed Central PMCID: PMC3341141 found at the end of this article. Epub 2012/03/14. eng.
107. Kroenke CH, Michael YL, Poole EM, Kwan ML, Nechuta S, Leas E, et al. Postdiagnosis social networks and breast cancer mortality in the after breast cancer pooling project. Cancer. 2017;123(7):1228–37. PubMed PMID: 27943274. Pubmed Central PMCID: PMC5360517. Epub 2016/12/13. eng.
108. Hudson P. A conceptual model and key variables for guiding supportive interventions for family caregivers of people receiving palliative care. Palliat Support Care. 2003;1(4):353–65. PubMed PMID: 16594225. Epub 2006/04/06. eng.
109. Wright LLM. Nurses and families: a guide to family assessment and intervention. Philadelphia: FA Davis; 2013.
110. Björneklett HG, Lindemalm C, Ojutkangas ML, Berglund A, Letocha H, Strang P, et al. A randomized controlled trial of a support group intervention on the quality of life and fatigue in women after primary treatment for early breast cancer. Support Care Cancer. 2012;20(12):3325–34. PubMed PMID: 22576981. Epub 2012/05/12. eng.
111. Schellekens MPJ, Tamagawa R, Labelle LE, Speca M, Stephen J, Drysdale E, et al. Mindfulness-based cancer recovery (MBCR) versus supportive expressive group therapy (SET) for distressed breast cancer survivors: evaluating mindfulness and social support as mediators. J Behav Med. 2017;40(3):414–22. PubMed PMID: 27722908. Pubmed Central PMCID: PMC5406481. Epub 2016/10/11. eng.
112. Wright LM, Leeahey A, Maureen. A guide to family assessment and intervention. 6th ed. Philadelphia: FA Davis Company; 2013.
113. Moore PM, Rivera S, Bravo-Soto GA, Olivares C, Lawrie TA. Communication skills training for healthcare professionals working with people who have cancer. Cochrane Database Syst Rev. 2018;7(7):CD003751. PubMed PMID: 30039853. Pubmed Central PMCID: PMC6513291 known. Camila Olivares: none known. Theresa A Lawrie: none known. Epub 2018/07/25. eng.
114. Banerjee SC, Manna R, Coyle N, Penn S, Gallegos TE, Zaider T, et al. The implementation and evaluation of a communication skills training program for oncology nurses. Transl Behav Med. 2017;7(3):615–23. PubMed PMID: 28211000. Pubmed Central PMCID: PMC5645276. Epub 2017/02/18. eng.
115. Northouse LL, Mood DW, Schafenacker A, Kalemkerian G, Zalupski M, LoRusso P, et al. Randomized clinical trial of a brief and extensive dyadic intervention for advanced cancer patients and their family caregivers. Psycho-Oncology. 2013;22(3):555–63. PubMed PMID: 22290823. Pubmed Central PMCID: PMC3387514. Epub 2012/02/01. eng.
116. Fujinami R, Sun V, Zachariah F, Uman G, Grant M, Ferrell B. Family caregivers' distress levels related to quality of life, burden, and preparedness. Psycho-Oncology. 2015;24(1):54–62. PubMed PMID: 24789500. Pubmed Central PMCID: PMC4216636. Epub 2014/05/03. eng.

117. Ferrell BR, Temel JS, Temin S, Smith TJ. Integration of palliative care into standard oncology care: ASCO clinical practice guideline update summary. J Oncol Pract. 2017;13(2):119–21. PubMed PMID: 28972832. Epub 2017/10/04. eng.
118. Hudson P, Remedios C, Zordan R, Thomas K, Clifton D, Crewdson M, et al. Guidelines for the psychosocial and bereavement support of family caregivers of palliative care patients. J Palliat Med. 2012;15(6):696–702. PubMed PMID: 22385026. Pubmed Central PMCID: PMC3362953. Epub 2012/03/06. eng.
119. Hudson P, Thomas T, Quinn K, Cockayne M, Braithwaite M. Teaching family carers about home-based palliative care: final results from a group education program. J Pain Symptom Manag. 2009;38(2):299–308. PubMed PMID: 19345553. Epub 2009/04/07. eng.
120. Hudson P, Trauer T, Kelly B, O'Connor M, Thomas K, Zordan R, et al. Reducing the psychological distress of family caregivers of home based palliative care patients: longer term effects from a randomised controlled trial. Psycho-Oncology. 2015;24(1):19–24. PubMed PMID: 25044819. Pubmed Central PMCID: PMC4309500. Epub 2014/07/22. eng.
121. Dionne-Odom JN, Azuero A, Lyons KD, Hull JG, Prescott AT, Tosteson T, et al. Family caregiver depressive symptom and grief outcomes from the ENABLE III randomized controlled trial. J Pain Symptom Manag. 2016;52(3):378–85. PubMed PMID: 27265814. Pubmed Central PMCID: PMC5023481. Epub 2016/06/07. eng.
122. Kavalieratos D, Corbelli J, Zhang D, Dionne-Odom JN, Ernecoff NC, Hanmer J, et al. Association between palliative care and patient and caregiver outcomes: a systematic review and meta-analysis. JAMA. 2016;316(20):2104–14. PubMed PMID: 27893131. Pubmed Central PMCID: PMC5226373. Epub 2016/11/29. eng.
123. Funk R, Cisneros C, Williams RC, Kendall J, Hamann HA. What happens after distress screening? Patterns of supportive care service utilization among oncology patients identified through a systematic screening protocol. Support Care Cancer. 2016;24(7):2861–8. PubMed PMID: 26838023. Epub 2016/02/04. eng.
124. Batson S, Greenall G, Hudson P. Review of the reporting of survival analyses within randomised controlled trials and the implications for meta-analysis. PLoS One. 2016;11(5):e0154870. PubMed PMID: 27149107. Pubmed Central PMCID: PMC4858202. Epub 2016/05/07. eng.
125. Wang M, Zhao J, Zhang L, Wei F, Lian Y, Wu Y, et al. Role of tumor microenvironment in tumorigenesis. J Cancer. 2017;8(5):761–73. PubMed PMID: 28382138. Pubmed Central PMCID: PMC5381164. Epub 2017/04/07. eng.
126. Andersen BL, Farrar WB, Golden-Kreutz D, Emery CF, Glaser R, Crespin T, et al. Distress reduction from a psychological intervention contributes to improved health for cancer patients. Brain Behav Immun. 2007;21(7):953–61. PubMed PMID: 17467230. Pubmed Central PMCID: PMC2039896. Epub 2007/05/01. eng.
127. Park H, Oh S, Noh Y, Kim JY, Kim JH. Heart rate variability as a marker of distress and recovery: the effect of brief supportive expressive group therapy with mindfulness in cancer patients. Integr Cancer Ther. 2018;17(3):825–31. PubMed PMID: 29417836. Pubmed Central PMCID: PMC6142099. Epub 2018/02/09. eng.
128. Carlson LE. Mindfulness-based interventions for coping with cancer. Ann N Y Acad Sci. 2016;1373(1):5–12. PubMed PMID: 26963792. Epub 2016/03/11. eng.
129. Carlson LE, Doll R, Stephen J, Faris P, Tamagawa R, Drysdale E, et al. Randomized controlled trial of mindfulness-based cancer recovery versus supportive expressive group therapy for distressed survivors of breast cancer. J Clin Oncol. 2013;31(25):3119–26. PubMed PMID: 23918953. Epub 2013/08/07. eng.
130. Björneklett HG, Rosenblad A, Lindemalm C, Ojutkangas ML, Letocha H, Strang P, et al. Long-term follow-up of a randomized study of support group intervention in women with primary breast cancer. J Psychosom Res. 2013;74(4):346–53. PubMed PMID: 23497838. Epub 2013/03/19. eng.

Psychological Healing and Leveraging the Placebo Effect

12

12.1 Introduction

The scientific community tends to consider the 'placebo effect' as nothing more than a nuisance to be controlled in randomized clinical trials. The placebo *effect* is regarded as a clinically measurable biological and behavioral response to the individual's *mistaken belief* in the sham treatment. It serves as a kind of benchmark against which the treatment under investigation is evaluated [1]. Typically, the magnitude of the effect size difference between treatment and placebo-related outcomes is used to determine treatment efficacy. Throughout the twentieth century, the placebo's healing effects have been dismissed as "immaterial" psychological effects; their belief-induced neurophysiological healing effects, ignored. In fact the actual placebo that has been hiding in plain sight is man's *belief* in his ability to be healed. Moreover the contextual factors in the clinical environment (such as the use of repeated words and procedural rituals) have also been found to trigger biological healing processes under certain conditions. Significantly, these healing capabilities may be activated without resorting to deceptive techniques [2]. Conversely analogous clinical research also has revealed how nocebo effects or negative expectations (beliefs) can contribute to poor clinical outcomes [3].

Today, clinical research is increasingly directed toward better understanding of the neurobiological processes underlying placebos, identifying psychosocial strategies to optimize the placebo (healing) effect and to enhance the efficacy of existing treatments. A concurrent effort is directed toward identifying psychosocial strategies to minimize nocebo effects in order to further improve treatment efficacy [4]. Activating either placebo or nocebo effects frequently occurs within the context of the nurse-patient relationship and clinical setting. Given frequent interactions with the patient before, during, and after treatment, it behooves nurses to learn how to leverage these innate healing processes in order to potentially optimize the patient's clinical outcomes while minimizing potentially deleterious clinical consequences of nocebo effects. This chapter examines the theoretical premises, scientific evidence, and therapeutic clinical applications associated with healing-inducing and worsening clinical outcomes.

12.2 Objectives

At the end of this chapter, the nurse will be able to:

1. Discuss the effects of cognitive expectations and conditioning on patient outcomes within the clinical context.
2. Leverage knowledge of cognitive expectations to foster healing outcomes in patients.
3. Describe unconscious conditioning and implications for a worsened healing outcome.
4. Use nursing strategies that can minimize the potentially deleterious effects (nocebo effects) of unconscious conditioning in the clinical setting.

Clinical Anecdote 12.1
Thanks to childhood illnesses, I came to believe that doctors would make me better whenever I was ill. So when I was first diagnosed with cancer of a particularly aggressive form, I remember being especially calm and very purposeful. I just 'knew' in my heart I would recover. Timely medical intervention and great medical and nursing care were the main keys to my current health, and I am most grateful. But I have also wondered whether my expectation of recovery assisted the treatment- due perhaps to my ability to remain calm. It is impossible to know whether that emotional equanimity born in the expectation of a positive clinical outcome, helped to minimize systemic inflammation. Or perhaps, this health-related belief enabled a greater cell mediated anti-cancer immune response. Perhaps it facilitated a more rapid recovery from various immuno-suppressed treatments which helped to eliminate roving cancer cells. It was certainly not the only explanation for my survival; but perhaps it was one contribution to a multi-modal multi targeted approach.

12.3 Definitions

People tend to hold positive or negative beliefs about illness, health, and treatment outcomes which shape their cognitive expectations regarding clinical outcomes [5]. Beliefs make sense of a clinical situation, such as cancer and its treatment, giving it greater clarity and purpose. Positive and negative health-related beliefs are infused with meaning and emotion associated with expectations for a future clinical improvement or a worsened outcome due to the treatment [4, 5].

Cognitive expectations refer to "specific cognitions about the likelihood of future events" that are held about the disease trajectory, treatment efficacy, the likelihood of side effects, and the individual's ability to influence future outcomes [4]. The placebo effect refers to the desired therapeutic outcomes triggered by positive expectations of a clinical benefit that typically involves treatment [5]. These healing-induced expectations have been shown to exert similar and even greater clinical benefit (for instance, symptom relief) compared to the corresponding effects of many administered anxiolytics and analgesics and/or depressive medications [6–8]. Conversely, the nocebo effect refers to adverse clinical outcomes triggered by negative beliefs about the treatment [5]. The activated interrelated psychological and neurobiological processes link the individual's positive or negative expectation with its corresponding clinical outcome.

12.4 How Cognitive Expectations Are Formed (See "Mechanisms" of Action in Sect. 12.6)

Consistent with social learning theory, these beliefs emanate from an array of sources including family stories, information from various sources, religious faith, and personal experience with previous illness and treatment, such as treatment efficacy, side effects, treatment failure, healthcare provider suggestions, social observation of someone else doing well or poorly on the same treatment, and the quality of the clinician-patient relationship [5, 9–11]. In addition cognitive expectations are affected by drug conditioning, unconscious conditioning, and genetics [12–14]. Whereas a positive expectation for a treatment may be shaped by previous positive health-related life experiences and/or favorable information from valued friends, family, and healthcare provider, negative expectations emanate from a prior negative clinical experience (unexpected side effects), discouraging verbal information about a clinical outcome from a healthcare provider, family member, or peer group; or information about treatment side effects during the consent process [3, 15, 16].

Both positive and negative expectations are mediated by underlying psycho-neurophysiological processes that drive clinical outcomes (i.e., placebo and nocebo effects) [5]. Cognitive expectations have been examined in terms of behavioral, physiological, endocrine, and immune parameters [11, 17–19].

Positive and Negative Expectations: Side Effects

Placebo/nocebo effects have been mainly observed in experimental and clinical research on treatment side effects, with important clinical implications.

Placebo Effects As many as 60% of individuals with various health conditions have induced desired clinical outcomes *without* a previous pharmacological intervention or administration of an inert substance [20]. The belief alone has induced the desired therapeutic outcome. Other placebo-designed human studies have produced significant healing effects across health-related conditions such as Parkinson's disease [21], heart surgery [19], oncology [22, 23], mental health problems [6], and/or medical treatments in which patients experienced a therapeutic reduction in pain, fatigue, anxiety, and depression, and for patients with Parkinson's, an improvement in motor function [11, 12, 23, 24].

Some evidence suggests that positive expectations modulate immune functioning as well. For instance, optimistic expectations were associated with activating cell-mediated immunity in first-year law students [25]. Although clinical research of patients with various medical conditions is needed, scientific experiments with both animals and humans and some patients suggest that positive conscious expectations not only reduce anxiety, pain, and depression or improve motor function in patients with Parkinson's disease, but likely also favorably modulate immunity, by reducing pro-inflammatory cytokines, reversing T-cell immunosuppression, and restoring natural killer T-cells that identify and destroy circulating tumor cells, bacteria, and viruses [5, 19, 26]. How these healing-inducing immune changes might be optimized to enhance clinical outcomes in patients with certain conditions is of growing scientific interest not only to medical researchers but healthcare providers in the clinical field.

Nocebo Effects According to Colloca et al. [5], the potential for a nocebo effect may emanate from a number of social learning contexts. Treatment side effects may be an outcome of the patients' initial expectation of adverse effects. This may be attributed to a previous "bad" treatment experience, a negative comment from family or healthcare providers, a discussion of potential treatment-related side effects through the process of informed consent, and or a significant side effect observed in a patient receiving the same treatment. In addition a number of nonspecific social and physical factors associated with the clinical context appear to impact treatment outcomes; and all these predisposing factors and health-related experiences have clinical implications for treatment adherence and the clinical strategies needed to manage them [5, 16, 27, 28]. Nocebo effects are shaped by both the negative information conveyed and the way the information was interpreted which can result in worsened clinical outcomes, poor quality of life, and low treatment adherence [16].

In an experimental study of negative expectations and pain, volunteers who expected to experience pain showed that a negative suggestion alone converted a painless tactile sensation into a perception of pain (allodynia) and the low-intensity painful stimuli into perceived high-intensity pain or hyperalgesia, underscoring the power of verbal suggestion as it relates to pain [29]. A systematic review of 73 clinical trials assessed 3 classes of anti-migraine medications (NSAIDs, triptans, and anticonvulsants) [30]. Findings showed that participants who had been assigned to the control (placebo) arm of the clinical trial nevertheless reported a high rate of adverse events, which also corresponded with the rates shown in the anti-migraine *treatment* group. Moreover the side effects reported by the placebo and treatment groups *were specific to each type of anti-migraine*

12.4 How Cognitive Expectations Are Formed

medication. This finding was also similar to another analysis of eight clinical trials that investigated the efficacy of statin medications [31]. Between 4% and 26% of the adults assigned to the control group reported side effects which also compelled many to drop out. The adverse effects in both control and treatment arms were significantly related, suggesting that these participants may have been influenced by the informed consent description of possible side effects [31]. A later meta-analysis revealed similar side effect correlations between placebo and treatment groups based on clinical trials assessing targeted or immunotherapy cancer drugs [32]. Given that the control group manifested adverse effects without exposure to the treatment, it also raises the concern whether the treatment's potential efficacy also may be *attenuated by the individual's negative expectations* likely derived from the informed consent process.

A more recent review of the side effects reported in the control and treatment arms of 88 clinical trials also indicated a high number of *nonspecific* side effects that appeared to be unrelated to the treatment itself. The nonspecific rate of side effects in each group was shown to be moderately to highly correlated, suggesting that nonspecific environmental factors in the clinical treatment context and possibly including disease-related symptoms may be producing a certain proportion of nocebo effects independent of the treatment itself [33].

These data highlight the clinical need to sensitively explore all possible patient concerns prior to treatment including the consent process in order to counter negative beliefs that may interfere with the goals of treatment [34, 35] (Review sections "Open/Hidden Clinical Condition" and "Promoting Cognitive Expectations: RCTs".

Clinical Anecdote 12.2
One example of a nocebo effect occurs when a patient has been previously told that inserting an intravenous in the arm may be painful which induces the expectation that it will be painful. And indeed the patient experiences greater pain than someone who had not been so informed. Had the nurse been cognizant of the power of words, she/he might have deliberately used a phrase such as "a remote possibility of a tiny pin prick" or even "barely a pinch" rather than using the word pain which would be suggestive of a higher level of acuity.

Cognitive Expectations Affect the Pharmacodynamics Associated with Drug Efficacy

Cognitive expectations based on verbal suggestions have been shown to modulate treatment efficacy for better or worse [12, 36, 37]. A within-group design assessed 3 different cognitive expectations of 22 volunteers administered remifentanil (an opioid medication) to relieve heat pain [12]. The experimental conditions consisted of (1) positive expectations of a clinical benefit induced by positive verbal suggestion, (2) no expected clinical outcome based on no verbal suggestion, and (3) negative expectation of pain based on verbal suggestion. The three conditions received the same dose and concentration of remifentanil.

The results showed that positive expectation of the drug's clinical benefit more than doubled its usual level of analgesic efficacy as measured by the "no expectation" condition [12]. The administered opioid analgesia produced a significantly higher drug efficacy over the drug's normal therapeutic effect when the volunteers were made aware of the clinical benefits of the medication as opposed to not informing them. Providing positive suggestions that induce positive expectations in support of the intended efficacy of an analgesic produces a greater treatment benefit. This finding is consistent with other experimental studies and does not depend on previous drug conditioning [37, 38].

Conversely, Bingel et al.'s [12] experimental study showed that holding negative expectations of the drug's efficacy (prompted by suggestions of increased pain) completely blocked the drug's analgesic efficacy. It resulted in a significant increase in pain intensity ratings that were similar to levels obtained at baseline (before the remifentanil was given) and were higher than the ratings from the group given remifentanil with "no expectation" of improvement (i.e., representing normal drug efficacy levels). Whereas functional magnetic resonance imaging showed that positive expectation corresponded with endogenous areas associated with modulation of pain, negative expectation showed activity in the hippocampus, suggesting two different areas of the brain which were activated by the two conditions. These findings have important potential clinical implications for patients on treatment that will be discussed in Sect. 12.7.

A nocebo effect can also occur as a clinical response to a previous medical treatment that failed to produce its intended clinical benefit resulting in a negative expectation that impedes the therapeutic benefit of a subsequent treatment [9, 39]. For example, patients who received an ineffective medication for depression subsequently experienced smaller effect size clinical improvements when a different medication was administered [40]. Although there are several possible explanations, one hypothesis is that one or more previous experiences of an adverse treatment may predispose the individual to negative treatment expectations resulting in *greater* anxiety or depressive symptomatology. Although more research is needed, the findings highlight the possibility that a chemotherapeutic agent that fails to achieve the desired clinical outcome might reduce the efficacy of a subsequent chemotherapy due to the patient's negatively held expectations. Similarly patients on chemotherapy who experience side effects of nausea or pain may be predisposed to repeat the experience due to their previously learned negative expectations.

Cognitive Expectations: Drug Conditioning

Drug conditioning occurs when a medication has been repeated more than once, embedding its pharmacodynamic neurophysiological pathways which terminate in its intended clinical outcome [11, 41]. Research findings have identified different ways that drug conditioning with an analgesic or narcotic may influence placebo and nocebo effects. Firstly, a drug repeated more than once with therapeutic effect has been shown to reinforce the patient's positive expectations for a healing response (based on principles of experiential and reinforcement learning) [42]. Secondly, studies have demonstrated that positive expectations combined with the therapeutic

12.4 How Cognitive Expectations Are Formed

Table 12.1 Positive cognitive expectation and drug conditioning effects [38]

- Interactional beliefs × drug effects
- Only possible when the drug conditioning is in the same direction as positive cognitive expectation of relief of a symptom/side effect
    Treatment efficacy ultimately depends on *the patient's cognitive expectation*

effects of a drug or conditioned drug can increase treatment efficacy (Table 12.1) [12, 43].

An experimental study also showed that a placebo analgesic was elicited (with a placebo "open" saline injection) on the third day after 2 days of morphine conditioning or NSAID conditioning [44]. The "open" injection refered to drawing the individual's attention to the placebo injection. The therapeutic expectation induced a significant reduction in pain even the day *after the drug was discontinued*. Cognitive *expectation* of pain relief was shown to stimulate endogenous opioid pathways previously embedded by morphine drug conditioning. Similarly cognitive expectation of pain relief also activated previously associated with the non-opioid NSAID analgesic, ketorolac was found to activate corresponding physiological pathways to induce a clinical benefit [44].

Notwithstanding the ethical breach in using a placebo (such as an open injection of saline), the findings raise the possibility that therapeutic expectations may be leveraged in clinical practice without deceit with respect to how narcotics or anxiolytics may be either reduced in dosage or discontinued without re-exacerbating symptoms [45]. Similarly the findings also underscore the clinical benefits of leveraging scientific knowledge that cognitive expectations with drug conditioning can increase treatment efficacy [37, 38, 46] (review Sect. 12.7).

Clinical Anecdote 12.3
J had taken paxel to manage her depression for 8 weeks and then decided to stop. Six weeks later, she felt her depressed mood returning and at her next clinic visit had her prescription renewed. In a telephone follow-up 10 days later, J told the nurse that she had felt better after taking only one pill! Normally a medication such as paxel requires a dosing period of up to a week or longer before the person begins to experience its therapeutic benefit. But is it possible that previous drug conditioning pathways were reactivated by J's positive expectation triggered by starting the medication again?

How to explain this unexpected clinical finding? The expectation of feeling better which was associated in the individual's mind with taking the drug (remembered wellness) activated underlying and embedded neuroendocrine pathways associated with the reward system [47]. Normally, the conditioned drug response decreases over time in the absence of the patient's re-exposure to the medication. Thus one hypothesis for the clinical finding above may have to do, in part, with the previously repeated exposure of the patient's neurobiology to the pharmacokinetics of the anxiolytic was now re-activated by the patient's *cognitive* expectations of symptom relief [5]. More clinical research in cancer care is needed to identify clinical situations in which the placebo effect may be optimized and the nocebo effect minimized.

Negative Expectations Our current understanding of negative expectations and drug conditioning comes mainly from randomized controlled trials evaluating the treatment efficacy of various pharmacological agents [14, 30, 32, 42]. In contrast to placebos and drug conditioning, experimental research has found that a negative expectation of a worse clinical outcome eradicated the therapeutic effects of a pain medication, such as remifentanil [12]. Similarly the therapeutic effects of a relaxation medication, carisoprodol was eradicated, when the participant was "falsely informed" it was a stimulant [38]. Unlike placebo effects, nocebo hyperalgesia can be achieved after just one negative suggestion without conditioning suggesting that it does not appear to require previous learning to evoke this adverse response. This finding highlights the importance of selecting words carefully in response to patient queries about an upcoming treatment or potential side effects [16, 29].

12.5 Unconscious Conditioning Associated with Treatment-Induced Immunosuppression

Some healing and nocebo responses may be unconsciously conditioned by nonspecific social and physical factors within the clinical environment [5, 14, 48]. *Unconscious neurobiological conditioning* occurs when a patient is repeatedly exposed to a conditioned stimulus (CS), such as a clinic *wall color, clinic smell, pill shape, taste,* or *repeated procedures* such as taking bloods, specific words, phrases, or rituals that may involve nurse behaviors (e.g., setting up an intravenous). The CS becomes unconsciously associated with the medical treatment (an unconditioned stimulus—US) that results in an unconditioned response (UCR) such as nausea or another treatment-related side effect. Eventually after a few repeat sessions, the CS can directly induce the nausea or immunosuppression which is now a conditioned response (CR) [14, 49].

A patient repeatedly exposed to the same olive green wall color in the clinic (CS) while receiving biweekly chemotherapy (US) may subsequently experience an unconditioned response to the chemotherapy (UCR), i.e., posttreatment nausea. After two or three repeat chemotherapies, the green wall color can now independently elicit nausea (CR) on arrival in the clinic [50, 51]. In addition the patient's pretreatment expectations about the side effects of chemotherapy also may be predictive of nocebo responses and interact with unconscious conditioning effects [51–53].

Experimental human studies have shown that immunosuppression can be conditioned by a nonspecific environmental cue within the clinical context (i.e., conditioned stimulus) [54]. A clinical study reported that patients on cyclophosphamide who had hospital bloods drawn just prior to the next chemotherapy showed anticipatory suppression of T-cell proliferative responses compared to their home blood samples. This finding appeared to correspond to a *conditioned*, unconsciously induced immunosuppressed response caused by physical or social environmental factors in the clinic [55].

Although the most likely explanation to account for a patient's immunosuppressed state prior to an upcoming treatment is the patient's naturally slow immune recovery, the patient's anxiety levels and expectations about the treatment should be assessed. If nothing clinically resonates, the possibility of unconscious conditioning should be considered. Immunosuppressed effects may result in delays in the patient's further treatment and is one of the main clinical concerns in caring for the patient's overall resilience and health during this phase of the cancer trajectory (see Sect. 12.7).

12.6 Mechanisms of Action: Psychosocial-Neurobiological Systems of Healing

The relationship between health-related cognitive expectations and desired clinical outcomes depends on a healthy brain, mediated by a complex network of interrelated psycho-neurophysiological and immune systems and pathways that implicate different paths depending on the medical condition, treatment, and desired clinical outcome. Individuals with compromised cognitive abilities due to severe brain injury, dementia, or Alzheimer's disease have been empirically shown *not to benefit* from placebo effects underscoring the importance of conscious beliefs and the brain's ability to make environmental-psychobiological connections [56–58].

Learning and Conditioning

According to learning theory, expectations are predicated on diverse and interactive learning processes such as cognitive learning, associated learning, experiential learning, instructional learning, and conditioning which account for placebo and nocebo responses [49, 50, 59]. For example, research findings suggest that *conscious* beliefs and *unconscious* conditioning interact in producing a clinical outcome [52]. What all these processes share in common is the link between social and physical environmental cues and the manifestation of specific clinical outcomes.

Clinical Anecdote 12.4
A classic example of experiential learning producing a placebo effect occurs when you have a cold causing general malaise, headache, and a sore throat. Feeling miserable you go to the family practice clinic, only to feel better the moment you are actually seated in front of the doctor who has asked you how you feel. The cognitive expectation that the doctor will make you better can be sufficient for you to experience, even temporarily, the sensation of feeling better.

The Brain's Reward System

The brain's reward system has been found to play a key role in the process of inducing healing-related (placebo effects) clinical outcomes [26, 37, 60]. *Conscious expectation* of a desired *positive* clinical outcome, particularly in stressful situations marked by uncertainty, triggers the downregulation of the sympathetic adrenal system and activates the reward circuitry producing a dopaminergic response which provides the sensation of anticipatory pleasure at a hoped-for albeit uncertain outcome [61]. Other mediators of the healing placebo response include endogenous opioids [44] and endocannabinoids [62, 63]. These mediators target specific biological systems associated with the desired clinical outcome.

Dopamine Release

Conscious expectation (the placebo) for a desired clinical outcome activates the release of dopamine in the ventral striatum (i.e., nucleus accumbens) which is associated with the brain's reward circuitry [64, 65]. The reward circuitry also includes the ventral tegmental area (VTA), dorsal striatum (caudate nucleus, putamen), substantia nigra, prefrontal cortex, anterior cingulate cortex, insular cortex, hippocampus, and ventral basal ganglia [61].

In an experimental study, positive expectations of clinical benefit from an experimental intervention for patients with Parkinson's caused a placebo-induced release of dopamine in the dorsal striatum resulting in better motor functioning [37]. Conversely, the expectation/placebo-associated neurophysiological pathways were shown to be disrupted in patients with Alzheimer's who were being treated with a combination of placebo-analgesic for pain [56]. Interestingly the patients with Alzheimer's who scored higher on a battery of prefrontal test scores required a higher dose of analgesic compared to those with the lowest scores. The higher prefrontal scores were attributed to the progressive reduction in the connectivity of prefrontal lobes with the rest of the regions in the brain, underscoring the role of cognition and prefrontal lobes in the placebo response. A desired placebo response depends on a functioning prefrontal cortical brain to induce the reward system which may explain in part why some individuals experience placebo effects and others do not [66].

Opioid and Related Pathways

When the *desired* outcome (i.e., the reward) is a reduction in pain, opioid and nonopioid systems are activated even in the absence of an actual pharmacological intervention [44, 67]. Activated descending opioid pathways emerge from the forebrain that regulates the sensation of pain starting at the level of the dorsal horn of the upper spinal cord [18]. Cognitive expectation of decreased pain results in the reduction of relevant neural activity in the upper spinal cord pathways enabling a reduction in pain sensation [4, 68]. This placebo-induced opioid release has also been reported in the anterior cingulate, orbitofrontal, and insular cortices, periaqueductal gray matter, nucleus accumbens, and amygdala [69, 70]. Notwithstanding, the placebo responses for pain are associated with both dopaminergic and opioid activity in the nucleus accumbens [70]. Cognitive expectations or beliefs in a clinical benefit are particularly effective in modulating physiological processes that are behaviorally experienced, such as anxiety, depressive symptoms, motor functions, as well as pain [37].

Neuroimaging and the Stress Response System and Immune Responses

Placebo-induced treatments have been shown to activate different regions of the brain in addition to those identified as part of the reward circuitry (described in sections "Dopamine Release" and "Opioid and Related Pathways"), specifically the ventromedial PFC, amygdala, HPA axis, ANS, and immune pathways [71]. From a clinical perspective, positive expectations downregulate the stress response system, mediated by neuroendocrinal and immune systems regulating homeostasis, healing, the body's defenses, and resilience [61]. Experimental data, based on a mouse model, also have shown significant causal links between activated dopaminergic neurons of the ventral tegmental area (VTA) and innate and adaptive immune responses to bacteria that were partially mediated by an activated SNS. These experimental data, which are difficult to replicate in humans, suggest endogenous bidirectional interactivity between conscious expectations, the dopaminergic neural reward circuitry, and, increasingly, immune functioning [26].

Although the therapeutic effects of cognitive expectations in the clinical field have been mainly demonstrated in terms of behavioral outcomes (i.e., pain, anxiety, depressed mood), the potential therapeutic effects on biological systems such as adaptive and innate immune functions are of increasing scientific interest [26, 60]. Restorative immune cell activity and function seem to occur as a consequence of the downregulation of the biological stress response system associated with cognitive expectation and activation of the reward systems. The reactivated cytotoxic natural killer cells may be part of a comprehensive healing-promoting approach with unique but also overlapping endpoints resulting in synergistic healing effects throughout the person.

Genes and the Placebo
Variations in placebo-induced responses across patients with the same medical condition have raised the possibility that genetic differences also may account for various placebo responses across people [71]. Hall's group and others seek to identify genetic correlates of the placebo response across clinical trials, the next scientific challenge in the field of placebos.

MOA and Nocebo Pathways

According to nocebo theory, beliefs about treatment-induced side effects trigger neuro*physiological and psychological* processes that result in the symptom worsening as cognitively expected [51, 72]. Mediating neurophysiological pathways connecting a nocebo expectation to its worsened clinical outcome has not been as well studied as placebo effects. What we are learning comes mainly from pain-related research [5].

Nocebo effects appear to suppress dopaminergic systems and the release of opioids [70]. Whereas cognitive expectations of pain relief are known to be mediated by the activation of μ-opioid pathways, expectations of increased pain activate the neuropeptide cholecystokinin (CCK) which *reduces* both opioid and dopamine release in the nucleus accumbens. The activation of CCK pathways appears to attenuate the reward circuitry that drives the placebo response. Moreover, the resultant hyperalgesia (i.e., increased perceived pain) has been associated with the activation of the HPA axis [72, 73].

CCK receptor antagonists such as benzodiazepine (for eg diazepam) block both nocebo-induced hyperalgesia (heightened pain) and the anxiety-induced HPA axis, suggesting that anxiety plays a role in hyperalgesia [72, 73]. Another CCK antagonist proglumide however was found to completely block nocebo hyperalgesia but not the activated HPA axis suggesting that CCK has a specific effect on nocebo-induced *pain increase* but perhaps not the anxiety component of the nocebo effect [72, 73].

Other areas of the brain that are co-activated by nocebo-induced expectations include the ACC, parietal operculum, thalamus, insula, and PFC [66]. Negative expectations or beliefs trigger the brain's sensory and cognitive circuits (i.e., activate the HPA axis and suppress the healing processes of the PNS) along neurobiological pathways that result in worsening effects such as greater anxiety, pain, or depressive mood [72, 73]. To the extent that these nocebo pathways and hormones such as CCK are known, it appears that both placebo and nocebo effects are likely mediated by the same neurophysiological systems and pathways with opposing neurotransmitters that culminate in their respective treatment effects [18].

Summary
This review highlights the various psychosocial, physical, and neurobiological factors that can trigger an individual's healing or provoke an adverse clinical outcome, with or without the conscious awareness of the patient, nurse, or other healthcare providers. Improved or worsened side effects may be determined by the patient's positive or negative expectations about a treatment outcome. An individual's positive expectations in association with drug conditioning can potentially optimize a patient's drug efficacy, which may be especially relevant in symptom management. And these desired clinical benefits may be further *amplified* by corresponding verbal suggestions in support of the treatment efficacy, by drawing the patient's attention to the drug being administered, and by

promoting the patient's positive expectations in the therapeutic direction of the treatment effect.

Other findings identify the clinical contexts that can lead to clinically worsened outcomes: the patient's own negative expectations, the process of informed consent, but also the words and behaviors of healthcare providers that sow doubt about the treatment's efficacy. What clinicians say or do modulate patient expectations concerning clinical outcomes and need to be carefully considered within the clinical setting in order to optimize treatment efficacy and reduce the possibility of unwanted side effects. As will be discussed in the next section, studies have identified the healing-promoting role of the healthcare (nurse)-patient relationship in promoting healing-inducing clinical outcomes.

Although medical scientists are investigating how unconscious conditioning may be leveraged to promote treatment efficacy, to date it is the immunosuppressive effects of certain anticancer treatments that are of most concern to nurses caring for oncology patients. In accordance with classical conditioning, it appears that the physical and social environment may trigger immunosuppressed effects between treatments or just prior to the next treatment on arrival to the clinic.

12.7 Nursing Approaches

The main nursing goals involve mobilizing relevant strategies in the clinical context in order to strengthen placebo or healing responses and counter the deleterious effects of nocebo responses. An expert consensus paper supports clinical practice that strives to optimize placebo effects in the clinical setting while minimizing nocebo effects in order to produce better treatment outcomes and fewer side effects in patients [34]. The expert panel recommends informing patients about placebo and nocebo effects as part of clinical treatment. Specifically, Evers et al.'s [34] recommendations include explaining the potential effects of placebos and how they may work in conjunction with a patient's medication in order to enhance treatment efficacy. In so doing, it may also help to reduce the incidence of nocebo effects in the clinical setting when patients understand the potential relationships between health-related beliefs and clinical outcomes.

The consensus paper also recommends providing workshops for healthcare providers to learn clinician-patient communication skills, relating especially to healing-inducing and nocebo-suppressing strategies [34]. These workshops should contain an educational component on the neurobiological processes involved in placebo/nocebo responses, social and physical environmental triggers, and the effect sizes and duration of effects. These recommendations are examined more closely as they can be easily incorporated into the nurse's daily practice (Table 12.2).

Table 12.2 Some strategies for enhancing the placebo effect and reducing the incidence of nocebo effects in patients, adapted from the expert consensus paper [34]

1. Explain the placebo/nocebo effects to patients and caregivers
a. *In the diagnostic phase and again just prior to anticancer treatment*, describe the placebo effect as a healing capability of all humans induced by positive clinical expectations. Explain that positive expectations can reduce symptom intensity by activating opioid pathways in the body for, e.g., pain intensity and inducing dopaminergic (reward) pathways that instill well-being. Explain that placebos plus the treatment *increase* drug efficacy. This discussion is also tailored to the patient's illness and corresponding expected treatment effects
b. *In the diagnostic phase and as clinically assessed afterward*, explain the relationship between *negative* beliefs about the treatment and its potential ability to induce adverse treatment effects, such as compromising treatment efficacy. This may be presented as part of a larger discussion in which patient concerns, fears, anxieties about the treatments, and use of coping skills are addressed. This discussion is also tailored to the patient's illness and treatment-related expected therapeutic effects
c. Describe the learning processes that link human beliefs with clinical outcomes and how they are translated into neurophysiological processes that tend to reflect our positive or negative beliefs about clinical outcomes
d. The consent process: Incorporate strategies to counter nocebo effects for, e.g., use of framing, while also promoting the clinical benefits of the treatment
2. Educate nurses and other healthcare providers on the team
a. Learn about positive/negative patient expectations, drug conditioning in relation to placebo and nocebo effects. Learn about the conscious and unconscious side effects of cancer-related treatment resulting in differential clinical outcomes, e.g. (side effects: immunosuppressed, nausea, pain)
b. Explore different nursing approaches to optimize placebo effects and reduce and/or overturn treatment-related side effects. Special attention should be given to nursing strategies that may be used to enhance placebo effects and reduce the incidence of nocebo effects around informed consent

The Quality of the Nurse-Patient Relationship
(Review Part IV Chap. 8)

The quality of the nurse-patient/caregiver relationship lies at the core of healing-inducing capabilities and is an integral part of the psychosocial and biological modulating influences on a patient's clinical outcomes [35, 74]. Clinical findings have highlighted the role *of mutual trust, warmth, empathy, and compassion* within the clinician-patient relationship in *creating dyadic conditions that can optimize* the patient's healing-related clinical outcomes [4, 34, 75]. Notwithstanding, the quality of the relationship can also serve as a nocebo when these properties of the relationship are lacking.

Research findings support the therapeutic value of creating a healing-inducing clinical environment based on the quality of the relationships among the nurse, patient, and caregiver [57, 74]. A RCT investigated whether placebo effects could be observed under different clinical conditions [58, 76]. Two hundred and sixty two adults with irritable bowel syndrome were randomly assigned to (1) a waitlist, (2) a placebo sham acupuncture group *with minimal contact* with the clinician, and (3) a placebo sham acupuncture with *a warm, attentive, and confident* clinician who engaged the patient in discussion regarding his knowledge and feelings about his illness. The interventions occurred twice a week for 3 or 6 weeks. The findings showed a global overall improvement in IBM symptoms and quality of life across the three conditions with a significant upward but differential trend ranging from (1) the lowest score (waitlist group) followed by (2) the intermediate higher score (the sham acupuncture with *minimal interaction* between the clinician and patient) to the (3) highest score (i.e., the sham acupuncture within the context of *a warm, empathetic, caring* interactive clinician-patient relationship). The quality of the clinician's relationship with the patient clearly served as a significant placebo or healing-inducing context in its own right [58]. This finding which lies at the theoretical core of nursing practice should be replicated in an RCT based on the nurse-patient relationship in cancer care.

A therapeutic nurse relationship with the patient (and caregiver), similar to that of the physician, is predicated on an authentic patient-centered relationship infused with compassion, warmth, competence, and a shared understanding of the patient's beliefs and expectations [75, 77, 78]. Within this relationship the nurse and patient share the clinical goal of optimizing the healing capabilities of the patient [58, 79].

Clinical Anecdote 12.5
When I first met with the oncologist, he discussed my illness, and all the treatment options that were possible. But he also stated something to the effect that together we would get through this: He would take care of the cancer, and my job was to strengthen my physical and psychological health so that my body could fight the cancer alongside the treatment. Although I did not realize it then: What he said constituted a 'placebo' that made me believe that I was going to get better!

Shared Beliefs
Beliefs serve as a prism through which a medical diagnosis such as cancer may be "subjectively interpreted and subsequently acted upon by both the patient and the nurse" for better or worse [47]. The quality of the nurse-patient or physician-patient relationship has been known to modulate the patient's cognitive expectations about a future clinical outcome. When the nurse and patient's beliefs are concordant or working together in the same positive direction, an important synergistic effect on the patient's healing capabilities is possible, even in the absence of a cure [47, 80, 81].

Fostering healing within the nurse-patient relationship includes the ability to convey warmth and demonstrated competence as part of the nurse's therapeutic relationship with the patient. An experimental study in which a histamine skin prick test was used to create an allergic reaction on the arm of volunteers to which an *inert cream* was applied showed that healthcare providers (HCPs) who exhibited warm and competent behaviors increased the volunteers' positive expectation that the *inert* cream would reduce the allergic reaction, with a subsequent better clinical "effect." In contrast, the HCPs' colder and/or less competent approach elicited negative expectations with a poorer therapeutic outcome [79].

Verbal Suggestions and Open/Closed Treatments
(Review Sect. 12.4)

The psychosocial clinical context has been shown to shape the patient's and caregiver's cognitive beliefs and expectations of either a therapeutic or adverse clinical outcome [28]. The power of verbal suggestions regarding the treatment by healthcare providers and nurses on subsequent patient outcomes cannot be underestimated in clinical practice. As Table 12.3 summarizes, a treatment-related healing effect is enhanced when the beliefs of the patient and nurse are both aligned in the same direction as the intended clinical treatment.

As the studies in this chapter have indicated, verbal information plays a significant role in influencing cognitive expectations of a positive treatment outcome or adverse effects [12]. When the individual's cognitive expectations *are in the same direction* as the pharmacological intent of the treatment, enhanced treatment efficacy is possible. For instance, positive information about the therapeutic effects of a medication such as a muscle relaxant (carisoprodol) *has been shown to* significantly *increase the absorption rate of the drug* compared to the two other control conditions [38].

When the expectation is at odds with the treatment intent, treatment efficacy is reduced. The findings from several studies suggest that a healthcare provider can *suppress* the actual pharmacodynamic drug effects that alleviate anxiety, depressive symptoms, or motor functions when giving information that *is contrary to a patient's therapeutic expectation* [82, 83]. Data from a few animal and human studies raise the added possibility that negative suggestions causing a lack of optimism, hope, or negative expectation for a therapeutic outcome may also impair normal immune functioning, including suppressing natural killer T-cells that identify and destroy some tumor cells, bacteria, and viruses [25, 26, 60]. More clinical research in this area would help to further inform nursing practice.

Table 12.3 Promoting healing within the nurse-patient relationship [4, 47, 78, 86]

Cognitive expectations—promoting healing outcomes
Depends on
• Patient *beliefs/expectations* about future clinical benefit (wellness), plus
• *Nurse beliefs, expectations, and behaviors relating to* the patient's future clinical benefit
In which
• Congruence between nurse and patient in the type, direction, and quality of beliefs is present
• The nurse's clinical behaviors to enhance the patient's positive clinical outcomes include (1) providing relevant information/suggestions about the goals and expected outcomes of the treatment and (2) informing the patient when the treatment is being administered
• Nurse-patient relationships are characterized by warmth, compassion, competence, and mutual trust
• The nurse also explains the goals, functions, and biopsychosocial processes of the placebo and nocebo and what the patient can do to promote the placebo effect and help to minimize the nocebo effect

12.7 Nursing Approaches

Even a discussion of the possible side effects of an upcoming treatment has been shown to be sufficient to convert a patient's anticipated therapeutic outcome into a worsened clinical result [28]. An informed consent session in which side effects are emphasized over expected clinical benefits of the treatment has been shown to induce treatment-related side effects [10, 16, 84, 85]. Analogously, a patient who has learned that the postoperative period may be painful is likely to experience greater pain.

Clinical Anecdote 12.6
At a clinic visit prior to starting chemotherapy, the oncologist wanted to review the treatment plan with me. Part of that discussion involved sharing that the preferred chemotherapy had an estimated 91% efficacy in eliminating the tumor. At first I was horrified. What is going to get rid of the remaining tumor cells, I wanted to understand. Your immune cells will. With exercise, a healthy diet and staying calm, your body defenses will do the rest. We were working together. The oncologist had taken time to provide relevant medical information that established an educated context for understanding my body and the tumor, the treatment expectations and the complementary roles of oncologist and patient in promoting my cognitive expectations. It was akin to the open treatment modality as discussed below.

Suggested Nurse Interventions [15, 87] (Review Section "Promoting Cognitive Expectations: RCTs") *Promote therapeutic benefits*: Sensitively assess the patient's expectations, concerns, and emotional distress [4, 34]. Strive to prevent or minimize negative expectations by describing the therapeutic benefits of the treatment, and use statistics in a way that tips the cognitive belief toward the unlikelihood of side effects, e.g., "85% of patients on this chemotherapy *do very well.*" Explain that medication is provided to enhance the likelihood of feeling well through chemotherapy (i.e., prophylactic medication to avoid side effects).

Educate Strengthen or support the patient's positive expectations by describing what a placebo is and that positive expectations aligned with the treatment actually enhance treatment efficacy. Provide the patient with relevant medical information about the disease and course of treatment and strategies the patient can use to strengthen resilience and healing through healthy lifestyle behaviors, coping strategies, and a meaningful life. Of course these suggestions must be tailored to the patient's physical and clinical status, but the healing-promoting approach remains the same until the end of life.

If the nurse disagrees with the patient's cognitive expectation of therapeutic benefit, support the patient's beliefs (hopes) while gently orienting the patient toward clinical reality. The nurse might say "We are both hoping for the very best outcome" and other comments such as "In any challenge in life, we do everything we can to support the best possible outcome while preparing for all eventualities." A more nuanced approach is one that my oncologist offered when my cancer was so advanced that there were no known protocols. He reminded me that we were a team; he would take care of the treatment (involving me as much as I wanted) while my goal was to strengthen my resilience and health to help fight the cancer.

Open/Hidden Clinical Condition

Open treatments occur when the patient *observes* the treatment being given *and is concurrently told* its therapeutic purpose. Conversely hidden treatments refer to the administration of a medication without the conscious awareness of the patient. A study of open/hidden treatment showed that patients with postoperative state anxiety *who were told they were currently receiving* an intravenous anxiolytic (diazepam) along with stated information about its intended therapeutic benefit significantly reduced anxiety levels, whereas those who were unaware that they had received the anxiolytic were still anxious 2 h later [37].

Similarly, postoperative patients in the recovery room who were informed they were currently receiving a medication for pain (morphine) showed *a more rapid and significant reduction* in pain levels compared to the "hidden treatment" group [37]. Furthermore, patients in the concealed group required significantly more narcotic to decrease the pain by at least 50%. The hidden treatment group was found to have a slower reduction in pain intensity over the next 4 hours, never achieving comparable low levels of pain relief compared to the open treatment group.

Clinical Anecdote 12.7
I was extremely groggy in the recovery room following surgery, wanting to sleep. Periodically I could hear the nurse calling my name, which took a lot of effort to respond to. 'Wake up, wake up, open your eyes,' she would say. Each time I was roused I was aware of tremendous pain, and would ask for medication, and then immediately I would fall back asleep, only to wake up again a while later asking for more medication. Invariably I would be told that I had received it and it was too soon for more. Yet I was still experiencing significant pain.

Studies illustrate that the combination of the patient's conscious awareness of the nurse currently administering a medication accompanied by the nurse's explanation of its therapeutic purpose, can trigger an *initial experience of symptom relief* (attributed to the placebo effect) which *occurs more rapidly and before* the medication itself normally produces a therapeutic effect. Thus clinical treatments for symptomatic relief given *openly* with the positive conscious awareness of the patient are more likely to be effective than treatments given without the patient's awareness [37, 48].

Colloca et al.'s [37] study also showed how an open versus hidden clinical approach in discontinuing a medication may produce adverse effects in patients. In the open treatment group, verbal information that the healthcare provider in the recovery room now intended to stop the morphine or anxiolytic resulted in increased pain or anxiety in patients. In contrast patients in the hidden condition (i.e., unaware of the cessation of the medication) resulted in less pain or anxiety.

These findings, taken together, indicate that the "open" goals of treatment must be in the same therapeutic direction as the desired clinical benefits held by the patient. When the verbal information opposes the individual's expectation creating heightened cognitive dissonance, the potential for a placebo effect will be eliminated, and the hidden condition by comparison will produce better placebo effects according to Babel's experimental findings [88]. That clinical knowledge has led to a possible, ethical nursing intervention that has been proposed in the placebo literature [45].

Suggested Interventions Promote open treatment approach: Direct the patient's attention to the medication's preparation and administration while informing the patient of hoped-for clinical goals of *the chemotherapy as well as any antiemetic, anxiolytic, and/or pain medications. Provide* pertinent information about each medication's therapeutic effects *during* its administration [37]. As part of boosting positive expectations, consider offering cognitive and behavioral coping skills to manage stress and relevant education about the underlying neurobiological healing-inducing processes, including immune responses, triggered by positive expectations that can result in symptom improvement and enhanced drug efficacy [25, 26, 37].

An unusual open-label clinical strategy involves patients *knowing* they are receiving actual placebos (i.e., inert substances or sham techniques) accompanied by an explanation of how positive cognitive expectations (with or without a placebo) can trigger a significant clinical improvement via conditioning of neurobiological processes that lead to desired clinical outcomes [4]. In a meta-analysis of 11 RCTs comparing patients in either open-label placebos (OLP) or no treatment, a significant overall therapeutic effect was shown for open-label placebos over the no-treatment group although risk of bias was moderately high [89]. The studies were based on patients with back pain, cancer-related fatigue, attention deficit hyperactivity, allergic rhinitis, major depression, irritable bowel syndrome, and menopausal hot flashes. The findings supported those of another similarly designed open-label placebo approach for fatigue in survivors of cancer, in which patients *knowingly* took two sugar pills a day which resulted in clinical benefit compared to usual treatment. This may be an effective strategy to consider clinically [90]. A randomized clinical trial to evaluate this clinical intervention for symptom management in patients with cancer would also inform the nurse's clinical practice.

Dose-Extending Placebo Another modification of the open-label approach concerns clinical decisions to discontinue a narcotic or analgesic treatment which might cause an immediate spike in subjective pain or anxiety [37]. Colloca et al. [45] proposed an informed consent strategy for relieving pain via a *"dose-extending" placebo*. In essence, the patient's consent is given to toggle between administering morphine and a placebo solution in order to optimize pain relief as the drug is being decreased under close nursing assessment, thereby minimizing the potential for nocebo responses. The intervention is based on previous clinical research in which patients receiving pain medication over 2 days and a placebo only on the third day showed continued analgesic effects [44]. Describe the strategy and its rationale to the patient, drawing on related research findings about placebos and their synergistic effects in combination with treatment that result in spillover effects. With the patient's consent, the nurse would toggle the placebo with the actual medication as the latter is being tapered out. This interesting strategy seems to have clinical merit and should be evaluated with a RCT in patients with cancer.

Promoting Cognitive Expectations: RCTs

RCTs that have investigated the effects of a patient's positive expectations of a therapeutic outcome in clinical oncology are still rare. Although not in the field of cancer care, a prospective RCT with a 6-month follow-up randomly assigned 124 patients awaiting coronary artery bypass graft surgery to 1 of 3 clinical interventions: (a) EXPECT in which the clinical intervention was designed to optimize the patient's positive expectations about life after surgery, (b) SUPPORT in which emotional support was offered, and (c) standard medical care (SMC) [19, 91, 92].

The EXPECT group showed significantly greater improvement (ie significant reduction) in disability, compared to the SMC group or SUPPORT group. At the 6-month follow-up, a trend still favored the EXPECT intervention ($p = 0.09$) with greater mental quality of life and fitness for work compared to the other conditions. Both the EXPECT and SUPPORT groups showed lower levels of pro-inflammatory cytokines after surgery compared to SMC and lower IL-6 levels in the EXPECT group suggesting a possible link to the reward circuitry and downregulation of the stress response system. The data also showed significantly lower adrenaline levels in both the EXPECT and SUPPORT groups compared with the SMC postoperatively. The findings provide further evidence of the importance of promoting the cognitive expectations of patients, which given the positive effects on immunity should be replicated in patients with cancer awaiting surgery.

Strategies to Minimize the Nocebo Effect

Nocebo effects appear to develop more easily than placebo effects and may be more difficult to eradicate [4, 50]. At a scheduled nurse appointment shortly after the diagnosis and before the first anticancer treatment, ask the patient what they know about *their* disease and their *expectations about its course and the treatment*. Address patient and family caregiver anxieties and worries [95]. Provide relevant information about the cancer and treatment goals and known efficacy (see below on framing). Clarify patient and caregiver concerns, misinformation, and negative thoughts about the cancer or treatment that could result in a nocebo effect [12]. Should the nurse identify negative expectations that could interfere with treatment efficacy, acknowledge the possibility of side effects by emphasizing the clinical benefits over the small likelihood of side effects and the measures taken to either prevent or mitigate their effect, for instance, patients usually take an antiemetic during and after treatment. Explain that a negative treatment expectation can worsen symptoms and even compromise treatment efficacy [4]. Propose use of positive self-talk and mindful meditation to reduce emotional reactivity to negative thoughts in at-risk patients [96–98].

Framing is an increasingly favored clinical strategy in which pretreatment information about side effects is presented within a larger clinical context of reviewing treatment goals and expected treatment benefits in relation to the patient's condition [84]. *Valence framing* refers to the use of statistically equivalent information which can be presented either within a *negative frame*, such as "Only 5% of people on this treatment report side effects," or a *positive frame*, such as "95% of patients take this medication without incident" [99]. Use of positive framing is increasingly recommended in order to minimize the potential salience of side effects in the patient's mind that may negatively inform his or her cognitive expectations of the treatment [16]. Framing side effects should consider using words such as "uncommon" and emphasizing the proportion of patients who *do not experience* these symptoms. In other words shift the conversation from a focus on the likelihood of side effects to the hoped-for clinical benefits of the treatment.

Managing Informed Consent

The process of informed consent in which the oncologist and nurse are ethically obliged to review the potential side effects of treatment with the patient is replete with nocebo-inducing possibilities, and the strategies outlined in the previous section are applicable in this very sensitive and consequential context. A pilot study investigated the effect of different ways to provide informed consent on treatment expectations. Their findings suggested that *framing and personalizing* the informed consent led to more positive treatment expectations and fewer decision-based conflicts [100]. However this study was based on healthy subjects asked to imagine their responses to either endocrine treatment or chemotherapy for breast cancer. When another study framed the side effects by emphasizing *the higher* percentage of patients who did not experience side effects (rather than the percent who did) using actual data, this positive framing strategy was shown to be effective during the session but was not sustained at the follow-up 24 h later [84, 85]. One clinical takeaway may be the need for a comprehensive approach using several strategies to counter nocebo responses and the importance of repeating these strategies just prior to and during each subsequent treatment. Hauser et al. [3] suggest emphasizing the benefits of the treatment, its goals, and general efficacy, as well as the fact that the majority of patients tolerate it without incident, and that the potential for side effects which may occur in a few patients is quickly addressed by appropriate medications. Future research might investigate the optimal structure of the consent session and the order of information provided about clinical benefits and side effects to ascertain whether structure and order influence the individual's healing-inhibiting or healing-enhancing effects.

Summary
The patient's positive *expectation for a clinical benefit* as well as drug efficacy can be improved with *these simple nursing interventions* that should become standard clinical practice to strengthen patients' cognitive expectations for a therapeutic benefit and to enhance drug *efficacy* [12, 15, 38, 43, 91]:

1. Emphasize that a given treatment is generally tolerated by most patients and that side effects tend to be "uncommon."

2. Draw the patient's attention to every medication about to be administered, by stating what it is and its intended clinical benefit (open treatment).
3. Offer positive verbal information about the therapeutic intent of the treatment *before and during* each administration to underscore the importance of maintaining a positive expectation regarding treatment efficacy (i.e., reducing the tumor size).
4. Educate patient and caregiver about the synergistic effects of therapeutic expectations and treatment efficacy.
5. Educate the patient and caregiver about the deleterious effects of negative expectations on treatment efficacy.
6. Ensure that healthcare provider and patient express or hold similar positive cognitive expectations of treatment to prevent nocebo effects.

Modulating Unconscious Conditioning (Review Sect. 12.5)

Unconscious conditioning may occur during chemotherapy and has important clinical implications for patients with cancer. When the treatment intent of the chemotherapy is the eradication of the disease but the side effect is immunosuppression, this is an obvious challenge for nurses striving to maintain the patients' resilience between chemotherapy sessions. As discussed in Sect. 12.5, nonspecific clinical, social, and environmental stimuli repeatedly observed by the patient at the time of chemotherapy may become unconsciously associated with the immunosuppressed side effects of the drug, triggering an immunosuppressed response in the clinic before chemotherapy, possibly delaying the next treatment [49, 55].

Immunosuppression also may be triggered by *memories* of the chemotherapy infusion or reactivated by similar environmental stimuli in the home that is evocative of the clinic conditioned stimulus, such as the same paint color. Moreover negative expectations and unconscious drug conditioning interact, resulting in increased behavioral side effects such as nausea and fatigue as well as immunosuppressed effects [52]. These side effects not only have been found to persist between treatments but years afterward, impeding the ability of the body to regain its full potential resilient capabilities [101]. More clinical research in this area is needed.

The immunosuppressed effects of unconscious conditioning in patients who have or had cancer is a particular nursing concern due to its negative effect on specific cytokines and T-cells that are normally recruited to hunt down and eradicate cancer cells. These include *the cytokine release of* IL-2, IFN-γ, natural killer cells, and cytotoxic T-cells [93, 102]. One hypothesis is that these behavioral and immunosuppressed effects are a consequence of negative conscious expectations and unconscious drug conditioning [14, 54]. Notwithstanding symptoms such as anxiety, fatigue, and nausea are empirically known to share an underlying inflammatory environment exacerbated by cancer- and treatment-related effects [103, 104]. Both processes likely interact.

These findings highlight *the importance* of introducing the placebo-promoting and nocebo-suppressing strategies described in the sections above to reduce the potential for nocebo responses at the time of informed consent, just prior to and during treatment, as well as during clinical interactions with the patient [4, 105]. But immunosuppressed side effects triggered by unconscious social-environmental stimuli are likely to be difficult for the nurse to identify and effectively reverse.

Nursing Suggestions Identify with the oncologist patients who are unusually and repeatedly immunosuppressed the morning of their next treatment (usually bloods are drawn before chemotherapy). This could be further resolved with a simple blood test taken during a home visit between treatments. If the home test reveals immune recovery that differs from the blood test taken in clinic just prior to his upcoming chemotherapy, a conditioned immunosuppressed state may exist.

If the patient is immunosuppressed at home between treatments with no immune recovery, another possibility that cannot be discounted, from an unconscious conditioning perspective, is that the conditioned clinical stimulus triggering immunosuppression in the clinical setting is similar to the triggering conditioned stimulus experienced at home. For instance, clinic walls and walls at home may share the same color and hue of wall paint. In this instance a home blood test would reveal little to no immune recovery. Or the patient uses a hospital bed at home that is reminiscent to the day bed used during cancer treatment may trigger an immunosuppressed response. Explore the possibility of patient intrusive ideation or patient memories of the chemotherapy experience between treatments which also may evoke a conditioned immunosuppressed response [106].

Consider using complementary therapies (CTs) that have been shown to strengthen immune cell functioning before, during, and after chemotherapy in clinically appropriate patients. These CTs may be feasible in patients for which immunosuppression *is an unwanted side effect, not a goal* of treatment. Therapies that elicit the relaxation response such as mindful meditation, yoga, and imagery have been shown to restore anticancer natural killer cell activity and IFN-γ functioning while suppressing the release of various inflammatory cytokines, cortisol and NFkB-related gene expression from roving leukocytes [107, 108]. Moderate exercise before, after, and even during the treatment phase is also recommended as recent research strongly indicates its role in enhancing immunosurveillance, including tracking and eliminating roving cancer cells [109, 110] (Part V Chap. 20). Last, consider therapeutic touch (TT), although much more clinical research is needed to provide credible scientific support for its potential immuno-protective effects during chemoradiation, as evidenced by findings from a controlled study of patients with cervical cancer [111]. One interesting PTSD study in soldiers suggested TT was helpful in controlling intrusive ideation [112] (Part IV, Chap. 17).

12.8 Final Comments

What nurses and other health providers say, how they say it, and what they do in the course of their work either promote or undermine healing capability. Studies have highlighted the *power of verbal suggestion* and open treatment, the value of framing especially during informed consent, and drug conditioning as a few of the interactive cognitive and neurobiological processes that may be leveraged to enhance treatment efficacy, promote positive cognitive expectations, and counter negative beliefs about a treatment outcome. Equally important is to minimize the possibility of unconscious conditioning of immunosuppressed and behavioral side effects associated with anticancer treatments in order to protect the individual's potential for healing and resilience.

References

1. Moerman DE, Jonas WB. Deconstructing the placebo effect and finding the meaning response. Ann Intern Med. 2002;136(6):471–6. PubMed PMID: 11900500. Epub 2002/03/20. eng.
2. Finniss DG, Kaptchuk TJ, Miller F, Benedetti F. Biological, clinical, and ethical advances of placebo effects. Lancet. 2010;375(9715):686–95. PubMed PMID: 20171404. Pubmed Central PMCID: PMC2832199. Epub 2010/02/23. eng.
3. Hauser W, Hansen E, Enck P. Nocebo phenomena in medicine: their relevance in everyday clinical practice. Deut Arzteblatt Int. 2012;109(26):459–65. PubMed PMID: 22833756. Pubmed Central PMCID: PMC3401955. Epub 2012/07/27. eng.
4. Petrie KJ, Rief W. Psychobiological mechanisms of placebo and nocebo effects: pathways to improve treatments and reduce side effects. Annu Rev Psychol. 2019;70:599–625. PubMed PMID: 30110575. Epub 2018/08/16. eng.
5. Colloca L, Barsky AJ. Placebo and nocebo effects. N Engl J Med. 2020;382(6):554–61. PubMed PMID: 32023375. Epub 2020/02/06. eng.
6. Weimer K, Colloca L, Enck P. Placebo effects in psychiatry: mediators and moderators. Lancet Psychiatry. 2015;2(3):246–57. PubMed PMID: 25815249. Pubmed Central PMCID: PMC4370177. Epub 2015/03/31. eng.
7. Gaab J. The placebo and its effects: a psychoneuroendocrinological perspective. Psychoneuroendocrinology. 2019;105:3–8. PubMed PMID: 30098833. Epub 2018/08/14. eng.
8. Häuser W, Sarzi-Puttini P, Tölle TR, Wolfe F. Placebo and nocebo responses in randomised controlled trials of drugs applying for approval for fibromyalgia syndrome treatment: systematic review and meta-analysis. Clin Exp Rheumatol. 2012;30(6):78–87. PubMed PMID: 23137770. Epub 2012/11/10. eng.
9. Zunhammer M, Ploner M, Engelbrecht C, Bock J, Kessner SS, Bingel U. The effects of treatment failure generalize across different routes of drug administration. Sci Transl Med. 2017;9:393. PubMed PMID: 28592563. Epub 2017/06/09. eng.
10. Faasse K, Parkes B, Kearney J, Petrie KJ. The influence of social modeling, gender, and empathy on treatment side effects. Ann Behav Med. 2018;52(7):560–70. PubMed PMID: 29860362. Epub 2018/06/04. eng.
11. Colloca L, Klinger R, Flor H, Bingel U. Placebo analgesia: psychological and neurobiological mechanisms. Pain. 2013;154(4):511–4. PubMed PMID: 23473783. Pubmed Central PMCID: PMC3626115. Epub 2013/03/12. eng.
12. Bingel U, Wanigasekera V, Wiech K, Ni Mhuircheartaigh R, Lee MC, Ploner M, et al. The effect of treatment expectation on drug efficacy: imaging the analgesic benefit of the opioid remifentanil. Sci Transl Med. 2011;3(70):70. PubMed PMID: 21325618. Epub 2011/02/18. eng.
13. Colloca L, Miller FG. How placebo responses are formed: a learning perspective. Philos Trans R Soc Lond Ser B Biol Sci. 2011;366:1859–69.
14. Kamen C, Tejani MA, Chandwani K, Janelsins M, Peoples AR, Roscoe JA, et al. Anticipatory nausea and vomiting due to chemotherapy. Eur J Pharmacol. 2014;722:172–9. PubMed PMID: 24157982. Pubmed Central PMCID: PMC3880638. Epub 2013/10/26. eng.
15. Bingel U. Avoiding nocebo effects to optimize treatment outcome. JAMA. 2014;312(7):693–4. PubMed PMID: 25003609. Epub 2014/07/09. eng.

16. Colloca L, Miller FG. The nocebo effect and its relevance for clinical practice. Psychosom Med. 2011;73(7):598–603. PubMed PMID: 21862825. Pubmed Central PMCID: PMC3167012. Epub 2011/08/25. eng.
17. Fricchione G, Stefano GB. Placebo neural systems: nitric oxide, morphine and the dopamine brain reward and motivation circuitries. Med Sci Monit. 2005;11(5):54–65. PubMed PMID: 15874901. Epub 2005/05/06. eng.
18. Rief W, Bingel U, Schedlowski M, Enck P. Mechanisms involved in placebo and nocebo responses and implications for drug trials. Clin Pharmacol Ther. 2011;90(5):722–6. PubMed PMID: 21975346. Epub 2011/10/07. eng.
19. Rief W, Shedden-Mora MC, Laferton JA, Auer C, Petrie KJ, Salzmann S, et al. Preoperative optimization of patient expectations improves long-term outcome in heart surgery patients: results of the randomized controlled PSY-HEART trial. BMC Med. 2017;15(1):4. PubMed PMID: 28069021. Pubmed Central PMCID: PMC5223324. Epub 2017/01/11. eng.
20. Lanotte M, Lopiano L, Torre E, Bergamasco B, Colloca L, Benedetti F. Expectation enhances autonomic responses to stimulation of the human subthalamic limbic region. Brain Behav Immun. 2005;19(6):500–9. PubMed PMID: 16055306. Epub 2005/08/02. eng.
21. Benedetti F, Colloca L, Torre E, Lanotte M, Melcarne A, Pesare M, et al. Placebo-responsive Parkinson patients show decreased activity in single neurons of subthalamic nucleus. Nat Neurosci. 2004;7(6):587–8. PubMed PMID: 15146189. Epub 2004/05/18. eng.
22. Chvetzoff G, Tannock IF. Placebo effects in oncology. J Natl Cancer Inst. 2003;95(1):19–29. PubMed PMID: 12509397. Epub 2003/01/02. eng.
23. de la Cruz M, Hui D, Parsons HA, Bruera E. Placebo and nocebo effects in randomized double-blind clinical trials of agents for the therapy for fatigue in patients with advanced cancer. Cancer. 2010;116(3):766–74. PubMed PMID: 19918921. Pubmed Central PMCID: PMC2815077. Epub 2009/11/18. eng.
24. Benedetti F, Pollo A, Lopiano L, Lanotte M, Vighetti S, Rainero I. Conscious expectation and unconscious conditioning in analgesic, motor, and hormonal placebo/nocebo responses. J Neurosci. 2003;23(10):4315–23. PubMed PMID: 12764120. Epub 2003/05/24. eng.
25. Segerstrom SC, Sephton SE. Optimistic expectancies and cell-mediated immunity: the role of positive affect. Psychol Sci. 2010;21(3):448–55. PubMed PMID: 20424083. Pubmed Central PMCID: PMC3933956. Epub 2010/04/29. eng.
26. Ben-Shaanan TL, Schiller M, Azulay-Debby H, Korin B, Boshnak N, Koren T, et al. Modulation of anti-tumor immunity by the brain's reward system. Nat Commun. 2018;9(1):2723. PubMed PMID: 30006573. Pubmed Central PMCID: PMC6045610. Epub 2018/07/15. eng.
27. Cohen S. The nocebo effect of informed consent. Bioethics. 2014;28(3):147–54. PubMed PMID: 22762392. Epub 2012/07/06. eng.
28. Colloca L, Finniss D. Nocebo effects, patient-clinician communication, and therapeutic outcomes. JAMA. 2012;307(6):567–8. PubMed PMID: 22318275. Pubmed Central PMCID: PMC6909539. Epub 2012/02/10. eng.
29. Colloca L, Sigaudo M, Benedetti F. The role of learning in nocebo and placebo effects. Pain. 2008;136(1-2):211–8. PubMed PMID: 18372113. Epub 2008/03/29. eng.
30. Amanzio M, Corazzini LL, Vase L, Benedetti F. A systematic review of adverse events in placebo groups of anti-migraine clinical trials. Pain. 2009;146(3):261–9. PubMed PMID: 19781854. Epub 2009/09/29. eng.
31. Rief W, Avorn J, Barsky AJ. Medication-attributed adverse effects in placebo groups: implications for assessment of adverse effects. Arch Intern Med. 2006;166(2):155–60. PubMed PMID: 16432082. Epub 2006/01/25. eng.
32. Chacón MR, Enrico DH, Burton J, Waisberg FD, Videla VM. Incidence of placebo adverse events in randomized clinical trials of targeted and immunotherapy cancer drugs in the adjuvant setting: a systematic review and meta-analysis. JAMA Netw Open. 2018;1(8):e185617. PubMed PMID: 30646278. Pubmed Central PMCID: PMC6324542. Epub 2019/01/16. eng.

33. Mahr A, Golmard C, Pham E, Iordache L, Deville L, Faure P. Types, frequencies, and burden of nonspecific adverse events of drugs: analysis of randomized placebo-controlled clinical trials. Pharmacoepidemiol Drug Saf. 2017;26(7):731–41. PubMed PMID: 28176407. Epub 2017/02/09. eng.
34. Evers AWM, Colloca L, Blease C, Annoni M, Atlas LY, Benedetti F, et al. Implications of placebo and nocebo effects for clinical practice: expert consensus. Psychother Psychosom. 2018;87(4):204–10. PubMed PMID: 29895014. Pubmed Central PMCID: PMC6191882. Epub 2018/06/13. eng.
35. Blasini M, Peiris N, Wright T, Colloca L. The role of patient-practitioner relationships in placebo and nocebo phenomena. Int Rev Neurobiol. 2018;139:211–31. PubMed PMID: 30146048. Pubmed Central PMCID: PMC6176716. Epub 2018/08/28. eng.
36. Faasse K, Petrie KJ. The nocebo effect: patient expectations and medication side effects. Postgrad Med J. 2013;89(1055):540–6. PubMed PMID: 23842213. Epub 2013/07/12. eng.
37. Colloca L, Lopiano L, Lanotte M, Benedetti F. Overt versus covert treatment for pain, anxiety, and Parkinson's disease. Lancet Neurol. 2004;3(11):679–84. PubMed PMID: 15488461. Epub 2004/10/19. eng.
38. Flaten MA, Simonsen T, Olsen H. Drug-related information generates placebo and nocebo responses that modify the drug response. Psychosom Med. 1999;61(2):250–5. PubMed PMID: 10204979. Epub 1999/04/16. eng.
39. Hunter AM, Cook IA, Tartter M, Sharma SK, Disse GD, Leuchter AF. Antidepressant treatment history and drug-placebo separation in a placebo-controlled trial in major depressive disorder. Psychopharmacology. 2015;232(20):3833–40. PubMed PMID: 26319158. Epub 2015/09/01. eng.
40. Hunter AM, Cook IA, Leuchter AF. Impact of antidepressant treatment history on clinical outcomes in placebo and medication treatment of major depression. J Clin Psychopharmacol. 2010;30(6):748–51. PubMed PMID: 21057245. Epub 2010/11/09. eng.
41. Brascher AK, Witthoft M, Becker S. The underestimated significance of conditioning in placebo hypoalgesia and nocebo hyperalgesia. Pain Res Manag. 2018;2018:6841985. PubMed PMID: 29670678. Pubmed Central PMCID: PMC5833150. Epub 2018/04/20. eng.
42. Amanzio M. Nocebo effects and psychotropic drug action. Expert Rev Clin Pharmacol. 2015;8(2):159–61. PubMed PMID: 25494811. Epub 2014/12/17. eng.
43. Vase L, Riley JL, Price DD. A comparison of placebo effects in clinical analgesic trials versus studies of placebo analgesia. Pain. 2002;99(3):443–52. PubMed PMID: 12406519. Epub 2002/10/31. eng.
44. Amanzio M, Benedetti F. Neuropharmacological dissection of placebo analgesia: expectation-activated opioid systems versus conditioning-activated specific subsystems. J Neurosci. 1999;19(1):484–94. PubMed PMID: 9870976. Epub 1998/12/31. eng.
45. Colloca L, Enck P, DeGrazia D. Relieving pain using dose-extending placebos: a scoping review. Pain. 2016;157(8):1590–8. PubMed PMID: 27023425. Pubmed Central PMCID: PMC5364523. Epub 2016/03/30. eng.
46. Bartels DJ, van Laarhoven AI, Haverkamp EA, Wilder-Smith OH, Donders AR, van Middendorp H, et al. Role of conditioning and verbal suggestion in placebo and nocebo effects on itch. PLoS One. 2014;9(3):e91727. PubMed PMID: 24646924. Pubmed Central PMCID: PMC3960153. Epub 2014/03/22. eng.
47. Benson H, Friedman R. Harnessing the power of the placebo effect and renaming it "remembered wellness". Annu Rev Med. 1996;47:193–9. PubMed PMID: 8712773.
48. Benedetti F, Amanzio M. The placebo response: how words and rituals change the patient's brain. Patient Educ Couns. 2011;84(3):413–9. PubMed PMID: 21621366. Epub 2011/05/31. eng.
49. Luckemann L, Unteroberdorster M, Kirchhof J, Schedlowski M, Hadamitzky M. Applications and limitations of behaviorally conditioned immunopharmacological responses. Neurobiol Learn Mem. 2017;142(A):91–8. PubMed PMID: 28216206. Epub 2017/02/22. eng.
50. Colloca L, Petrovic P, Wager TD, Ingvar M, Benedetti F. How the number of learning trials affects placebo and nocebo responses. Pain. 2010;151(2):430–9. PubMed PMID: 20817355. Pubmed Central PMCID: PMC2955814. Epub 2010/09/08. eng.

References

51. Roscoe JA, Bushunow P, Morrow GR, Hickok JT, Kuebler PJ, Jacobs A, et al. Patient expectation is a strong predictor of severe nausea after chemotherapy: a University of Rochester Community Clinical Oncology Program study of patients with breast carcinoma. Cancer. 2004;101(11):2701–8. PubMed PMID: 15517574. Epub 2004/11/02. eng.
52. Kirsch I, Kong J, Sadler P, Spaeth R, Cook A, Kaptchuk T, et al. Expectancy and conditioning in placebo analgesia: separate or connected processes? Psychol Conscious. 2014;1(1):51–9. PubMed PMID: 25093194. Pubmed Central PMCID: PMC4118664. Epub 2014/08/06. eng.
53. Montgomery GH, Tomoyasu N, Bovbjerg DH, Andrykowski MA, Currie VE, Jacobsen PB, et al. Patients' pretreatment expectations of chemotherapy-related nausea are an independent predictor of anticipatory nausea. Ann Behav Med. 1998;20(2):104–9. PubMed PMID: 9989316. Epub 1999/02/16. eng.
54. Goebel MU, Trebst AE, Steiner J, Xie YF, Exton MS, Frede S, et al. Behavioral conditioning of immunosuppression is possible in humans. FASEB J. 2002;16(14):1869–73. PubMed PMID: 12468450. Epub 2002/12/07. eng.
55. Bovbjerg DH, Redd WH, Maier LA, Holland JC, Lesko LM, Niedzwiecki D, et al. Anticipatory immune suppression and nausea in women receiving cyclic chemotherapy for ovarian cancer. J Consult Clin Psychol. 1990;58(2):153–7. PubMed PMID: 2335631. Epub 1990/04/01. eng.
56. Benedetti F, Arduino C, Costa S, Vighetti S, Tarenzi L, Rainero I, et al. Loss of expectation-related mechanisms in Alzheimer's disease makes analgesic therapies less effective. Pain. 2006;121(1-2):133–44. PubMed PMID: 16473462. Epub 2006/02/14. eng.
57. Benedetti F. Placebo and the new physiology of the doctor-patient relationship. Physiol Rev. 2013;93(3):1207–46. PubMed PMID: 23899563. Pubmed Central PMCID: PMC3962549. Epub 2013/08/01. eng.
58. Kaptchuk TJ, Kelley JM, Conboy LA, Davis RB, Kerr CE, Jacobson EE, et al. Components of placebo effect: randomised controlled trial in patients with irritable bowel syndrome. BMJ. 2008;336(7651):999–1003. PubMed PMID: 18390493. Pubmed Central PMCID: PMC2364862. Epub 2008/04/09. eng.
59. López FJ, Alonso R, Luque D. Rapid top-down control of behavior due to propositional knowledge in human associative learning. PLoS One. 2016;11(11):e0167115. PubMed PMID: 27893814. Pubmed Central PMCID: PMC5125669. Epub 2016/11/29. eng.
60. Ben-Shaanan TL, Azulay-Debby H, Dubovik T, Starosvetsky E, Korin B, Schiller M, et al. Activation of the reward system boosts innate and adaptive immunity. Nat Med. 2016;22(8):940–4. PubMed PMID: 27376577. Epub 2016/07/05. eng.
61. Dutcher JM, Creswell JD. The role of brain reward pathways in stress resilience and health. Neurosci Biobehav Rev. 2018;95:559–67. PubMed PMID: 30477985. Epub 2018/11/28. eng.
62. Benedetti F, Amanzio M, Rosato R, Blanchard C. Nonopioid placebo analgesia is mediated by CB1 cannabinoid receptors. Nat Med. 2011;17(10):1228–30. PubMed PMID: 21963514. Epub 2011/10/04. eng.
63. Benedetti F, Carlino E, Pollo A. How placebos change the patient's brain. Neuropsychopharmacology. 2011;36(1):339–54. PubMed PMID: 20592717. Pubmed Central PMCID: PMC3055515. Epub 2010/07/02. eng.
64. de la Fuente-Fernandez R, Ruth TJ, Sossi V, Schulzer M, Calne DB, Stoessl AJ. Expectation and dopamine release: mechanism of the placebo effect in Parkinson's disease. Science. 2001;293(5532):1164–6. PubMed PMID: 11498597. Epub 2001/08/11. eng.
65. de la Fuente-Fernandez R, Schulzer M, Stoessl AJ. Placebo mechanisms and reward circuitry: clues from Parkinson's disease. Biol Psychiatry. 2004;56(2):67–71. PubMed PMID: 15231437. Epub 2004/07/03. eng.
66. Enck P, Benedetti F, Schedlowski M. New insights into the placebo and nocebo responses. Neuron. 2008;59(2):195–206. PubMed PMID: 18667148. Epub 2008/08/01. eng.
67. Benedetti F, Mayberg HS, Wager TD, Stohler CS, Zubieta JK. Neurobiological mechanisms of the placebo effect. J Neurosci. 2005;25(45):10390–402. PubMed PMID: 16280578. Epub 2005/11/11. eng.
68. Eippert F, Finsterbusch J, Bingel U, Büchel C. Direct evidence for spinal cord involvement in placebo analgesia. Science. 2009;326(5951):404. PubMed PMID: 19833962. Epub 2009/10/17. eng.

69. Scott DJ, Stohler CS, Egnatuk CM, Wang H, Koeppe RA, Zubieta JK. Individual differences in reward responding explain placebo-induced expectations and effects. Neuron. 2007;55(2):325–36. PubMed PMID: 17640532. Epub 2007/07/21. eng.
70. Scott DJ, Stohler CS, Egnatuk CM, Wang H, Koeppe RA, Zubieta JK. Placebo and nocebo effects are defined by opposite opioid and dopaminergic responses. Arch Gen Psychiatry. 2008;65(2):220–31. PubMed PMID: 18250260. Epub 2008/02/06. eng.
71. Hall KT, Loscalzo J, Kaptchuk T. Pharmacogenomics and the placebo response. ACS Chem Neurosci. 2018;9(4):633–5. PubMed PMID: 29498823. Pubmed Central PMCID: PMC6309549. Epub 2018/03/03. eng.
72. Benedetti F, Amanzio M, Vighetti S, Asteggiano G. The biochemical and neuroendocrine bases of the hyperalgesic nocebo effect. J Neurosci. 2006;26(46):12014–22. PubMed PMID: 17108175. Pubmed Central PMCID: PMC6674855. Epub 2006/11/17. eng.
73. Benedetti F, Lanotte M, Lopiano L, Colloca L. When words are painful: unraveling the mechanisms of the nocebo effect. Neuroscience. 2007;147(2):260–71. PubMed PMID: 17379417. Epub 2007/03/24. eng.
74. Thorne SE, Kuo M, Armstrong EA, McPherson G, Harris SR, Hislop TG. 'Being known': patients' perspectives of the dynamics of human connection in cancer care. Psycho-Oncology. 2000;14(10):887–98. PubMed PMID: 16200520. Epub 2005/10/04. eng.
75. Durkin J, Usher K, Jackson D. Embodying compassion: a systematic review of the views of nurses and patients. J Clin Nurs. 2019;28(9-10):1380–92. PubMed PMID: 30485579. Epub 2018/11/30. eng.
76. Kaptchuk TJ, Friedlander E, Kelley JM, Sanchez MN, Kokkotou E, Singer JP, et al. Placebos without deception: a randomized controlled trial in irritable bowel syndrome. PLoS One. 2010;5(12):e15591. PubMed PMID: 21203519. Pubmed Central PMCID: PMC3008733. Epub 2011/01/05. eng.
77. Edvardsson D, Watt E, Pearse F. Patient experiences of caring and person-centeredness are associated with perceived nursing care quality. J Adv Nurs. 2017;73:217–27.
78. Durkin J, Jackson D, Usher K. Defining compassion in a hospital setting: consensus on the characteristics that comprise compassion from researchers in the field. Contemp Nurse. 2020;56(2):146–59. PubMed PMID: 32420794. Epub 2020/05/19. eng.
79. Howe LC, Goyer JP, Crum AJ. Harnessing the placebo effect: exploring the influence of physician characteristics on placebo response. Health Psychol. 2017;36(11):1074–82. PubMed PMID: 28277699. Pubmed Central PMCID: PMC7608626. Epub 2017/03/10. eng.
80. Leuchter AF, Hunter AM, Tartter M, Cook IA. Role of pill-taking, expectation and therapeutic alliance in the placebo response in clinical trials for major depression. Br J Psychiatry. 2014;205(6):443–9. PubMed PMID: 25213159. Pubmed Central PMCID: PMC4248233 support from the National Institutes of Health, Wyeth Pharmaceuticals, Novartis Pharmaceuticals, Seaside Therapeutics, Genentech, Shire Pharmaceuticals, Neuronetics, Eli Lilly and Company, and Neurosigma. He has served as a consultant to NeoSync Inc., Brain Cells, Inc., Taisho Pharmaceuticals, Eli Lilly and Company, and Aspect Medical Systems/Covidien. He is Chief Scientific Officer of Brain Biomarker Analytics LLC (BBA). He owns stock options in NeoSync, Inc. and has equity interest in BBA. I.A.C., within the past 5 years, has received research support from Aspect Medical Systems/Covidien, National Institutes of Health, Neuronetics and Shire; he has been on the speakers' bureau for Neuronetics and the Medical Education Speakers Network; he has been an advisor/consultant/reviewer for Allergan, Covidien, Pfizer, Neuronetics, NeuroSigma, NIH (ITVS), US Department of Defense, US Department of Justice, VA (DSMB); his biomedical intellectual property is assigned to the Regents of the University of California, and he owns stock options in NeuroSigma. Epub 2014/09/13. eng.
81. Remen RN. Kitchen table wisdom: stories that heal. New York: Riverhead Books; 2006.
82. Kaptchuk TJ, Stason WB, Davis RB, Legedza AR, Schnyer RN, Kerr CE, et al. Sham device v inert pill: randomised controlled trial of two placebo treatments. BMJ. 2006;332(7538):391–7. PubMed PMID: 16452103. Pubmed Central PMCID: PMC1370970. Epub 2006/02/03. eng.

References

83. Bingel U, Colloca L, Vase L. Mechanisms and clinical implications of the placebo effect: is there a potential for the elderly? A mini-review. Gerontology. 2011;57(4):354–63. PubMed PMID: 20975261. Pubmed Central PMCID: PMC3130981. Epub 2010/10/27. eng.
84. Faasse K, Huynh A, Pearson S, Geers AL, Helfer SG, Colagiuri B. The influence of side effect information framing on nocebo effects. Ann Behav Med. 2019;53(7):621–9. PubMed PMID: 30204841. Epub 2018/09/12. eng.
85. Faasse K, Martin LR. The power of labeling in nocebo effects. Int Rev Neurobiol. 2018;139:379–406. PubMed PMID: 30146055. Epub 2018/08/28. eng.
86. Benson H, Stark M. Timeless healing: the power and biology of belief. New York: Simon & Schuster; 1997.
87. Jacobsen J, Kvale E, Rabow M, Rinaldi S, Cohen S, Weissman D, et al. Helping patients with serious illness live well through the promotion of adaptive coping: a report from the improving outpatient palliative care (IPAL-OP) initiative. J Palliat Med. 2014;17(4):463–8. PubMed PMID: 24579823. Epub 2014/03/04. eng.
88. Babel P, Adamczyk W, Swider K, Bajcar EA, Kicman P, Lisinska N. How classical conditioning shapes placebo analgesia: hidden versus open conditioning. Pain Med. 2018;19(6):1156–69. PubMed PMID: 29016984. Epub 2017/10/11. eng.
89. von Wernsdorff M, Loef M, Tuschen-Caffier B, Schmidt S. Effects of open-label placebos in clinical trials: a systematic review and meta-analysis. Sci Rep. 2021;11(1):3855. PubMed PMID: 33594150. Pubmed Central PMCID: PMC7887232. Epub 2021/02/18. eng.
90. Hoenemeyer TW, Kaptchuk TJ, Mehta TS, Fontaine KR. Open-label placebo treatment for cancer-related fatigue: a randomized-controlled clinical trial. Sci Rep. 2018;8(1):2784. PubMed PMID: 29426869. Pubmed Central PMCID: PMC5807541. Epub 2018/02/11. eng.
91. Webster RK, Weinman J, Rubin GJ. Medicine-related beliefs predict attribution of symptoms to a sham medicine: a prospective study. Br J Health Psychol. 2018;23(2):436–54. PubMed PMID: 29405507. Pubmed Central PMCID: PMC5900880. Epub 2018/02/07. eng.
92. Salzmann S, Euteneuer F, Laferton JAC, Auer CJ, Shedden-Mora MC, Schedlowski M, et al. Effects of preoperative psychological interventions on catecholamine and cortisol levels after surgery in coronary artery bypass graft patients: the randomized controlled PSY-HEART Trial. Psychosom Med. 2017;79(7):806–14. PubMed PMID: 28846584. Epub 2017/08/29. eng.
93. Wang M, Zhao J, Zhang L, Wei F, Lian Y, Wu Y, et al. Role of tumor microenvironment in tumorigenesis. J Cancer. 2017;8(5):761–73. PubMed PMID: 28382138. Pubmed Central PMCID: PMC5381164. Epub 2017/04/07. eng.
94. Ramirez MF, Ai D, Bauer M, Vauthey JN, Gottumukkala V, Kee S, et al. Innate immune function after breast, lung, and colorectal cancer surgery. J Surg Res. 2015;194(1):185–93. PubMed PMID: 25475022. Epub 2014/12/06. eng.
95. Vanbockstael J, Coquan E, Gouerant S, Allouache D, Faveyrial A, Noal S, et al. How to improve the prevention of chemotherapy-induced nausea and vomiting? The French NAVI study. Support Care Cancer. 2016;24(3):1131–8. PubMed PMID: 26268784. Epub 2015/08/14. eng.
96. Carlson LE, Zelinski E, Toivonen K, Flynn M, Qureshi M, Piedalue KA, et al. Mind-body therapies in cancer: what is the latest evidence? Curr Oncol Rep. 2017;19(10):67. PubMed PMID: 28822063. Epub 2017/08/20. eng.
97. Meichenbaum D. A clinical handbook for assessing and treating adults with post-traumatic stress disorder (PTSD). Waterloo: Institute Press; 1994.
98. Du S, Hu L, Dong J, Xu G, Jin S, Zhang H, et al. Patient education programs for cancer-related fatigue: a systematic review. Patient Educ Couns. 2015;98(11):1308–19. PubMed PMID: 26072422. Epub 2015/06/15. eng.
99. Devlin EJ, Whitford HS, Denson LA. The impact of valence framing on response expectancies of side effects and subsequent experiences: a randomised controlled trial. Psychol Health. 2019;34(11):1358–77. PubMed PMID: 31132015. Epub 2019/05/28. eng.

100. Heisig SR, Shedden-Mora MC, Hidalgo P, Nestoriuc Y. Framing and personalizing informed consent to prevent negative expectations: an experimental pilot study. Health Psychol. 2015;34(10):1033–7. PubMed PMID: 25689300. Epub 2015/02/18. eng.
101. Ebede CC, Jang Y, Escalante CP. Cancer-related fatigue in cancer survivorship. Med Clin North Am. 2017;101(6):1085–97. PubMed PMID: 28992856. Epub 2017/10/11. eng.
102. Lutgendorf SK, Andersen BL. Biobehavioral approaches to cancer progression and survival: mechanisms and interventions. Am Psychol. 2015;70(2):186–97. PubMed PMID: 25730724. Pubmed Central PMCID: PMC4347942. Epub 2015/03/03. eng.
103. Miller AH, Ancoli-Israel S, Bower JE, Capuron L, Irwin MR. Neuroendocrine-immune mechanisms of behavioral comorbidities in patients with cancer. J Clin Oncol. 2008;26(6):971–82. PubMed PMID: 18281672. Pubmed Central PMCID: 2770012.
104. Miller AH, Maletic V, Raison CL. Inflammation and its discontents: the role of cytokines in the pathophysiology of major depression. Biol Psychiatry. 2009;65(9):732–41. PubMed PMID: 19150053. Pubmed Central PMCID: PMC2680424. Epub 2009/01/20. eng.
105. Devlin EJ, Denson LA, Whitford HS. Cancer treatment side effects: a meta-analysis of the relationship between response expectancies and experience. J Pain Symptom Manag. 2017;54(2):245–58. PubMed PMID: 28533160. Epub 2017/05/24. eng.
106. Pacheco-Lopez G, Engler H, Niemi MB, Schedlowski M. Expectations and associations that heal: immunomodulatory placebo effects and its neurobiology. Brain Behav Immun. 2006;20(5):430–46. PubMed PMID: 16887325.
107. Bhasin MK, Dusek JA, Chang BH, Joseph MG, Denninger JW, Fricchione GL, et al. Relaxation response induces temporal transcriptome changes in energy metabolism, insulin secretion and inflammatory pathways. PLoS One. 2013;8(5):e62817. PubMed PMID: 23650531. Pubmed Central PMCID: PMC3641112. Epub 2013/05/08. eng.
108. Antoni MH, Lutgendorf SK, Blomberg B, Carver CS, Lechner S, Diaz A, et al. Cognitive-behavioral stress management reverses anxiety-related leukocyte transcriptional dynamics. Biol Psychiatry. 2012;71(4):366–72. PubMed PMID: 22088795. Pubmed Central PMCID: PMC3264698. Epub 2011/11/18. eng.
109. Campbell JP, Turner JE. Debunking the myth of exercise-induced immune suppression: redefining the impact of exercise on immunological health across the lifespan. Front Immunol. 2018;9:648. PubMed PMID: 29713319. Pubmed Central PMCID: PMC5911985. Epub 2018/05/02. eng.
110. Nieman DC, Wentz LM. The compelling link between physical activity and the body's defense system. J Sport Health Sci. 2019;8(3):201–17. PubMed PMID: 31193280. Pubmed Central PMCID: PMC6523821. Epub 2019/06/14. eng.
111. Lutgendorf SK, Mullen-Houser E, Russell D, Degeest K, Jacobson G, Hart L, et al. Preservation of immune function in cervical cancer patients during chemoradiation using a novel integrative approach. Brain Behav Immun. 2010;24(8):1231–40. PubMed PMID: 20600809. Pubmed Central PMCID: PMC3010350. Epub 2010/07/06. eng.
112. Reeve K, Black PA, Huang J. Examining the impact of a Healing Touch intervention to reduce posttraumatic stress disorder symptoms in combat veterans. Psychol Trauma. 2020;12(8):897–903. PubMed PMID: 33346680. Epub 2020/12/22. eng.

Mindfulness-Based Practice and Eliciting the Relaxation Response

13.1 Introduction

At stressful moments along the cancer and recovery continuum, individuals may struggle to effectively manage various side effects and symptoms. Distress, anxiety, a depressive mood, and fears of a cancer recurrence are widely shared responses to cancer-related stresses across all phases of the disease, treatment, and transition to survivorship [1–3]. Behavioral side effects such as persistent fatigue, insomnia, or pain as well as treatment-related physical disfigurement can exacerbate distress [4–8]. Cognition-related difficulties due to the residual effects of various chemotherapies and/or cranial radiation are known to occur during and after the end of treatment [9]. Chemotherapeutic agents not only increase the production of *peripheral* pro-inflammatory cytokines but many cross the blood-brain barrier, contributing directly to cognitive difficulties. Often referred to as "chemobrain," these cognitive impairments may be characterized by problems with verbal memory, critical thinking skills, and concentration [9, 10].

To prevent, improve, or counteract the deleterious effects of these cancer-related experiences, a growing body of clinical research indicates that mindfulness-related practices, such as Benson's relaxation response technique, can trigger psychological and biological processes of healing, enhancing overall resilience and well-being [11–13].

13.2 Objectives

At the end of this chapter, you will be able to:
1. Describe the purpose and functions of mindfulness-related relaxation response techniques.
2. Discuss the relationship between mindfulness and meditative techniques.

3. Identify various mindful meditative techniques and their impact on indicators of stress, resilience, and healing.
4. Practice and implement the steps involved in eliciting the relaxation response technique in clinical practice.

Clinical Anecdote 13.1
Betty and Jack had been married for over 40 years. They were one another's best friend. As Betty herself rationalized, "We are old, and God must take us one day- but does it have to be so soon?," smiling at the irony. As Jack's cancer progressed to the terminal phase, he became more philosophical and accepting of his impending death. But Betty faltered. She became depressed and tearful, even as she could see that her husband was calm and comfortable and ready to make his farewells. Jack confided to the nurse that seeing his wife so distraught was deeply upsetting; nothing he said seemed to comfort her. Betty confided to the nurse that she did not know how to help her husband anymore, which caused her enormous distress. In the beginning of his illness, she had cared for him at home, relying on her sense of humor to remind her husband that life was still about living. But now, she saw life being slowly extinguished, and she was beside herself.

The nurse wondered whether doing something together, such as Benson's relaxation response technique, might be therapeutic for the couple. It tended to have a calming and ofttimes spiritual effect. Both were willing to try. So she led them through each simple step and thereafter regularly dropped by Jack's hospital room in order to accompany him and his wife in eliciting the relaxation response. After Jack passed away, Betty sought out the nurse to thank her for her suggestion. Meditating together had brought back memories of doing things together—but was all the more precious because she was able to do this one last activity with and for her husband. The experience had been spiritually powerful because they had been able to reconnect through this deeply meaningful experience.

13.3 Definitions

State and Trait Mindfulness Various types of meditation share the essential component of "mindfulness" [14]. "State" mindfulness refers to present-focused, moment-by-moment, nonjudgmental total awareness of thoughts, feelings, and sensations *that are cultivated in* meditative practices [15]. Regular engagement in present-oriented mindfulness through daily meditative practices is thought to enhance one's ability to be mindful in everyday life, which is referred to as "trait" mindfulness (TM) [16]. Regular mindful meditation practice is thought to strengthen state mindfulness which eventually transforms into trait mindfulness [16]. *TM is about being mindful in everyday life and is associated with an intensified nonjudgmental, nonreactive awareness* of thoughts, feelings, sensations, and external stimuli that are often associated with distress. Thus repeated state mindfulness and trait mindfulness lead to increased *self-regulatory attention* mediated by a sense of openness, kindness, curiosity, and acceptance [15, 17, 18].

Mindfulness consists of three main elements: (1) intention refers to the principle guiding how one wishes to live one's life exemplified by the focus of practice; (2) attention refers to being mindful in the present and is cultivated through repeated practices of redirecting conscious attention to the present focus; and (3) an attitude of curiosity, acceptance, and kindness [11, 15, 19]. Thoughts, sensations, and emotional stimuli in the present that enter into one's consciousness are acknowledged without emotional reactivity, judgment, or cognitive elaboration, such as engaging in internal convoluted discussion about the incoming stimuli. Rather the individual adopts an open, curious and accepting outlook that is thought to lead to greater patience, calmness, self-reflection, loving-kindness, compassion toward self and others, and attentiveness and acceptance [17, 20].

Meditation is an ancient practice of Eastern and Middle Eastern cultures, philosophies, and religions, most notably Hinduism and Buddhism. Meditation may be defined as a deeply contemplative process in which the practitioner focuses exclusively on his breath or a saying of his choice, for the purpose of staying in the moment even while acknowledging distractible thoughts and feelings without emotional reactivity or cognitive elaboration, before returning to the object of his focus. Thoughts and sensations in the present are acknowledged in a nonjudgmental, open, curious, and accepting manner (which is part of mindfulness).

13.4 Mindful Meditation

Mindful meditative practices are self-induced behaviors activated by present-focused, interrelated processes of mindfulness and meditation in which the conscious mind experiences a heightened awareness of emotions, memories, thoughts, sensations, and intentions. This multifaceted awareness comes from external factors mediated through the senses such as physical sensations as well as internal factors, such as thoughts, emotions, or sensations associated with interoceptive signaling. Modes of practice include mindful meditation (MM), different yoga practices, tai chi, qi gong, Benson's relaxation response technique, as well as Carlson's mindfulness-based cancer recovery (MBCR), derived from Kabat-Zinn's mindfulness-based stress reduction (MBSR) program [11, 14, 15, 21, 22]. Each is distinguished by their respective behavioral approach for entering a mindful meditative state. Mindful meditation practices have become mainstream in the west, the subject of numerous scientific investigations in healthy volunteers as well as in patients with cancer. The beneficial results have increasingly testified to their overall contribution in strengthening resilience, reducing stress, and inducing psychological, neurophysiological, metabolic, and molecular restorative (healing) processes [23–25]. MM practices have a positive and comprehensive effect on the mind and body, by reducing emotional distress and enhancing attention regulation, emotional regulation, body awareness, and healing processes, even when disease is present [26]. Eliciting the relaxation response like mindful meditation and other mindful techniques has a top-down effect on the whole being.

Two meditative practices are frequently associated with patients with cancer and their caregivers.

Benson's Relaxation Response (RR) Technique

The RR technique was developed by Benson and colleagues at Harvard University for use in clinical practice and resembles *concentration meditation* practices [12, 14, 27]. The individual or group technique is a simplified version of Kabat-Zinn's mindfulness-based stress reduction program and is analogous to brief meditation practices [28]. The technique similarly involves diaphragmatic breathing, focusing on a word, mantra, or repetitive prayer in order to refrain from emotional reactivity to outside distractions and internal thoughts and sensations during RR [22]. It is a self-induced, biological, and emotional response that downregulates the biological stress response system and activates physiological, metabolic, and molecular processes of healing and resilience in a timely, dose-dependent manner. In so doing, it enhances mindfulness, reduces emotional distress, and improves emotional regulation, cognitive clarity, attentiveness, mood, and concentration, making it particularly suitable as a potential therapeutic intervention in clinical practice [12, 28–30]. The RR has been utilized at the bedside and during treatment for patients with cancer and their family caregivers due to the ease with which it may be taught and implemented in clinical settings [31]. More clinical research based on this technique for healing-promoting purposes in patients with cancer and family caregivers at different phases of the continuum is needed due especially to its ease of use in in-hospital units.

Mindfulness-Based Cancer Recovery (MBCR)

The MBCR intervention was adapted for individuals with cancer and survivors from Kabat-Zinn's mindfulness-based stress reduction (MBSR) intervention [15, 32]. Both are well-known and validated programs generally offered to groups and standardized via a manualized program. The MBCRs and MBSRs main practice-related components are mindfulness or conscious awareness in the present moment and a nonjudgmental and open manner that may be developed through repeated practices of mindful meditation, gentle yoga, and other related exercises of the program. For instance, MBSR/MBCR includes a relaxing body scan, sitting and walking loving-kindness practices, and gentle hatha yoga for the purpose of developing greater mindfulness (dispositional mindfulness) in everyday life. The program comprises 90-minute sessions each week over 8 weeks and a 6-hour workshop between the sixth and seventh practice sessions [32, 33]. Sessions consist of group discussion and practical exercises to illustrate key concepts, a review of weekly progress, and discussion of potential obstacles to practice. Participants are asked to engage in MM every day at home between group sessions.

This intervention has been found to be effective in reducing symptoms of stress, fatigue, and sleep problems and improving feelings of being supported, mood, and quality of life. The intervention has also been shown to down regulate the biological stress response system and normalize stress induced biomarkers in patients or survivors of breast cancer [32, 34, 35]. More studies on the effects of mindfulness meditation on immune parameters would deepen our understanding of the effects of MM on innate and cell-mediated immunity and elucidate the potential of MM as an adjunct therapy during and after treatment to protect, buffer, and even strengthen immune activity during and after treatment.

13.5 Mechanism of Action

As will become evident in the section on research findings, the mechanism of action of MM involves complex interrelated biological systems of neural endocrine, physiological, and immune pathways and molecular signaling pathways associated with (1) attention regulation (anterior cingulate cortex), (2) body awareness (insula, temporoparietal junction), (3) emotion regulation implicating critical thinking and reappraisal (the lateral prefrontal cortex modulating the activity of the amygdala), (4) exposure/extinction/reconsolidation (ventromedial prefrontal cortex, hippocampus, and amygdala), (5) cognitive reevaluation ("activation" of the dorsal medial prefrontal cortex or "diminished activity" in prefrontal regions), and (6) flexible self-concept (prefrontal median cortex, posterior cingulate cortex, insula, temporoparietal junction) [30, 36].

Mindful meditation practices also induce the downregulation of the neurophysiological stress response system (i.e., the HPA, ANS, and SAM axes). This enables the reemergence of healing processes such as the PNS and vagal nerve and the restoration of many psychological, neurophysiological, immunological, metabolic, molecular, and behavioral indicators of resilience. In so doing, MM lowers metabolic energy consumption to basal physiological levels [23, 37–39].

13.6 Research Findings

Systematic reviews of MM and RR in healthy and cancer populations highlight healing- and resilient-promoting effects on psychological, cognitive, physiological, molecular, and metabolic processes and neural structural systems with clinical implications for nurses wanting to restore healing processes, reduce intrusive ideation and emotional distress, and strengthen resilient capabilities of patients and their informal caregivers throughout the cancer and recovery experience [21, 24, 25, 40, 41].

Mindful Techniques on Neural Structural Regions
(Review Fox [42])

Various meditation-based approaches exert similar but also differential effects on the neuroanatomy of the individual. A recent meta-analysis revealed differential *activation and deactivation* of neuroanatomical regions of the brain as a function of the type of meditation that was practiced [42]. Fox and colleagues compared and contrasted the effects of four types of meditation on the brain: focused attention meditation, mantra meditation, open monitoring practice, and loving-kindness and compassion meditation. Different brain sites appeared to be recruited by different mindful practices (see Fox et al. [42] article for the deactivated sites based on meditation type).

Although each meditation has a distinct purpose, the findings revealed overlapping as well as distinct effects of the four types on the brain. For instance, focused attention meditation, open monitoring practice, and loving-kindness and compassion meditation (but not the mantra meditation) activated the anterior insular cortex. The anterior insula is involved in conscious awareness of the body's internal states, integrating various interoceptive signals with higher-order attentional goals and emotional states. This awareness without emotional reactivity is central to restoring emotional equanimity.

Focused attention meditation, mantra meditation, and open monitoring practice meditation (but not the loving-kindness and compassion meditation) were found to activate the posterior dorsolateral prefrontal cortex (PFC) and premotor and supplementary motor cortices which are involved not only in motor activities but *higher-order cognitive functions and attention regulation* such as memory and working memory, attention control, reasoning, and mental imagery [42]. Moreover, the focused attention meditation and the open monitoring practice meditations were shown to activate neuronal clusters in the dorsal anterior, mid-cingulate cortex along the periphery of the supplementary motor regions as well as the dorsal anterior cingulate cortex (ACC), which among the latter's diverse functions include attention and emotion regulation, as well as self-monitoring behaviors [42].

Finally, open monitoring meditation and loving-kindness meditation were observed to activate regions within the frontal-polar cortex and rostro-lateral PFC. This region is associated with meta (conscious)-awareness and metacognitive capability. These activated areas are associated with heightened awareness of an experience and greater cognitive awareness such as being cognizant that one's mind is wandering [42]. The findings from this meta-analysis highlight the possibility that in the future, different meditation approaches may be purposefully selected to help patients, depending on their behavioral difficulties, due to their specific effects on the brain's neuroanatomy.

Another systematic review examined the effects of the 8-week mindfulness-based stress reduction (MBSR) and mindfulness-based cognitive therapy (MBCT) programs on brain function and structure, based on 21 functional magnetic resonance imaging (fMRI) studies and 7 MRI studies [43]. The findings showed that mindfulness tasks were related to the activation, connectivity, and increased volume of the prefrontal cortex (PFC), cingulate cortex, insula, and hippocampus in previously stressed, anxious, and/or healthy participants. Conversely, mindfulness tasks also decreased the amygdala's functional capability (i.e., reduced emotional reactivity) and restored functional connectivity with the prefrontal cortex, which normally modulates the amygdala's response to stressful stimuli. These findings are consistent with downregulation of the stress response system and improved emotion regulation. The systematic review identified the main brain areas associated with enhanced functional and structural changes in long-term meditators: (a) a PFC associated with increased meta-awareness and reappraisal), (b) the sensory cortices and insula related to body awareness, (c) the hippocampus associated with improved memory processes, and (d) the cingulate cortex related to self- and emotion regulation). However, as previously demonstrated, neuronal effects varied as a function of the differences in goals and activities associated with different mindfulness approaches [42].

Finally, a study of the effect of mindful meditation on sensory processes of pain using neuroimaging showed that mindfulness meditation was associated with neuroplastic modifications in the anterior cingulate cortex (associated with functions of attention) and anterior insular cortices (associated with the sensation or perception of pain) and the orbitofrontal cortex (involved in reframing sensory experiences of pain) [44]. MM appeared to have restorative neurophysiological effects on parts of the brain associated with reducing pain sensation, enhancing emotion regulation, and improving cognitive reappraisal, critical thinking, and memory processes.

Physiological Outcomes

The relaxation response technique (RR), mindful meditation (MM), yoga, and various forms of meditation which includes reciting the rosary have been shown to restore physiological functioning as measured by heart rate, blood pressure, low-density lipoprotein (LDL), high-density lipoprotein (HDL), and cortisol levels [13, 23, 45]. Mindfulness-based stress reduction programs have also been shown to regulate the cortisol response associated with wakening, which is blunted in many survivors of breast cancer due to chronic stress [33, 46]. In fact, RR appears to enhance synchronicity across various circadian body rhythms, thereby helping to restore internal physiological coherence and a more effective utilization of energy [12, 25, 27, 47].

Other noted physiological changes include a reduction in oxygen consumption and carbon dioxide elimination, an increase in heart rate variability, and fractional exhaled nitric oxide, an indicator of vascular dilatation. These physiological parameters are experienced in hypometabolic and relaxed states of being [12, 23]. Increased heart rate variability refers to "an increase in low frequency oscillations of the heart rate which tend to be at optimal functioning in infants, but gradually becomes more irregular and less effective as we are exposed to stresses over the developmental lifespan" [48].

Immune Functions

Mindfulness-based stress reduction (MBSR) programs also appear to reduce some inflammatory biomarkers in survivors of breast cancer [49]. A 6-week MBSR program based on 322 cancer survivors produced significant improvements in TNF-α and IL-6 levels between 6 and 12 weeks after the program ended, compared to usual care. These cytokines may serve as immune markers of recovery [49]. Because human B-cells express TNF-α and IL-6, the researchers suggest that the MBSR intervention may normalize these cytokine levels by strengthening B-cells given that these survivors also experienced enhanced well-being. Other cancer-related research, however, has associated increased levels of TNF-α in patients with *cancer progression and metastases* in which TNF secretion emanates from cancer cells and/or tumor-associated macrophages. Under these clinical conditions, TNF exerts a pro-tumorigenic role [50]. The finding highlights the importance of understanding the different patterns of cytokine responses at each stage of the cancer illness and survivorship along with the goals of mindfulness practices.

Mindfulness-based stress reduction (MBSR) practice was studied in relation to immune functioning, quality of life, and coping effectiveness [51]. Forty-four newly diagnosed early-stage post surgery individuals with breast cancer and no further treatment were self-selected into the 8-week MBSR group and 31 into the control group. At baseline both the MBSR and control groups had reduced levels of natural killer cell activity (NKCA) and IFN-γ and increased levels of IL-4, IL-6, and IL-10 (i.e., inflammatory cytokines) and elevated cortisol levels. Compared to controls, the MBSR increased natural killer cell activity and reduced IFN-γ, IL-4, IL-10, and IL-6 and cortisol levels to within their normal parametric ranges. Moreover, the MBSR women also reported a significant improvement in quality of life and coping effectiveness compared to controls. Conversely the control group continued to decrease NKCA and IFN-γ production and increase the levels of inflammatory cytokines [51].

A systematic review of mindful meditation in relation to the immune system suggests possible beneficial effects on cell-mediated immunity, inflammatory factors, and aging, although the results were mired by high heterogeneity across studies. RCTs based on more rigorous designs and an adequate sample size are needed to investigate the MBSR-induced effects on resilience across diverse cancers at different phases of the continuum [52].

Molecular Changes

In a randomized controlled trial, a mindfulness-based stress reduction program reported a significant decrease in gene expression associated with the inflammatory transcription factor, nuclear factor kappa B (NF$_K$B) in older adults after cancer treatment, and a downward trend in C-reactive protein levels over time [53]. Whereas baseline measures demonstrated a significant positive relationship between loneliness and NF$_K$B gene expression in circulating leukocytes, post intervention, loneliness was significantly reduced and NF$_K$B, downregulated. NF$_K$B is a major pro-inflammatory transcription factor associated with chronic inflammation and cancer [54]. A related RCT of young breast cancer survivors indicated that mindful meditation similarly induced a significant reduction in pro-inflammatory gene expression and in inflammatory signaling, including NF_KB activity after the intervention [55]. Secondary outcomes also showed significant corresponding improvements in fatigue, sleep disturbance, positive affect, peace, and meaning, although these positive clinical changes were not sustained 3 months later, with the exception of psychological distress which was still reduced.

Benson's relaxation response (RR) technique was similarly shown to produce significant changes in gene expression associated with improved energy metabolism, mitochondrial functioning, insulin secretion, and telomere maintenance [23, 25]. Conversely, RR was shown to downregulate the expression of genes associated with pro-inflammatory pathways including the NFkB transcription factor [23, 53]. In fact 38 genes linked to stress-induced pathways related to inflammation, dysregulated immune responses, mRNA processing, and T-cell signaling were shown to be suppressed [23].

In summary, empirical findings strongly suggest that MM or RR strategies can reverse many stress-induced psychological, cognitive, immune, physiological, and genomic impairments in postsurgical cancer patients, early-stage breast cancer patients, survivors, and lonely individuals [25, 53]. Although we still do not know to what extent these changes actually contribute to survival, empirical evidence strongly suggests that MM can improve overall resilience and, by extension, quality of life.

Psychological and Behavioral Outcomes

MM practices also produce clinical improvements in affect, mood, and emotional stress. A meta-analysis of 29 RCTs with 3476 cancer patients and survivors showed that mindfulness interventions significantly reduced depression, anxiety, fatigue, and perceived stress, and improved post-traumatic growth, quality of life, and mindfulness compared to controls [34]. Mindfulness-based art therapy (MBAT) had the strongest downregulating effects on anxiety and depression, followed by mindfulness-based stress reduction programs. The MM interventions were effective across patients with different cancers, strongly suggesting that MM should be considered as a complementary therapy for managing cancer- and treatment-related symptoms and side effects.

Other meta-analyses similarly supported the use of mindfulness-based interventions for anxiety, depression, fatigue, sleep disturbances, and pain as well as for attenuating fear of a cancer recurrence, with commensurate improvements in emotional well-being, quality of life, physical functions, and physical health in patients with cancer including breast and lung cancers and survivors [35, 56–59]. However, the effects on pain, sleep, and spirituality only trended toward significance in some studies [56, 57]. Even brief 13-minute daily meditations for 8 weeks resulted in significant reductions in negative mood and state anxiety and significant improvements in attention and overall emotional regulation [28].

Five RCTs reported significant reductions in hostility, unhappiness, loneliness, intrusive ideation, and emotional distress as well as significant improvements in quality of life, post-traumatic growth, spirituality meaning, and perceived support compared to controls in patients with breast cancer and older adults [32, 53, 55, 60, 61]. For instance, MBCR was shown to significantly enhance perceptions of social support, in part, by reducing a sense of loneliness and by increasing feelings of spirituality, meaning, and a sense of connectedness to something greater than oneself [11]. A secondary analysis of Carlson's study similarly revealed that the meditation group effectively reduced stress-related symptoms and mood disturbances while improving quality of life and, significantly, increasing perceptions of support compared to the group that received a supportive expressive intervention [62]. The effects of mindfulness on *caregivers of patients* with cancer also demonstrated similar stress-relieving benefits [63].

Not all research findings are positive. Goyal's systematic review and meta-analyses suggested that mindful meditation programs do not significantly enhance mental health-related quality of life or improve feelings of emotional distress. These unexpected findings may have to do with weakly designed studies, the lack of standardized programs, and issues around randomization and sample size, dosing, and duration. The inconsistent results across studies call for more rigorous designs, use of a control group, and standardized MM practices and measures to be used in future studies of cancer populations other than breast cancer and at diagnostic and treatment phases.

Cognitive Functions

Many patients experience acute or chronic problems with memory, critical thinking, and attention focusing [10, 64]. These difficulties have been attributed to various anticancer treatments such as chemotherapy or cranial radiation therapy causing a pro-inflammatory immune response, emotional distress, and fatigue [65]. An enhanced ability to focus attention through mindfulness practices is thought to improve critical thinking capabilities such as problem-solving, decision-making, cognitive analysis, as well as making relevant inferences and positive reappraisals [66, 67].

A study investigated the effects of mindfulness training on processes of appraisal given that mindfulness involves creating *a state of non-appraisal* [66]. In a controlled study, 44 participants were randomized to (1) a mindful training program (for a total of only 40 min), (2) a thought suppression condition, or (3) a mind wandering condition participants were asked to practice for 1 week. The mindfulness group had significantly higher levels of state mindfulness compared to the other groups. Results did not show significant differences between groups in levels of cognitive reappraisal perhaps due to the small sample and the very brief duration of the mindfulness intervention [66].

However, a path analysis of all study participants showed that the highest "state mindfulness" levels at T1 were significantly associated with the highest levels of positive reappraisal a week later at T2. Increased non-emotional reactivity was also significantly related to increased cognitive reappraisal ($r = 0.43$, $p = 0.003$). Also, greater dispositional mindfulness at T1 (i.e., trait mindfulness) was significantly associated with greater state mindfulness at T1 ($r = 0.43$, $p = 0.003$) and greater change scores in positive reappraisal from T1 to T2 ($r = 0.41$, $p = 0.005$). Participants who received the 1-week mindfulness training also showed a higher score on non-emotional reactivity at T2, compared to T1 scores ($t(14) = 2.2.18$, $p = 0.047$). These findings are consistent with other cross-sectional studies in which mindfulness was shown to be related to differential aspects of critical thinking [68, 69]. Whereas this small body of studies suggests that mindfulness training contributes to emotion regulation and different components of critical thinking, more rigorously designed RCTs based on the recommended 8-week mindfulness course would provide better evidentiary data to inform the nature of these relationships.

Mindfulness meditation practices have also been shown to enhance *creative approaches* that are instrumental in solving "insight" problems [67]. People who were mindful in everyday life (i.e., trait mindfulness) were better able to solve problems based on sudden creative insights. Moreover, insight problem-solving capabilities were also improved by state mindfulness practices of meditation. Mindfulness practices *avoid cognitive elaborations of* thoughts, feelings, or sensations, which tend to block the potential for generating creative insights to solve problems. (Conversely, non-insight problems are those that depend on logical steps toward finding solutions to problems.)

More recently, MM was shown to enhance "decentering" processes during meditative practice and afterward in everyday life [70]. Decentering is the ability to consider thoughts more objectively, almost disassociated from subjective experience, as "events" rather than reflections of external reality or of oneself, which impedes thinking at a more elevated cognitive perspective [71]. Key interrelated components of decentering are:

1. Meta-awareness or conscious awareness of thoughts, sensations, and feelings being in the moment as process.
2. Dis-identification from internal experiences in which, for instance, the person can separate an internal experience from the self. It has also been described as experiencing one's sensations, feelings, and thoughts from a more "objective" perspective, for instance, it is the difference between stating that "I am sad" and "there is this feeling of sadness" as if it is disconnected from the self.

3. The third component relates to decreased emotional reactivity. Decentering processes have been described as the "ability to step outside of one's immediate experience, thereby changing the very nature of that experience" [71]. Decentering is thought to serve as a substrate for a number of therapeutic psychological interventions.

To summarize, mindfulness has been shown to reduce intrusive thoughts and enhance emotional self-regulation; mindful meditation may enable better cognitive abilities by activating the neural circuits responsible for executive functions and critical thinking while deactivating other, interfering neural pathways such as those associated with a hyperbolic amygdala [42, 65].

Clinical Anecdote 13.2
As a cancer survivor, I lived with daily physical reminders of my cancer experience. Most disturbing, however, were the mild cognitive changes: difficulty retrieving words or coming up with a customary timely response, the ability to rapidly retrieve facts in conversation, and to concentrate for prolonged periods, all of which my family and friends laughingly dismissed as 'old age'. I knew what I was experiencing was different.

I lived with this self awareness until one day, as part of my clinical mandate to develop an integrative program for patients with lung cancer and their loved ones, my readings led to research on mindful meditation and the relaxation response. I decided to test these practices first hand and enrolled in a 6-week program for health practitioners at the university. Within a couple of weeks, I experienced unexpected changes in myself- I felt much better overall- more energy, a lighter mood and most critically the fog in my brain seemed to have dissipated. I was able to concentrate much better and to think more clearly. As with any therapeutic modality, what works for one person may not be as effective for another. The key is to know the clinical evidence and then to make these mindful practices available to patients and their caregivers.

13.7 MM as a Self-Care Skill for Nurses

The therapeutic effects of the relaxation response technique or mindful meditation on the overall stress of nurses and aids working in a highly charged environment are mainly known from pilot studies [17, 72, 73]. Orellano-Rios' pre-/post-pilot study of a mindfulness intervention with 28 health professionals (19/28 were nurses) suggested improvements in emotional exhaustion, personal accomplishment, anxiety, and emotion regulation. The intervention was based on the key elements of mindfulness, "mette or loving-kindness," and the cultivation of tonglen meditation. Mette or loving-kindness meditation focuses on feelings of "impartial kindness, warmth and benevolence" [72]. Tonglen meditation has to do with *directing one's attention* toward the "source of inner warmth" and with maintaining feelings of kindness toward others. Tonglen meditation inhales inner acceptance of negative stimuli and exhales with feelings of kindness and compassion.

Other pilot studies suggest that MM programs have a beneficial, dosing effect on nurses' health and by extension even patient satisfaction. For instance, Horner's mindfulness training pilot study reported improvements in burnout, stress, mindfulness, and, significantly, patient satisfaction, suggesting unsurprisingly that the nurse's well-being is connected to patient satisfaction with care. Other studies of mindfulness practices with nurses report similar findings [74]. However one mindful meditation study for nurses in a PICU showed a significant reduction in the nurses' level of perceived stress but no significant changes in feelings of burnout and depersonalization [75]. A pilot waitlist randomized controlled study of the effects of an 8-week Benson relaxation response technique revealed nonsignificant changes in depression, anxiety, work-related stress, and well-being in 46 nurses working in cardiac units, although these nurses expressed competence and interest in teaching RR to patients [17]. Following an instructor-led session at work, nurses were encouraged to practice RR twice a day for an estimated 10–20 min, significantly less time than other mindful meditation practices [32]. The fact that it was a voluntary activity in which the length of time meditating could have varied may account for the nonsignificant effects. The high nurse adherence rate to the mindfulness sessions was likely due to the program being offered in the workplace. Future studies are needed based on rigorously designed randomized controlled trials to clarify the clinical benefits for nurses as well as patients.

In Summary
The majority of mindfulness-related studies are based on patients with breast cancer and healthy volunteers and, more infrequently, patients with prostate cancer, lung cancer, and other cancers [76]. These studies include RCTs but also nonrandomized studies based on small samples. More rigorously designed studies assessing cognitive, behavioral, physiological, and immune functions before, during, and after anticancer treatments as well as in survivorship are needed. Clinical issues such as dosing, frequency, duration, and standardization of the mindfulness programs across studies would further inform the findings. There may be synergistic effects in combining MM/RR with other complementary strategies as observed in some studies based on MBSR.

13.8 Nursing Implications

Mindful meditation practices have been shown to improve a number of emotional, physical, and cognitive-related symptoms in patients with mostly breast and prostate cancers as well as in survivors, although further research would be useful based on other cancer types [56, 76, 77].

Suggested Approaches

1. Incorporate RR as a complementary therapy within the treatment plan starting from diagnosis, prior to surgery, or just before and during chemotherapy to promote better symptom management such as less breakthrough nausea, lack of appetite, or other side effects of the treatment [78].
2. Consider MM or RR as nonpharmacological strategies to reduce emotional distress and facilitate emotional regulation.
3. Consider MM or RR to facilitate or improve cognitive thinking, attention focus, positive reappraisal, creative problem-solving, and overall quality of life particularly in the survivorship phase [32, 66, 67]. The ability to maintain emotion regulation impacts cognitive capabilities to reappraise situations and problem-solve effectively which can also boost feelings of self-efficacy.
4. As part of a nursing approach to enhance the patient's skills in seeking and maintaining relevant supportive relationships, consider introducing RR with the patient, family caregiver, and/or significant other as one strategy for strengthening perceived patient-caregiver-family support. Schellekens [79] secondary analysis of Carlson's study suggested that the enhanced support experienced by cancer survivors in the mindful meditation group mediated the relationship between the mindful meditation intervention and psychological distress. The support was attributed to the caring- and compassionate-inducing exercises that were an integral part of the MM intervention, led by caring facilitators. MM may have a role to play in strengthening the supportive bonds of patients and their informal caregivers and may help alleviate feelings of loneliness in some patients.
5. Consider introducing RR or MM in patients who are struggling to find meaning or acceptance in their cancer. Carlson's findings of spiritual and personal growth evidenced weeks after the MM course was over suggest that patients who have difficulty coming to terms with cancer or a shortened life may find their way to acceptance via the quiet introspective practices of mindful meditation.
6. Encourage patients and caregivers to incorporate MM or RR into their daily routine. Although the duration of most manualized MM or RR programs is between 8 and 12 weeks long, both have shown evidence of a dose response—the longer you practice (each day normally for 20–30 min), the more comprehensive and sustaining the benefits [31]. But for the hesitant novice practitioner, you might suggest starting with even 10 min a day and then gradually lengthening the time dedicated to the practice.
7. Finally the RR technique may be easily taught at the bedside or in the clinic by the nurse. Please contact the Benson Henry Institute at Harvard University to register for workshops on RR (https://bensonhenryinstitute.org/). Review strategies to elicit the relaxation response in Benson and Stuart [31]. RR can be applied in many clinical and home situations and is of potential benefit not only for the well-being and resilience of patients and caregivers, but for

nurses and other healthcare providers. A few focused breaths to rid oneself of work-related worries, and to become more fully present for each patient and loved one, is an effective centering activity that nurses may use just prior to seeing the next patient [14].

13.9 Final Thoughts

Each time I have been invited to speak to students about the benefits of mindful meditation or the relaxation response, two concerns have inevitably been raised—the first being a lack of time. It would take too much time to teach and/or accompany patients in eliciting the relaxation response. Eliciting the relaxation response is an extremely simple technique that downregulates an individual's biological stress response system *within mere minutes*. And every minute thereafter invested in this exercise provides healing- and resilient-promoting effects in a dose-dependent manner for the patient and the nurse who accompanies him/her. RR is a self-induced healing approach that nurses should consider teaching their patients *at the first or second clinic visit*, encouraging them to continue at home as a self-empowering strategy to control anxiety and depression and to reduce the intensity of intrusive negative thoughts that compromise the person's resilience. The nurse may provide 10-minute "booster" sessions each time she or he meets the patient in clinic as a supportive strategy and to encourage continuity. The mindfulness-based cancer recovery (MBCR) and Kabat-Zinn's mindfulness-based stress reduction (MBSR) program are most appropriate for cancer survivors given the 8 weekly sessions and multimodal activities involved to successfully complete their programs.

The second concern that is frequently expressed is how to reconcile recommending the RR or MM when "one *neither believes in it nor has benefited from using it*." To individuals who hold these convictions, as colleagues in a science-based profession, I encourage you to dive into the clinical research data. The scientific evidence shared in this chapter alone indicates that RR and mindful meditation can improve the healing and resilient capabilities of most individuals, including patients with cancer during and after treatment, although research based on more rigorous designs is needed particularly in the field of oncology [4, 80].

Whether or not we personally "believe" in a given treatment, is not the clinical touchstone; it is the converging scientific evidence of a potentially effective intervention that does no harm. Just as antibiotics or various chemotherapies have differential effects on people depending on their biological makeup, the same may be true of RR. As health-promoting professionals, we are ethically bound to inform the patient about evidence-based interventions that may ease distress and other symptoms. Our personal opinion about a given therapy should not impede our ability to suggest, educate, and lead willing patients in this evidence-based strategy. And then let the patient and family caregiver decide what works for them!

Appendix: MBSR. Psychosocial and Behavioral Interventions—Mindful Meditation (MM), Relaxation Response Technique (RR), Mindfulness-Based Stress Reduction Intervention (MBSR), and Mindfulness-Based Cancer Recovery (MBCR)

Author	Purpose/intervention	Study design	Sample/phase of disease	Outcomes
Andersen et al. [81]	(1) Part of larger study that assessed MBSR on psychological and somatic symptoms (2) the purpose was to evaluate effects of MBSR on secondary outcome: sleep quality Intervention Psychoeducation on stress responses, mindfulness meditation (body scan, sitting/walking meditation, and gentle yoga), encouraged to practice at home for 45 min daily	RCT RA to (a) MBSR—8 weekly 2-h program including a 5-h silent retreat ($n = 168$) (b) Usual care ($n = 168$)	336 breast cancer patients I–III, 3–18 months postsurgery	(1) Mean sleep problems were significantly lowered in MBSR group than controls (2) Quantile regression analyses showed significant benefits for subjects with the greatest sleep problems (3) After 12 months NS between group differences based on intention to treat analysis Conclusion: MBSR was most effective immediately after the intervention, which then decreased over time

Carlson et al. [32]	To assess effects of mindfulness-based cancer recovery (MBCR) versus supportive expressive group therapy (SET) in distressed breast cancer survivors Interventions (a) MBCR for patients with cancer and adapted from MBSR [15] (b) SET Goals to enhance mutual support, family support, increase openness and emotional expression, increase coping skills, strengthen doctor-patient relationship, discuss feelings about death and dying	RCT RA to (a) MBCR (b) SET Assessed at baseline, postintervention, 6, 12 months later	252 Stage I–III distressed breast cancer survivors	(1) Postintervention, MBCR group had significant reduction in mood disturbance (i.e., in fatigue, anxiety, and confusion) ($p = 0.001$–0.03) over SET group (2) MBCR evidenced significant decrease over baseline in stress symptoms tension, sympathetic arousal, and cognitive symptoms) compared to SET with medium effect sizes (3) MBCR also demonstrated significant improvement in emotional and functional quality of life, emotional, affective and positive social support, spirituality (feelings of peace and meaning in life), and posttraumatic growth (appreciation for life and ability to see new possibilities) (4) Effect sizes for time × group interactions were small to medium: most benefits maintained over 12 months Conclusion: Findings suggest that the adapted MBCR may be most appropriate for use in patients with cancer (5) Overall findings suggest the effectiveness of the intervention to restore to normal parameters or heal survivors

(continued)

Appendix (continued)

Author	Purpose/intervention	Study design	Sample/phase of disease	Outcomes
Schellekens et al. [79]	Effectiveness of a change in mindfulness and/or social support mediated the effect of MBCR [32] compared to SET in survivors of breast cancer Intervention MBCR_Contact Carlson [11]	RA to (a) MBCR ($n = 69$) (b) SET ($n = 70$) This mediation study was embedded in a multisite RCT that examined the effects of MBCR and SET on 271 distressed cancer survivors Current study used the pre- (Time 1) and postintervention (Time 2) data of survivors RA to either group for the mediation analysis	Distressed breast cancer survivors of stage I, II, or III (see [32])	(1) MBCR participants significantly improved mood disturbance, stress symptoms, social support but not on quality of life or mindfulness compared to SET participants (2) Increased social support partially mediated the impact of MBCR on mood disturbance and stress symptoms (3) No group differences on mindfulness or quality of life observed (4) Findings showed that increased social support was related to greater improvement in mood and stress after MBCR compared to support groups, but not mindfulness Conclusion This suggests a more important role for social support in enhancing outcomes in MBCR than previously considered More research needed but suggests the MBCR may provide a safe environment in which participants may support and be studies

Study	Objective/Intervention	Design	Population	Results/Conclusion
Schellekens et al. [62]	To investigate effectiveness of MBCR to decrease emotional distress in patients with lung cancer and/or their caregivers Intervention Schellekens et al. [82] (see Table 2, p. 5) (1) 8 weekly sessions of 2.5 h, plus one 6-h silent session, plus 45 min a day MM practice at home (2) learned about stress, grief, and invited to share experiences	Multicentered, parallel group RCT RA to (1) 31 patients and 21 partners to respective MBCR plus usual care groups (2) 32 patients and 23 partners to usual care (i.e., tx, supportive care, medical consultations) assessments at: baseline, postintervention, and 3-month follow-up	(1) Patients in curative and noncurative stages of lung cancer (2) Patients and partners could participate in the same group or separately as preferred	(1) MBSR patients had significantly reduced emotional distress ($d = 0.69$, $p = 0.008$) compared to usual care (2) Individuals with higher distress scores at baseline benefited most from the intervention (3) Patients in MBSR also showed improvements in quality of life, mindfulness skills, self-compassion, and rumination compared to those in usual care alone (4) Partners had no significant differences between the intervention and usual care groups Conclusion (1) Psychological distress is significantly improved following this intervention in patients but not partners (2) More research is needed to understand the needs of partners of lung cancer patients (3) This study needs to be replicated in a more rigorous, adequately powered RCT (4) The clinical benefits for patients suggest that an MM expert plus a nurse could cofacilitate this intervention
Haller et al. [83]	To update evidence for mindfulness-based stress reduction (MBSR) and mindfulness-based cognitive therapy (MBCT) in women with breast cancer Primary outcome: Quality of life Secondary outcomes: fatigue, sleep, stress, depression, anxiety, safety	Meta-analysis Using 10 RCTs (1709 participants)	Women with breast cancer	(1) Compared to usual care, significant postintervention effects for MBSR/MBCT were shown for quality of life, fatigue, sleep, stress, anxiety, and depression (2) Up to 6 months after baseline significant small effects findings were found for: anxiety, depression (3) Up to 12 months after baseline only anxiety remained significantly improved (4) Average effects were all below the threshold of minimal clinically important differences Conclusion Meta-analysis indicates short-term benefits of mindfulness-based interventions, though the clinical relevance remains unclear

(continued)

Appendix (continued)

Author	Purpose/intervention	Study design	Sample/phase of disease	Outcomes
Hall et al. [8]	To evaluate mind-body (M-B) approaches on fear of cancer recurrence (FOCR) Interventions included one therapy ($k = 9$) or in combination ($k = 10$) (a) Mindfulness-based stress reduction (MBSR) (b) Relaxation with cognitive behavioral, relaxation and meditation movement (tai chi, qigong, yoga), meditation and other CTs, psychoeducational, TCM ($k = 1$) (c) CBT skills, therapies that include spirituality, meaning, existential therapy, meaning therapy, expressive arts in oncology patients	Systematic review and meta-analysis Duration of interventions varied Ranged from 9 days to 12 months Cochrane criteria used to assess bias	19 RCTs (pooled $N = 2806$) Patients had breast ($k = 11$, 84%), prostate ($k = 3$, 16%), gynecological ($k = 1$, 5%), melanoma ($k = 1$, 5%) cancers Treatment status (a) 5 studies had patients undergoing active treatment (26%) (b) 14 studies (74%) had patients who had finished treatment for early-stage disease or were being actively watched	(1) Types of interventions (a) Interventions with only one MB strategy ($k = 9$) or included multiple M-B elements ($k = 10$) (b) CBT skills ($k = 11$, 58%) were most common MB component (c) Meditation practices ($k = 10$, 53%) (d) Relaxation exercises ($k = 4$, 21%) (2) Re analyses from preintervention to postintervention (median 2 months) (a) Small-to-medium pooled effect sizes were found (Hedges $g = -0.36$, 95% CI = -0.49 to -0.23, $P < 0.001$) (b) Significant heterogeneity ($I^2 = 47.99$) (3) Re analyses from preintervention to follow-up (median 8 months) (a) Pooled effect size was significant at ($g = -0.31$, 95% CI = -0.47 to -0.16, $P = 0.001$) Conclusion (1) Effective in reducing emotional distress with small to moderate effect size reductions across studies (2) But heterogeneity across studies also present ($I^2 = 63.36$) (3) 84% of patients had breast cancer intervention: needs to be reproduced in patients with other cancers (4) Given the high proportion of patients who dropped out of the intervention, an analysis of causes needed before mounting another study

Reich et al. [49]	To assess effectiveness of mindfulness-based stress reduction (breast cancer) (MBSR(BC)) on normalizing levels of inflammatory biomarkers in recovering breast cancer survivors Intervention (1) 2-hour weekly sessions for 6 weeks (ii) goal is to reduce specific symptoms of new survivors of breast cancer (3) used manuals and discs to facilitate home practice (iv) components included: MM, 4 practice techniques, group processes and elements of self-regulation of attention, nonjudgmental acceptance of present experience [15]	Substudy of RCT RA to (a) MBSR(BC): 6-week program (b) Usual care (UC) Assessments made at baseline, 6, and 12 weeks	322 recovering breast cancer survivors	(1) Linear mixed methods were used to assess 6 cytokine levels over baseline, 6 and 12 months: IL-1B, IL-6, IL-10, tumor necrosis factor (TNF)-α, transforming growth factor (TGF)B1, soluble tumor necrosis factor receptor (sTNFR)-1 Results (1) IL-10, Il-1B, TGF-B1 were not detected at rates greater than 50% and due to low prevalence, were not included in future analyses (2) Results showed that TNF-α and IL-6 increased during the follow-up period, i.e., between 6 and 12 weeks rather than during the MBSR(BC) training period (baseline to 6 weeks) compared to usual care (3) sTNFR-1 levels did not change across 12-week period Conclusion Findings suggest that intervention appeared to increase TNF-α and IL-6 which may be markers of recovery and that B cell changes may be a part of the immune recovery

(continued)

Appendix (continued)

Author	Purpose/intervention	Study design	Sample/phase of disease	Outcomes
Dusek et al. [25]	To test hypothesis that eliciting the relaxation response technique (RR) results in gene expression changes that can be used to measure physiological responses to RR in an unbiased manner. Intervention RR can be elicited by repeating a word, sound, phrase, prayer, or focusing on one's breath, disregarding intrusive everyday thoughts. Can be elicited via various meditation modalities, repetitive prayer, yoga, tai chi, breathing exercises, progressive muscle relation, biofeedback, guided imagery	8-week prospective, crossover design assessing blood transcriptional profiles of (a) 19 healthy long-term practitioners of daily RR (Group M) (b) 19 healthy comparison (Group N1) (c) 20 N1 Comparison group then reassessed after completing an 8-week RR training, i.e., became novice practitioners (Group N2)	Healthy volunteers	(1) Group M expressed 2209 genes compared to group N1 (controls) ($p < 0.05$) (2) Group N2 (the novice practitioners) expressed 1561 genes compared to their pretraining baseline (N1) ($p < 0.05$) (3) 433/2209 expressed genes from Group M and 433/1561 expressed genes from novice Group N2 were shared by both groups (4) Gene ontology analysis and gene set enrichment analyses showed significant improvements in (a) cell metabolism (b) oxidative phosphorylation (c) generation of reactive oxygen species and response to oxidative stress in long-term and short-term practitioners of daily RR practice that may counter cellular damage induced by chronic stress Conclusion (1) Evidence that RR in a dose-dependent manner may elicit gene expression changes in practitioners that ultimately impact health outcomes (2) Appears to be a simplified yet effective MM modality for patients and caregivers

Bhasin et al. [23]	Assessed effects of the relaxation response technique meditative practices on gene expression in expert and novice practitioners before and after 8 weeks of training	8-week prospective, crossover design assessing blood transcriptional profiles of
		(a) 26 Meditative (M) group (4–20 years)
		(b) 26 Novice group at baseline (N1)
		(c) 26 After 8 weeks of training (N2)
			Healthy volunteers	(1) RR induced changes in short- and long-term MM practitioners of significant gene expression M > N2 > N1
				(2) MM upregulated (increased) expression of gene sets associated with:
				  (a) Mitochondrial ATP synthase (i.e., improved energy metabolism and mitochondrial function)
				  (b) Improved insulin secretion
				  (c) Improved telomere maintenance
				  (d) Increased FeNO levels associated with vessel dilation and relaxation
				(3) MM downregulated gene sets associated with inflammation and stress-related pathways
				  (a) NFKB pathways related genes (pro-inflammatory transcription factor)
				  (b) 38 genes linked to inflammation, immune response, T cell signaling, and other stress-related pathways
				Summary
				Group M with the longest RR experience had the most healing-inducing, health-inducing changes in gene expression, followed by the N2 group, with N1 group (baseline) showing no changes
				Conclusion: Strengthened biological resilience and health
				  (a) RR elicitation counters stress that causes damaging molecular and cell effects
				  (b) Regulates inflammatory pathways by upregulating anti-inflammatory gene expression
				  (c) RR has a role to play in facilitating resilience and healing in patients with cancer and their stressed caregivers

(continued)

Appendix (continued)

Author	Purpose/intervention	Study design	Sample/phase of disease	Outcomes
Nissen et al. [84]	To investigate the effect of an internet delivered mindfulness-based cognitive therapy (MBCT) intervention for survivors of breast and prostate cancer Intervention (1) Home-based; 8 weekly modules with written materials, audio exercises, videos of patients with experts, weekly diary submitted to therapist for feedback (2) content adapted to cancer-based issues	RCT RA to (1) intervention (2) usual care wait list	1282 cancer survivors screened Final: Survivors of breast cancer ($n = 137$) and prostate ($n = 13$) and RA	(1) Significant effects of MBCT compared to usual care for: (a) anxiety (Cohen's $d = 0.45$, $p = 0.017$) (b) depressive symptoms ($d = 0.40$, $p = 0.024$) (c) effects maintained at 6 months for anxiety ($d = 0.40$, $p = 0.029$) (d) NS for depressive symptoms ($d = 0.28$, $p = 0.131$) Conclusion Appears to be effective as an internet-delivered mindfulness cognitive intervention

Bower et al. [55]	Investigated a mindfulness awareness practice (MAP) intervention for women survivors younger than 50 Intervention (1) 6 weekly, 2-hour sessions (2) included mindfulness exercises, relaxation, psychoeducational sessions (3) also problem solving at adherence to MM at home, managing difficult thoughts and emotions, pain and acquiring loving kindness	RCT with RA (1) intervention (2) usual care Based on linear mixed models	Survivors of breast cancer (stages 0 to III)	(1) MAP intervention significantly reduced perceived stress MAPS Mean: 14.25 (1.04) vs Controls Mean: 19.15 (1.14), $p = 0.004$ (2) MAP significantly reduced downregulation of pro-inflammatory genes ($p = 0.009$ (Fig. 3, p. 14) (a) MAP significantly reduced NFKB activity ($p = 0.0016$); increased activity of anti-inflammatory glucocorticoid receptor R ($p = 0.018$) and increased activity of transcription factors implicated in type 1 interferon signaling ($p = 0.007$) (3) participants who practiced more at home evidenced significant improvement over their baseline measure for IL-6 Conclusion Intervention was effective for a short-time posttreatment

(continued)

Appendix (continued)

Author	Purpose/intervention	Study design	Sample/phase of disease	Outcomes
Zhang et al. [85]	To evaluate effectiveness of mindfulness-based stress reduction (MBSR) in breast cancer during and after treatment for breast cancer	Systemic review and meta-analysis of 13 RCTs following Cochrane handbook-based criteria	$N = 1505$ survivors of breast cancer	(1) Significant findings of MBSR compared to usual care related to (a) Physical functioning (SMD = 0.28, 95% CI, 0.07–0.04, $p = 0.008$) (b) Cognitive function (SMD = 1.48, 95% CI, 0.34–2.61, $p = 0.01$) (c) Fatigue (SMD = −0.66, 95% CI −1.11 to −0.20, $p = 0.004$) (d) Emotional well-being (SMD = 1.01, 95% CI, 0.35–1.67, $p = 0.003$) (e) Anxiety (SMD = −0.54, 95% CI, −1.01 to −0.07, $p = 0.02$) (f) Depression (SMD = −0.61, 95% CI, −1.11 to −0.11, $p = 0.02$) (g) Stress (SMD = −0.48, 95% CI, −0.81 to −0.15, $p = 0.004$) (h) Distress (SMD = −0.56, 95% CI, −0.85 to −0.26, $p = 0.0002$) (2) NS findings for pain, sleep quality, global quality of life ($p > 0.05$) based on inadequate evidence Conclusion Evidence of therapeutic benefits for survivors of breast cancer Studies of generally low quality with substantial heterogeneity across studies

Lengacher et al. [61]	To evaluate efficacy of mindfulness-based stress reduction intervention in improving physical and psychological symptoms and quality of life among breast cancer survivors Intervention Consisted of (a) Meeting specific needs, concerns and symptoms (b) Education and materials, practice sessions of meditative techniques for sitting and walking, and gentle yoga and body scan (c) Discussion of barriers to daily practice, and supportive interactions within the group	RCT 322 survivors with breast cancer RA to (a) 6-week intervention of MBSR (b) Usual care	322 breast cancer survivors	Assessed immediately after 6-week intervention (1) Anxiety, overall fear of recurrence, fear of recurrence of problems, fatigue severity, and fatigue interference significantly improved at 12 weeks compared to usual care based on effect size difference using Cohen's d (a) Anxiety $d = 0.27$, 95% CI, 0.06–0.47, $p = 0.007$ (b) Fear of recurrence $d = 0.28$, 95% CI, 0.08–0.48, $p = 0.001$ (c) Problems with fear of recurrence $d = 0.35$, 95% CI, 0.15–0.56, $p = 0.001$ (d) Fatigue severity $d = 0.27$ 95% CI, 0.07–0.47, $p = 0.002$ (e) Fatigue interference $d = 0.23$ 96% CI, 0.02–0.43, $p = 0.006$ (2) Overall effect size was largest for fear of recurrence problems ($d = 0.35$) and fatigue severity ($d = 0.27$) (3) Survivors with the highest stress at baseline evidenced the greatest benefit from the intervention (4) NS for pain severity and pain interference

(continued)

Appendix (continued)

Author	Purpose/intervention	Study design	Sample/phase of disease	Outcomes
Chang et al. [86]	Assessed the psychological and biological effects of the RR response between long-term (M) and short-term (N2) practitioners of RR RR intervention Novices received training to elicit the RR for 8 weeks which included (a) Diaphragmatic breathing (b) Body scan Mantra repetition (c) Mindfulness meditation passively ignoring intrusive thoughts (d) 20-min audio so subjects could practice daily at home	8-week prospective, crossover design (a) 28 meditative (M) group (4–20 years) (b) 28 novice group at baseline (N1) (c) 28 After 8 weeks of training (N2)	Healthy volunteers	(1) Long-term M group had significantly lower levels of emotional distress than novices at baseline (N1) (2) Post 8 weeks of RR training, the N2 novice group showed significantly lower levels of psychological distress comparable to long-term practitioners (3) After listening to a RR CD, M > N2 showed significantly greater immediate decreases in psychological distress (4) In M group: reduction in psychological distress was related to a reduction in biological measures of stress hormones after controlling for baseline values (5) In the N2 group: a NS correlation between psychological distress and biological indicators of stress Conclusion Only years of RR practice may significantly reduce psychological distress and biological distress, although distress can be improved

References

1. Riba MB, Donovan KA, Andersen B, Braun I, Breitbart WS, Brewer BW, et al. Distress management, version 3.2019, NCCN clinical practice guidelines in oncology. JNCCN. 2019;17(10):1229–49. PubMed PMID: 31590149. Pubmed Central PMCID: PMC6907687. Epub 2019/10/08. eng.
2. Sharpe L, Curran L, Butow P, Thewes B. Fear of cancer recurrence and death anxiety. Psycho-Oncology. 2018;27(11):2559–65. PubMed PMID: 29843188. Epub 2018/05/31. eng.
3. Ferrell BR, Twaddle ML, Melnick A, Meier DE. National consensus project clinical practice guidelines for quality palliative care guidelines. J Palliat Med. 2018;21(12):1684–9. PubMed PMID: 30179523. Epub 2018/09/05. eng.
4. Treanor CJ, McMenamin UC, O'Neill RF, Cardwell CR, Clarke MJ, Cantwell M, et al. Non-pharmacological interventions for cognitive impairment due to systemic cancer treatment. Cochrane Database Syst Rev. 2016;16(8):CD011325. PubMed PMID: 27529826. Epub 2016/08/17. eng.
5. Lehmann V, Hagedoorn M, Gerhardt CA, Fults M, Olshefski RS, Sanderman R, et al. Body issues, sexual satisfaction, and relationship status satisfaction in long-term childhood cancer survivors and healthy controls. Psycho-Oncology. 2016;25(2):210–6. PubMed PMID: 25959111. Epub 2015/05/12. eng.
6. Chirico A, Lucidi F, Mallia L, D'Aiuto M, Merluzzi TV. Indicators of distress in newly diagnosed breast cancer patients. PeerJ. 2015;3:e1107. PubMed PMID: 26244115. Pubmed Central PMCID: PMC4517964. Epub 2015/08/06. eng.
7. Keeley V. Advances in understanding and management of lymphoedema (cancer, primary). Curr Opin Support Palliat Care. 2017;11(4):355–60. PubMed PMID: 28984676. Epub 2017/10/07. eng.
8. Hall DL, Luberto CM, Philpotts LL, Song R, Park ER, Yeh GY. Mind-body interventions for fear of cancer recurrence: a systematic review and meta-analysis. Psycho-Oncology. 2018;27(11):2546–58. PubMed PMID: 29744965. Pubmed Central PMCID: PMC6488231. Epub 2018/05/11. eng.
9. Wigmore P. The effect of systemic chemotherapy on neurogenesis, plasticity and memory. Curr Top Behav Neurosci. 2013;15:211–40. PubMed PMID: 23239468. Epub 2012/12/15. eng.
10. Lindner OC, Mayes A, McCabe MG, Talmi D. Acute memory deficits in chemotherapy-treated adults. Memory. 2017;2017:1–13. PubMed PMID: 28285570. Epub 2017/03/14. eng.
11. Carlson LE. Mindfulness-based interventions for coping with cancer. Ann N Y Acad Sci. 2016;1373(1):5–12. PubMed PMID: 26963792. Epub 2016/03/11. eng.
12. Dusek JA, Benson H. Mind-body medicine: a model of the comparative clinical impact of the acute stress and relaxation responses. Minn Med. 2009;92(5):47–50. PubMed PMID: 19552264. Pubmed Central PMCID: PMC2724877. Epub 2009/06/26. eng.
13. Carlson LE. Distress management through mind-body therapies in oncology. J Natl Cancer Inst Monogr. 2017;2017:52. PubMed PMID: 29140490. Epub 2017/11/16. eng.
14. Manuello J, Vercelli U, Nani A, Costa T, Cauda F. Mindfulness meditation and consciousness: an integrative neuroscientific perspective. Conscious Cogn. 2016;40:67–78. PubMed PMID: 26752605. Epub 2016/01/12. eng.
15. Kabat ZJ. Full catastrophe living: using the wisdom of your body and mind to face stress, pain and illness. New York: Delacourt; 1990.
16. Kiken LG, Garland EL, Bluth K, Palsson OS, Gaylord SA. From a state to a trait: trajectories of state mindfulness in meditation during intervention predict changes in trait mindfulness. Personal Individ Differ. 2015;81:41–6. PubMed PMID: 25914434. Pubmed Central PMCID: PMC4404745. Epub 2015/04/29. eng.
17. Calder CC. The effects of the relaxation response on nurses' level of anxiety, depression, well-being, work-related stress, and confidence to teach patients. J Holist Nurs. 2017;35(4):318–27. PubMed PMID: 28720029. Epub 2017/07/20. eng.

18. Botha E, Gwin T, Purpora C. The effectiveness of mindfulness based programs in reducing stress experienced by nurses in adult hospital settings: a systematic review of quantitative evidence protocol. JBI Database System Rev Implement Rep. 2015;13(10):21–9. PubMed PMID: 26571279. Epub 2015/11/17. eng.
19. Carlson LE, Tamagawa R, Stephen J, Doll R, Faris P, Dirkse D, et al. Tailoring mind-body therapies to individual needs: patients' program preference and psychological traits as moderators of the effects of mindfulness-based cancer recovery and supportive-expressive therapy in distressed breast cancer survivors. J Natl Cancer Inst Monogr. 2014;2014(50):308–14. PubMed PMID: 25749597. Epub 2015/03/10. eng.
20. Bishop S. Mindfulness: a proposed operational definition. Clin Psychol. 2004;11(3):230–41.
21. Grecucci A, Pappaianni E, Siugzdaite R, Theuninck A, Job R. Mindful emotion regulation: exploring the neurocognitive mechanisms behind mindfulness. Biomed Res Int. 2015;2015:670724. PubMed PMID: 26137490. Pubmed Central PMCID: PMC4475519. Epub 2015/07/03. eng.
22. Benson H. The relaxation response. New York: HarperCollins; 2000.
23. Bhasin MK, Dusek JA, Chang BH, Joseph MG, Denninger JW, Fricchione GL, et al. Relaxation response induces temporal transcriptome changes in energy metabolism, insulin secretion and inflammatory pathways. PLoS One. 2013;8(5):e62817. PubMed PMID: 23650531. Pubmed Central PMCID: PMC3641112. Epub 2013/05/08. eng.
24. Lazar SW, Bush G, Gollub RL, Fricchione GL, Khalsa G, Benson H. Functional brain mapping of the relaxation response and meditation. Neuroreport. 2000;11(7):1581–5. PubMed PMID: 10841380. Epub 2000/06/07. eng.
25. Dusek JA, Otu HH, Wohlhueter AL, Bhasin M, Zerbini LF, Joseph MG, et al. Genomic counter-stress changes induced by the relaxation response. PLoS One. 2008;3(7):e2576. PubMed PMID: 18596974. Pubmed Central PMCID: PMC2432467. Epub 2008/07/04. eng.
26. Saatcioglu F. Regulation of gene expression by yoga, meditation and related practices: a review of recent studies. Asian J Psychiatr. 2013;6(1):74–7. PubMed PMID: 23380323. Epub 2013/02/06. eng.
27. Dusek JA, Hibberd PL, Buczynski B, Chang BH, Dusek KC, Johnston JM, et al. Stress management versus lifestyle modification on systolic hypertension and medication elimination: a randomized trial. J Altern Complement Med. 2008;14(2):129–38. PubMed PMID: 18315510.
28. Basso JC, McHale A, Ende V, Oberlin DJ, Suzuki WA. Brief, daily meditation enhances attention, memory, mood, and emotional regulation in non-experienced meditators. Behav Brain Res. 2019;356:208–20. PubMed PMID: 30153464. Epub 2018/08/29. eng.
29. Holzel BK, Carmody J, Evans KC, Hoge EA, Dusek JA, Morgan L, et al. Stress reduction correlates with structural changes in the amygdala. Soc Cogn Affect Neurosci. 2010;5(1):11–7. PubMed PMID: 19776221. Pubmed Central PMCID: PMC2840837. Epub 2009/09/25. eng.
30. Holzel BK, Lazar SW, Gard T, Schuman-Olivier Z, Vago DR, Ott U. How does mindfulness meditation work? Proposing mechanisms of action from a conceptual and neural perspective. Perspect Psychol Sci. 2011;6(6):537–59. PubMed PMID: 26168376. Epub 2011/11/01. eng.
31. Benson H, Stuart E. The wellness book: the comprehensive guide to maintaining health and treating stress-related illness. New York: Simon and Schuster; 1992.
32. Carlson LE, Tamagawa R, Stephen J, Drysdale E, Zhong L, Speca M. Randomized-controlled trial of mindfulness-based cancer recovery versus supportive expressive group therapy among distressed breast cancer survivors (MINDSET): long-term follow-up results. Psycho-Oncology. 2016;25(7):750–9. PubMed PMID: 27193737. Epub 2016/05/20. eng.
33. Carlson LE, Doll R, Stephen J, Faris P, Tamagawa R, Drysdale E, et al. Randomized controlled trial of Mindfulness-based cancer recovery versus supportive expressive group therapy for distressed survivors of breast cancer. J Clin Oncol. 2013;31(25):3119–26. PubMed PMID: 23918953. Epub 2013/08/07. eng.
34. Xunlin NG, Lau Y, Klainin-Yobas P. The effectiveness of mindfulness-based interventions among cancer patients and survivors: a systematic review and meta-analysis. Support Care Cancer. 2020;28(4):1563–78. PubMed PMID: 31834518. Epub 2019/12/14. eng.

35. Cillessen L, Johannsen M, Speckens AEM, Zachariae R. Mindfulness-based interventions for psychological and physical health outcomes in cancer patients and survivors: a systematic review and meta-analysis of randomized controlled trials. Psycho-Oncology. 2019;28(12):2257–69. PubMed PMID: 31464026. Pubmed Central PMCID: PMC6916350. Epub 2019/08/30. eng.
36. Ngô TL. Review of the effects of mindfulness meditation on mental and physical health and its mechanisms of action. Sante Ment Que. 2013;38(2):19–34. PubMed PMID: 24719001. Epub 2014/04/11. Revue des effets de la méditation de pleine conscience sur la santé mentale et physique et sur ses mécanismes d'action. fre.
37. Sternberg EM, Chrousos GP, Wilder RL, Gold PW. The stress response and the regulation of inflammatory disease. Ann Intern Med. 1992;117(10):854–66. PubMed PMID: 1416562.
38. Thayer JF, Sternberg E. Beyond heart rate variability: vagal regulation of allostatic systems. Ann N Y Acad Sci. 2006;1088:361–72. PubMed PMID: 17192580.
39. Thayer JF, Sternberg EM. Neural aspects of immunomodulation: focus on the vagus nerve. Brain Behav Immun. 2010;24(8):1223–8. Pubmed Central PMCID: PMC2949498. Epub 2010/08/03. eng.
40. Shennan C, Payne S, Fenlon D. What is the evidence for the use of mindfulness-based interventions in cancer care? A review. Psycho-Oncology. 2011;20(7):681–97. PubMed PMID: 20690112. Epub 2010/08/07. eng.
41. Morean DF, O'Dwyer L, Cherney LR. Therapies for cognitive deficits associated with chemotherapy for breast cancer: a systematic review of objective outcomes. Arch Phys Med Rehabil. 2015;96(10):1880–97. PubMed PMID: 26026579. Epub 2015/06/01. eng.
42. Fox KC, Dixon ML, Nijeboer S, Girn M, Floman JL, Lifshitz M, et al. Functional neuroanatomy of meditation: a review and meta-analysis of 78 functional neuroimaging investigations. Neurosci Biobehav Rev. 2016;65:208–28. PubMed PMID: 27032724. Epub 2016/04/02. eng.
43. Gotink RA, Meijboom R, Vernooij MW, Smits M, Hunink MG. 8-week mindfulness based stress reduction induces brain changes similar to traditional long-term meditation practice - a systematic review. Brain Cogn. 2016;108:32–41. PubMed PMID: 27429096. Epub 2016/07/19. eng.
44. Zeidan F, Martucci KT, Kraft RA, Gordon NS, McHaffie JG, Coghill RC. Brain mechanisms supporting the modulation of pain by mindfulness meditation. J Neurosci. 2011;31(14):5540–8. PubMed PMID: 21471390. Pubmed Central PMCID: PMC3090218. Epub 2011/04/08. eng.
45. Carlson LE, Speca M, Faris P, Patel KD. One year pre-post intervention follow-up of psychological, immune, endocrine and blood pressure outcomes of mindfulness-based stress reduction (MBSR) in breast and prostate cancer outpatients. Brain Behav Immun. 2007;21(8):1038–49. PubMed PMID: 17521871. Epub 2007/05/25. eng.
46. Matousek RH, Pruessner JC, Dobkin PL. Changes in the cortisol awakening response (CAR) following participation in mindfulness-based stress reduction in women who completed treatment for breast cancer. Complement Ther Clin Pract. 2011;17(2):65–70. PubMed PMID: 21457893. Epub 2011/04/05. eng.
47. Bernardi L, Sleight P, Bandinelli G, Cencetti S, Fattorini L, Wdowczyc-Szulc J, et al. Effect of rosary prayer and yoga mantras on autonomic cardiovascular rhythms: comparative study. BMJ. 2001;323(7327):1446–9. PubMed PMID: 11751348. Pubmed Central PMCID: 61046.
48. Servan-Schreiber D. Anticancer: a new way of life. Toronto: HarperCollins; 2007.
49. Reich RR, Lengacher CA, Alinat CB, Kip KE, Paterson C, Ramesar S, et al. Mindfulness-based stress reduction in post-treatment breast cancer patients: immediate and sustained effects across multiple symptom clusters. J Pain Symptom Manag. 2017;53(1):85–95. PubMed PMID: 27720794. Pubmed Central PMCID: PMC7771358. Epub 2016/10/11. eng.
50. Cruceriu D, Baldasici O, Balacescu O, Berindan-Neagoe I. The dual role of tumor necrosis factor-alpha (TNF-α) in breast cancer: molecular insights and therapeutic approaches. Cell Oncol. 2020;43(1):1–18. PubMed PMID: 31900901. Epub 2020/01/05. eng.
51. Witek-Janusek L, Albuquerque K, Chroniak KR, Chroniak C, Durazo-Arvizu R, Mathews HL. Effect of mindfulness based stress reduction on immune function, quality of life and

coping in women newly diagnosed with early stage breast cancer. Brain Behav Immun. 2008;22(6):969–81. PubMed PMID: 18359186. Pubmed Central PMCID: PMC2586059. Epub 2008/03/25. eng.
52. Black DS, Slavich GM. Mindfulness meditation and the immune system: a systematic review of randomized controlled trials. Ann N Y Acad Sci. 2016;1373(1):13–24. PubMed PMID: 26799456. Pubmed Central PMCID: PMC4940234. Epub 2016/01/23. eng.
53. Creswell JD, Irwin MR, Burklund LJ, Lieberman MD, Arevalo JM, Ma J, et al. Mindfulness-based stress reduction training reduces loneliness and pro-inflammatory gene expression in older adults: a small randomized controlled trial. Brain Behav Immun. 2012;26(7):1095–101. PubMed PMID: 22820409. Pubmed Central PMCID: PMC3635809. Epub 2012/07/24. eng.
54. Liu T, Zhang L, Joo D, Sun SC. NF-κB signaling in inflammation. Signal Transduct Target Ther. 2017;2:17023. PubMed PMID: 29158945. Pubmed Central PMCID: PMC5661633. Epub 2017/11/22. eng.
55. Bower JE, Crosswell AD, Stanton AL, Crespi CM, Winston D, Arevalo J, et al. Mindfulness meditation for younger breast cancer survivors: a randomized controlled trial. Cancer. 2015;121(8):1231–40. PubMed PMID: 25537522. Pubmed Central PMCID: PMC4393338. Epub 2014/12/30. eng.
56. Zhang MF, Wen YS, Liu WY, Peng LF, Wu XD, Liu QW. Effectiveness of mindfulness-based therapy for reducing anxiety and depression in patients with cancer: a meta-analysis. Medicine. 2015;94(45):e0897. PubMed PMID: 26559246. Epub 2015/11/13. eng.
57. Huang HP, He M, Wang HY, Zhou M. A meta-analysis of the benefits of mindfulness-based stress reduction (MBSR) on psychological function among breast cancer (BC) survivors. Breast Cancer. 2016;23(4):568–76. PubMed PMID: 25820148. Epub 2015/03/31. eng.
58. Ngamkham S, Holden JE, Smith EL. A systematic review: mindfulness intervention for cancer-related pain. Asia Pac J Oncol Nurs. 2019;6(2):161–9. PubMed PMID: 30931361. Pubmed Central PMCID: PMC6371675. Epub 2019/04/02. eng.
59. Xie C, Dong B, Wang L, Jing X, Wu Y, Lin L, et al. Mindfulness-based stress reduction can alleviate cancer- related fatigue: a meta-analysis. J Psychosom Res. 2020;130:109916. PubMed PMID: 31927347. Epub 2020/01/14. eng.
60. Henderson VP, Clemow L, Massion AO, Hurley TG, Druker S, Hebert JR. The effects of mindfulness-based stress reduction on psychosocial outcomes and quality of life in early-stage breast cancer patients: a randomized trial. Breast Cancer Res Treat. 2012;131(1):99–109. PubMed PMID: 21901389. Pubmed Central PMCID: PMC3784652. Epub 2011/09/09. eng.
61. Lengacher CA, Reich RR, Paterson CL, Ramesar S, Park JY, Alinat C, et al. Examination of broad symptom improvement resulting from mindfulness-based stress reduction in breast cancer survivors: a randomized controlled trial. J Clin Oncol. 2016;34(24):2827–34. PubMed PMID: 27247219. Pubmed Central PMCID: PMC5012660 online at www.jco.org. Author contributions are found at the end of this article. Epub 2016/06/02. eng.
62. Schellekens MPJ, Tamagawa R, Labelle LE, Speca M, Stephen J, Drysdale E, et al. Mindfulness-based cancer recovery (MBCR) versus supportive expressive group therapy (SET) for distressed breast cancer survivors: evaluating mindfulness and social support as mediators. J Behav Med. 2017;40(3):414–22. PubMed PMID: 27722908. Pubmed Central PMCID: PMC5406481. Epub 2016/10/11. eng.
63. Li G, Yuan H, Zhang W. The effects of mindfulness-based stress reduction for family caregivers: systematic review. Arch Psychiatr Nurs. 2016;30(2):292–9. PubMed PMID: 26992885. Epub 2016/03/20. eng.
64. Dumas JA, Makarewicz J, Schaubhut GJ, Devins R, Albert K, Dittus K, et al. Chemotherapy altered brain functional connectivity in women with breast cancer: a pilot study. Brain Imaging Behav. 2013;7(4):524–32. PubMed PMID: 23852814. Pubmed Central PMCID: PMC3852152. Epub 2013/07/16. eng.
65. Biegler KA, Chaoul MA, Cohen L. Cancer, cognitive impairment, and meditation. Acta Oncol. 2009;48(1):18–26. PubMed PMID: 19031161. Epub 2008/11/26. eng.
66. Garland EL, Hanley A, Farb NA, Froeliger BE. State mindfulness during meditation predicts enhanced cognitive reappraisal. Mindfulness. 2015;6(2):234–42. PubMed PMID: 26085851. Pubmed Central PMCID: PMC4465118. Epub 2015/06/19. Eng.

67. Ostafin BD, Kassman KT. Stepping out of history: mindfulness improves insight problem solving. Conscious Cogn. 2012;21(2):1031–6. PubMed PMID: 22483682. Epub 2012/04/10. eng.
68. Hanley A, Garland EL, Black DS. Use of mindful reappraisal coping among meditation practitioners. J Clin Psychol. 2014;70(3):294–301. PubMed PMID: 23818289. Epub 2013/07/03. eng.
69. Noone C, Bunting B, Hogan MJ. Does mindfulness enhance critical thinking? Evidence for the mediating effects of executive functioning in the relationship between mindfulness and critical thinking. Front Psychol. 2015;6:2043. PubMed PMID: 26834669. Pubmed Central PMCID: PMC4717844. Epub 2016/02/03. eng.
70. Shoham A, Goldstein P, Oren R, Spivak D, Bernstein A. Decentering in the process of cultivating mindfulness: an experience-sampling study in time and context. J Consult Clin Psychol. 2017;85(2):123–34. PubMed PMID: 28134540. Epub 2017/01/31. eng.
71. Bernstein A, Hadash Y, Lichtash Y, Tanay G, Shepherd K, Fresco DM. Decentering and related constructs: a critical review and metacognitive processes model. Perspect Psychol Sci. 2015;10(5):599–617. PubMed PMID: 26385999. Pubmed Central PMCID: PMC5103165. Epub 2015/09/20. eng.
72. Orellana-Rios CL, Radbruch L, Kern M, Regel YU, Anton A, Sinclair S, et al. Mindfulness and compassion-oriented practices at work reduce distress and enhance self-care of palliative care teams: a mixed-method evaluation of an "on the job" program. BMC Palliat Care. 2017;17(1):3. PubMed PMID: 28683799. Pubmed Central PMCID: PMC5501358. Epub 2017/07/08. eng.
73. Moody K, Kramer D, Santizo RO, Magro L, Wyshogrod D, Ambrosio J, et al. Helping the helpers: mindfulness training for burnout in pediatric oncology–a pilot program. J Pediatr Oncol Nurs. 2013;30(5):275–84. PubMed PMID: 24101747. Epub 2013/10/09. eng.
74. Bazarko D, Cate RA, Azocar F, Kreitzer MJ. The impact of an innovative mindfulness-based stress reduction program on the health and well-being of nurses employed in a corporate setting. J Work Behav Health. 2013;28(2):107–33. PubMed PMID: 23667348. Pubmed Central PMCID: PMC3646311. Epub 2013/05/15. eng.
75. Gauthier T, Meyer RM, Grefe D, Gold JI. An on-the-job mindfulness-based intervention for pediatric ICU nurses: a pilot. J Pediatr Nurs. 2015;30(2):402–9. PubMed PMID: 25450445. Epub 2014/12/03. eng.
76. Carlson LE, Zelinski E, Toivonen K, Flynn M, Qureshi M, Piedalue KA, et al. Mind-body therapies in cancer: what is the latest evidence? Curr Oncol Rep. 2017;19(10):67. PubMed PMID: 28822063. Epub 2017/08/20. eng.
77. Goyal M, Singh S, Sibinga EM, Gould NF, Rowland-Seymour A, Sharma R, et al. Meditation programs for psychological stress and well-being: a systematic review and meta-analysis. JAMA Intern Med. 2014;174(3):357–68. PubMed PMID: 24395196. Pubmed Central PMCID: PMC4142584. Epub 2014/01/08. eng.
78. Harorani M, Davodabady F, Farahani Z, Hezave AK, Rafiei F. The effect of Benson's relaxation response on sleep quality and anorexia in cancer patients undergoing chemotherapy: a randomized controlled trial. Complement Ther Med. 2020;50:102344. PubMed PMID: 32444038. Epub 2020/05/24. eng.
79. Schellekens MPJ, van den Hurk DGM, Prins JB, Donders ART, Molema J, Dekhuijzen R, et al. Mindfulness-based stress reduction added to care as usual for lung cancer patients and/or their partners: a multicentre randomized controlled trial. Psycho-Oncology. 2017;26(12):2118–26. PubMed PMID: 28337821. Epub 2017/03/25. eng.
80. Treanor CJ, Santin O, Prue G, Coleman H, Cardwell CR, O'Halloran P, et al. Psychosocial interventions for informal caregivers of people living with cancer. Cochrane Database Syst Rev. 2019;6(6):CD009912. PubMed PMID: 31204791. Pubmed Central PMCID: PMC6573123. Epub 2019/06/18. eng.
81. Andersen SR, Wurtzen H, Steding-Jessen M, Christensen J, Andersen KK, Flyger H, et al. Effect of mindfulness-based stress reduction on sleep quality: results of a randomized trial among Danish breast cancer patients. Acta Oncol. 2013;52(2):336–44. PubMed PMID: 23282113. Epub 2013/01/04. eng.

82. Schellekens MP, van den Hurk DG, Prins JB, Molema J, Donders AR, Woertman WH, et al. Study protocol of a randomized controlled trial comparing Mindfulness-Based Stress Reduction with treatment as usual in reducing psychological distress in patients with lung cancer and their partners: the MILON study. BMC Cancer. 2014;14:3. Pubmed Central PMCID: PMC3893473. Epub 2014/01/07. eng.
83. Haller H, Winkler MM, Klose P, Dobos G, Kümmel S, Cramer H. Mindfulness-based interventions for women with breast cancer: an updated systematic review and meta-analysis. Acta Oncol. 2017;56(12):1665–76. PubMed PMID: 28686520. Epub 2017/07/08. eng.
84. Nissen ER, O'Connor M, Kaldo V, Højris I, Borre M, Zachariae R, et al. Internet-delivered mindfulness-based cognitive therapy for anxiety and depression in cancer survivors: a randomized controlled trial. Psycho-Oncology. 2020;29(1):68–75. PubMed PMID: 31600414. Pubmed Central PMCID: PMC7004073. Epub 2019/10/11. eng.
85. Zhang Q, Zhao H, Zheng Y. Effectiveness of mindfulness-based stress reduction (MBSR) on symptom variables and health-related quality of life in breast cancer patients-a systematic review and meta-analysis. Support Care Cancer. 2019;27(3):771–81. PubMed PMID: 30488223. Epub 2018/11/30. eng.
86. Chang BH, Dusek JA, Benson H. Psychobiological changes from relaxation response elicitation: long-term practitioners vs. novices. Psychosomatics. 2011;52(6):550–9. PubMed PMID: 22054625. Epub 2011/11/08. eng.

Physical Touch and Healing Touch

14.1 Introduction

Physical touch, healing touch, and reiki are healing-promoting nursing interventions that are distinguishable from one another in their therapeutic intent and functions. These therapies are thought to foster healing and resilience through the activation of neural-physiological pathways and/or manipulation of energy fields [1]. From a whole-person perspective, it may be argued that the quality, intensity, and type of physical touch triggers relevant neurobiological pathways throughout the individual, whereas a biofield modality such as healing touch or reiki stimulates endogenous energy fields in the recipient (patient) and provider (nurse). As the human organism is replete with metabolic and other forms of energy, it is likely that both physical touch and healing touch impact different forms of human energy and physiological processes. The manner in which touch is conveyed in practice is a function of the nurse's own personal experiences, theoretical understanding of the goals and intent of the touch modality, and skillfulness within the clinical context. Each modality, first Physical Touch and its different forms of physical touch, followed by the biofield modalities of healing touch and reiki will be considered separately in this chapter.

14.2 Objectives

At the end of this chapter, you will be able to:

1. Distinguish the goals and practices between physical touch and healing touch or reiki.
2. Discuss the clinical evidence in relation to each modality.
3. Consider how attachment and embodiment theories may be interconnected and serve as a theoretical framework for the effects of physical touch on growth, development, and healing.

4. Consider the roles of electromagnetic and subtle energy fields in relation to biofield modalities.
5. Identify the clinical contexts in which the use of physical touch and/or healing touch may optimize the healing and well-being of patients with cancer or their caregivers.

14.3 Physical Touch

Definitions

Physical Touch

Physical touch refers to the various ways in which humans establish a physical connection, typically by holding hands, stroking the other person's arm, massaging a back, hugging or kissing, or gently laying a hand upon a patient's arm. The form of touch and how it is experienced and interpreted is a function of the quality and composition of the dyadic relationship and the purpose and context within which it takes place. It is the most fundamental method of social and nonverbal human communication used to calm, reassure, nurture, and potentially heal one another throughout the lifespan [2–4].

Touch may be characterized by *its communicative intent* which refers to the goal or purpose for human connection transmitted to another through the quality of the physical touch [5–7]. We use touch to *convey* feelings, emotions, and meanings to convey mutual understanding and regard within a relational predicate [4]. Humans appear to possess an innate ability to understand the various meanings inherent in a touch [8].

The main forms of *physical touch* to be addressed in the first half of this chapter include (1) the nurse's use of affective gentle touch, comfort touch, and procedural touch and (2) affectionate touch experienced within close patient-partner or familial relationships. Thus the nurse may use affective, comfort, and procedural touch with patients as an intentional therapeutic intervention. In addition, the nurse may encourage the use of affectionate touch between patient and family caregiver to strengthen their relationship and its potential therapeutic benefits for both patient and family caregiver.

Affective Touch

The intention of affective touch is to convey caring and an emotional connection with the patient [9, 10]. It refers to a gentle, tactile pleasant touch containing an emotional component within a "cognitive-relational" human context [11–13]. Affective touch includes a range of therapeutic intents such as conveying reassurance, comfort, emotional support, and understanding of the patient's experience. Affective touch involves gentle caresses with a slow and soft hand for the purpose of providing reassurance, support, and a meaningful connection with the patient [14, 15]. It is sometimes described as effleurage [16]. Affective touch activates low-threshold mechanoreceptors lodged in the cutaneous layer of the hairy skin that are innervated by C-afferent nerve fibers [13]. A nurse's affective touch conveys compassion, warmth, and positive emotions that are experienced by both the nurse and patient within a therapeutic nurse-patient clinical context [17].

Comfort Touch
The intent of this touch is to convey a sense of security, presence, and compassion. It provides a reassuring physical connection in stressful situations between the nurse's hand and the patient's covered arm, for instance. Comfort touch conveys to patients that they are not alone in their pain or suffering and are understood [17, 18]. Human separation and attachment needs may be mitigated by comfort touch which has a particular resonance for patients with serious illnesses, such as cancer [5]. A frightened patient may ask the nurse to hold his or her hand during a procedure. But it is the sensitive nurse who can correctly interpret nonverbal cues in order to ask permission and confidently take the patient's hand to provide the needed comfort and reassurance. The intentional quality of touch can assuage patient fear and also relieve feelings of distress and frustration.

Tactile Touch or Effleurage
The intent of tactile touch, also known as effleurage, is to stimulate the parasympathetic healing response in order to promote healing processes throughout the whole person. It involves gentle but slow and firm circular massage with the palm of the hand and flat closed fingers, and has been applied in patients in palliative care as well as patients on chemotherapy, in critical intensive care and geriatric care [19–21].

Procedural Touch
This form of physical touch may be described as incidental physical contact in which the nurse performs a clinical function that may involve a task-oriented touch [15, 22]. Examples include providing physical assistance with activities of daily living and carrying out various medical procedures such as changing dressings and starting IVs. As such, it may fail to convey the quality of human connection that is essential for well-being and growth. However, when procedural touch occurs within a meaningful and connected nurse-patient relationship, it has been perceived as compassionate behavior [17, 18].

Affectionate Touch
Touch aimed at conveying affection, love, closeness, intimacy, fondness, and appreciation is generally experienced within family relationships, partnerships, and marital relationships and is mediated by low-threshold, unmyelinated C-afferent nerve fibers [3]. Affectionate touch behaviors include hand holding, kissing, hugging, and caressing one another. Nurses may strengthen *patient-caregiver* relationships by encouraging affectionate touch within the dyad to convey affection which has been shown to positively enhance relational, physical, and psychological well-being [3].

In Summary
These forms of physical touch are characterized by provider intent within the social context of the nurse-patient relationship or patient-caregiver relationship.

14.4 Contextual Factors

The quality, duration, frequency, and firmness of the touch can convey different meanings mediated by the patient's emotional state, appraisal of the touch, prior experiential attachment and socio-relational experiences, clinical context, therapeutic intent of the nurse or family caregiver, and the extent to which a meaningful relationship between the nurse and patient or the patient and family caregiver has been established [13, 16]. Personal, relational, and cultural factors all have a modulating effect on the recipient's interpretation of the touch whether the provider is the family caregiver or the nurse [23, 24].

Context Matters: Physical contact may convey nurturing, caring, and comfort within the context of a connected nurse-patient relationship, or it may convey indifference in the absence of a meaningful therapeutic relationship [17, 18, 25, 26]. Or physical touch may be associated with feelings of caution and distrust by both caregiver and patient. The MeToo movement has contributed to behavioral ambivalence, underscoring the fact that to be therapeutic, the nurse's physical touch must occur within a meaningful clinical context involving a "neutral" part of the patient's body that reassures rather than confuses the patient and accompanied by the patient's permission [25].

Clinical Anecdote 14.1
After the fifth or sixth course of chemotherapy, the veins of K's only available arm were exhausted by the numerous blood tests, intravenous procedures, and the toxic effects of chemotherapy. The process of inserting the intravenous line had become a psychological and physical ordeal that filled her with dread. On this particular occasion, three nurses had tried unsuccessfully to insert the IV—each one in good faith taking K's arm rather brusquely, tapping rather forcefully on the intended sites as if willing the veins to comply. The stronger they tapped, the greater the nurses' frustration and impatience, and the faster the veins hastened a retreat. And finally the third nurse stated: "I think Serena should have a go."

Serena was well known among patients for her unique approach to intravenous insertions. She approached each IV from an extremely centered place; she was intentional and radiated an aura of quiet, gentle confidence, despite the surrounding commotion of the clinic. Serena walked slowly, purposefully toward K, pulled up a chair and sat down in front of her. She extended K's arm slowly toward her, very lightly passing the palm of her hand over possible sites she was considering. Her touch was gentle and reassuring. And K's whole body just relaxed. She inserted the IV on her first try, as she had always done.

In this clinical anecdote, the nurse utilized an intentional gentle touch which conveyed the clear message that we were going to figure this out *together*. Nurse Serena was working *with* K not for K. Utilizing a gentle touch is described in the Korean literature as caregiving behavior known as Yaksom, which refers to intentional touching to soothe and comfort. Yaksom has been empirically shown to enhance psychological bonding between mother and infant but also, as illustrated by the anecdote above, between patient and nurse [14].

14.5 Attachment and Embodiment Theories (Review [27, 28])

Two theories elucidate the significance of physical touch to the well-being of the whole person.

Attachment theory posits that a parent's touch in infancy through childhood is a human imperative for successful bonding, healthy neurobiological and behavioral growth of the individual, and the development of healthy personal relationships throughout the lifespan [27, 29, 30]. Humans have an innate "psychobiological system" that drives the desire for physical and social proximity with significant others in order to feel secure, especially during stressful times [28]. Starting from infancy, emotional bonds are thought to stimulate mental representations that shape relationships of the self with others and facilitate a growing understanding of the world, others, and the self. These cognitive models help the individual to predict, interact, and control his/her expanding environment, influencing thoughts, feelings, and behaviors in adult relationships [27]. Attachment-seeking behaviors that converge with caregiving behaviors offer human closeness and comfort (often expressed by the quality of the physical touch). According to Lenzi and colleagues caregiving systems interact with the psychoneural physiology of attachment through different qualities of physical touching starting in infancy and continuing throughout life [31].

Embodiment Theory Whereas attachment theory is anchored in assumptions of internal representations, embodiment theory is predicated on growing neurobiological systems that underlie social or relational interactions in the environment with respect to cognition, physical sensations (such as physical touch), and feelings (emotions) [27]. Embodiment theory argues that interactions between cognition (via perception, thought, and the senses) and bodily experiences in relation to others facilitate the development of attachment and meaningful relationships. Thus social resources such as social soothing, interpersonal warmth, and support seeking promote and are promoted by the individual's neurobiological-brain-body interactions with the environment [27]. These interactions are also shaped by social thermoregulating relationships which are implicated in the development of social cognition, attachment behaviors, feelings, and nonsexual physical touch. Social thermoregulation refers to behaviors, for instance, from parents, the nurse, or caregiver, that lessen the stress of exposure to the cold, loss of body heat, thereby protecting homeostatic energy for growth and survival [27].

By extension we may include social regulating behaviors of affective touch, comfort touch, and affectionate touch within the context of a therapeutic nurse-patient or patient-family caregiver relationship which reduce stress and enhance psychological well-being. Together these biobehavioral-environmental interactions contribute to the development of *relationship cognition* and influence processes of healing, growth, and development [27].

Relationship Cognition Interrelated thoughts, feelings, physical sensations, and behaviors of individuals dynamically influence one another within the context of a relationship [3, 32]. Cognition refers to thoughts, perceptions, judgment, and critical thinking. Relational cognition has to do *with thinking* about the behaviors, physical sensations, and emotions that emerge within a dyadic encounter. These relational-cognitive processes interpret the significance of received physical touch, and in reciprocal fashion, the nature of the physical touch also impacts relational-cognitive processes.

14.6 Buffering and Main Effects

Jakubiak's and Feeney's model proposes that affectionate touch induces buffering effects in stressful situations and main effects independently of stress due, in part, to the relational-cognitive and neurobiological changes that occur after touch has been encoded and transmitted to the brain, to be processed by C-afferent pathways, which subsequently influence relational, psychological, and physical well-being. Whereas Jakubiak's theoretical model was mainly based on the effects of affectionate touch on physical, relational, and psychological well-being, research also indicates that other forms of touch, in particular affective touch, trigger these same pathways and induce buffering and/or main effects even when the provider such as a nurse is not a close partner or friend [2, 11, 16]. Affective touch and affectionate touch are thought to be modulated by cognition and shape social functioning within a specified relationship, such as the nurse-patient or patient-informal caregiver relationship [12].

14.7 Neurobiological Processes of Physical Touch

Pressure, vibration, temperature, and pain activate low-threshold mechanoreceptors (LTM) embedded in the skin and joints that are associated with distinct receptors which "encode" incoming stimuli. One touch-sensitive group of LTM receptors is innervated by high-velocity myelinated A_β-afferent nerves that are rapidly processed by the cerebral cortex in order to expedite urgent human responses [13].

The skin also is a critical organ through which unmyelinated C-tactile afferents process touch-related experiences that influence the way the individual thinks, feels, and interacts with another based on the quality of touch [11, 13]. Touch within the large area of human hairy skin activates unmyelinated LTM fibers known as C-tactile afferents (CTs) that are part of the somatic sensory system [2]. Whereas the myelinated afferents are involved in discriminative aspects of touch (such as texture, type of touch), unmyelinated C afferents are most involved in affiliate aspects.

Gentle touch, light touch, pleasant touch, affective touch, and affectionate touch activate and transmit information carried by the C afferents to the brain where it is interpreted in brain areas mainly associated with the reward circuitry, social processing, empathy, and emotions [2]. C afferents have a conduction velocity that is much slower than the myelinated pathways but are distinguished by a wider band of mechano-sensations.

Brain areas associated with interpreting C-afferent fibers innervated by touch include the orbitofrontal cortex, pregenual anterior cingulate cortex, posterior insular cortex, superior temporal sulcus, caudate cortex and the amygdala [2]. The insular cortex is thought to be associated with emotional, hormonal, and affiliative responses to touch that convey nurturing and social grooming [4]. The insular cortex can process converging signals from touch and other sensory processes that lead to emotional responses.

These and other findings appear to support the contention that affective touch contains an emotional component [9, 10]. The affective touch hypothesis posits that C-tactile afferents increase emotional reactions in response to physical closeness to a "friendly person" bestowing feelings of pleasure and security, which suggest that these feelings may be evoked outside a close partner or family relationship [12]. Current thinking is that the activated unmyelinated C-tactile afferents may also induce the need for physical touch which is a nurturing behavior across the lifespan, enabling healthy development, healing, and resilience [2].

Downregulating Biological Stress Response System Interpersonal touch facilitates overall development, neurophysiological healing- and resilient-promoting neurophysiological processes [2, 8]. Findings suggest that affective touch, comfort touch, and moderate massage attenuate the stress-activated HPA axis and SNS, enabling the reemergence of healing processes of the PNS and vagal nerve [33]. Moderate tactile pressure in particular appears to activate pressure receptors and vagal activity causing increased relational, psychological, and physical well-being, relaxation, and emotional equanimity [3].

14.8 Experimental Research

Touch and Healthy Volunteers

Experiments suggest that healthy individuals can identify the emotion conveyed by the quality of the touch on their arm [34, 35]. Anger, disgust, fear, love, gratitude, and sympathy were correctly identified between 48 and 83% of the time without observing the person doing the touching. Observers to this interpersonal touch were also able to identify the emotion caused by each type of touch, validating the volunteers' responses [35]. This study was replicated with the same results [34]. The use of touch as a clinical strategy within a meaningful clinical context may serve as a powerful modality of therapeutic communication whether or not the patient is able to observe the touch behavior. The findings have clear clinical implications for critically ill or dying individuals.

Affective Touch An experimental study with 22 healthy adults based on functional magnetic resonance imaging (fMRI) showed that manually stroking the arm or palm led to changes in a network of brain areas that activated the right posterior superior temporal sulcus and the medial prefrontal cortex (mPFC)/dorso-anterior cingulate cortex (dACC), which amplify social and cognitive perceptions [9]. Connectivity analyses among the key nodes of the social brain (mPFC/Acc, insula, and amygdala) appeared to show co-activation in processing the touch-activated C afferents lending further support to the involvement of social cognition and emotions in relation to touch [9].

A meta-analysis of 13 studies investigated the effects of affective touch in terms of sex differences [12]. More females than male participants reported that affective touch exerted "pleasant" effects. The findings were hypothesized to be related to the nurturing and caregiving roles of females. However, the small number of eligible studies signifies the need for more clinical research.

The effects of moderate- versus light-pressure massage on the parasympathetic response were assessed in 20 healthy adult volunteers who were randomized to either a moderate-pressure or light-pressure massage [33]. EKG readings taken at baseline, during the 15-minute massage and post massage, were used to obtain measures of heart rate variability (HRV), specifically the high-frequency (HF, such as 0.15–0.4 Hz) and low-frequency (LF, such as 0.04–0.15 Hz) components in order to assess the LF/HF ratio of sympatho-vagal balance [36]. Heart rate variability has been used as an estimate of cardiac autonomic regulation; it refers to the variation in the length of time (i.e., interval) between two consecutive heartbeats and is often used as a measure of stress, optimal wholeness, and healing although it is not without methodological issues [36, 37]. Because fluctuations may be imperceptible to the human eye, specialized technology is used to obtain the readings. Whereas increased LF/HF reflects low vagal activity (i.e., increased sympathetic activity), a decreased LF/HF ratio suggests an increased parasympathetic modulating tone.

The results for the moderate-pressure massage showed an increase in HF which decreased the LF/HF ratio suggesting a parasympathetic nervous system response due to an increase in activity of the efferent vagal nerve [33]. The increased HF indicated a shift from sympathetic to parasympathetic activity denoting the reemergence of healing, restorative processes. Conversely light-pressure massage was associated with an increase in SNS activity characterized by a decreased HF and an increased LF/HF ratio. The therapeutic effects of physical touch appeared to vary according to the intensity of applied pressure, frequency, duration, body site, and timing. The effectiveness of moderate- pressure massage was supported by other studies in which moderate- pressure massage was related to significant improvements in systolic and diastolic blood pressure, respiratory rates, and quality of sleep as well as decreased pain in critically ill patients compared to controls [16]. In all these studies, the duration of effects was not assessed or tended to be short-lived.

The effects of the velocity of gentle touch on people's sense of social affiliation or belonging have also been investigated [38]. Eighty-four volunteers participated in a two (ostracism: "excluded" versus "included") by two (touch velocity: "slow" versus "fast") experimental design based on a "game" that examined the relationship between gentle touch and social belonging. The "ostracized" participants reported feeling distressed after the game. However the distress was significantly reduced although not completely eliminated in the group that received the slow affective touch intervention compared to the group with the fast "neutral" touch. These findings are particularly relevant to patients with cancer who experience psychological feelings of being separated from their social network by the clinical implications of the cancer threat on a potentially shortened life. A sensitive nurse may help to alleviate that feeling of social isolation with a simple gentle touch within a relevant clinical context.

Affectionate Touch (AF) Touch that conveys warmth and emotional support from a close relationship has been shown to down regulate stress-related physiological mediators and promote well-being. An experimental study in which 34 happy married couples were randomized either to a "warm touch" or a "no touch" intervention between married couples over 4 weeks showed significant reductions in alpha-amylase levels and increased salivary oxytocin in both men and women in the warm touch group compared to the control group. However, only the husbands showed a significant reduction post treatment in 24-hour systolic pressure, suggesting a difference between men and women in response to affectionate touch [39].

Another experimental study demonstrated how a partner's touch was more effective at decreasing stress-induced heart rate and cortisol levels in women compared either to their partner's verbal support or doing nothing [40]. The physical touch within a dyad appeared to protect or buffer the effects of stress-induced neurobiological responses which have clinical implications for nurses working with patients and informal caregivers in cancer care. For example, the nurse might encourage the caregiver's physical expression of caring and connectedness with the patient through physical gestures of affectionate or gentle touch and hand holding by explaining these empirically known therapeutic effects.

As implied by previous studies, the quality of the touch is an important factor in stressful situations. A within-subject experimental study of pain perceptions based on the effects of supportive touch (that is, passive presence, gentle stroking, and/or hand holding conditions) was investigated in 51 romantic partners [41]. The main participant of the dyad received painful heat that was administered to three different areas of the left leg. The three touch conditions were found to decrease pain-related skin conductance ratings in both men and women. Skin conductance ratings refer to changes in the skin's electrical conductance due to many factors such as psychological stress, an unexpected event, or heightened emotion. All three supportive conditions were shown to decrease perceptions of pain in women over baseline, although not in men.

Significantly, hand holding had the largest effect size reduction on perceived pain and also appeared to reduce skin conductance ratings in the supportive partner as well. Individual differences in interpersonal synchrony ratings appeared to be related to the partner's dispositional empathy [41]. Synchronous ratings corresponded with high perceived empathy within the dyad. The experimental results highlight, in part, the value of social context within which touch takes place.

Perceptions of mutual support, quality of the relationship, attachment styles, gender, as well as empathic tendencies in the partners may also be factors in how partner touch is interpreted and pain is perceived. The findings have clinical applicability for nurses in cancer care by highlighting examples of supportive behaviors, such as hand holding within the couple dynamic that may facilitate more effective coping.

Physiological Studies Affectionate touch and moderate-pressure massage have been shown to increase oxytocin and endogenous opioids, especially beta-endorphins, which are associated with an activated opioid system [3]. Both interact with the stress response system. Evidence suggests that these hormones downregulate neurobiological stress-related systems that subsequently reduce anxiety and pain and promote well-being. Experimentally induced oxytocin has been associated with an increased sense of trust in human subjects, which enhances social bonding even in the absence of stress, thereby promoting positive relational behaviors [42]. Examples of positive relational behaviors include mutual respect, trust, honesty, feeling valued, support, and empathy.

Endogenous opioids produce analgesic effects and also have been shown to activate the mesolimbic dopaminergic system (i.e., reward circuitry) which enhances the cognitive expectation of a positive clinical outcome, thereby inducing the downregulation of the biological stress response system (i.e., HPA axis and ANS) [3] (review also Part IV Chap. 12). Consequently an opioid pathway and likely oxytocin are thought to mediate the relationship between touch and well-being. Massage also has been associated with increased serotonin and dopamine levels (as well as a reduction in substance P) which are also associated with reward mechanisms that promote well-being and reduce the perception of pain [3, 8]. Substance P is a neurotransmitter that modulates the perception of pain.

14.9 Clinical Research Findings

Touch appears to be an essential facilitator of development and growth, healing, and well-being via its positive effects on both interpersonal relationships and intrapersonal neurobiological processes [8, 26, 43, 44]. This section examines the effects of different forms of touch used by nurses and other therapists in the clinical setting and the effects of affectionate touch between patient-caregiver relationships or between loved ones.

Physical Touch Within the Context of the Nurse-Patient Relationship

Affective touch is thought to strengthen the sense of mutual connectedness between nurse and patient, thereby enhancing patient security [17]. Well-designed studies of the therapeutic effects of a nurse's touch on distressed patients are underrepresented.

An early qualitative study explored the use and meaning of touch in caring for patients with cancer [45]. Patterns of touch were analyzed using videotapes of nurses caring for patients as well as audiotapes of selected nurses with patients. Types of touch that were observed included comforting, connecting, working, orienting, and social touch and fell into either task-oriented or affective touch categories. The different types of touch were associated with verbal and/or nonverbal behaviors and associated meanings.

In an early between-subjects study design, the effects of the nurses' touch/no touch on males and females during preoperative teaching were assessed [46]. Overall, the men and women in the touch condition expressed more positive reactions to the upcoming surgery than the no touch group. Women in the touch group, in particular, experienced significant pre- and postoperative affective, behavioral, and physiological benefits associated with the nurse's touch compared to the no touch controls. In the recovery room, the females in the touch group had a significantly lower systolic blood pressure than females in the control group. These women were significantly less anxious about the surgery, potential complications, or an "unpleasant" hospital stay following the pre-op teaching. In contrast, males in the touch condition were more anxious than the males in the control group. For example, males in the touch group recorded higher systole ratings than the control males, postoperatively. Within the touch group, males were more anxious than females. Conversely, within the no touch control group, females were significantly more anxious than males [46].

Women and men may respond differently to a nurse's touch when the patient is in a clearly *dependent* role. Women being nurturers may also be more comfortable with tactile displays than men and consequently interpret these behaviors as being supportive rather than perceiving these behaviors negatively as the men may have in this study. The findings suggest the importance of asking permission to touch a patient's hand or arm, especially a male patient, and to sensitively evaluate its impact on the patient who for many personal reasons may not feel comfortable, regardless of the therapeutic intent of the touch. This study also highlights the importance of the clinical context such as the patient's condition, symptom presentation or medical information (e.g., a bad diagnosis, disease progression), and clinical expectations of treatment to consider within which the therapeutic intent of physical touch is more likely to occur. These findings have been subsequently supported by a recent meta-analysis of 13 studies that also revealed a sex difference in the response to affective touch with females reporting more favorable touch-related ratings than males [12].

A qualitative study examined nurses' touch and its relationship with compassion toward patients, and how patients perceived both, based on a secondary analysis of 12 interviews with 4 nurses and 8 patients from the hospital emergency, palliative, oncology, surgical, and rehabilitation units and community centers [17]. Nurses described their use of physical touch in terms of (1) the intent or motivation, (2) the desired outcome for the patient, and (3) their use of clinical observation to assess beneficial clinical changes in the patients and to identify those patients who were not optimally served by the nurse's touch, respecting the fact that patients perceive touch differently. The nurses' physical touch of the patient was also *contextualized* by the nurses' competence, knowledge, and verbal/nonverbal communications, key components of a quality nurse-patient relationship. Patients appeared to experience the nurse's compassion through touch that conveyed comfort, safety, and relief from distress, predicated on an authentic connection between nurse and patient [17].

Clinical situations that connected touch and compassion in the mind of the patient included the nurse brushing a critically ill patient's hair or holding the patient's hand with tenderness and carefulness. The quality of the touch was as significant to the patient as the act itself [17]. Patient interviews also revealed that the patients' use of the word "touch" or "cling to" served as metaphors to denote the patients' sense of connection to their nurse, inferring that a strong bond between them existed. These findings highlight the importance of a quality nurse-patient relationship in optimizing the clinical benefits of touch, in particular how the nurse's behaviors may be conveyed and understood by patients as compassionate.

Other studies have explored the potential effectiveness of effleurage or tactile touch in critically ill patients. A controlled study of 44 Swedish patients in the intensive care showed that a 5-day, hourly tactile touch intervention delivered by trained nurses significantly reduced levels of anxiety and stabilized the heart rate compared to patients in the standard care group [21]. In a within-group pre-/post-test study of the effectiveness of 10-minute hand effleurage given by trained volunteers on patients receiving chemotherapy, the findings similarly produced significant reductions in systolic blood pressure, anxiety and pain according to visual analogue scales [19]. The use of trained volunteers also raises the possibility that predisposed family caregivers might be trained by nurses to provide hand effleurage to their loved one.

The tactile touch intervention appeared to help downregulate the biological stress response system, enabling the reemergence of the parasympathetic nervous system. Tactile touch may be effective in promoting overall resilience in critically ill patients with cancer. Randomized controlled trials are needed to provide evidentiary support for the deliberate use of physical touch as a complementary therapeutic healing modality in the comprehensive care of critically ill patients with advanced cancer.

Thirty-four breast cancer survivors were randomly assigned to a classical massage intervention (two 30-minute massages/week for 5 weeks) at least 3 months after all medical treatments were completed. Results showed improved levels of depression and anxious depression compared to usual care, although a more rigorous adequately powered controlled trial would inform these results [47]. Classical massage might be a therapeutic option that nurses should discuss with survivors experiencing mood changes.

Finally, the effects of massage therapy (gentle effleurage, petrissage and the myofascial trigger points) compared to simple touch (light placement of hands at different areas of the body) on moderate-to-severe pain and symptom distress were investigated in 380 patients with advanced cancer [48]. Both the massage intervention and the simple touch intervention significantly improved mood and reduced moderate-to-severe pain experienced by patients with advanced cancer, although massage produced larger, albeit, non-sustainable effects. A nurse's attention and simple touch may be just as therapeutic as massage in certain illness-related contexts that warrant further systematic inquiry.

Immune Function Studies have also investigated the effects of massage or tactile touch interventions on the immune functions of patients with cancer with inconclusive results. A controlled study investigated the effects of massage and also progressive relaxation interventions compared to usual care in 58 survivors of breast cancer [49]. The massage and relaxation interventions were each administered for 30 min, 3 times/week for 5 weeks. Dopamine, natural killer cells, and lymphocytes progressively increased from the first to the last day of the study in the massage group compared to the relaxation and usual care groups. Significantly the interventions *started 3 months or later after the end of anticancer treatment*. These results essentially supported findings from their earlier RCT which reported significant increases over the course of the intervention in natural killer cell numbers and lymphocytes as well as in urinary dopamine and serotonin, with a significant decrease in depression and hostility compared to controls [50]. The frequency and duration of the massage are important considerations in producing therapeutic outcomes although long-term effects are unknown.

A RCT of 30 women with breast cancer investigated the effects *of full-body*, tactile touch *during radiation treatment* on circulating lymphocytes compared to usual care based on a *single* 20-minute intervention [51]. The findings showed that the tactile touch intervention not only reduced heart rate and systolic blood pressure, but appeared to decrease the rate of "deterioration" of natural killer cell activity typically associated with radiation therapy compared to controls. Tactile touch was defined as full-body, light-pressure effleurage. The timing of the single intervention with respect to the therapeutic course of the radiation treatment is not mentioned. Other findings based on massage and gentle or light touch have failed to observe immune-based clinical benefits, underscoring the importance of conducting more rigorous trials in order to determine their clinical impact across the treatment and recovery trajectory [16, 52].

In Summary
Overall, moderate-pressure massage and tactile touch appear to promote healing processes with potential benefits for the patient with cancer [49, 50]. The inconsistent immune responses to massage may be the consequence of generally poor methodological studies with small samples, and interventions that have yet to determine the appropriate frequency, duration, and optimal timing for the massage intervention as a function of the treatment and type of cancer.

The apparent short-term improvements in both psychological and physiological outcomes suggest that the therapeutic effects of physical touch within the nurse-patient relationship based on well-designed and powered clinical studies are urgently needed. The intensity, frequency, location, and different types of touch across various cancer types, stages, and the treatment and recovery continuum have yet to be fully addressed.

Facilitating Affectionate Touch Within a Close Patient-Family Caregiver Relationship

Jakubiak's model proposes that affectionate touch as evidenced by a hug, kiss, or gentle stroking within the context of a close relationship, such as the patient-caregiver relationship, induces or reinforces positive cognitive-relational changes such as feelings of security and trust within the dyad due to the recipient's accurate interpretation of the provider's hugs, caresses, or kisses. Affectionate touch reaffirms, strengthens, and/or increases affiliative seeking behaviors within the relationship. However, studies of affectionate touch within the patient and family caregiver relationship in cancer care were not located.

Physical touch between parents has been shown to produce positive well-being and adaptive behavioral and physiological synchrony and to enhance family-, paternal-, and maternal-infant bonds of attachment [43, 44]. Affectionate touch between a couple has been shown to significantly increase levels of oxytocin, which is thought to strengthen the emotional bonds between partners or spouses [4].

Clinical Anecdote 14.2
A couple were in a dressing cubicle of the recovery room, the husband in a patient gown awaiting the orderly to take him to the operating room for major cancer surgery. His wife was beside him holding his hand and supportively describing how smoothly the *whole procedure would be. She explained that the IV inserted in the OR theater typically occurs while the patient is being distracted by other things going on so that he would be unlikely to notice. Before he knew it, the operation would be over. As his wife offered further reassurances relating to the recovery room experience, she could see her husband begin to noticeably relax, even as he continued to hold onto her hand. In that moment a nurse passed in the corridor, saw the couple, and called out, "Why you two look like newly married kids," and then kept going, momentarily disrupting a moment of intimacy between the couple at a high stress moment in their lives.*

Supportive gentle touch has been shown to activate u-opioid receptors in the nucleus accumbens core (NAc) and frontal cortices of men [53]. The NAc part of the ventral striatum, located in the basal ganglia, is associated with *motivation and emotional* processes. Significantly NAc is also associated with the brain's reward pathways and dopamine receptors which have been implicated *in cognitive expectations and healing processes* [54] (review Chap. 12). As previously discussed in the chapter on placebo/nocebo effects, negative expectations borne of anxiety and fear can result in greater intensity of pain and anxiety [55, 56]. As well intended as the nurse in the clinical anecdote surely was, perhaps in the future, more nurses will intervene *prior to the date of surgery* to alleviate couple anxiety, provide emotional support, allay patient concerns, highlight the therapeutic goals of the surgery supported by relevant information to promote positive expectations of the surgery, and perhaps offer a gentle touch [57].

An experimental study of 16 married couples involved the wife being told of a potential electric shock under three conditions: (1) holding her husband's hand, (2) holding a male experimenter's hand, and (3) holding no hand [58]. The findings using functional magnetic resonance imaging (fMRI) indicated that when the wife held her husband's hand, the neurobiological stress response and emotional reactivity were more attenuated compared to holding a male experimenter's hand. Moreover, the beneficial effects of holding the husband's hand were also a function of the quality of the marital relationship. Hand holding within a higher-quality marital relationship was associated with less threat-associated neural activation in the hypothalamus, right anterior insula, and superior frontal gyrus, whereas this was not observed holding the hand of the experimenter.

Finally, the effect of touch in combination with empathy may induce dyadic physiological synchrony as assessed by an experimental study of romantic partners. Each romantic partner was randomly assigned either to serve as (1) the recipient of the pain/no pain condition (pain receiver) or (2) the partner who touches/does not touch their partner (i.e., the recipient) during the experiments (i.e., pain observer) [59]. The EKG recordings and respiratory rate showed that the partner's touch (hand holding) during the pain/no pain conditions appeared to enhance interpersonal respiratory synchrony, including increased heart rate synchrony under the pain condition. Moreover, high partner empathy combined with touch also appeared to enhance physiological synchrony. However, the recipient's pain did not induce physiological synchrony without the observer's touch. Based on other findings on the therapeutic effects of social touch, i.e., hand holding and affective touch, the partner's touch and empathy during the pain condition also appeared to trigger a reduction of perceived pain in the recipient [4]. More clinical research on the effects of physical touch within the patient-caregiver relationship may further inform the nurse's clinical strategies to strengthen the patient-caregiver relationship and their therapeutic use of dyadic touch.

14.10 Nursing Implications

Affective touch, tactile touch (pressure touch or massage), and comfort touch are an integral part of compassionate care and meaningful communication in nursing practice [17, 60, 61]. The nurse's intent, the emotional connection between nurse and patient, and the nurse's clinical knowledge and competence are all important factors in the patient's interpretation of the nurse's physical touch in response to his or her distress (review Part IV Chap. 8).

Similarly, the studies on touch within the context of partner relationships may serve as a useful frame of reference for the nurse to consider clinical strategies to promote affectionate touch within the patient-caregiver relationship. These studies provide a stepping stone toward the development of clinically relevant nurse interventions that support affectionate touch between patient and caregiver, thereby enhancing mutual support within the dyad or married couple. The findings suggest the value of encouraging dyadic hand holding, gentle hand or arm stroking, and providing back, foot, and/or hand massage in order to promote patient and even dyadic well-being.

Nursing Take-aways

1. Physical touch is optimized by the quality of the nurse-patient relationship and the nurse's therapeutic intent within the context of the patient's clinical condition. The nurse's intent is connected to the type of physical touch to be used.
2. *Comfort touch and affective touch* can alleviate an individual's emotional distress in relation to a health-related situation [13, 26].
3. *Tactile touch* which requires gentle but firm circular strokes with the palm of the hand and closed fingers (often called effleurage) may be effective in activating a parasympathetic healing response in critically ill patients [19, 21].
4. *Affectionate touch* expressed by hugs, kissing, and gentle caresses within the patient-family caregiver relationship can alleviate stress within the dyad and may potentially also strengthen the partnership relationship. Accordingly, affectionate touch should be encouraged by the nurse given evidence of its healing effects [3].
5. Physical touch is generally preceded by asking the individual's permission and by ongoing, sensitive assessments of male and female responses to touch in general given gender-related differences in perceptions of touch [17, 61].
6. The quality, intensity, timing, and duration of touch are all important factors the nurse must consider. Assess the quality of the skin for excess bruises, fragile veins, new spots, or lumps. Critically, avoid implementing all touch-related activities including massage, anywhere in the vicinity of the tumor, port-a-catheter sites, intravenous sites, or other inserted medical devices. Also avoid lymph pathways, legs, and arms with lymph edema or susceptible to lymph edema due to the extraction of lymph nodes during surgery.
7. All forms of moderate and especially deep *kneading* should be avoided on the core body.
8. Review do's and don'ts of applying moderate-pressure massage especially in supportive cancer care [62].

Given the clinical finding that effleurage can be effective in reducing the biological stress response and triggering healing processes, nurses need to reappropriate this legacy of nursing practice by acquiring the skills of foot, back, head, and hand massage from certified nurse specialists, so that healing and resilience in patients across the stages of cancer and recovery may be enhanced. Advanced practice nurses specialized in cancer care are strongly encouraged to get certified in massage techniques through massage programs in various cancer centers, such as Sloan Kettering, whether or not the nurse incorporates massage in his or her practice. Learning principles of massage may be useful for teaching simple massage techniques to partners caring for their loved ones; it can comfort caregivers with the knowledge that they can enhance the patient's physical comfort and well-being with physical touch; and in so doing, the caregiver may reassure the patient that he or she is loved and cared for and meaningfully connected with loved ones. Learning the principles and caveats of massage can also be helpful in vetting potential massage therapists outside the cancer facility who the cancer patient or survivor may want to engage for therapeutic sessions and who may not be aware of the do's and don'ts of massage in people who have or had cancer.

Clinical Anecdote 14.3
Shortly after a port-a cath was inserted just below my right clavicle for maintenance treatments I was gifted a massage to celebrate the end of treatment. For all intents and purposes, I was cancer free (that is, the tumor was undetectable). Before the massage therapist started, I had requested that only my head, arms and legs be massaged. But during an arm massage the therapist went as high as the location of the portacath and began to lightly touch it- for a brief milli-second- It was enough time to realize the educational role nurses must play in all modalities of physical touch.

More studies in which the nurse uses affective touch, comfort touch, and tactile touch to alleviate both physical and psychic pain at the bedside are needed. A nurse's touch that responds to patient cues can enhance a sense of connectedness, spirituality, and well-being and convey a *shared understanding* of the human condition between the nurse and patient [22, 26]. In so doing, the nurse's touch may momentarily ease suffering, in part by down regulating the patient's heightened emotional reactions [5]. In a reciprocal manner, the nurse often experiences a sense of well-being and satisfaction at being able to effectively comfort the patient with a timely touch on the arm.

However, not all nurses are able to convey the therapeutic meanings inherent in physical touch. Routasalo and colleagues have hypothesized that the quality of the nurse's physical touch is linked to experiential learning and attachment capabilities which the nurse brings to bear in her or his caregiving behaviors. Both influence their therapeutic work with patients, impacting for better or worse the potential for physical, emotional, cognitive, social, and physiological healing and resilience in patients.

Clinical Anecdote 14.4
G reported to the recovery room, in the early morning of her scheduled cancer surgery. She was given a brown paper bag, directed to a changing room and locker, and then told to wait on top of a transport bed in a small room adjacent to the recovery room. G was left alone. A few minutes or so later, a nurse arrived and exchanged a few administrative words, and then an orderly wheeled G to a darkish corridor just outside the operating theater where again she was left alone. G may have sat on this patient transport bed for a good 20 min. What she vividly remembers was the number of times she toyed with the idea of just hopping off the bed and walking away. She was frightened, about to undergo a life-changing operation and feeling extremely vulnerable.

A nurse's ability to extend a meaningful touch that conveys comfort, reassurance, and succor to the patient depends on many factors, including the extent to which the nurse also may be *negatively* affected by the stressful burden of work-related demands and/or burnout [63].

14.11 Final Comments

This first half of the chapter offers preliminary evidence of the importance of the nurse's touch across various clinical situations to alleviate distress and promote emotional regulation and physiological healing in patients (and caregivers) within the nurse-patient or patient-caregiver relationship. Although studies based on touch within the patient-caregiver relationship in cancer care were not widely found, the experimental studies and clinical research with other critically ill patients and even healthy volunteers strongly suggest the importance of physical touch in cancer care.

The studies, to date, on physical touch are mostly clinical studies with small samples or experimental studies with volunteers, providing a kind of proof of concept that must be replicated with more rigorous designs and adequate samples. The studies in this chapter may serve as a clinical impetus to further investigate the therapeutic effects of these different forms of physical touch particularly in the clinical setting of patients with cancer and caregivers. From a nursing perspective, more rigorous clinical trials and qualitative studies of affective, comfort, and tactile touch are required to assess their therapeutic effects across the cancer continuum.

14.12 Biofield Modalities: Therapeutic Touch (TT), Healing Touch, and Reiki

Therapeutic touch, healing touch, and reiki are energy-driven healing modalities in which the nurse's intent is to restore or alter energy fields by laying hands on or just above the individual's body for the purpose of healing [64–66]. The intent of healing touch is described as rebalancing or clearing the individual's energy fields in order to facilitate well-being and health [67]. Therapeutic touch is described as a healing practice in which the nurse moves her/his hands through energy fields in order to assess and "treat" energy imbalances [68, 69]. Reiki is a Japanese energy healing approach that touches the individual's body in order to create optimal conditions for healing the body's systems [70, 71]. These related and overlapping techniques continue to be regarded by most healthcare providers with considerable clinical skepticism. At best, these biomodalities are considered placebos. Yet recent clinical research suggests that these biofield modalities may be helpful for oncology patients who do not tolerate being either touched or massaged and who do not appear to clinically benefit from conventional anxiolytics or pain analgesia [72].

Clinical Anecdote 14.5
Ms X was in the terminal phase of her life, and despite being heavily sedated for pain, she was clearly suffering. Ms X would recoil and cry out each time the nurse gently touched her or tried to reposition her body. Her husband sat helplessly nearby watching her immobile body curled into a fetal position, her upper body moving slightly with each breath, the only signs of life. As a last resort, a nurse with only level one or two training in healing touch was asked to see the patient. And as she practiced, Ms X incredibly began to visibly relax and even to extend her legs into a seemingly more comfortable position.

Definitions

Einstein's principles of quantum physics in which humans are recognized as unitary beings of complex energy fields and networks have been propounded by nurse theorists such as Martha Rogers [73, 74]. Therapeutic touch (TT), healing touch (HT), and reiki (R) emanate from ancient healing practices based on intentional, energy-mobilizing, biofield modalities. The healer uses her or his hands as a mediator of energy to remove energy-related blockages and to restore energy flow and energy balance in and around the patient in order to reduce symptomatic sensations and to enhance healing processes and overall health [72, 75]. The practitioner typically positions his or her hands above the patient's body (therapeutic touch) or very lightly on and above the body (healing touch) or on the body (reiki) in order to rebalance his or her energy fields depending on the healing modality. Light touch is used to identify areas of energy imbalance, experienced by the healer as a change in temperature, vibration, and texture [76]. The three principles of TT are compassion, willingness to heal another, and nonattachment to the outcome [77]. TT, reiki, and healing touch are considered safe interventions with the possible exception of using these modalities with patients with psychotic disorders [72].

The Electromagnetic Field
The human biofield *refers to* "an endogenous, complex and dynamic *electromagnetic field*" [78]. *It consists of* numerous integrated waves of different frequencies generated by the myriad oscillators of the human organism which underlie self-organization and drive bio-regulation of the human organism at the molecular, cellular, and ligand-receptor biological interactional levels [79, 80]. The patterns of endogenous vibrations have been found to vary and these vibrations create electromagnetic radiation [79]. Moreover a chemical change in a molecule appears to change the pattern of its vibration and thus the emitted electromagnetic frequency pattern. This type of tangible or *veritable* energy may be measured in frequencies and wavelengths such as "magnetism," in mechanical vibrations (e.g., sound) and in radiation from the "electromagnetic spectrum" [65]. For instance, an

electrocardiogram (ECG) measures the pattern of electromagnetic fields created by the heart; and an electroencephalogram (EEG) captures the electromagnetic pattern of the brain [81, 82].

Electromagnetic radiation is thought to be associated with the different structural parts of the cell such as the proteins, glycoproteins, and lipids, but also the genetic mechanisms and transduction communications such as signaling pathways, between the nucleus and cell membrane [83]. Transduction here refers to the process of a cell surface receptor binding with its circulating ligand (such as cortisol) in order *to convert its* energy to another form within the cytoplasm which is then conveyed to DNA for transcription. The "material" structures of the body such as cells and tissues and their endogenous electromagnetic field are thought to comprise an inseparable whole [79, 83]. For instance, a magnetic resonance imaging (MRI) scan uses the body's *own magnetic field* as well as the machine's magnet and radio waves to produce clear images of soft body tissues [84].

Experiments have shown how waves interact based on Newtonian physics: whereas some waves may be enhanced, others cancel each other out [85]. Thrane and Cohen posit that these patterns may explain the interactional pattern between two human magnetic fields with results predicated on any touch-related intervention.

"Subtle" Energy

This energy type refers to difficult-to-measure "nonphysical" energy within and surrounding the human being [65]. Across cultures, subtle energy has been popularly known as the life force, vital energy, spiritual entity (western cultures), pana (India), and tai chi or qi (Chinese). According to Monzillo these terms reflect an underlying belief that humans are not just "matter" but are infused with and emit energy which may become "blocked," depleted, or imbalanced, causing illness.

Healing touch or reiki is thought to foster healing when a nurse healer mobilizes external subtle energy fields and intentionally transmits energy to the patient or individual. Humans may also mobilize their own subtle energy fields to induce innate healing via practices such as qigong, tai chi, or yoga [82]. As every cell in the human body is known to vibrate with its own electromagnetic energy field, it is possible that what is referred to as spiritual or subtle energy is energy-induced sensations that have been generated from our thoughts, beliefs, and feelings [86].

Medical scientists are considering the possibility that electromagnetic human energy may be manipulated in the near future for the purpose of enhancing, replacing, or complementing pharmacological interventions [79]. As research is at the beginning of this new medical frontier, the relationship between endogenous and exogenous energy fields remains to be elucidated. We still do not understand the underlying mechanism of how an externally mobilized energy force directed at an endogenous energy field can result in rebalancing an individual's energy field to restore healing processes.

14.13 Conceptual Underpinnings

To date there is no confirmed theory that explains how any of nursing's biofield modalities function, although the theory of quantum physics may inform our understanding of how these modalities might function [85]. Quantum physics investigates small particles of atoms such as protons, neutrons, electrons, and neutrinos and their behavior in order to describe the interactions between matter and energy. An estimated 99% of the human body is composed of atoms (https://www.symmetrymagazine.org/article/the-particle-physics-of-you#, Accessed April 28 2021). The behavior of these particles is extremely unpredictable. For instance, they have been shown to be in more than one place *at the same time*, which theorists contend is a necessary function and for which S. Laroche and D Wineland won the Nobel Prize (Nobelprize.org 2012).

One theoretical contention is that these particles are intrinsic to the human being's multidimensional energy fields and are also in continuous relationship with the environment. In keeping with principles of nature, the complex human organism is driven toward reestablishing biological order via healing processes sustained by energy [77]. When individuals experience illness, their energy resources may be blocked, depleted, or out of balance. According to Hanley, TT is an energy process reflective of the interactional human-environment that helps the individual "bring order out of the disorder caused by the illness" [77].

The energy of healing touch, therapeutic touch, and reiki is thought to be transmitted bidirectionally between therapist and patient, but is mainly directed toward the patient via the *intentional use* of the therapists' energy flow. These healing modalities are thought to regulate the energy field around the patient's body and the *chakras or subtle energy centers*, controlling energy transfer from the external to the internal environment of the patient, via the deliberate movements of the therapist's hands [65]. Restoring the patient's flow and balance of the energy field is thought to facilitate the restoration of the patient's neurobiological healing processes.

Clinical Anecdote 14.6
In the spring of 2005, I was enjoying the life-affirming offerings of a one-week hike with friends through the Pyrenees mountains. On this particular day, our hiking path led us to the top of a mountain ridge enveloped by undulating mauve and green mountain peaks. My only complaint was a bum knee that had blown up after three days of arduous ascents and rocky descents, along tricky pathways that meandered across brooks, forests and meadows.

At the summit, a rambling stone wall presented the perfect opportunity to give my sore knee a timely respite. I stretched my leg along its surface to absorb the soothing rays of a scorching sun. Chatting away to a pal beside me, I was suddenly startled by a laser- like jet of heat cutting through the centre of my knee, and turned sharply to discover a member of our group with his hands about 6–7 inches above my knee. Crimson cheeks betrayed his embarrassment at my profound surprise.

'I was just trying to help,' he said. *While I clearly remember the heat from his 'intention', my knee nonetheless continued to be problematic for the rest of the rather challenging hike. My determination to continue the hike may have inhibited the possibility for further healing. I will never know. But the strange sensation in my knee has remained all these years as a mystery, that appeared to emanate from his hands, without touching me. It was in retrospect my first encounter with a biofield modality.*

14.14 Research Findings

Reviews of the potential effects of therapeutic touch or reiki on psychological, physical, and physiological outcomes in different patient and practitioner populations have shown mixed results [70, 87–89]. Meta-analyses are lacking due to few well-designed RCTs. The majority of studies tend to be pilot or feasibility studies with small convenience samples, lacking both blinding and a control group. Notwithstanding, a few systematic reviews have identified moderate-to-strongly designed studies according to CONSORT and/or JADAD guidelines [70, 88–90].

Given the questionable research methods against a backdrop of considerable scientific skepticism, the studies of reiki or therapeutic touch that were selected for this chapter met the following inclusion criteria: (a) RCT, crossover or experimental design, (b) samples of at least 20 individuals per group, (c) only one biotherapy assessed in a given study with experienced practitioners, (d) a control group and/or sham placebo group, included (e) at least single blinding, and (f) no distant healing. These criteria meant that studies based on cancer patients were sacrificed so that studies with a stronger research design could serve as the basis for better evaluat the potential efficacy of the biofield modality.

Symptom Relief

Depression A few studies have shown significant improvements in the psychological symptoms of individuals with various chronic conditions including cancer. For instance, in a randomized, three-arm, single-blinded, and placebo-controlled trial, 90 elderly volunteers with depression and no previous experience with reiki who lived in a nursing home were randomly assigned to receive either (1) reiki given by a reiki master ($n = 30$), (2) sham reiki given by nurses without reiki training but believing they were doing reiki ($n = 30$), or (3) control group ($n = 30$) [91]. The reiki intervention consisted of eight weekly sessions of 45–60 min. There was a significant decrease in depression scores for participants in the reiki group over baseline scores at 4, 8, and 12 weeks posttreatment (all $p < 0.001$), as well as compared to either the sham or control groups at the 4-, 8-, and 12-week assessments (all $p < 0.001$) indicating a significant duration of reiki effects for at least 4 weeks post-intervention. Reiki may be an effective therapeutic for depression in the elderly; The research design should be replicated to assess the effectiveness of reiki in depressed patients with cancer.

Depression and Physiological Indicators A block randomized controlled trial assessed the effects of healing touch or relaxation on cellular immune functioning and depressed mood in 60 women with cervical cancer, who were randomly assigned to 1 of 3 conditions: (1) the five techniques of healing touch (HT), (2) relaxation training (RT), and (3) usual care [92]. During the 6-week chemoradiation treatment, patients received either HT or RT immediately following radiation therapy. The healing touch or relaxation training sessions lasted 20–30 min and were given 4 times a week for 6 weeks. Patients were assessed with validated psychosocial instruments and blood work before treatment at baseline and at weeks 4 and 6.

The HT intervention had a significant effect in *minimizing* the decline of natural killer cell cytotoxicity (NKCC) during the course of chemoradiation [92]. The HT group also showed a significant reduction in depressed mood (based on two measures of depression: the CESD and POMS) compared to the RT and usual care groups ($p < 0.05$). In contrast, the RT and usual care groups showed a significant *decrease* in NKCC during chemoradiation (based on a group by time interaction, $p = 0.018$). NS differences were obtained for measures of quality of life, fatigue, or clinically related toxicities.

An HT intervention during chemoradiation may help to buffer the toxic effects of chemoradiation on cellular immunity and depressed mood. The fact that participants learned their group assignment after randomization may have played a role in the clinical outcomes. The study should be replicated with an added sham HT placebo group, control group, and double blinding if possible (researchers/experimenters and participants) to the goals of treatment and group assignments.

Pain, Anxiety, and Depression A randomized, single-blinded placebo-controlled study assessed the clinical effects of reiki in 120 stressed patients with chronic illnesses which included patients with cancer (8%) [93]. Patients were randomly assigned to one of four treatment groups: (1) reiki ($n = 30$), (2) sham reiki placebo ($n = 30$), (3) progressive muscle relaxation, and (4) control group ($n = 30$). Full-body reiki was administered by three reiki masters in 30-min sessions, *twice weekly for 5 weeks*. The sham reiki was given by four assistants with no reiki experience. Compared to all the other groups, reiki was significantly more effective in reducing pain, depression, and state/trait anxiety. A within-group analysis of the reiki group showed that more men than women experienced a reduction in depression but more women than men experienced an increased sense of faith. Reiki also was found to significantly improve self-esteem and showed a nonsignificant improvement in sense of personal control. Reiki may be a useful complementary therapy for patients with cancer afflicted by anxiety, depression, and pain.

Post-traumatic Stress and Intrusive Ideation A 22% incidence of post-traumatic stress disorder has been reported in individuals 6 months after a diagnosis of cancer compared to 6%, 4 years later [94]. Intrusive ideation and avoidant behaviors are well-documented reactions to traumatizing events that have been observed in patients with cancer, particularly in response to a life-threatening diagnosis or cancer recurrence. These intrusive and avoidant behaviors have also been observed in response to life-threatening events, such as war [94]. A two-armed, randomized controlled crossover waitlist trial assessed the effects of healing touch on combat veterans suffering from PTSD [95]. Symptoms included re-experiencing the traumatic events, use of cognitive and behavioral avoidance of known trauma triggers, and hyper-emotional reactivity. In phase 1 of the study, 40 war veterans were randomly assigned to receive(1) the intervention ($n = 20$), healing touch plus standard care followed by a transfer to the standard care control condition, and (2) the standard control condition ($n = 19$) (one participant dropped out), consisted of standard care followed by a transfer to the experimental condition.

Healing touch (HT) was administered by a certified healing therapist in ten weekly treatments of 60 min during which two different HT protocols were delivered (see [95]). Standard care consisted of medications, psychotherapy, relaxation, meditation, archery, or yoga. PTSD was assessed with the PTSD checklist (PCL-5) based on the DSM-5 medical manual of mental health disorders (PCL-5) (https://www.ptsd.va.gov/professional/assessment/adult-sr/ptsd-checklist. Accessed 30 April, 2021). The PCL-5 has a score range between 0 and 80. A score ≥ 33 indicates a provisional diagnosis of PTSD; a change score of 5 points indicates a clinical response to treatment; a change ≥ 10 indicates a clinically meaningful improvement. The intervention plus standard care significantly reduced symptom severity with a clinically significant decrease (18.11 points) that was sustainable at a follow-up assessment 3 months later [95]. Whereas the authors recommend further study with a larger sample, the findings suggest that healing touch may be helpful for patients experiencing emotional distress accompanied by intrusive ideation and should be studied in a cancer population based on a rigorous adequately powered design that includes a sham healing placebo group, standard care group, and the intervention group given by a certified healing therapist.

Quality of Life (QOL)

In a randomized, double-blinded, placebo-controlled study, 116 in-hospital patients on isolation with blood cancer were randomized to receive either (1) reiki given by a reiki master ($n = 58$) or (2) sham reiki ($n = 42$) given by sham therapists, that is, not qualified in reiki [96]. Reiki was given twice weekly for 4 weeks, each session lasting 60 min. Reiki was shown to significantly increase overall quality of life over baseline, including the QOL dimensions of physical, environmental, and social QOL, though not psychological QOL. In addition, the reiki group scored higher on overall QOL and the social relations dimension, compared to the sham reiki group, suggesting that reiki may be a useful therapeutic intervention for enhancing well-being in hospitalized patients with blood cancer. The analyses did not address the fact that 16 patients died following recruitment into the sham reiki group and whether they differed from the participants who remained in the study. A future RCT with a larger powered sample to accommodate the number of statistical analyses done would further inform the use of reiki for patients with blood cancer.

Well-Being and Comfort A double-blinded RCT assessed the effect of reiki on the well-being of 189 patients receiving chemotherapy. Patients were assigned to (1) the reiki intervention, (2) sham reiki, and (3) standard care [97]. Reiki was provided by a nurse who was a reiki master, in a single, 20-min intervention. Sham reiki was provided by a nurse who was told what positions to follow during the sham intervention and to use cognitive distraction such as counting backward and making a shopping list.

Both the reiki and sham interventions demonstrated significant improvements over baseline measures for comfort and well-being. There were nonsignificant differences between the two groups on patient comfort and well-being posttreatment. The nonsignificant difference between the reiki and sham modalities raises at least three possible explanations. First, the nonsignificant difference between the single reiki and sham reiki suggests that the improvement in well-being and comfort might be caused more by the individual's *cognitive expectations of a* clinical benefit in both the sham and reiki groups (review Chap. 12). Second, the effects of both the reiki and sham reiki interventions might be attributed to gentle touch which has been shown to trigger therapeutic effects along C-tactile afferents, as described in the previous section on physical touch [98]. Third, the nonsignificant finding may highlight the need for more than one reiki session in order to produce a dosing effect, as evidenced by other studies [95]. As well as only a 20-min session, it is unclear whether the reiki intervention included all its therapeutic components. Notwithstanding, other studies based on one reiki session have been found to be effective [99], suggesting that other factors, such as the purpose of the intervention, the clinical condition, length of time of the session, and/or the physiological and clinical measures, must be taken into consideration.

Healthcare Providers and Reiki

Healthcare provider (HCP) burnout is a frequently discussed concern of nurses in practice [100, 101]. Burnout is an energy-depleting condition distinguished by emotional exhaustion, reduced feelings of personal accomplishment, and a sense of depersonalization. A placebo-controlled, repeated-measures crossover, single-blinded randomized trial assessed the effects of reiki versus sham reiki on a number of physiological variables associated with burnout syndrome [71]. An experienced level 3 reiki therapist carried out the intervention in the reiki group, whereas a nurse without any experience in reiki used the same hand positions without intention in the sham reiki group. Both groups completed one session taking an estimated 30 min.

Results showed that after reiki, the standard deviation of the normal-to-normal intervals of time between heart beats (SDNN) and temperature, but not cortisol, was significantly *higher* than after sham reiki. The SDNN is a measure of heart rate variability (HRV). Conversely, the low-frequency (LF) component associated with sympathetic activity was significantly lower than the LF measured from the sham reiki group.

The significantly *higher* SDNN (i.e., greater variation in milliseconds in the R-R intervals), along with the *significantly decreased* LF (i.e., lower sympathetic activity), indicated that the autonomic nervous system had been shifted toward the parasympathetic nervous system (PNS) which increased HRV [71]. A lower HRV occurs with increased anxiety or stress which over time poses an increased risk for health problems, including early death. The study appears to demonstrate the possible effects of an energy modality on human physiology, and specifically the cardiac system, which depends on its endogenous electromagnetic field to function properly throughout the human body. Reiki may be a useful intervention for healthcare providers who are suffering from burnout. Although participants were blinded to the treatment assignment, it is possible that at least some participants recognized the reiki and sham reiki practices. Further study is required to determine the dosing effects of any biofield modality in terms of the length of each session and the number of sessions required to sustain a therapeutic effect after treatment.

Clinical Anecdote 14.7

The ICU once called our team with an unusual request. A patient with advanced cancer on a ventilator was "fighting" the intubation. She was restless and agitated. Although she was receiving sedation and her husband was trying to reassure his wife, she was unable to settle. So as a last-gap measure, the ICU nurse suggested the surprising option of healing touch. She was just about to launch into an explanation of the intervention, when the husband interjected. He had heard about healing touch and was willing to try anything to help his wife. By drawing the curtains around the patient's bed, the nurse created an intimate space between herself and the patient in order to enable healing capabilities. Within a few moments of the nurse's interventions, the patient's breathing fell in synchrony with the respirator's rate, and she fell asleep.

Experimental Animal Research

Although findings from animal studies do not necessarily translate to humans, one study highlighted some interesting potential effects of therapeutic touch. Gronowicz and colleagues assessed evidence of metastasis and immune cell changes *in mice* assigned to the therapeutic touch intervention, mock treatment, or controls. The therapeutic touch group showed significantly less evidence of metastasis than the mock treatment group. Whereas cancer was associated with the significant increase of 11 cytokines in the control group, the TT group appeared to show a significant decrease in cytokines such as IL-1a, MIG, IL-1b, and MIP-2. Moreover, the TT group of mice also showed a significant reduction in the percentage of macrophages and pro-inflammatory cytokines which have been associated with tumor progression in breast cancer patients [102]. Other experimental biological studies appear to show the same positive effects of therapeutic touch on normal human cells and osteosarcoma [65]. These findings are interesting in that they were also obtained independent of placebo effects typically associated with cognitive expectations.

14.15 Clinical Research Caveats

How biofield therapies directly or indirectly affect the human mind and body in order to promote healing and resilience remains unclear. One hypothesis that appears to have little to do with the energy-driven hypotheses of biofield modalities is that healing touch and reiki are "placebo" interventions in which healing-promoting pathways are mobilized by the patient's *cognitive expectation* (beliefs) of therapeutic benefits. This perspective does not explain the changes at the cellular level that experimental studies of human cells and rodents have demonstrated. Nor does it explain the significant differences between healing touch and sham touch as the studies above have reported. But it is conceivable that conscious expectations of patients may in fact synergize or optimize the effects of a biofield modality in consciously aware individuals.

This brings me to the clinical issue of using therapeutic touch to relieve pain across all stages of development. One study that was located failed to show any effects of therapeutic touch in preterm infants during a painful heel prick [103]. From a cognitive expectation perspective, this intervention *would not be* expected to result in significant clinical benefits. From a procedural perspective, a therapeutic touch intervention *would also not be* expected to result in clinical benefits for a heel prick that generally produces a short-lived painful sensation. The ephemeral nature of the painful procedure would appear to be fundamentally incompatible with a TT approach. Therapeutic touch and healing touch generally require more than one session of 20–45 min each, which precludes its usefulness in assuaging a briefly painful heel prick [92, 95]. Moreover, the clinical environment also would not have been conducive to a TT intervention in which a barrier between the TT therapist and the baby existed with only openings for the TT's arms and hands, thereby disrupting putative energy fields according to current scientific understanding of electromagnetic biofields [79, 101, 104]. A soothing parent using cuddling and gentle and affectionate touching would heal a crying infant's experience of pain much more effectively.

As findings from the studies above suggest, reiki, healing touch, and therapeutic touch effects appear to be dose-dependent, usually requiring more than one session to elicit a healing response. These modalities may be most effective in improving symptoms associated with critical and chronic illness and the side effects of medical treatment in which it might be argued that energy dysregulation is likely present [71]. As in all potential treatments, there must be a fit among the health-related condition, the clinical goals of the intended clinical modality, and an enabling clinical environment.

Clinical studies of biofield modalities require more well-designed, double-blinded, adequately powered, randomized controlled trials that include a sham placebo and a reiki master or therapeutic touch-certified expert to carry out the biofield intervention in a clinical environment which enables the therapist's use of all needed components of the intervention to unblock and facilitate energy flow according to their respective healing modality.

14.16 Final Thoughts

This review finds that reiki, healing touch, and therapeutic touch may be effective for managing symptoms of pain, anxiety, depression, and intrusive ideation in individuals with chronic conditions including cancer. Rigorously designed studies with adequately sized samples and a sham as well as control group would strengthen the potential interpretation of the findings. Clinical investigations are needed to determine the medical conditions for which therapeutic touch, healing touch, or reiki would be a potentially effective adjunct treatment. The potential effects of these biofield modalities on the individual's physiological parameters and especially immune functioning in patients with cancer is an interesting area with obvious clinical implications for immunosuppressed patients undergoing treatment [79, 92].

Other areas of critical inquiry concern whether reiki or healing touch could potentially reduce the amount of medication or provide synergistic effects with conventional medicine in order to alleviate pain, anxiety, and other symptoms in cancer patients [95]. Finally, TT and reiki may be a useful healing intervention to reduce stress in nurses [1].

Appendix: Mind-Body (MBSR). Psychosocial Interventions—Multimodal Interventions—Mind-body (MBSR), Energy, and Other CTs

Author	Purpose/intervention	Study design	Sample/phase of disease	Outcomes
Hall et al. [105]	To evaluate mind-body (M-B) approaches on fear of cancer recurrence (FOCR) Interventions included one therapy ($k = 9$) or in combination ($k = 10$) (a) mindfulness-based stress reduction (MBSR) (b) relaxation with cognitive behavioral, relaxation and meditation movement (tai chi, qigong, yoga), meditation and other CTs, psychoeducational, TCM ($k = 1$) (c) CBT skills, therapies that include spirituality, meaning, existential therapy, meaning therapy, expressive arts in oncology patients	Systematic review and meta-analysis Duration of interventions varied Ranged from 9 days to 12 months Cochrane criteria used to assess bias	19 RCTs (pooled $N = 2806$) Patients had breast ($k = 11$, 84%), prostate ($k = 3$, 16%), gynecological ($k = 1$, 5%), melanoma ($k = 1$, 5%) cancers Treatment status (a) 5 studies had patients undergoing active treatment (26%) (b) 14 studies (74%) had patients who had finished treatment for early-stage disease or were being actively watched	(1) Types of interventions (a) Interventions with only one MB strategy ($k = 9$) or included multiple M-B elements ($k = 10$) (b) CBT skills ($k = 11$, 58%) were most common MB component (c) Meditation practices ($k = 10$, 53%) (d) Relaxation exercises ($k = 4$, 21%) (2) Re analyses from preintervention to postintervention (median 2 months) (a) Small-to-medium pooled effect sizes were found (Hedges $g = -0.36$, 95% CI= -0.49 to -0.23, ($P < 0.001$) (b) Significant heterogeneity ($I^2 = 47.99$) (3) Re analyses from preintervention to follow-up (median 8 months) (a) Pooled effect size was significant at ($g = -0.31$, 95% CI = -0.47 to -0.16, $P = 0.001$) Conclusion (1) Effective in reducing emotional distress with small to moderate effect size reductions across studies (2) But heterogeneity across studies also present ($I^2 = 63.36$) (3) 84% of patients had breast cancer intervention: needs to be reproduced in patients with other cancers (4) Given the high proportion of patients who dropped out of the intervention, an analysis of causes needed before mounting another study

(continued)

Appendix: Continued

Author	Purpose/intervention	Study design	Sample/phase of disease	Outcomes
Lee et al. [106]	Assess effects of massage therapy on cancer pain	Meta-analysis Used a random effects model for analysis Used PEDro scale and Cochrane risk of bias for study quality in meta-analysis; Chi-square and Higgins I^2 tests to assess heterogeneity of the data	(a) 12 studies with 559 participants (9 RCTs and 3 nonrandomized controlled clinical trials) (b) included studies with all types of cancer, breast cancer, digestive cancer	(1) Types of massage in final sample Body massage ($k = 7$), foot reflexology ($k = 4$), and aroma massage ($k = 2$) (2) Overall effect of massage on cancer pain (12 studies) (a) The effect of massage therapy on cancer pain was significant at (SMD −1.25, 95% CI −1.63 to −0.87), $P < 0.00001$ (3) Effects of massage therapy according to cause of pain (subgroup meta-analysis) (a) Massage had a significant inverse effect on treatment-related cancer pain especially postsurgery (3 studies) (SMD −1.86 (95% CI −2.78 to −0.94), $P < 0.0001$)

Massage. Complementary therapies (CTs) on symptom distress in patients with cancer and caregivers: mind-body, energy, and other CTs

Lee et al. [106]	(b) Massage had a significant inverse effect on cancer pain after chemotherapy ($k = 3$ studies) (SMD -0.98 (95% CI -1.69 to -0.26), $P = 0.007$ (c) Massage had a significant negative effect on cancer pain related to metastases ($k = 3$) (SMD -1.29 (95% CI -1.64 to -0.95), $P < 0.00001$ (d) Massage showed a significant negative effect on cancer pain associated with symptom cluster ($k = 4$) (SMD -1.08 (95% CI -1.47 to -0.70), $P < 0.00001$) (4) Effects of massage therapy according to cancer type A sub-meta-analysis showed that the effects of massage on all types of cancer were significant ($k = 7$) (SMD -1.11 (95% CI -1.50 to -0.71), $P < 0.00001$). Subanalyses showed that massage therapy was particularly effective in reducing pain in patients with breast cancer and digestive cancer (5) Effects of massage therapy according to massage type (a) Body massage ($k = 7$) had significant effects on cancer related pain (SMD -1.11 (95% CL -1.50 to -0.71) ($P < 0.00001$) (b) Foot reflexology ($k = 4$) was significantly effective (SMD -1.46 (95% CI -2.45 to -0.47), $P = 0.004$ (c) Aroma massage showed significant effects in 2 studies: (SMD -1.26 (95% CI -1.83 to -0.69) $P < 0.0001$) Conclusion Quality of studies ranged from 5-9 according to PEDRO scoring; 9 studies were deemed high quality (score ≥ 6) Cochrane risk of bias varied widely across studies

(continued)

Appendix: Continued

Author	Purpose/intervention	Study design	Sample/phase of disease	Outcomes
Kinkead et al. [107]	To investigate effect of Swedish massage (SMT) compared to light touch (LT) and waitlist controls (WLC) on persistent cancer-related fatigue in survivors of breast cancer Intervention 45 min/session every week for 6 weeks	Early phase single masked, 3-arm 6-week study	57/66 women with past stage 0–III breast cancer who had received surgery, radiation, and/or chemotherapy/chemoprevention	(1) Based on the multidimensional fatigue scale (MFI) at 6 weeks postintervention (a) SMT (M: −16.50 (6.37), $n = 20$) vs LT (M: −8.06 (6.50), $n = 20$) vs WLC (M: +5.88 (6.48), $n = 17$): treatment by time: $p < 0.0001$ The SMT was more effective in reducing fatigue after 6 weekly sessions than the other two modalities (2) Based on the NIH-PROMIS fatigue scale at 6 weeks (a) SMT (M: 5.49 (2.53)) vs LT (M: −3.24 (2.57)) vs WLC (M: −0.06 (1.88)): treatment by time: $p < 0.0008$ Conclusion SMT produced clinically significant reduction in fatigue, though duration of effects unclear

Reflexology. Complementary therapies (CTs) on symptom distress in patients with cancer and caregivers: mind-body, energy, and other CTs

| Tarrasch et al. [108] | To assess effects of reflexology treatment on quality of life, sleep disturbances, and fatigue in patients with breast cancer undergoing radiation therapy. Intervention 1/week × 10 weeks, 30 min/session 5–6 weeks coincided with radiation therapy plus 4–5 weeks after the end of radiation | Women self-assigned to (1) reflexology (2) controls | 58/72 women stages I–II | (1) Fatigue outcomes
  (a) Significant interaction between group and time (F(2, 10) = 4.50, p = 0.001). Fatigue levels significantly increased in controls over time whereas no increase in fatigue levels observed in reflexology group
(2) Quality of life
  (a) Significant interactional effect between group and time (F(2, 112) = 4.06, p = 0.02). Source of interaction derived from significant decrease in QOL in controls over time, i.e., T2 (p = 0.01) and T3 (p = 0.03) whereas quality of life in reflexology group improved
(3) Quality of sleep
  (a) Significant interactional effects between group and time (F(2, 112) = 3.44, p = 0.04). Source of interaction derived from improved sleep in reflexology group and decrease, then slight increase in controls
(4) Pain
  (a) Analysis of current pain nonsignificant F(2, 112) = 1.95, p = 0.15, i.e., no significant differences in pain in the reflexology group; pain increased in controls between T1 and T2 (p = 0.01), between T2 and T3 (p = 0.03)
  (b) Analysis of average pain in the previous week NS between group and time (f(2, 112) = 2.31, p = 0.10); average pain level also increased in controls between T1 and T2 (p = 0.03) and declined between T2 and T3 (p = 0.02)
  (c) Analysis of maximum pain in previous week Showed significant interactions between group and time F(2, 112) = 3.81, p = 0.03. Significant increase between T1 and T2 (p = 0.003) and T2 and T3 (p = 0.05) in worst pain observed in control group
Conclusion
(1) Reflexology may exert positive effect on pain, quality of sleep, fatigue, and quality of life in patients with breast cancer during radiation therapy
(2) whereas women self-selected into groups may be seen to be a bias of study—the fact that they showed significant improvement suggests the value of this intervention for all patients who want it |

(continued)

Appendix: Continued

Author	Purpose/intervention	Study design	Sample/phase of disease	Outcomes

Mantoudi et al. [109]	Effects of reflexology versus relaxation on pain, anxiety, depression, and quality of life	Sample was randomly assigned to
		(a) reflexology group ($n = 40$)
		(b) relaxation group ($n = 40$) and used an experimental design Number of sessions for each group was 6, 30 min weekly sessions
		Assessments made at baseline, 4th, and 6th week of interventions
			88 distressed patients with cancer	(1) Reflexology and relaxation groups showed significant improvements in anxiety and depression at week 4
				  (a) Reflexology and relaxation groups; NS difference at baseline for anxiety ($p = 0.796$) and depression ($p = 0.459$)
				  (b) At week 4 both groups significantly reduced levels of anxiety and depression over baseline scores ($p = <0.001$)
				(2) Anxiety: percent changes from baseline to week 4 and to week 6
				  (a) The reflexology group showed a greater percent reduction in anxiety levels at week 4 than the relaxation group, though not attaining significance ($p = 0.06$)
				  (b) The reflexology group showed a greater significant percent reduction in anxiety at week 6 compared to the relaxation group ($p = 0.005$)
				(3) Depression: percent changes from baseline to week 4 and to week 6:
				  (a) Reflexology showed a significant and greater reduction in depression scores compared to relaxation at week 4 ($p = 0.0.006$)
				  (b) Reflexology also showed a greater reduction in depression scores compared to relaxation, at week 6, which was significant at $p = 0.001$
				(4) Physical health: percent change from baseline to week 4, and to week 6
				  (a) The percent changes for both groups were similar and not significantly different at week 4 ($p = 0.149$)
				  (b) The percent changes at week 6 showed significant improvement of reflexology group compared to relaxation group at $p < 0.001$
				(5) Mental health: percent change from baseline to week 4, and to week 6
				  (a) Mental health changes for both groups were similar at week 4, and nonsignificantly different $p = 0.244$
				  (b) At week 6, mental health changes were greater for the reflexology group than the relaxation group, attaining significance at $p = 0.017$

Mantoudi et al. [109]				(6) Pain scores percent change from baseline to week 4, and to week 6 (a) Percent change from baseline to week 4 was similar for both groups evidenced by NS difference ($p = 0.536$) (b) Percent change from baseline to week 6 showed a reduced pain score for the reflexology group compared to the relaxation group, which did not attain significance ($p = 0.207$) Conclusion (1) No control group, underpowered sample size for number of variables (2) Potential trends in the effects of both reflexology and relaxation on the well-being of cancer patients that need to be investigated with a more rigorously designed RCT (3) The results from this study have a high risk of bias
Toygar et al. [110]	To investigate effects of foot reflexology on anxiety and sleep in informal caregivers of patients with cancer Intervention 3 consecutive days following hospitalization 30 min sessions Reflexology: pressed on reflexology points on sole of foot Placebo Gently rubbed sole of foot	RCT—double-blind placebo-controlled study RA to (1) intervention (2) placebo	66 Caregivers of patients on a university oncology unit	(1) Baseline scores for state anxiety and sleep at baseline were NS (2) Posttreatment: sleep (a) reflexology (M: 441.82 (±35.51)) vs placebo (M 409.55 (±50.08)), $p = 0.001$ (3) Posttreatment: anxiety (a) reflexology (M: 38.91 (±5.63)) vs placebo (M: 46.30 (±11.29)), $p = 0.004$ Reflexology compared to placebo had a greater effect on reducing anxiety in informal caregivers Conclusion (1) Reflexology was effective in reducing anxiety and improving quality of sleep of informal caregivers (2) Need a control group to strengthen design (3) Differences between the two groups in marital status

(continued)

Appendix: Continued

Author	Purpose/intervention	Study design	Sample/phase of disease	Outcomes
Music. Complementary therapies (CTs) on symptom distress in patients with cancer and caregivers: mind-body, energy, and other CTs				
Bradt et al. [111]	To assess and compare effects of music therapy and music medicine interventions on psychological and physical outcomes in people with cancer Interventions (a) music therapy interventions by trained music therapists (b) music medicine interventions based on listening to prerecorded music offered by oncology team	Cochrane library systematic review/meta-analysis 52 RCT and quasi-randomized trials	3731 people with cancer based on 52 trials (a) 23 trials as music therapy (b) 29 trials as music medicine	(1) Music interventions appear to significantly reduce anxiety in patients with cancer (i.e., with an average reduction in anxiety of 8.54 units ($P < 0.0001$) based on the Spielberger state anxiety Inventory (SSAI) (2) 13 studies ($n = 1028$) showed a significant reduction in Trait anxiety using Spielberger ($P < 0.00001$) (3) Other anxiety scales yielded moderate to strong inverse effects with low quality evidence (4) 7 studies ($n = 723$) showed moderately strong positive effects on depression based on low quality evidence, and to be regarded with caution (5) NS effects of music interventions on mood or distress (6) Music may lead to small decreases in heart rate, respiratory rate, blood pressure, but not oxygen saturation (7) 7 studies ($n = 528$) reported a large pain reducing effect, but evidence again of low quality ($p = 0.001$) (8) Effects on quality of life uncertain given the large confidence interval and low quality evidence (9) Comparison between music therapy and music medicine based on 3 studies ($n = 132$) suggests moderate effects of music therapy over music medicine on quality of life, but evidence is low quality Conclusion: High bias risk across studies

Acupuncture. Complementary therapies (CTs) on symptom distress in patients with cancer and caregivers: mind-body, energy, and other CTs

Chiu et al. [112]	To assess the effects of acupuncture on cancer-related pain, chemotherapy-related pain (CT), radiation therapy-induced pain (RT), surgery-induced pain (ST), and hormone therapy-induced pain (HT)	(a) Systematic review and RCTs for meta-analysis (b) Used a random effect model for analysis (c) Cochrane statistic Q assessed between study heterogeneity and I^2, the magnitude of heterogeneity ($I^2 \leq 50\%$ sig. little heterogeneity observed)	29 studies ($n = 2213$) used in qualitative synthesis 36 studies for meta-analysis Studies based on patients with a wide range of cancers	(1) Overall effect of acupuncture on cancer-related pain Analysis showed that acupuncture had a significant small effect size reduction on cancer-related pain: -0.45 (95% CI= -0.63 to -0.26). Significant heterogeneity was present ($Q < -96.17$, $P < 0.001$; $I^2 =$ 63.6%) (2) Effect of acupuncture on malignancy-related pain ($k = 17$ trials) Pooled weighted mean effect size was moderate at -0.71 and significant based on 95% CI = -0.94 to -0.48. The Cochran's Q statistic (24.39) and I^2 values indicate trend to homogeneity ($P = 0.08$) among the 17 trials (3) Effect of acupuncture on CT or RT-induced pain ($k = 11$) No evidence of therapeutic effect of acupuncture on either CT or RT-induced pain ($g = -0.05$, 95% CI= -0.33 to 0.24) Heterogeneity also found ($Q = 21.35$, $P = 0.02$, $I^2 = 53.15$)
Chiu et al. [112]				(4) Effect of acupuncture on surgery-induced pain ($k = 5$) Pooled weighted mean effect size was significant at -0.40 (95% CI = -0.69 to -0.10). The Q statistic and I^2 indicate homogeneity among the trials ($Q = 5.95$; $P = 0.20$, $I^2 = 32.9$) (5) The treatment effects of acupuncture compared to sham acupuncture showed a greater effect size which was still NS ($g = -0.64$, 95% CI = -1.55 to 0.27) Heterogeneity also present ($Q = 12.84$, $P = 0.002$, $I^2 = 84.42$) Conclusion (a) Notwithstanding the substantial heterogeneity among studies, this meta-analysis provided evidence of the differential effects of acupuncture on pain, by grouping acupuncture studies according to the type of cancer-related pain (b) Most of the studies however lack description of the actual procedure for conducting acupuncture (c) Various forms of sham acupuncture for controls were used (d) Underlying biological processes remain unknown, but may vary according to the cancer type

(continued)

Appendix: Continued

Author	Purpose/intervention	Study design	Sample/phase of disease	Outcomes
Anderson and Taylor [113]	To evaluate effect of healing touch as an adjunct supportive intervention	Systematic review of randomized controlled trials JADAD score is used to assess methodological quality—5 points total (a) description of trial as randomized +1 if method described; −1 for inappropriate method (b) blinding subjects gets 1 point (c) 1 point for details about withdrawals/dropouts (d) 1 point Blinding of evaluator	5 RCTs included in review/327 excluded Of 5 included (1) 4 used a parallel group design (2) one used a crossover design	(1) Quality scores ranged from 2 to 5/5 (2) Post-White (crossover design) diverse cancer patients, with a 2/5 JADAD score (a) Healing touch intervention showed significant reduction in respiratory rate, heart rate, BP, current pain, and total mood disturbance and fatigue over baseline (b) Healing touch more effective than presence in decreasing levels of respiratory rate and heart rate (3) Cook et al. parallel, 2 groups breast or gynecological ca, blinding with 5/5 jadad (a) Significant increase in overall functional score, emotional role functioning, mental health, health transition with healing touch compared to controls (b) Significant increases also with Mock healing touch in: health transition, physical functioning Conclusion Nonconclusive, poor quality evidence The lack of protocols or manuals to standardize the healing touch intervention, heterogenous cancer groups, lack of standard measures across studies, one study lacked a control group

Acupuncture vs CBT. Psychosocial interventions: mind-body, energy, and other CTs

Garland et al. [114]	Effects of acupuncture compared to CBT on insomnia Interventions CBT-I: 5 weekly sessions plus 2 biweekly sessions: first session = 60 min; other sessions = 30 min each (1) manualized multicomponents (see supplementary Materials online for the protocol) (2) sleep restriction strategies, stimulus control, cognitive restructuring, address sleep-related anxiety, relaxation training, education about healthy sleep hygiene	Pragmatic study design based on a dual-center, parallel group randomized comparative, effectiveness trial A pragmatic trial design used to inform the patient/clinical decisions in real world PI, coinvestigators, statistician were blinded to RA: Patients, research staff, and treatment therapists were not blinded RCT compared 8 weeks of acupuncture ($n = 80$) with 8 weeks of cognitive–behavioral therapy ($n = 80$) tailored for insomnia (CBT-I)	$N = 160$ men and women survivors of cancer	(1) At 8 weeks posttreatment CBT-I showed a larger and significant effect size reduction (M: −10.91; 95% CI, −11.97 to −9.85) compared to acupuncture (M: −8.31; 95% CI = −9.36 to −7.26) with a between-group difference of 2.60 points (Cohen $d = 0.32$, $p < 0.001$) (2) Both the acupuncture and CBT-I surpassed the clinically meaningful change value of 8 points (3) Both maintained improvements in insomnia at 20 weeks with a significant mean difference still favoring CBT-i (M: 2.53; 95% CI, 1.03–4.02, $P = 0.001$, $d = 0.31$) (4) CBT-I also showed significantly better overall sleep quality ($p = 0.009$), faster sleep onset ($p < 0.001$), reduced waking after sleep onset ($p = 0.002$), and improved sleep efficiency ($p < 0.001$) (5) Acupuncture also was found to increase total sleep time over CBT-I ($P = 0.003$) (6) Although baseline pain was generally low, acupuncture was found to be more effective than CBT-I in reducing pain intensity posttreatment (M: 0.49, 95% CI, −0.95 to −0.02) Conclusion CBT-I appeared to be most effective. Future trials may benefit from adequately powered trials with a control group also included

(continued)

Appendix: Continued

Author	Purpose/intervention	Study design	Sample/phase of disease	Outcomes
Healing touch. Psychosocial interventions: mind-body, energy, and other CTs				
Reeve et al. [95]	To assess the effect of healing touch (HT) to reduce symptom severity by a minimum of 18 points after 10 treatments as measured by the military's self-report measure of PTSD symptom severity (PCL-5) Standard care: Consisted of medication, psychotherapy, plus relaxation, meditation, archery, or yoga HT-10 weekly treatments for 10 weeks, 60 min/session	2-armed randomized crossover waitlist-controlled study Groups (1) HT plus standard care (n = 19) (2) standard care (n = 20)	Combat veterans	(1) The HT group's mean reduction in symptom severity was clinically significant at 18.11 points compared to a reduction of 5.57 points for standard care Conclusion Initial data suggests that healing touch may be a helpful treatment option as an adjunct to standard therapy

Appendix: Mind-Body (MBSR). Psychosocial Interventions—Multimodal… 391

Healing touch. Complementary therapies (CTs) on symptom distress in patients with cancer and caregivers: mind-body, energy and other CTs

Lutgendorf et al. [92]	To evaluate the effects of a complementary therapy, healing touch (HT) compared to relaxation training (RT) and usual care (UC) on (a) protecting cellular immunity, (b) improving mood and quality of life, (c) reducing treatment-associated toxicities and treatment delays in patients receiving chemoradiation (see Part IV Chap. 6 for a description of HT)	Prospective RCT RA to (a) HT (b) RT (c) UC Patients in HT or RT group received 4 weekly individual sessions immediately after radiation during their 6-week chemoradiation treatment MDs and lab personnel blinded to treatment, but it does not state whether research assistants were blinded to goals of treatment Data assessed at baseline, and weeks 4 and 6	60 women with stages 1B1 to IVA cervical cancer receiving chemoradiation	(1) HT patients showed minimal decrease in natural killer cell cytotoxicity (NKCC) over the treatment course (2) RT and UC patients showed significant declines during chemoradiation (group by time interaction: $p = 0.018$) (3) HT patients showed greater reductions in 2 different indicators of depressed mood: (CESD depressed mood subscale, POMS depression scale) compared to RT or UC (group X time interactions: $p < 0.05$) (4) NS between group differences in QOL, treatment delays, or clinically rated toxicities (5) NS effects of HT on fatigue, toxicities, treatment delays, QOL Conclusion (1) HT appears to moderate effects of chemo radiation on depressed mood and cellular immunity (2) did not use a sham placebo (3) lack of patient blinding, unavoidable Relatively small samples may have underrepresented actual significant findings (type 2 error)

References

1. Kramer D. Energetic modalities as a self-care technique to reduce stress in nursing students. J Holist Nurs. 2018;36(4):366–73. PubMed PMID: 29205082. Epub 2017/12/06. eng.
2. Kerr F, Wiechula R, Feo R, Schultz T, Kitson A. Neurophysiology of human touch and eye gaze in therapeutic relationships and healing: a scoping review. JBI Database System Rev Implement Rep. 2019;17(2):209–47. PubMed PMID: 30730854. Pubmed Central PMCID: PMC6382052 Systematic Reviews and Implementation Reports. Epub 2019/02/08. eng.
3. Jakubiak BK, Feeney BC. Affectionate touch to promote relational, psychological, and physical well-being in adulthood: a theoretical model and review of the research. Personal Soc Psychol Rev. 2017;21(3):228–52. PubMed PMID: 27225036. Epub 2016/05/27. eng.
4. Gallace A, Spence C. The science of interpersonal touch: an overview. Neurosci Biobehav Rev. 2010;34(2):246–59. PubMed PMID: 18992276. Epub 2008/11/11. eng.
5. Fricchione GL. Illness and the origin of caring. J Med Humanit. 1993;14(1):15–21. PubMed PMID: 11612936. Epub 1993/04/01. eng.
6. Schwartz SA. Therapeutic intention: into the next generation. Exp Dermatol. 2017;13(3):158–62. PubMed PMID: 28433646. Epub 2017/04/24. eng.
7. Cascio CJ, Moore D, McGlone F. Social touch and human development. Dev Cogn Neurosci. 2019;35:5–11. PubMed PMID: 29731417. Pubmed Central PMCID: PMC6968965. Epub 2018/05/08. eng.
8. Field T. Touch for socioemotional and physical well being: a review. Dev Rev. 2010;30:367–83.
9. Gordon I, Voos AC, Bennett RH, Bolling DZ, Pelphrey KA, Kaiser MD. Brain mechanisms for processing affective touch. Hum Brain Mapp. 2013;34(4):914–22. PubMed PMID: 22125232. Pubmed Central PMCID: PMC6869848. Epub 2011/11/30. eng.
10. Gordon I, Zagoory-Sharon O, Leckman JF, Feldman R. Oxytocin, cortisol, and triadic family interactions. Physiol Behav. 2010;101(5):679–84. PubMed PMID: 20723553. Epub 2010/08/21. eng.
11. Morrison I. Keep calm and cuddle on: social touch as a stress buffer. Adapt Hum Behav Physiol. 2016;2:344–62.
12. Russo V, Ottaviani C, Spitoni GF. Affective touch: a meta-analysis on sex differences. Neurosci Biobehav Rev. 2020;108:445–52. PubMed PMID: 31614152. Epub 2019/10/16. eng.
13. McGlone F, Wessberg J, Olausson H. Discriminative and affective touch: sensing and feeling. Neuron. 2014;82(4):737–55. PubMed PMID: 24853935. Epub 2014/05/24. eng.
14. Kim J. A concept analysis on the use of Yakson in the NICU. J Obstet Gynecol Neonatal Nurs. 2016;45(6):836–41. PubMed PMID: 27718367. Epub 2016/10/09. eng.
15. Fredriksson L. Modes of relating in a caring conversation: a research synthesis on presence, touch and listening. J Adv Nurs. 1999;30(5):1167–76. PubMed PMID: 10564416. Epub 1999/11/17. eng.
16. Papathanassoglou ED, Mpouzika MD. Interpersonal touch: physiological effects in critical care. Biol Res Nurs. 2012;14(4):431–43. PubMed PMID: 22773451. Epub 2012/07/10. eng.
17. Durkin J, Jackson D, Usher K. The expression and receipt of compassion through touch in a health setting: a qualitative study. J Adv Nurs. 2021;77:1980–91.
18. Durkin J, Jackson D, Usher K. Defining compassion in a hospital setting: consensus on the characteristics that comprise compassion from researchers in the field. Contemp Nurse. 2020;56(2):146–59.
19. Gensic ME, Smith BR, LaBarbera DM. The effects of effleurage hand massage on anxiety and pain in patients undergoing chemotherapy. JAAPA. 2017;30(2):36–8. PubMed PMID: 28098671. Epub 2017/01/19. eng.
20. Ferrell-Torry AT, Glick OJ. The use of therapeutic massage as a nursing intervention to modify anxiety and the perception of cancer pain. Cancer Nurs. 1993;16(2):93–101. PubMed PMID: 8477405. Epub 1993/04/01. eng.

21. Henricson M, Ersson A, Määttä S, Segesten K, Berglund AL. The outcome of tactile touch on stress parameters in intensive care: a randomized controlled trial. Complement Ther Clin Pract. 2008;14(4):244–54. PubMed PMID: 18940711. Epub 2008/10/23. eng.
22. Chang SO. The conceptual structure of physical touch in caring. J Adv Nurs. 2001;33(6):820–7. PubMed PMID: 11298220. Epub 2001/04/12. eng.
23. Pedrazza M, Berlanda S, Trifiletti E, Minuzzo S. Variables of individual difference and the experience of touch in nursing. West J Nurs Res. 2018;40(11):1614–37. PubMed PMID: 28459179. Epub 2017/05/02. eng.
24. Beltrán MI, Dijkerman HC, Keizer A. Affective touch experiences across the lifespan: development of the tactile biography questionnaire and the mediating role of attachment style. PLoS One. 2020;15(10):e0241041. PubMed PMID: 33112898. Pubmed Central PMCID: PMC7592771. Epub 2020/10/29. eng.
25. Jones T, Glover L. Exploring the psychological processes underlying touch: lessons from the alexander technique. Clin Psychol Psychother. 2014;21(2):140–53. PubMed PMID: 23129565. Epub 2012/11/07. eng.
26. Connor A, Howett M. A conceptual model of intentional comfort touch. J Holist Nurs. 2009;27(2):127–35. PubMed PMID: 19443699. Epub 2009/05/16. eng.
27. Beckes L, Tops M. Toward a radically embodied neuroscience of attachment and relationships. Front Hum Neurosci. 2015;9:266. PubMed PMID: 26052276. Pubmed Central PMCID: PMC4439542. Epub 2015/06/09. eng.
28. Mikulincer M, P RS. Enhancing the "broaden and build" cycle of attachment security in adulthood: from the laboratory to relational contexts and societal systems. Int J Environ Res Public Health. 2020;17(6):32244872. Pubmed Central PMCID: PMC7143531. Epub 2020/04/05. eng.
29. Mikulincer M, Shaver PR. Attachment orientations and emotion regulation. Curr Opin Psychol. 2019;25:6–10. PubMed PMID: 29494853. Epub 2018/03/02. eng.
30. Mikulincer M, Shaver PR. Attachment, group-related processes, and psychotherapy. Int J Group Psychother. 2007;57(2):233–45. PubMed PMID: 17419673. Epub 2007/04/11. eng.
31. Lenzi D, Trentini C, Tambelli R, Pantano P. Neural basis of attachment-caregiving systems interaction: insights from neuroimaging studies. Front Psychol. 2015;6:1241. PubMed PMID: 26379578. Pubmed Central PMCID: PMC4547017. Epub 2015/09/18. eng.
32. Clark-Polner E, Clark MS. Understanding and accounting for relational context is critical for social neuroscience. Front Hum Neurosci. 2014;8:127. PubMed PMID: 24723868. Pubmed Central PMCID: PMC3971189. Epub 2014/04/12. eng.
33. Diego MA, Field T. Moderate pressure massage elicits a parasympathetic nervous system response. Int J Neurosci. 2009;119(5):630–8. PubMed PMID: 19283590. Epub 2009/03/14. eng.
34. Hertenstein MJ, Holmes R, McCullough M, Keltner D. The communication of emotion via touch. Emotion. 2009;9(4):566–73. PubMed PMID: 19653781. Epub 2009/08/06. eng.
35. Hertenstein MJ, Keltner D, App B, Bulleit BA, Jaskolka AR. Touch communicates distinct emotions. Emotion. 2006;6(3):528–33. PubMed PMID: 16938094. Epub 2006/08/30. eng.
36. Heathers JA. Everything Hertz: methodological issues in short-term frequency-domain HRV. Front Physiol. 2014;5:177. PubMed PMID: 24847279. Pubmed Central PMCID: PMC4019878. Epub 2014/05/23. eng.
37. Bernardi L, Sleight P, Bandinelli G, Cencetti S, Fattorini L, Wdowczyc-Szulc J, et al. Effect of rosary prayer and yoga mantras on autonomic cardiovascular rhythms: comparative study. BMJ. 2001;323(7327):1446–9. PubMed PMID: 11751348. Pubmed Central PMCID: 61046.
38. von Mohr M, Kirsch LP, Fotopoulou A. The soothing function of touch: affective touch reduces feelings of social exclusion. Sci Rep. 2017;7(1):13516. PubMed PMID: 29044137. Pubmed Central PMCID: PMC5647341. Epub 2017/10/19. eng.
39. Holt-Lunstad J, Birmingham WA, Light KC. Influence of a "warm touch" support enhancement intervention among married couples on ambulatory blood pressure, oxytocin, alpha amylase, and cortisol. Psychosom Med. 2008;70(9):976–85. PubMed PMID: 18842740. Epub 2008/10/10. eng.

40. Ditzen B, Neumann ID, Bodenmann G, von Dawans B, Turner RA, Ehlert U, et al. Effects of different kinds of couple interaction on cortisol and heart rate responses to stress in women. Psychoneuroendocrinology. 2007;32(5):565–74. PubMed PMID: 17499441. Epub 2007/05/15. eng.
41. Reddan MC, Young H, Falkner J, López-Solà M, Wager TD. Touch and social support influence interpersonal synchrony and pain. Soc Cogn Affect Neurosci. 2020;15(10):1064–75. PubMed PMID: 32301998. Pubmed Central PMCID: PMC7657460. Epub 2020/04/18. eng.
42. Olff M, Frijling JL, Kubzansky LD, Bradley B, Ellenbogen MA, Cardoso C, et al. The role of oxytocin in social bonding, stress regulation and mental health: an update on the moderating effects of context and interindividual differences. Psychoneuroendocrinology. 2013;38(9):1883–94. PubMed PMID: 23856187. Epub 2013/07/17. eng.
43. Feldman R, Rosenthal Z, Eidelman AI. Maternal-preterm skin-to-skin contact enhances child physiologic organization and cognitive control across the first 10 years of life. Biol Psychiatry. 2014;75(1):56–64. PubMed PMID: 24094511. Epub 2013/10/08. eng.
44. Feldman R, Singer M, Zagoory O. Touch attenuates infants' physiological reactivity to stress. Dev Sci. 2010;13(2):271–8. PubMed PMID: 20136923. Epub 2010/02/09. eng.
45. Bottorff JL. The use and meaning of touch in caring for patients with cancer. Oncol Nurs Forum. 1993;20(10):1531–8. PubMed PMID: 8278279. Epub 1993/11/01. eng.
46. Whitcher SJ, Fisher JD. Multidimensional reaction to therapeutic touch in a hospital setting. J Pers Soc Psychol. 1979;37(1):87–96. PubMed PMID: 458550. Epub 1979/01/01. eng.
47. Krohn M, Listing M, Tjahjono G, Reisshauer A, Peters E, Klapp BF, et al. Depression, mood, stress, and Th1/Th2 immune balance in primary breast cancer patients undergoing classical massage therapy. Support Care Cancer. 2011;19(9):1303–11. PubMed PMID: 20644965. Epub 2010/07/21. eng.
48. Kutner JS, Smith MC, Corbin L, Hemphill L, Benton K, Mellis BK, et al. Massage therapy versus simple touch to improve pain and mood in patients with advanced cancer: a randomized trial. Ann Intern Med. 2008;149(6):369–79. PubMed PMID: 18794556. Pubmed Central PMCID: PMC2631433. Epub 2008/09/17. eng.
49. Hernandez-Reif M, Field T, Ironson G, Beutler J, Vera Y, Hurley J, et al. Natural killer cells and lymphocytes increase in women with breast cancer following massage therapy. Int J Neurosci. 2005;115(4):495–510. PubMed PMID: 15809216.
50. Hernandez-Reif M, Ironson G, Field T, Hurley J, Katz G, Diego M, et al. Breast cancer patients have improved immune and neuroendocrine functions following massage therapy. J Psychosom Res. 2004;57(1):45–52. PubMed PMID: 15256294. Epub 2004/07/17. eng.
51. Billhult A, Lindholm C, Gunnarsson R, Stener-Victorin E. The effect of massage on immune function and stress in women with breast cancer–a randomized controlled trial. Auton Neurosci. 2009;150(1-2):111–5. PubMed PMID: 19376750. Epub 2009/04/21. eng.
52. Billhult A, Lindholm C, Gunnarsson R, Stener-Victorin E. The effect of massage on cellular immunity, endocrine and psychological factors in women with breast cancer–a randomized controlled clinical trial. Auton Neurosci. 2008;140(1-2):88–95. PubMed PMID: 18474451. Epub 2008/05/14. eng.
53. Nummenmaa L, Tuominen L, Dunbar R, Hirvonen J, Manninen S, Arponen E, et al. Social touch modulates endogenous μ-opioid system activity in humans. NeuroImage. 2016;138:242–7. PubMed PMID: 27238727. Epub 2016/05/31. eng.
54. Dutcher JM, Creswell JD. The role of brain reward pathways in stress resilience and health. Neurosci Biobehav Rev. 2018;95:559–67. PubMed PMID: 30477985. Epub 2018/11/28. eng.
55. Carlino EFE, Benedetti F. Pain and the context. Nat Rev Rheumatol. 2014;10:348–55.
56. Colloca L, Lopiano L, Lanotte M, Benedetti F. Overt versus covert treatment for pain, anxiety, and Parkinson's disease. Lancet Neurol. 2004;3(11):679–84. PubMed PMID: 15488461. Epub 2004/10/19. eng.
57. Petrie KJ, Rief W. Psychobiological mechanisms of placebo and nocebo effects: pathways to improve treatments and reduce side effects. Annu Rev Psychol. 2019;70:599–625. PubMed PMID: 30110575. Epub 2018/08/16. eng.

58. Coan JA, Schaefer HS, Davidson RJ. Lending a hand: social regulation of the neural response to threat. Psychol Sci. 2006;17(12):1032–9. PubMed PMID: 17201784. Epub 2007/01/05. eng.
59. Goldstein P, Weissman-Fogel I, Shamay-Tsoory SG. The role of touch in regulating inter-partner physiological coupling during empathy for pain. Sci Rep. 2017;7(1):3252. PubMed PMID: 28607375. Pubmed Central PMCID: PMC5468314. Epub 2017/06/14. eng.
60. Routasalo P. Physical touch in nursing studies: a literature review. J Adv Nurs. 1999;30(4):843–50. PubMed PMID: 10520096. Epub 1999/10/16. eng.
61. Durkin J, Usher K, Jackson D. Embodying compassion: a systematic review of the views of nurses and patients. J Clin Nurs. 2019;28(9-10):1380–92. PubMed PMID: 30485579. Epub 2018/11/30. eng.
62. Collinge W, MacDonald G, Walton T. Massage in supportive cancer care. Semin Oncol Nurs. 2012;28(1):45–54. PubMed PMID: 22281309. Epub 2012/01/28. eng.
63. White EM, Aiken LH, Sloane DM, McHugh MD. Nursing home work environment, care quality, registered nurse burnout and job dissatisfaction. Geriatr Nurs. 2019;41(2):158–64. PubMed PMID: 31488333. Epub 2019/09/07. eng.
64. Coakley AB, Barron AM. Energy therapies in oncology nursing. Semin Oncol Nurs. 2012;28(1):55–63. PubMed PMID: 22281310. Epub 2012/01/28. eng.
65. Monzillo E, Gronowicz G. New insights on therapeutic touch: a discussion of experimental methodology and design that resulted in significant effects on normal human cells and osteosarcoma. Exp Dermatol. 2011;7(1):44–51. PubMed PMID: 21194672. Epub 2011/01/05. eng.
66. Jackson E, Kelley M, McNeil P, Meyer E, Schlegel L, Eaton M. Does therapeutic touch help reduce pain and anxiety in patients with cancer? Clin J Oncol Nurs. 2008;12(1):113–20. PubMed PMID: 18258581. Epub 2008/02/09. eng.
67. Maville JA, Bowen JE, Benham G. Effect of healing touch on stress perception and biological correlates. Holist Nurs Pract. 2008;22(2):103–10. PubMed PMID: 18317289. Epub 2008/03/05. eng.
68. Krieger D. The therapeutic touch: how to use your hands to help or heal. New York: Prentice Hall Press; 1986.
69. Krieger D. Dolores Krieger, RN, PhD healing with therapeutic touch. Interview by Bonnie Horrigan. Altern Ther Health Med. 1998;4(1):86–92. PubMed PMID: 9439024. Epub 1998/01/24. eng.
70. van der Vaart S, Gijsen VM, de Wildt SN, Koren G. A systematic review of the therapeutic effects of Reiki. J Altern Complement Med. 2009;15(11):1157–69. PubMed PMID: 19922247. Epub 2009/11/20. eng.
71. Diaz-Rodriguez L, Arroyo-Morales M, Fernandez-de-las-Penas C, Garcia-Lafuente F, Garcia-Royo C, Tomas-Rojas I. Immediate effects of reiki on heart rate variability, cortisol levels, and body temperature in health care professionals with burnout. Biol Res Nurs. 2011;13(4):376–82. PubMed PMID: 21821642. Epub 2011/08/09. eng.
72. Armstrong K, Lanni T Jr, Anderson MM, Patricolo GE. Integrative medicine and the oncology patient: options and benefits. Support Care Cancer. 2018;26(7):2267–73. PubMed PMID: 29396594. Epub 2018/02/06. eng.
73. Malinski V. Models and theories focused on human existence and universal energy. Sudbury: Jones and Bartlett Learning; 2011.
74. Malinski VM. Rogerian science-based nursing theories. Nurs Sci Q. 2006;19(1):7–12. PubMed PMID: 16407593. Epub 2006/01/13. eng.
75. Hammerschlag R, Marx BL, Aickin M. Nontouch biofield therapy: a systematic review of human randomized controlled trials reporting use of only nonphysical contact treatment. J Altern Complement Med. 2014;20(12):881–92. PubMed PMID: 25181286. Epub 2014/09/03. eng.
76. Post-White J, Kinney ME, Savik K, Gau JB, Wilcox C, Lerner I. Therapeutic massage and healing touch improve symptoms in cancer. Integr Cancer Ther. 2003;2(4):332–44. PubMed PMID: 14713325. Epub 2004/01/10. eng.
77. Kunz D, Krieger D. The spiritual dimensions of therapeutic touch. Rochester: Bear; 2004.

78. Rubik B. The biofield hypothesis: its biophysical basis and role in medicine. J Altern Complement Med. 2002;8(6):703–17. PubMed PMID: 12614524.
79. Jaross W. Hypothesis on interactions of macromolecules based on molecular vibration patterns in cells and tissues. Front Biosci. 2018;23:940–6. PubMed PMID: 28930582. Epub 2017/09/21. eng.
80. Kučera O, Cifra M. Radiofrequency and microwave interactions between biomolecular systems. J Biol Phys. 2016;42(1):1–8. PubMed PMID: 26174548. Pubmed Central PMCID: PMC4713408. Epub 2015/07/16. eng.
81. Jain S, Hammerschlag R, Mills P, Cohen L, Krieger R, Vieten C, et al. Clinical studies of biofield therapies: summary, methodological challenges, and recommendations. Glob Adv Health Med. 2015;4(Suppl):58–66. PubMed PMID: 26665043. Pubmed Central PMCID: PMC4654788. Epub 2015/12/15. eng.
82. Jain S, Mills PJ. Biofield therapies: helpful or full of hype? A best evidence synthesis. Int J Behav Med. 2010;17(1):1–16. PubMed PMID: 19856109. Pubmed Central PMCID: PMC2816237. Epub 2009/10/27. eng.
83. Skarja M, Jerman I, Ruzic R, Leskovar RT, Jejcic L. Electric field absorption and emission as an indicator of active electromagnetic nature of organisms–preliminary report. Electromagn Biol Med. 2009;28(1):85–95. PubMed PMID: 19337899. Epub 2009/04/02. eng.
84. Berger A. Magnetic resonance imaging. BMJ. 2002;324(7328):35. PubMed PMID: 11777806. Pubmed Central PMCID: PMC1121941. Epub 2002/01/05. eng.
85. Thrane S, Cohen SM. Effect of Reiki therapy on pain and anxiety in adults: an in-depth literature review of randomized trials with effect size calculations. Pain Manag Nurs. 2014;15(4):897–908. PubMed PMID: 24582620. Pubmed Central PMCID: PMC4147026. Epub 2014/03/04. eng.
86. Servan-Schreiber D. Anticancer: a new way of life. Toronto: HarperCollins; 2007.
87. McManus DE. Reiki is better than placebo and has broad potential as a complementary health therapy. J Evid-Based Complement Alternat Med. 2017;22(4):1051–7. PubMed PMID: 28874060. Pubmed Central PMCID: PMC5871310. Epub 2017/09/07. eng.
88. Baldwin AL, Hammerschlag R. Biofield-based therapies: a systematic review of physiological effects on practitioners during healing. Exp Dermatol. 2014;10(3):150–61. PubMed PMID: 24767262. Epub 2014/04/29. eng.
89. Baldwin AL, Vitale A, Brownell E, Scicinski J, Kearns M, Rand W. The touchstone process: an ongoing critical evaluation of reiki in the scientific literature. Holist Nurs Pract. 2010;24(5):260–76. PubMed PMID: 20706088. Epub 2010/08/14. eng.
90. Lee MS, Pittler MH, Ernst E. Effects of reiki in clinical practice: a systematic review of randomised clinical trials. Int J Clin Pract. 2008;62(6):947–54. PubMed PMID: 18410352. Epub 2008/04/16. eng.
91. Erdogan Z, Cinar S. The effect of reiki on depression in elderly people living in nursing home. Indian J Tradit Knowl. 2016;15(1):35–40.
92. Lutgendorf SK, Mullen-Houser E, Russell D, Degeest K, Jacobson G, Hart L, et al. Preservation of immune function in cervical cancer patients during chemoradiation using a novel integrative approach. Brain Behav Immun. 2010;24(8):1231–40. PubMed PMID: 20600809. Pubmed Central PMCID: PMC3010350. Epub 2010/07/06. eng.
93. Dressen L, Singg S. Effects of reiki on pain and selected affective and personality variables of chronically ill patients. Subtle Energ Energ Med. 1998;9(1):51–82.
94. Chan CMH, Ng CG, Taib NA, Wee LH, Krupat E, Meyer F. Course and predictors of post-traumatic stress disorder in a cohort of psychologically distressed patients with cancer: a 4-year follow-up study. Cancer. 2018;124(2):406–16. PubMed PMID: 29152719. Epub 2017/11/21. eng.
95. Reeve K, Black PA, Huang J. Examining the impact of a healing touch intervention to reduce posttraumatic stress disorder symptoms in combat veterans. Psychol Trauma. 2020;12(8):897–903. PubMed PMID: 33346680. Epub 2020/12/22. eng.

96. Alarcao Z, Fonseca JRS. The effect of reiki therapy on quality of life of patients with blood cancer: results from a randomized controlled trial. Eur J Integr Med. 2016;8:239–49.
97. Catlin A, Taylor-Ford RL. Investigation of standard care versus sham Reiki placebo versus actual Reiki therapy to enhance comfort and well-being in a chemotherapy infusion center. Oncol Nurs Forum. 2011;38(3):212–20. PubMed PMID: 21531671. Epub 2011/05/03. eng.
98. Weze C, Leathard HL, Grange J, Tiplady P, Stevens G. Healing by gentle touch ameliorates stress and other symptoms in people suffering with mental health disorders or psychological stress. Evid Based Complement Alternat Med. 2007;4(1):115–23. PubMed PMID: 17342249. Pubmed Central PMCID: PMC1810357. Epub 2007/03/08. eng.
99. Díaz-Rodríguez L, Arroyo-Morales M, Fernández-de-las-Peñas C, García-Lafuente F, García-Royo C, Tomás-Rojas I. Immediate effects of reiki on heart rate variability, cortisol levels, and body temperature in health care professionals with burnout. Biol Res Nurs. 2011;13(4):376–82. PubMed PMID: 21821642. Epub 2011/08/09. eng.
100. Canadas-De la Fuente GA, Gomez-Urquiza JL, Ortega-Campos EM, Canadas GR, Albendin-Garcia L, De la Fuente Solana EI. Prevalence of burnout syndrome in oncology nursing: a meta-analytic study. Psycho-Oncology. 2018;27(5):1426–33. PubMed PMID: 29314432. Epub 2018/01/10. eng.
101. Welp A, Meier LL, Manser T. The interplay between teamwork, clinicians' emotional exhaustion, and clinician-rated patient safety: a longitudinal study. Crit Care. 2016;20(1):110. PubMed PMID: 27095501. Pubmed Central PMCID: PMC4837537. Epub 2016/04/21. eng.
102. Gronowicz G, Secor ER Jr, Flynn JR, Jellison ER, Kuhn LT. Therapeutic touch has significant effects on mouse breast cancer metastasis and immune responses but not primary tumor size. Evid Based Complement Alternat Med. 2015;2015:926565. PubMed PMID: 26113869. Pubmed Central PMCID: PMC4465772. Epub 2015/06/27. eng.
103. Johnston C, Campbell-Yeo M, Rich B, Whitley J, Filion F, Cogan J, et al. Therapeutic touch is not therapeutic for procedural pain in very preterm neonates: a randomized trial. Clin J Pain. 2013;29(9):824–9. PubMed PMID: 23817594. Epub 2013/07/03. eng.
104. Hanley MA, Coppa D, Shields D. A practice-based theory of healing through therapeutic touch: advancing holistic nursing practice. J Holist Nurs. 2017;35(4):369–81. PubMed PMID: 28821217. Epub 2017/08/20. eng.
105. Hall DL, Luberto CM, Philpotts LL, Song R, Park ER, Yeh GY. Mind-body interventions for fear of cancer recurrence: a systematic review and meta-analysis. Psycho-Oncology. 2018;27(11):2546–58. PubMed PMID: 29744965. Pubmed Central PMCID: PMC6488231. Epub 2018/05/11. eng.
106. Lee SH, Kim JY, Yeo S, Kim SH, Lim S. Meta-analysis of massage therapy on cancer pain. Integr Cancer Ther. 2015;14(4):297–304. PubMed PMID: 25784669. Epub 2015/03/19. eng.
107. Kinkead B, Schettler PJ, Larson ER, Carroll D, Sharenko M, Nettles J, et al. Massage therapy decreases cancer-related fatigue: results from a randomized early phase trial. Cancer. 2018;124(3):546–54. PubMed PMID: 29044466. Pubmed Central PMCID: PMC5780237. Epub 2017/10/19. eng.
108. Tarrasch R, Carmel-Neiderman NN, Ben-Ami S, Kaufman B, Pfeffer R, Ben-David M, et al. The effect of reflexology on the pain-insomnia-fatigue disturbance cluster of breast cancer patients during adjuvant radiation therapy. J Altern Complement Med. 2018;24(1):62–8. PubMed PMID: 28440664. Epub 2017/04/26. eng.
109. Mantoudi A, Parpa E, Tsilika E, Batistaki C, Nikoloudi M, Kouloulias V, et al. Complementary therapies for patients with cancer: reflexology and relaxation in integrative palliative care. A randomized controlled comparative study. J Altern Complement Med. 2020;26(9):792–8. PubMed PMID: 32924560. Epub 2020/09/15. eng.
110. Toygar I, Yeşilbalkan OU, Malseven YG, Sönmez E. Effect of reflexology on anxiety and sleep of informal cancer caregiver: randomized controlled trial. Complement Ther Clin Pract. 2020;39:101143. PubMed PMID: 32379631. Epub 2020/05/08. eng.

111. Bradt J, Dileo C, Magill L, Teague A. Music interventions for improving psychological and physical outcomes in cancer patients. Cochrane Database Syst Rev. 2016;8:CD006911. PubMed PMID: 27524661. Epub 2016/08/16. eng.
112. Chiu HY, Hsieh YJ, Tsai PS. Systematic review and meta-analysis of acupuncture to reduce cancer-related pain. Eur J Cancer Care. 2017;26:2. PubMed PMID: 26853524. Epub 2016/02/09. eng.
113. Anderson JG, Taylor AG. Effects of healing touch in clinical practice: a systematic review of randomized clinical trials. J Holist Nurs. 2011;29(3):221–8. PubMed PMID: 21228402. Epub 2011/01/14. eng.
114. Garland SN, Xie SX, DuHamel K, Bao T, Li Q, Barg FK, et al. Acupuncture versus cognitive behavioral therapy for insomnia in cancer survivors: a randomized clinical trial. J Natl Cancer Inst. 2019;111(12):1323–31. PubMed PMID: 31081899. Pubmed Central PMCID: PMC6910189. Epub 2019/05/14. eng.

Part V
Nursing Approaches

Introduction

Part V addresses the main health-related concerns of patients and caregivers in respective chapters across the diagnostic (Chap. 15), treatment (Chap. 16), transition to survivorship (Chap. 17), and end-of-life (Chap. 18) phases. Psychosocial interventions based on evidence from clinical trials, systematic reviews, and or meta-analysis are also proposed. Last, the feasibility of using the Stress, Healing and Resilience Model of Whole Person Care across clinical cancer settings is addressed (Chap. 19). Although Part V is discussed in terms of the different phases of the cancer and recovery experience, nursing should be conceptualized as a *continuous whole-person approach* with the family caregiver from diagnosis through survivorship and/or end of life in which psychosocial nursing interventions are directed toward reducing emotional distress, promoting healing, strengthening resilience capabilities, and improving healthy lifestyles and well-being even in the absence of a cure. Through these clinical objectives, the nurse supports the medical goals of treatment by increasing the likelihood of the patients' ability to tolerate and complete treatment and potentially enhance treatment efficacy (review Chap. 12). Psychosocial nursing interventions may enhance the patients' and family caregivers' ability to live well with the disease as a chronic illness, thrive in a healthy survivorship, and face the end of life in acceptance and serenity. These objectives are enabled by the quality of the therapeutic nurse-patient relationship *across the continuum*.

The emotional distress of patients and caregivers may ebb and flow depending on the stage of disease, treatment, and clinical results, but it always hovers in some form, posing a potential physical threat to the patients' and family caregivers' future health [1, 2]. An estimated 20–52% of patients report high levels of distress depending on the stage and type of cancer and its cancer- and treatment-related symptoms and side effects [1, 3]. An estimated 10–60% of caregivers experience similar anxiety, depression, grief, and poor physical health across the continuum, which may exceed that of patients, especially toward the terminal phase (e.g., [4, 5]). Given the emotional interdependence between patients and caregivers which impact their respective psychological and physical health, it is incumbent upon nurses to address the psychological and physical needs of both at all phases, starting at diagnosis and continuing throughout the course of the disease and/or transitioning to survivorship [6].

Patient Centered Findings from meta-analyses and clinical trials that have assessed the effectiveness of *patient-centered* psychosocial interventions across the disease and recovery continuum have generally reported positive patient outcomes with respect to quality of life, anxiety, depression, and the marital relationship [7–9]. Patient-centered therapeutic interventions consisted of providing relevant information, enhancing supportive relationships [10], coping skills training [11], meaning-making [12], mindfulness-based cancer recovery intervention [13], mindfulness-based stress reduction (MBSR) [14], different modalities of meditation [15], various strategies for symptom management (e.g., [16]), and/or self-management strategies [17]. Ascertaining the most appropriate intervention(s) depended on the goals of care, the behavioral and physiological target(s), and preferences of the patient.

Patient-Caregiver Focus When patients are accompanied by the family caregiver, clinical interventions tend to focus on the patient, based on the partially misplaced assumption that helping the patient helps the caregiver. Too often, the unique and mounting psychological, physical, and informational needs of the caregiver are inadequately managed as the caregiving burden increases with progression of the disease [18]. The few studies reporting caregiver as well as patient improvements may reflect the extent to which the clinical interventions addressed their *shared* concerns [19]. This clinical finding underscores the importance of doing a nursing assessment of the patient and the caregiver and, if clinically warranted, providing separate and tailored interventions with the patient and caregiver.

Caregiver Focus In the year following a cancer diagnosis, findings suggest that as patient well-being improves, caregiver health declines [20]. Although caregiver needs clearly increase as the patients' cancer progresses toward its terminal phase, the findings also highlight the *unique* experiences of family caregivers as well as the interdependence between the patient and caregiver [21]. Clinical interventions that do not address caregiver concerns earlier in the disease trajectory may undermine the health of both patient and caregiver.

Practice-Related Challenges Many nurses try to set aside meaningful time for patients and their family caregivers, particularly at distressing moments. But the clinical reality is that the unique needs of the whole patient and caregiver tend to be sacrificed by nursing goals that are predominantly centered on treatment, side effects, and symptoms (Chap. 19). The reasons are multifactorial. Most of all, enabling the psychosocial clinical expertise of nursing staff tends to be lacking. Staff schedules rarely build in quality time for nurses with advanced degrees to address the unique needs of patients and caregivers (e.g., [22]). Although the psychosocial interventions discussed in Part IV all fall within the purview of advanced nursing practice, the oncology literature suggests that most clinic nurses would benefit from additional training not only in these psychosocial nursing strategies, but in the skills of communication, the essential clinical predicate for developing further psychosocial expertise (e.g., [18, 23]). It is hoped that Part V, which offers nurses an essential repository of clinical interventions supported by the latest scientific findings consistent with the conceptual model, will help to foster a shift in nursing goals and objectives toward clinical interventions that address the psychosocial needs of the whole individual.

References

1. Riba MB, Donovan KA, Andersen B, Braun I, Breitbart WS, Brewer BW, et al. Distress management, version 3.2019, NCCN clinical practice guidelines in oncology. J Natl Compr Canc Netw 2019;17(10):1229–49; PubMed PMID: 31590149. Pubmed Central PMCID: PMC6907687. Epub 2019/10/08. eng.
2. Hagedoorn M, Sanderman R, Bolks HN, Tuinstra J, Coyne JC. Distress in couples coping with cancer: a meta-analysis and critical review of role and gender effects. Psychol Bull 2008;134(1):1–30; PubMed PMID: 18193993. Epub 2008/01/16. eng.
3. Dans M, Smith T, Back A, Baker JN, Bauman JR, Beck AC, et al. NCCN guidelines insights: palliative care, version 2.2017. J Natl Compr Canc Netw 2017;15(8):989–97; PubMed PMID: 28784860. Epub 2017/08/09. eng.
4. Ahn S, Romo RD, Campbell CL. A systematic review of interventions for family caregivers who care for patients with advanced cancer at home. Patient Educ Couns. 2020;103:1518–30; PubMed PMID: 32201172. Epub 2020/03/24. eng.
5. Dionne-Odom JN, Azuero A, Lyons KD, Hull JG, Prescott AT, Tosteson T, et al. Family caregiver depressive symptom and grief outcomes from the ENABLE III randomized controlled trial. J Pain Symptom Manage 2016;52(3):378–85; PubMed PMID: 27265814. Pubmed Central PMCID: PMC5023481. Epub 2016/06/07. eng.
6. Ferrell BR, Twaddle ML, Melnick A, Meier DE. National consensus project clinical practice guidelines for quality palliative care guidelines, 4th edition. J Palliat Med 2018;21(12):1684–9; PubMed PMID: 30179523. Epub 2018/09/05. eng.

7. Hu Y, Liu T, Li F. Association between dyadic interventions and outcomes in cancer patients: a meta-analysis Support Care Cancer 2019;27(3):745–61; PubMed PMID: 30604008. Epub 2019/01/04. eng.
8. Kalter J, Verdonck-de Leeuw IM, Sweegers MG, Aaronson NK, Jacobsen PB, Newton RU, et al. Effects and moderators of psychosocial interventions on quality of life, and emotional and social function in patients with cancer: an individual patient data meta-analysis of 22 RCTs. Psychooncology 2018;27(4):1150–61; PubMed PMID: 29361206. Pubmed Central PMCID: PMC5947559. Epub 2018/01/24. eng.
9. Salsman JM, Pustejovsky JE, Schueller SM, Hernandez R, Berendsen M, McLouth LES, et al. Psychosocial interventions for cancer survivors: a meta-analysis of effects on positive affect. J Cancer Surviv. 2019;13(6):943–55; PubMed PMID: 31741250. Pubmed Central PMCID: PMC7330880. Epub 2019/11/20. eng.
10. Andersen BL, Farrar WB, Golden-Kreutz D, Emery CF, Glaser R, Crespin T, et al. Distress reduction from a psychological intervention contributes to improved health for cancer patients. Brain Behav Immun 2007;21(7):953–61; PubMed PMID: 17467230. Pubmed Central PMCID: PMC2039896. Epub 2007/05/01. eng.
11. Cohen L, Parker PA, Vence L, Savary C, Kentor D, Pettaway C, et al. Presurgical stress management improves postoperative immune function in men with prostate cancer undergoing radical prostatectomy. Psychosom Med 2011;73(3):218–25; PubMed PMID: 21257977. Epub 2011/01/25. eng.
12. Lee V, Cohen SR, Edgar L, Laizner AM, Gagnon AJ. Meaning-making and psychological adjustment to cancer: development of an intervention and pilot results. Oncol Nurs Forum 2006;33(2):291–302; PubMed PMID: 16518445. Epub 2006/03/07. eng.
13. Carlson LE, Tamagawa R, Stephen J, Drysdale E, Zhong L, Speca M. Randomized-controlled trial of mindfulness-based cancer recovery versus supportive expressive group therapy among distressed breast cancer survivors (MINDSET): long-term follow-up results. Psychooncology 2016;25(7):750–9; PubMed PMID: 27193737. Epub 2016/05/20. eng.
14. Reich RR, Lengacher CA, Alinat CB, Kip KE, Paterson C, Ramesar S, et al. Mindfulness-based stress reduction in post-treatment breast cancer patients: immediate and sustained effects across multiple symptom clusters. J Pain Symptom Manage 2017;53(1):85–95; PubMed PMID: 27720794. Epub 2016/10/11. eng.
15. Bhasin MK, Dusek JA, Chang BH, Joseph MG, Denninger JW, Fricchione GL, et al. Relaxation response induces temporal transcriptome changes in energy metabolism, insulin secretion and inflammatory pathways. PLoS One 2013;8(5):e62817; PubMed PMID: 23650531. Pubmed Central PMCID: PMC3641112. Epub 2013/05/08. eng.
16. Lau BHP, Chow AYM, Ng TK, Fung YL, Lam TC, So TH, et al. Comparing the efficacy of integrative body-mind-spirit intervention with cognitive behavioral therapy in patient-caregiver parallel groups for lung cancer patients using a randomized controlled trial. J Psychosoc Oncol 2020;38(4):389–405; PubMed PMID: 32146876. Epub 2020/03/10. eng.
17. McCorkle R, Ercolano E, Lazenby M, Schulman-Green D, Schilling LS, Lorig K, et al. Self-management: enabling and empowering patients living with cancer as a chronic illness. CA Cancer J Clin 2011;61(1):50–62; PubMed PMID: 21205833. Pubmed Central PMCID: PMC3058905. Epub 2011/01/06. eng.
18. Dionne-Odom JN, Azuero A, Lyons KD, Hull JG, Tosteson T, Li Z, et al. Benefits of early versus delayed palliative care to informal family caregivers of patients with advanced cancer: outcomes from the ENABLE III randomized controlled trial. J Clin Oncol 2015;33(13):1446–52; PubMed PMID: 25800762. Pubmed Central PMCID: PMC4404423. Epub 2015/03/25. eng.
19. Northouse LL, Mood DW, Schafenacker A, Kalemkerian G, Zalupski M, LoRusso P, et al. Randomized clinical trial of a brief and extensive dyadic intervention for advanced cancer patients and their family caregivers. Psychooncology 2013;22(3):555–63; PubMed PMID: 22290823. Pubmed Central PMCID: PMC3387514. Epub 2012/02/01. eng.

20. Shaffer KM, Kim Y, Carver CS. Physical and mental health trajectories of cancer patients and caregivers across the year post-diagnosis: a dyadic investigation. Psychol Health 2016;31(6):655–74; PubMed PMID: 26680247. Pubmed Central PMCID: PMC4930392. Epub 2015/12/19. eng.
21. Kershaw T, Ellis KR, Yoon H, Schafenacker A, Katapodi M, Northouse L. The interdependence of advanced cancer patients' and their family caregivers' mental health, physical health, and self-efficacy over time. Ann Behav Med 2015;49(6):901–11; PubMed PMID: 26489843. Pubmed Central PMCID: PMC4825326. Epub 2015/10/23. eng.
22. Molin J, Lindgren B, Graneheim U, Ringner A. Time together: a nursing intervention in psychiatric inpatient care-feasibility and effects. Int J Ment Health Nurs 2018;27(6):1698–708.
23. Banerjee SC, Manna R, Coyle N, Penn S, Gallegos TE, Zaider T, et al. The implementation and evaluation of a communication skills training program for oncology nurses. Transl Behav Med 2017;7(3):615–23; PubMed PMID: 28211000. Pubmed Central PMCID: PMC5645276. Epub 2017/02/18. eng.

The Diagnostic Phase 15

15.1 Introduction

Cancer signifies a threat to life, an insidious presence that surreptitiously takes hold initially beyond conscious awareness. Once diagnosed, cancer generally is a source of considerable emotional distress. At first people may not know what to think and may be numb to the clinical implications of the diagnosis. Some patients respond to the diagnosis with a sense of futility, their personal resources unable to rise to this potentially life-threatening challenge nor find the hope within to fuel their beliefs in a healthy future. Most individuals successfully face down the terrifying specter, by taking matters calmly, 1 day at a time. Even these patients and their caregivers may benefit from resilient-promoting psychosocial as well as physical interventions to strengthen their overall fitness for treatment. It may also facilitate their subsequent ability to adapt successfully to related threats and stresses along the illness and recovery continuum. No matter how resilient an individual may appear on the surface, know that all are deeply affected by the realization that cancer constitutes an assault to the person's sense of self, the world he has always known, and his potential ability to live a long, healthy life.

This chapter explores the impact of a cancer diagnosis on the whole individual and their loved ones and reviews the goals of pretreatment programs aimed at strengthening the overall resilience of the individual and where applicable the caregiver.

15.2 Objectives

At the end of this chapter, you will be able to:

1. Identify the effects of a diagnosis of cancer on the individual.
2. Analyze the potential efficacy of the clinical interventions within the context of the patient's clinical status.

3. Discuss various one-on-one strategies for patients and the family caregiver as well as possible group workshops that may strengthen resilience and promote healing processes.

Clinical Anecdote 15.1
In 2004, when I was first diagnosed with cancer, no one talked about healing or resilience. The talk was about medical treatment to eliminate the disease. There were no nursing goals specifically aimed at the whole person beyond the procedures surrounding the administration of the treatments. The only appointments were with the oncologist, the surgeon and rotating clinic nurses on the day of chemotherapy. Thankfully, my oncologist appeared to practice more comprehensively. He wanted me to understand that he would be in charge of my tumour, if I would be in charge of my health by walking every day, and eating nutritionally. And, as I have previously mentioned, the oncologist asked me whether I would like to read some of the recent research findings and then meet to discuss the treatment options based on the findings and feedback from his colleagues across Canada and the US. In so doing, he reminded me that I was not helpless, and could be an active agent in my own recovery.

15.3 Definitions: The Diagnostic Prehabilitation Phase

The diagnostic phase varies in duration but typically starts with the cancer diagnosis and culminates in the first cancer treatment. It refers to the patient-centered health-related process of investigating and assessing (1) the patient's clinical information and past history and (2) the results from relevant tests, diagnostic procedures, the latest scientific evidence, and clinical guidelines that determine the course of treatment to eliminate or effectively manage the condition as a chronic illness. From a nursing perspective, it refers to the first critical opportunity to develop a therapeutic nurse-patient (and family care giver) relationship. It is the phase in which the nurse gets to know the whole person in terms of their life before the diagnosis, their life goals, assumptions and beliefs about the world and the self; their beliefs (anxieties and fears) about their diagnosis, coping capabilities, personal and social resources and lifestyle behaviors. It is the clinical basis for developing tailored interventions to promote the healing and resilient capabilities of the whole person before starting treatment.

Significantly, the diagnostic period is also referred to as the prehabilitation phase during which cancer patients participate in preparatory programs to strengthen their physical and psychological resilience in advance of the health-related challenges they must manage throughout the acute treatment phase [1]. The goals of prehabilitation programs include enhancing treatment tolerability, adherence to treatment, reducing the incidence or severity of treatment-related side effects, and improving health-related outcomes and quality of life [1–4]. Programs usually focus on physical exercise, muscle strengthening exercises, and/or promoting an appropriate diet and nutrition. Increasingly this phase also includes promoting coping strategies to manage stressors as a function of the type and stage of cancer, clinical status, impending treatment and patient preferences (e.g., [5]). The prehabilitation phase is conceptualized as the first phase *in a continuum of rehabilitation care* throughout all stages of the illness and into survivorship in which interventions are tailored to the individual needs of the patient and caregiver ([1], p. 14).

15.4 Emotional Distress (Review Part II Chap. 3; Part IV Chaps. 9 and 10)

Uncertainty, fear, and disrupted personal/family and work-related roles are typical of the diagnostic phase, with an estimated 22–58% of patients experiencing emotional distress [6, 7]. Cancer-related distress refers to "a multifactorial unpleasant experience" of a psychological (i.e., cognitive, behavioral, emotional), social, spiritual, and physical nature that can impede the ability to cope effectively with cancer, its physical symptoms, and its treatment [8]. Distress may be conceptualized along a continuum, ranging from "common normal feelings of vulnerability, sadness and fears to problems that become disabling, such as depression, anxiety, panic, social isolation, and existential and spiritual crisis" ([8], p. 2).

Patients may find themselves in what Weisman and Worden [9] have described as an "existential plight" which may be experienced at pivotal moments throughout the disease and treatment course (e.g., [10]). An existential crisis is generally triggered by threatening or shattered assumptions about the self, the self in relation to others and the world, leaving the individual, at least temporarily, estranged from his or her inner self as well as others [11]. Everything that has defined the patient up to the diagnosis and given life meaning and purpose may now have been thrust into psychological jeopardy (review Chap. 10).

A cancer diagnosis may produce uncontrollable and disturbing thoughts that feed the patient's anxiety and depressive mood swings, as the mind struggles to come to terms with the diagnosis [12]. Intrusive ideation, if temporary, serves as the mind's cognitive process (via accommodation and assimilation) of integrating a traumatic event into an adapted sense of self [11, 13]. When prolonged, intrusive ideation undermines the person's ability to maintain emotional equanimity, think clearly, or experience a health-promoting good night's sleep. Prolonged emotional distress impairs the ability to cognitively process medical information or draw on reasoning processes to make informed decisions about a course of treatment (review Part III Chap. 6; Part IV Chap. 10). Some patients may display signs of avoidance, an unwillingness, for instance, to take appropriate medical and nursing actions.

Acute and chronic stresses have been shown to cause structural remodeling in the regions of the prefrontal cortex (PFC), amygdala, and hippocampus mediated in part by elevated glucocorticoids and other mediators [14]. Loss of structural volume and dendritic shortening in the PFC and hippocampus, and dendritic growth in the amygdala cause changes in normal behavior and functions, as manifested by increased anxiety (amygdala), impaired learning and memory formation (hippocampus), and diminished acuity in critical thinking capability (PFC) [14]. These alterations generally tend to be temporary and are restored to nearly normal structures and functions when stress ends. For this reason nurses play a critical role in assessing and introducing various strategies that can facilitate the downregulation of emotional distress at this early phase in the continuum.

Factors Underlying Patient and Caregiver Distress

Perhaps for the first time, the individual (and family) are forced to confront the possible mortality of the self or a loved one [15]. Emotional distress may be caused by the uncertainty surrounding the prognosis and disease trajectory, personal doubts concerning the medical treatment, the lack of needed support, the fear of suffering, and multiple imagined and impending losses [15, 16]. A perceived lack of personal control over the illness and the treatment may contribute to a sense of helplessness, a loss of self-identity, and a demoralized self [7, 17, 18]. For most resilient patients, however, the disrupted beliefs tend to be temporary, with the traumatic diagnosis ultimately serving as the impetus for self-reflection, growth-enhancing, and health-promoting behaviors [19]. Those patients tend to perceive cancer as a challenge, bringing all their personal and social resources to the task of somehow overcoming the disease or living well with it [12].

15.5 Physical Functioning, Fitness, and Activity
(Review Part V Chap. 16)

Emotional distress may be accompanied by an array of physical symptoms, impaired functions, or capabilities which also negatively impact quality of life. A prospective study of 942 newly diagnosed people with cancer showed that the overall level of physical activity before a diagnosis of cancer was significantly decreased following the diagnosis in individuals with breast, prostate, skin, and colorectal cancer [20]. In particular, individuals who had engaged in *vigorous* pre-diagnosis activity were shown to significantly reduce their physical activity following the diagnosis, especially in individuals with skin and prostate cancers. There were nonsignificant differences in levels of *moderate* physical activity before and after diagnosis. Other studies based on similar evidence strongly recommend that patients engage in physical exercise as early as possible after diagnosis and to continue throughout treatment and into survivorship (e.g., [21]).

In addition, sedentary behaviors also were found to be increased post diagnosis, especially in women over 60 and in individuals who were professionally inactive [20]. Even individuals who tended to be less sedentary before diagnosis also became more sedentary. Given the resilient-promoting and health-promoting effects of physical activity on physical, mental, and immune functioning, these findings underscore the clinical imperative of assessing a newly diagnosed patient's physical and sedentary activities before and after diagnosis in terms of the type of activity, frequency and duration of activity/day per week, as well as the level of physical intensity [22].

15.6 Neurophysiological Dysregulation (Review Part III Chaps. 6 and 7)

All behavior, at its core, is biology. Emotionally distressing thoughts, feelings, and behaviors constitute the outer manifestation of underlying neurobiological maladjustments. Left untreated, the dysregulated HPA axis and sympatho-adrenomedullary (SAM) pathways inhibit the activities of the parasympathetic nervous system (PNS) and vagal nerve associated with healing processes [14]. This can lead to an increase in systemic inflammation and, critically for newly diagnosed patients with cancer, immunosuppression of natural killer cells, cytotoxic T-cells, and interferons (IFN) that normally track down and eliminate cancer cells in a process known as immunosurveillance. Prolonged stress downregulates expression of anticancer-related genes and produces higher levels of reactive oxygen species (ROS) resulting in oxidative stress that exceeds the body's antioxidant capabilities, further exposing the person to a systemic inflammatory environment conducive to cancer growth, progression and metastases [23, 24].

Knowing the deleterious consequences of acute and prolonged stress on the individual's underlying neurobiology enables us to better understand, indeed visualize, the potential short- and long-term threats of emotional distress to the patient's whole being. This serves as a clinical impetus for developing healing- and resilient-promoting interventions early in the illness and treatment trajectory that may counter some of the neurobiological damage caused by prolonged psychological and physical stress.

Although emotional distress appears to be greatest at diagnosis, it may be exacerbated by various cancer- and treatment-related stressors encountered along the continuum. Areas of known vulnerability include the perisurgical phase, prior to and during chemotherapy and onco-radiation, the transition to survivorship, and during the end-of-life phase, underscoring the clinical imperative of providing continuity of care by regularly supporting and helping patients and caregivers to acquire needed capabilities and resources.

15.7 Clinical Research Findings: Prehabilitation Interventions

In principle prehabilitation interventions are aimed at enhancing the psychological and physical health of patients prior to upcoming cancer-related treatment in the hope of reducing posttreatment complications and side effects (e.g., [25]). Most studies to date appear to consist of physical fitness-related exercise, diet or nutrition, and/or psychological interventions.

Presurgery

Multimodal Interventions

A systematic review and meta-analysis of 18 randomized controlled trials recently evaluated the effectiveness of prehabilitation programs for newly diagnosed individuals with cancer compared to usual care [4]. The programs comprised one or more components of psychological support, education, and/or exercise. The results showed pelvic floor muscle training was significantly associated with continence at 3 months although pad use at 6 months was not significantly reduced in patients with prostate cancer. Presurgical exercise was associated with a significant reduction in days in hospital and a significant decrease in the odds of surgical complications in patients with lung cancer. Psychological interventions significantly improved mood, physical well-being, and immune functions in patients with prostate cancer, and also decreased fatigue and improved psychological outcomes in women with breast cancer. The findings must be regarded with caution due to the high risk of bias across the studies. More studies with stronger designs and methodology based on the same and different cancer types are needed to evaluate the efficacy of these psychosocial and other prehabilitation programs.

A systematic review and meta-analysis of 33 studies ($N = 3962$) assessed the effects of prehabilitation interventions for older patients awaiting elective abdominal cancer surgery [26]. Interventions included nutrition, exercise, psychological "input," smoking cessation, and/or multimodal interventions of two or more of these interventions [26]. Although 30/33 studies showed moderate-to-high risk of bias, the findings suggested that exercise, nutrition, and a multimodal approach may reduce post treatment abdominal complications or morbidity.

A 2-session pre-/post-stress management intervention with 159 patients undergoing radical prostatectomy was reported to significantly increase mood, physical well-being, and immune functioning, with significantly greater natural killer cell cytotoxicity, circulating IL-2 and tumor necrosis factor-alpha cytokines, after surgery compared to a 2-day supportive attention intervention or usual care. However the data were limited by a high risk of bias [3]. The intervention consisted of breathing exercises, relaxation skills, acquiring problem-solving and support-seeking skills, and discussing realistic expectations. Booster sessions occurred on the day of surgery and 48 h postsurgery. In summary a multimodal psychosocial and behavioral approach appeared to produce important pre- and posttreatment clinical benefits. Despite the moderate-to-high risk of bias, the results across other studies were consistently in the same positive clinical direction, highlighting the need for better, more rigorously designed RCTs [4].

Exercise

The efficacy of prehabilitation *exercise* programs with respect to pre-/post-intra-abdominal surgery has also been investigated. A meta-analysis of nine RCTs ($N =435$) based on presurgical exercise programs showed a significant reduction in postoperative complications following intra-abdominal surgery [27]. Exercises included breathing-related muscle training, aerobic exercise, and/or resistance training. Patients awaiting surgery had colorectal, abdominal, upper gastrointestinal, and liver cancers and obesity.

Another study examined the effects of an exercise program running simultaneously with preoperative chemotherapy or chemoradiation in preparation for pancreatic cancer surgery. The single-arm, within-group study of 50 patients participated in a prehabilitation home-based exercise program, consisting of more than 60 min each week in moderate-to-intense aerobic exercise plus other less intense physical activity and more than 60 min each week in strengthening exercises until the presurgical assessment [28]. Participants made significant improvements in various measures of physical function and health-related quality of life (HRQOL) [28]. For instance, the 6-minute walk test (MWT) and the gait speed (GS) significantly improved at follow-up over baseline measures. The significant improvement in the 6-minute walk was related to self-reported and significant increases in aerobic exercise, moderate-to-vigorous physical activity, and light physical activity. The increase in weekly light physical activity was associated with a significant increase in HRQOL. In contrast, an increase in weekly sedentary activity was associated with a significant decrease in HRQOL, underscoring the importance of encouraging patients to engage in physical exercise to improve physical function and quality of life.

Diet/Nutrition
Compared to exercise, there is relatively little research during the prehabilitation phase of the effects of nutrition or nutritional supplements on patient fitness, immune functioning, or other clinical outcomes known to be influenced by nutritional intake [29, 30]. A scoping review was carried out to determine (1) the composition of current prehabilitation programs and (2) more specifically the proportion of these programs that included a nutritional component. One hundred and ten quantitative and qualitative studies met inclusion criteria. Only 49% of the studies consisted of multimodal programs, and 44% had exercise programs that prepared patients for surgery [31]. Of 110 studies only 34% had a nutritional component, and of these, two-thirds did not evaluate the impact of the nutrition intervention on measurable and appropriate outcomes. Standard tools for nutritional assessments appeared to be lacking.

Last, in a double-blind RCT, 48 individuals awaiting colorectal cancer surgery were randomized to receive either (1) personalized nutrition counseling plus whey protein supplements or (2) personalized nutrition counseling plus a nonnutritive "placebo" [32]. The significant mean improvement in functional walking before surgery compared to the placebo group was clinically significant. Four weeks postsurgery revealed comparable recovery rates. The intervention began 4 weeks prior to surgery and continued for 4 weeks afterward. This pilot study suggested that the whey protein supplement appeared to be a significant factor in the patients' improvement in functional walking, highlighting the potential clinical benefits of preoperative nutritional supplementation. The findings also underscore the importance of nurses consulting with the dietician and oncologist regarding the need for tailored health-promoting diets and or nutritional supplements to optimize the physical fitness of all pre surgical patients.

Exercise and Nutrition
A meta-analysis of five RCTs and four cohort studies ($N = 914$) investigated the effects of 438 patients who received a prehabilitation program (i.e., nutrition alone) or multimodal (nutrition plus exercise) compared to 476 patients who received

usual care [33]. Both prehabilitation programs significantly reduced the length of time in hospital by 2 days compared to usual care, suggesting that nutrition alone as well as the multimodal condition buffered the patient against postoperative complications. Individual studies reported that multimodal prehabilitation (nutrition plus exercise) significantly improved the 6-minute walk (a marker usually used to assess the effects of exercise or physical fitness) [33]. Among the recommendations for future study, Gillis and colleagues suggest that outcome measures should assess the individual's physical resilience in terms of (1) length of time to recover from postoperative complications and (2) length of time to return to activities of daily living and/or start adjuvant chemotherapy.

Pooled data from two RCTs and a cohort study ($n = 202$) also examined the effectiveness of a prehabilitation exercise and nutrition program for patients awaiting colorectal surgery [34]. Patients with stage III cancer showed a significant improvement in disease-free survival (DFS) compared to patients on usual care, based on a hazard ratio, after controlling for cancer stage and confounding variables. In the main, exercise and nutrition were shown to be important components of prehabilitation programs to strengthen overall resilience in patients awaiting surgery. The effectiveness of prehabilitation programs based on exercise and nutrition should also be evaluated in patients before and after receiving chemotherapy and radiation oncology treatment.

Psychosocial Interventions

The role of psychosocial interventions to promote resilience in pretreatment patients by enhancing cognitive-behavioral coping skills is gaining clinical recognition (e.g., [3]). In a Cochrane review of 30 trials, psychosocial interventions that took place over the course of the 12 months after diagnosis produced a small significant improvement in quality of life in newly diagnosed patients with various cancers based on cancer-specific measures [35]. Whereas psychological distress appeared to improve based on measures of "mood," measures of anxiety and depression produced nonsignificant findings. These discrepancies may be attributed to methodological issues across studies, but it also highlights the importance of developing *tailored* interventions and selecting measures that reflect the psychological concerns under study.

A small effect size improvement in quality of life (QOL) was also observed when cancer-specific measures of QOL were used [35]. Nurse-administered face-to-face interventions and by telephone that consisted of psychoeducational information provided within a supportive nurse-patient relationship showed a significant small effect size increase in quality of life in patients with breast cancer [35]. Although it is unclear what constituted the key components of a "supportive nurse-patient dialogue" across the studies, addressing psychological distress in the prehabilitation phase is a clinical imperative.

Cognitive-Behavioral Therapy A Cochrane review based on a meta-analysis of 28 RCTs with 3940 patients with breast cancer showed that cognitive-behavioral therapy rather than psychotherapy appeared to be most effective in reducing anxiety, depression, and mood disturbance in a group of women after a diagnosis of cancer [36] (review Appendix in Chap. 9). However the timing of the interventions and the duration and frequency were not reported. The high risk of bias due to the heterogeneity of the studies indicates the need for more rigorously designed RCTs to evaluate the clinical effectiveness of the intervention in the prehabilitation phase.

Another Cochrane review of psychosocial interventions for patients with head and neck cancer based on seven RCTs and quasi-RCTs revealed a lack of therapeutic benefit based on measures of global quality of life [37]. Neither anxiety nor depression levels improve post intervention. The findings may be attributed in part to the high risk of bias reported across the studies. But another important factor may be the type of cancer the newly diagnosed patients and their caregivers must face. Because the actual timing, duration, and content of the psychosocial interventions were not easily retrievable from the Cochrane review, future clinical interventions might benefit from carrying out qualitative studies first in order to develop a deeper understanding of what patients with different types of cancer and caregivers need from healthcare workers during this highly distressing phase.

Summary The majority of prehabilitation studies consist mainly of exercise and/or diet/nutrition counselling and, increasingly, psychoeducation. Most vary in terms of their content. In the main, prehabilitation programs administered shortly after diagnosis and before treatment that focus on strengthening physical fitness and enhancing diet and nutrition appear to provide clinical benefits for patients, with some studies even attributing these programs to long-term survivability effects, for instance, in colorectal patients [34].

A handful of studies were located that focused on psychosocial interventions, but none appeared to be purposefully integrated into a comprehensive program aimed at enhancing physical, nutritional, and *psychosocial* resilience *prior* to the start of treatment. Most prehabilitation studies tend to focus on preparing patients for surgery. More programs are needed for patients about to start chemotherapy and other anticancer treatments.

The overall poor-quality evidence in support of these preparatory programs for patients underscores the need for well-designed studies of patients with the same cancer type to evaluate specifically tailored health-promoting interventions. In this first generally brief phase of the cancer and treatment continuum, no interventions were located that focused on the family caregiver. Pretreatment programs were delivered one on one or in groups with some telephone-/Internet-delivered components. Given this critical phase in the illness and recovery trajectory, more rigorously designed nursing studies of psychosocial interventions to promote the healing and resiliient capabilities of patients and caregivers is a clinical imperative.

15.8 Nursing Implications

The main goal of the prehabilitation phase is to strengthen overall psychosocial and physical resilience and the health potential of the patient during the period leading up to the start of his or her treatment. The intent is to put the patient in an optimal condition or overall state of readiness to successfully meet the physical and psychosocial challenges that characterize the treatment phase.

This chapter discusses the key components involved in providing comprehensive nursing care. It covers:

8.1. Nursing assessment
8.2. Therapeutic nurse-patient relationship (review Part IV Chap. 8)
8.3. Information related to emotional distress, the illness, and treatment
8.4. Patient beliefs and expectations about clinical outcomes
8.5. Cognitive-behavioral coping and meaning-making strategies (review Part IV Chaps. 9 and 10; Appendix in Chap. 10; Appendix B)
8.6. Self-management information and skills to handle practical problems expected to arise from the upcoming treatment (review Part IV Chap. 9; Appendices A and B)
8.7. Relevant information about healthy lifestyle behaviors (review Part V Chap. 16; Appendix C)
8.8. Supportive relationships between the patient and family caregiver (and family) (Part IV Chaps. 8 and 11; Appendix B)

These nursing objectives may serve as a nursing template for practice, to be revisited over the course of the continuum, but especially at stressful cancer- or treatment-related points along the continuum.

Clinical Anecdote 15.2
The literature talks a lot about the emotional distress associated with cancer-related symptoms at the time of a diagnosis [38]. *Symptoms were not my immediate concern at first. It was discovering that my cancer was a true interloper, showing up without any apparent forewarning. Or rather that I had been so pre-occupied with just getting through each day that I had not paid sufficient attention to subtle signs. My mind had been somehow lulled into a false sense of security, distracted by the day to day responsibilities of daily life. And all the while, and likely because of all of that, cancer was stealthily rooting itself, growing and proliferating. By the time I was diagnosed, I was stage 4 with a poor prognosis.*

Nursing Assessment (Review Part IV Chaps. 9–11)

Over the first couple of meetings, *a baseline assessment* can provide invaluable information about the patient and caregiver, often serving as a therapeutic process in its own right, by engaging the patient/caregiver in a discussion about his or her thoughts, feelings, and behaviors relating to the reasons that brought the patient to clinic but extending beyond to topics that reveal the whole person (who now happens to have cancer) (Table 15.1). Along the way, gather information about current and past sources and levels of distress; current and past social, cognitive-emotional,

15.8 Nursing Implications

Table 15.1 Nursing assessment

Areas	
1. Emotional distress (screen using distress thermometer)	Review Part II Chap. 3
1.1 Causes and concerns (e.g., cancer- and/or treatment-related stressors)	
1.2 Perceived as challenge or threat [8, 39]	
2.0 Patient/caregiver expectations or beliefs about cancer; the treatment and survivorship: presence of distorted beliefs about cancer or treatment [40, 41]	Review Part IV Chaps. 9, 10, and 12
3.0 Before vs. current use of cognitive, behavioral coping responses to manage stressors	Review Part IV Chap. 9
3.1 Effective/not effective: explain	
3.2 Lessons learned to carry forward to current clinical situation [42–44]	
4.0 Personal resources: self-efficacy, sense of optimism, religiosity/spirituality, resilience	Review Part IV Chap. 9
4.1 Perception of personal resources before/after cancer-related stressor (high, medium, low). Please elaborate [45–48]	
5.0 Explore patient and caregiver sources and examples of supportive relationships in terms of emotional, instrumental, informational, and appraisal support and sense of security, before/after cancer	Review Part IV Chap. 11
5.1 Does the individual have a confidant(s)	
5.2 Support-related needs of the patient from caregiver, the nurse, and other members of the team, going forward	
5.3 Support-related needs of the caregiver from the nurse, the team, family, patient [49, 50]	
6.0 Is patient/caregiver *seeking meaning or coming to terms with the clinical* reality of cancer, i.e., meaning found?	Review Part IV Chap. 10
6.1 Who has helped/is helping patient seeking to make sense of the diagnosis, cancer recurrence, etc.	
6.2 Assumptions (beliefs) about the world (just, predictable, controllability)	
6.3 Values that guide choices in life (education, career, family, life partner, leisure time)	
6.4 Values also may include dependability, concern for others, sense of purpose, integrity, humor, loyalty, determination [45, 48, 51, 52]	
7.0 What gives life meaning in everyday life? Changes attributed to cancer/treatment?	Review Part IV Chap. 10
8.0 Lifestyle behaviors (describe in terms of typical nutrition/diet, physical activity, use of drugs, alcohol, smoking, sleep habits, and duration of sleep vs. wakefulness during night)	Review WCRF/AICR 2018 or its latest online cancer update publications (CUP)
8.1 Itemize the meals and snacks/day × 1 week	
8.2 Ask whether patient has referral to oncology nutritionist and follow up [22]	
9.0 Use of complementary therapies (meditation, yoga, other)	Review Part IV Chaps. 13 and 14
10.0 Patient/caregiver other concerns, needs from nurse	

physical/mental resilient capabilities, coping responses, supportive relationships, and lifestyle behaviors (diet, nutrition, physical activity, weight); and sources of meaning in his or her life [1, 8, 22]. Frame questions from a neutral perspective; avoid the use of negative terms such as the word "problem" which tends to be prominent in medical screening or assessment tools (see below). Begin by ascertaining whether the patient or caregiver have top of mind concerns. In no particular order invite the person to talk about his life before cancer, and what has been most meaningful in his life, the values and assumptions he has held. And the impact of the diagnosis on his life (career, family, future plans and goals).

Obtain information about what the patient and caregiver understand about cancer, its treatment, and their corresponding beliefs and expectations. Assess the patient's current and past emotion-regulating coping responses to stressful experiences. Explore perceived personal resources such as sense of self-efficacy and optimism (e.g., how would you describe yourself before and after the cancer diagnosis: as a person who sees a glass half full or empty, optimistic or cynical; a problem solver who also reaches out for help in new situations). Explore the sources and types of support patient and caregiver value/receive, including their perceptions of their intimate/important relationships. Inquire about the use of health-related resources (e.g., Internet sites, community center, massage therapist, and other complementary therapies) and what they have learned from them or how they have benefited. Review their lifestyle behaviors to ascertain what areas may also be enhanced by a health-promoting discussion [22].

An assessment also should capture values and beliefs or assumptions that have guided the individual throughout his life and how if at all these have changed since the diagnosis (Part IV Chap. 10). "What values and beliefs have guided the choices you have made in relation to yourself (e.g., education, career, choice of a partner, decision to have or not have a family)?" "What has been most meaningful in your life over the years before and after the diagnosis (may prompt family, friends, close partnership, religion/spirituality)?" This information provides important insights about the individual and some of the factors that could contribute to or alleviate distress.

Emotional Distress (Review Part II Chap. 3)

Cancer may be a symptom of previously experienced and unsuccessfully managed acute and chronic stresses that now have culminated into a life-threatening biological stressor in itself [14]. Emotional distress, anxiety, depression, and existential suffering in addition to the physical presence of the tumor must be regarded as a simultaneous biological as well as behavioral threat to the individual's healing and resilient capabilities and to the goals of medical treatment (review Part III Chaps. 6 and 7). Emotional distress may be difficult to overcome in people who have little faith in the proposed medical treatment; have difficulty adjusting psychologically to the diagnosis; and have pessimist personalities, high death anxiety, poor decision-making capabilities, and poor beliefs about their self-efficacy in this new clinical experience [7, 53]. The nurse's assessment should reveal key issues potentially impacting the individual's healing and resilient capabilities in the face of adversity.

According to NCCN guidelines, the level of emotional distress and its causes based on a 10-point rating scale must be assessed ([8], p. 8) (review Part II Chap. 3).

A *problem* list may help identify areas contributing to distress which may then be assessed in greater depth. The areas include practical "problems," family "problems," emotional "problems," spiritual/religious concerns, and physical "problems." I suggest substituting "possible areas of concern" or "challenges" for "problems" and even completing this assessment as part of the one-on-one interview (rather than as a self-completed questionnaire) in which you may further reframe the "problem list" in terms of "open questions" such as: "Tell me about your family and how you are all functioning these days—the strengths and challenges you see." An additional area to assess would be the presence of intrusive thoughts and avoidant behaviors triggered by the cancer or upcoming treatment [54].

Establishing a Nurse-Patient/Caregiver Relationship (Review Part IV Chap. 8)

It is within the context of a therapeutic nurse-patient relationship that healing-promoting and resilient-strengthening strategies may be introduced, discussed, scientifically justified, and encouraged. Establish a therapeutic nurse-patient relationship that is sustainable throughout the disease and recovery continuum. Although the majority of patients and caregivers are resilient, most nonetheless experience periodic distress at various points of vulnerability throughout the cancer experience, no more so than at the diagnosis. It may be particularly distressing as the patient must form new health-related relationships, make sense of the new clinical demands and expectations about managing their health, prepare for the treatment phase, and make informed decisions about treatment within the larger context of the stressful disruptions in their life to family, career, and related roles.

Patients have stated that they need to be understood, validated, and known by their healthcare providers as individuals, treated with respect through honest and compassionate communication, and provided the guidance they need to successfully navigate this phase of the illness trajectory [55]. They ask for illness- and treatment-related content to be delivered at the patient's rate of cognitive processing rather than all at once, and shared in simple language [55, 56]. They would like to feel that their preferences and needs are acknowledged and, as feasible, acted upon. Being present with *regular* relevant nurse-patient/caregiver interactions is key to developing and sustaining a meaningful, therapeutic relationship.

Both oncologist and nurse should be present at the initial meeting to discuss the diagnosis. The objectives are to listen, respond to questions, provide reassurance and compassion, and outline a few next steps to provide a meaningful context. Invite the patient's and caregiver's concerns and questions. "It is a lot to take in. Don't worry if you miss anything today." "We will be there for you every step of the way." "If there is a nagging concern after you leave, the nurse will give you her or his coordinates." "We will discuss more at next week's meeting …." The goal is to provide reassurance and comfort that the oncologist, nurse, and team will be there to help the patient. In response to concerns about treatment efficacy, reassure the patient and caregiver, for instance, "If one medication doesn't seem to be working as well as we would like, our approach is to try others; and everyday more treatments using new molecules are being released into the market."

Clarify the goals and roles of the different members of the team. Make a distinction between the role of the oncologist who will be more focused on treatments to eliminate the disease and the nurse whose goal is to strengthen healing and resilient capabilities to support the goals of treatment and to protect or strengthen their current health. Encourage the patient to reach out with any concerns anytime. Use touch as a means of connecting or deepening the bond between patient and nurse particularly at moments of observed patient vulnerability (review Part IV Chap. 14). Set a follow up appointment in which the patient, caregiver and nurse can start the nursing assessment, get to know one another and discuss resilient- promoting interventions or strategies. It is impossible to address everything in one setting. Select those aspects of the nursing assessment that will provide a solid initial snapshot of the patient and family caregiver in particular related to stress, coping, personal resources, support, beliefs and assumptions about the cancer, and lifestyle behaviors.

Provide Relevant Information

Patients and caregivers require different types of information depending on the clinical context. In principle both require information emanating from their stated health- and treatment-related concerns. Ask for the patient's and caregiver's preferences regarding the nature of the information and the amount they prefer as neither patient nor caregiver may be ready to absorb detailed information. In keeping with this rule of thumb, offer a general overview of what to expect, the nature of the illness, the treatment course, and the normal procedural flow in the treatment center which may help to enhance the patient's sense of control over this new clinical experience.

Philosophy of Care

Orient the family to the philosophy of the oncology team with respect to the care of patients and family such as principles of continuity of care across the continuum. Outline in general terms the different phases of the continuum, from the goals of the diagnostic phase through treatment. (A discussion about survivorship and/or supportive care may be incorporated later, as relevant.) Emphasize in greater detail the goals of the prehabilitation phase, the recommended programs, and healthcare workers who are likely to be involved in optimizing their health readiness for treatment. Again check in with the patient and caregiver and go at their own speed, stopping to answer questions throughout.

Roles and Functions

Explain the different roles and functions of the team members and especially the nurse and oncologist. Describe how clinical decisions are made and the patient's and/or caregiver's involvement, ascertaining their preferences. Describe what a clinic visit usually entails, such as getting bloods done, seeing the doctor/nurse, and then the treatment, and what to do in an emergency and important telephone/email contact nurse/oncologist information. Orient the patient to areas of the hospital they are most likely to access on a regular basis, such as the locations of the medical appointments, clinic infusion center, and where bloods are taken. Again do not flood the patient and caregiver with too much information at once; go at their pace as a function of stated interest, preference, or need.

Accessing Reliable Health-Related Resources
Most patients and caregivers go to the Internet for information about their cancer. Suggest team-vetted websites such as the MD Anderson Cancer Center (mdanderson.org) and the British Columbia Cancer Agency (bccancer.bc.ca). Critically, explain that cancer statistics provide average statistics rather than capturing an individual's unique response to treatment which depends on multiple factors. Invite the patient and caregiver to discuss their findings with the nurse or physician. Explain also that new drugs and interventions that target specific biological molecules are always being produced and in fact their efficacy may not be reflected by the *current* statistics on the Internet.

Information About the Cancer and Treatment (Review Chap. 12)
Discuss the biological links between cancer and emotional distress and conversely the relationship between emotional well-being and healing and resilient capabilities that can support the goals of anticancer treatment. Use relevant, gentle humor such as "You know cancer just hates it when you are calm!" It can be rather effective in sending an important message. As these patients are especially vulnerable, providing information in a light-hearted way can sometimes convey to the patient the importance of reducing stress but in a compassionate manner. Comments that anthropomorphize cancer can actually make cancer less threatening, transforming cancer from the insidious unknown to something tangible, and therefore more manageable and potentially less psychologically threatening. It can sometimes be a good way to introduce this topic for the first time, but can be used at any vulnerable moment when the patient is feeling fragile.

Clinical Anecdote 15.3
Mrs T. had an aggressive cancer. She desperately hoped to go to Costa Rica one last time, but was very fearful of leaving her medical team behind even as they felt it would "do her a lot of good." We discussed the best and worst possible consequences about going: the best, seeing her family again, and the worst, feeling sick and being far from home. Then we talked about the fact that she felt good right now, she would not miss a treatment, and a good hospital was located near her family home. But she was still worried. So I blurted out, "You know what I think? You tell that cancer you are going home to visit with or without it!" And this individual laughed and laughed, and said, "What a good idea!" Sadly she never made it, but I felt that for those few moments, she had laughed at cancer, and it had made her feel better.

Cognitive Beliefs and Expectations (Review Part IV Chap. 12)

Enhancing Positive Expectations About Treatment
A small but growing body of experimental and clinical studies have shown that a patient's positive expectations for a treatment outcome, particularly related to symptoms, can significantly increase the efficacy of treatment, reduce symptoms of pain

and anxiety, and even reduce the likelihood of breakthrough chemotherapy-related symptoms such as nausea [57, 58]. Chapter 12 reviews this literature and also describes a number of recommended strategies nurses can use during the process of obtaining informed consent as well as immediately prior to the patient's cancer-related surgery, radiation therapy, and/or chemotherapy. These strategies include reviewing the positive aspects of a given treatment with the patient and caregiver, framing side effects from a positive perspective (e.g., 95% of patients like you taking this treatment have experienced no ill effects, rather than emphasizing the 5% who did). Just prior to giving a treatment, the nurse should ensure that the patient's attention is on the medication (such as an intravenous) about to be administered with a brief recapitulation of its therapeutic goals.

Counter Negative Treatment Expectations
Negative beliefs or expected poor clinical outcomes (nocebo effect) may adversely impact the patient's clinical decisions about treatment. Critically, negative beliefs also activate the biological stress response system which suppresses physiological healing processes and critical anticancer immune functions (e.g., [59, 60]).

The nocebo effects induced by negative beliefs about the treatment are also known to trigger corresponding neurophysiological pathways that can result in the expected poor outcome. Negative expectations can lead to unwelcomed emotional, psychological, physiological, and immune consequences (nocebo effects). It can potentially inhibit the absorption rate of given medications, thereby compromising treatment efficacy, and contribute to poor symptom management and quality of life [61]. These beliefs also may influence a patient's clinical decisions, including whether or not to adhere to treatment.

Negative beliefs about the treatment may belie depression that requires medical intervention. A patient who believes he will not get better may inadvertently suppress immune functioning and especially the natural killer cells and cytotoxic T-cells and certain cytokines needed to track and eliminate the cancer (e.g., [62]). Because of the empirically known interdependent relationship between the patient and family caregiver, negative or distorted beliefs by the caregiver must also be addressed.

Suggested Strategies A medical and social history may reveal incidents in the individual's past that have contributed to these beliefs. Explore the patient's rationale for the beliefs. Share relevant medical information, reiterate *the positive goals* of the treatment, and emphasize that the vast majority of patients tolerate the treatment well, to encourage a more neutral or even more positive reappraisal of the goals of treatment. In addition, draw the patient's attention to the medication as it is being administered. Review Part IV Chap. 12 which provides suggested interventions to minimize negative beliefs and promote positive cognitive expectations about the treatment during informed consent and at the time of a drug's infusion [60, 63].

Clinical Anecdote 15.4
You know, this chemotherapy has the highest known efficacy with more than 97% of patients who have <u>your</u> cancer, responding well. You mentioned that you are worried about nausea. The vast majority of folks today do not experience this because all our patients receive an anti nausea medication before the chemo starts. I will tell you when the anti emetic is being administered so you will know that you are getting it. Let's review some things you can do to counter the fatigue that some patients have noted for a few days during treatment. Daily walks, use of the relaxation response technique, food high in protein, and vegetables that boost immune functioning can help with that, and of course a positive mood and positive self-talk. And of course avoid stress which in itself can deplete your energy resources. So try and do fun things during times in the day when you do feel more energetic.

As Ren and Xu [64] recommend, be truthful, balanced, and as positive as possible in giving information to minimize nocebo effects and enhance the possibility of placebo effects. Reframe information about negative effects in a way that increases patient expectation that things will go at least better than expected!

Strategies to Redress Distorted Beliefs (Review Part IV Chap. 9)
Distorted beliefs about a diagnosis may be characterized by hyperbolic and exaggerated ideations that tend to reflect patient or caregiver fear and anxiety. These distorted beliefs are akin to a nocebo that can interfere with the intended goals of treatment. Patients can benefit from the nurse's sensitive exploration of *distorted beliefs*, *hyperbolic generalizations*, and *catastrophic thinking* [41].

The main nursing goal is to uncover the potential drivers of the individual's generalizations, adverse metaphors, and distorted beliefs which interfere with the ability to adapt and strengthen overall resilience. Share relevant clinical information and scientific facts, offer alternative interpretations, reduce generalizations into smaller components, working with the individual to sort out fact from belief, what can be changed (clinical outcome) versus what cannot. Dispelling a myth about cancer such as "it kills everyone" or the treatment "makes you sicker" often just requires relevant information, grounded in scientific fact in order to foster more positive cognitive reappraisals.

Notwithstanding, nurse strategies may also involve engaging the individual in a process known as "cognitive restructuring" (i.e., working with the individual through Socratic questioning in which the nurse facilitates a process of making links between positive or negative beliefs and their impact on the individual's emotions and behavior and vice versa in an exercise to demonstrate reciprocal interdependent effects that lie within the individual's control) [40, 41]. The aim is to encourage a more neutral or even more positive reappraisal. The nurse draws the patient's attention to the impact of positive thinking on his or her emotions and behaviors. In so doing, the patient can experience a greater sense of personal control, which is also empowering and can enhance overall well-being (Part IV Chap. 9, section "The Nurse's Essential "Resilient-Promoting Toolbox""). An important aspect of cognitive restructuring is helping the individual to distinguish between a belief and a fact [40].

Another nursing strategy involves "breaking down" generalizations or metaphors into smaller, manageable versus unmanageable parts, prioritizing the resulting manageable components, and then finding appropriate solutions for each one (Part IV Chap. 9, section "The Nurse's Essential "Resilient-Promoting Toolbox""").

Enhancing Cognitive-Behavioral and Meaning-Making Coping Strategies (Review Part IV Chaps. 9 and 10; Appendix in Chap. 9; Appendix in Chap. 10; Appendix B)

Coping efforts typically involve four main components for promoting resilience in the face of adversity: problem-focused, emotion-focused, meaning-focused, and behavioral coping strategies. This section highlights various nursing strategies that may be utilized to facilitate the patient's resilient capabilities as a function of his or her concerns and distress. Critically it serves as a psychosocial repository of nurse interventions. That said, these interventions call upon the nurse to acquire the clinical expertise for each one via learning workshops, clinical stages with clinical experts, and/or by taking relevant clinical courses on psychosocial interventions (Chap. 19).

Problem-Focused Coping Strategies [39, 40]

The main problem-solving coping strategy consists of (1) a practical problem arising from the cancer or treatment, (2) a desired outcome, (3) an action plan tailored to the problem, (4) the patient's ownership of the problem, and (5) implementation and evaluation of effectiveness. The goals are to find a solution to the stated problem and enable patient or caregiver adherence.

Facilitating problem-solving approaches involves drawing on a number of strategies (Part IV Chap. 9, section "Facilitating Self-Management Strategies"). Encourage an exploration of the identified threat or problem from different perspectives, including the individual's perceived causes for the problem. As needed, break down the threat into smaller manageable parts; identify what can and cannot be changed; eliminate what is no longer a threat or concern and encourage individual to define the problem (Part IV Chap. 9, section "The Nurse's Essential "Resilient-Promoting Toolbox""). Define the goal or desired outcome. Use reframing and encourage reappraisals based on relevant information. Encourage "brainstorming" to identify the patient's preferred strategy for realizing the desired outcome. Once these components have been clearly delineated, the nurse and patient move to the action plan, implementation, and finally the reevaluation phase. Examples include adopting strategies for reducing emotional stress by developing an action plan to integrate these activities into their routine or daily life.

15.8 Nursing Implications

Emotion-Focused Strategies (Part IV Chaps. 9–11; Part V Chaps. 16 and 18; Review Appendix B)

Promote emotion-regulating strategies of the individual with cancer and their family caregiver:

1. Normalize worries: For instance, 'It's okay to worry, we all do when confronting something challenging in our life, so long as it does not immobilize us'. (If your assessment suggests emotional distress a deeper discussion involving the impact the diagnosis has had on the patient's (and caregiver's) life, thoughts, beliefs, feelings, and supportive relationship with the family (family caregiver) is warranted).
2. Encourage positive emotions: Invite the patient and family caregiver to make the most of each day by doing something that makes *their heart sing*, working on a beloved hobby, going to the theater, listening to favorite music, celebrating family occasions, spending time with friends, and *then sharing* these positive events at the next clinic visit which also creates feelings of well-being in the telling and contributes to quality of life [42, 65].
3. Support hope within a clinically realistic context (e.g., "We are *both* wishing for the best outcome, and together we can do things to optimize your health") (e.g., daily walks or practicing the relaxation response technique to lower stress and activate immune cells that hunt down and eliminate cancer cells) [65, 66] (review Part IV Chap. 9).
4. Encourage the use of distraction behaviors (seeing a movie) (e.g., [65, 67]).
5. Encourage a focus on the present (e.g., [68]) (review Appendix B). Human beings have a tendency to live in the future or the past, without realizing it. In so doing we often miss the immense riches that await us in the present such as the warmth and love of friendships and family, the magic of a sunrise or sunset, a great book, a wonderful concert, or a walk through nature. Too often our minds are somewhere along a future horizon or a remembered past. Encourage the patient to reorient thoughts to the present, rather than the past or future, in order to experience the silver linings that await in the here and now that also helps maintain emotional equanimity. When we truly live in the present which demands our total attention, it is difficult to remain distressed.

Meaning-Focused Coping Strategies [45]
(Review Part IV Chaps. 9 and 10)

For most resilient newly diagnosed patients, the disrupted beliefs about the world and the self tend to be temporary, with the traumatic diagnosis ultimately serving as the impetus for self-reflection, adaptive coping, and growth-promoting behaviors [19, 48]. Those patients tend to perceive cancer as a challenge, bringing all their personal and social resources to the task of somehow overcoming the disease or living well with it.

Making Sense of the Cancer Diagnosis Patients may express feelings of "why me" or interpret the diagnosis of cancer as a punishment from "above." Others experience intrusive ideation, a cognitive perseveration of thoughts about cancer or dying. Each in his/her own way is seeking to make sense of what has happened [45,

69]. Everything that had defined the patient up to the diagnosis and given life meaning and purpose may now have been thrust into psychological upheaval.

Sometimes making sense of a cancer diagnosis is facilitated through patient discussions with their supportive relationships who are in themselves an important source of meaning, but in addition have been shown to foster reappraisal and other coping capabilities in the patient [70, 71]. Some patients may reach for a steady ballast found in a personal philosophy of life, in spiritual connections experienced within the context of a formal religion, nature, or any deeply felt, meaningful activity that connects the person to something beyond the self. It may be a love of music, volunteering, painting or hockey, saying the rosary in church, or something else [45, 48, 72]. Sometimes, self-awareness evolves and a transformed self emerges later in the illness trajectory. *However, seeking* meaning in a cancer diagnosis when *prolonged* is maladaptive and perpetuates feelings of anxiety or even a demoralized depressive state [45, 48].

Encourage the individual's *narrative* about life before cancer, eliciting his thoughts, feelings, and behaviors leading up to the diagnosis and immediately afterward which may help the patient to cognitively process what has happened (e.g., [12, 73, 74]). Through a guided narrative, the threat of cancer may be reframed or positively reappraised within a more purposeful context that lends meaning to this experience. For many, cancer may serve as a silver lining in that some individuals would never have imagined taking time out from work to do things that are dear to them, but they never had time to do such as travel more, paint, write, and spend more time with family.

For patients who continue to struggle, the nurse may suggest, at a certain point, that "bad things do happen to good people," for no apparent reason (see Part IV Chap. 10) and that the "secret" to living well with cancer is accepting it and finding meaning in one's current life. You also might raise for discussion one of the main takeaways of V Frankl's book [75] on the search for meaning: the essence being that we have a choice to perseverate on things we want but cannot change or to change our response to adverse circumstances in order to make the most of the life we have right now. These supportive interventions may be revisited over regular clinic appointments.

Meaning in Life After a Diagnosis Another meaning-related concern of the newly diagnosed is the quest for meaning *in life after the diagnosis*. Patients may have accepted the reality of the cancer, but it has left their life fearful and bereft of meaning and purpose. The cancer diagnosis may generate an existential crisis with the belief that one's self has been forever altered and one's existence threatened (e.g., [74]). A qualitative study of support groups for newly diagnosed women with breast cancer found that women derived a greater sense of control and found meaning in their life through connecting with other newly diagnosed women [76]. These discussions facilitated problem-solving behaviors regarding issues surrounding the diagnosis and treatment; it provided a collaborative environment in which to review priorities and values that touched upon their meaningful relationships; it facilitated better management of their emotions and encouraged planning for and doing meaningful activities. These discussions facilitated their ability to find meaning in their daily life. These findings suggest that a psychosocial intervention is an essential component of the prehabilitation phase (e.g., [76]).

In addition to promoting a problem-focused coping approach, the nurse may also promote the patient's use of emotion-focused and meaning-making coping strategies that enable a reduction in emotional distress while also reframing the diagnosis through facts, information, cognitive restructuring, and breaking generalizations into smaller more manageable components to promote a cognitive shift toward more neutral or positive reappraisals of the possibilities for meaning in life. (Review Chaps. 9 and 10; Appendix B for nursing strategies.) You might also invite the patient to share meaningful experiences in life before cancer and to consider that these meaningful experiences might still be possible even likely in their current life. The nurse may also consider implementing a meaning-making intervention [74]. This nurse-developed intervention for patients with cancer may be conducted at clinic visits or by the bedside.

Clinical Anecdote 15.5
Previously, I have described the meaningful encounter I had with a supportive care physician who dropped by to see me on the unit as I was recuperating from an operation. He stayed maybe 20 min, but that discussion still resonates deeply. Somehow through our conversation about a much loved symphony, memories of the sound of the music and the images of a flowing river, lifted my spirits and intensified my immanent sense of connectedness with nature. Our conversation reminded me of the deeply felt experiences still possible in the moment that gave me hope. And, a bit like Humpty Dumpty, it helped to put my self together again.

Part IV Chap. 10 on meaning discusses in depth the various strategies that may be used to foster meaning and acceptance. An important facet of advanced nursing practice is to be well rounded as a whole person with diverse interests that enable the nurse to engage in topics of shared interest with the patient which can momentarily distract the patient's mind from his worries or provide a deeper more meaningful discussion about spiritual matters or topics of hope and meaning in our lives every day.

Facilitate Deliberate Rumination (See Part IV Chap. 10)
Intrusive ideation refers to repeated unwanted thoughts which are the mind's efforts to cognitively process the traumatic event yet can perpetuate emotional distress [77, 78]. Unabated intrusive ideation and avoidance may exacerbate emotional distress and interfere with healing- and health-promoting behaviors in the prehabilitation

phase. Conversely deliberate rumination refers to *the purposeful analysis* of thoughts and feelings related to the stressor event that involves narrative sharing around the source and triggers of the stressor event [12, 79]. Deliberate rumination facilitates the patient's ability to regain "personal control" over uncontrollable thoughts via an intentional examination of the unwanted ideation within a more "controlled" environment, for instance, through a series of nurse-led questions about the quality, intensity, frequency, duration, triggers, and subject matter of the unwanted ideation. The "controlled" and repeated discussions about the event facilitate cognitive processing or coming to terms with the event [78].

You might begin by asking the patient to share his thoughts about the source of distress—the nature of the intrusive thoughts. Ask the individual to identify the precipitating factors of the intrusive ideation, the time of day when they mostly manifest, and their potential significance [41]. Ask the individual to consider personal concerns (e.g., fears) that may be driving these uncontrollable thoughts; and then break those into manageable parts, dispelling, for instance, the misguided beliefs and myths that may be the source of the disturbing thoughts.

Each time the individual talks about the unwanted thoughts their traumatizing effects may diminish, reflecting cognitive processing. Deliberate rumination may reduce the presence and or intensity of intrusive thoughts, but it may also lead patients to accept and/or come to terms with the traumatic diagnosis. *Benson's relaxation response technique* [80] may serve as an apt strategy *to accompany deliberate rumination* due to its goal of reducing the intensity of emotional reactivity in response to unwanted ideation (review Part IV Chap. 13). Interestingly, healing touch has been shown to be effective as part of a multimodal approach to post-traumatic stress ideation (review Part IV Chap. 14).

A Cautionary Note Prolonged intrusive thoughts ultimately interfere with growth-promoting capabilities such as the ability to reframe the diagnosis as a potential opportunity; to live a less stressful, more fulfilling life; or to imagine what such a life might look like. Patients who remain psychologically stuck would benefit from the aid of a psychologist and/or the physician due to its stress-inducing effects on the biology and emotions of the patient.

Promote Behavioral Coping Strategies (See Part IV Chap. 13)
Meditative practices such as Benson's relaxation response technique, mindful meditation, yoga, and qigong have been shown to effectively downregulate the biological stress response system and reduce feelings of anxiety, depressed mood, and distress. Significantly these practices appear to reduce the practitioner's emotional reactivity to intrusive ideation.

The relaxation response technique, for instance, is extremely simple to implement in the clinic, by the hospital bedside, or at home: Consider explaining its purpose, function, clinical benefits, and dosing effect, and demonstrate the technique. Encourage the newly diagnosed person and family member to practice, together if possible, at least once a day increasing from 10 to 30 min each session [81–84]. Each clinic visit or bedside visit in which the nurse proposes to accompany the patient and loved one in the RR can facilitate the integration of this technique into their daily routine while validating the potential therapeutic benefits. These few minutes also may have a healing and restorative effect on the nurse (e.g., [85]).

RR practices heighten the individual's awareness of sensations, feelings, and thoughts, and the practitioner of the technique learns how to ignore or become detached emotionally from intrusive and unwanted ideation which interferes with emotional equanimity [86]. It also facilitates reorientation of the mind to the present. Please review Benson and Stuart's *The Wellness Book* (Chap. 4, p. 33) to become familiar with the steps to follow.

Encourage physical activity/exercise such as moderate-to-brisk walking or cycling or skiing which are widely known strategies to reduce emotional distress, but also critically to strengthen physical fitness in order to more effectively tolerate the upcoming treatment [22]. Explain the physiological relationship of exercise on anticancer immune system functioning [87]. Explore the physical activity that is preferred by the patient and caregiver, while encouraging the exercises proposed in an enrolled prehabilitation program.

Self-Management Interventions (Review Part IV Chap. 9; Appendices A and B)

As nursing conceptualizations of prehabilitation programs continue to evolve, self-management interventions for both the patient and family caregiver have increasingly been recognized as important problem-solving skills to master at the beginning of the cancer and treatment continuum [88]. Given the increased complexity of cancer care, the clinical goal is to enhance the patient's and/or caregiver's level of self-efficacy in order to manage practical problems that may arise between treatments or hospital visits. Consequently, it is essential that the patient or caregiver takes ownership of each step of the collaboratively agreed-upon self-management strategy, with the support of the nurse [39, 89].

To date, self-management interventions have been mostly offered to patients with advanced disease and family caregivers starting in the early diagnostic and treatment phases of supportive care (e.g., [90, 91]).

Strengthening Supportive Relationships (Review Part III Chap. 6; Part IV Chap. 11; Appendix B)

The scientific consensus is that informal support is a significant predictor of survival and an essential resource that strengthens resilience throughout the illness and recovery trajectory [92, 93]. An important nursing objective is to identify, enhance, and strengthen the quality of support, existing between the patient and his or her significant others. An initial strategy is to engage the patient and family caregiver in an informal discussion of behaviors they feel are supportive and the role of support in helping one another cope with moments of stress they may experience (e.g., [71, 94]).

Engage the patient and family member in a conversation regarding the meaning of support, inviting each to illustrate with examples the "most supportive" and "least supportive" behaviors, and why. Ask the patient and family to share their thoughts about the types of support each person *needs* from one another to feel supported going forward. Encourage the patient and family to share their ideas about ways to obtain and retain emotional and instrumental support from one another and from the family [95, 96]. Illustrate your discussion with examples. For instance, suggest that rather than second guessing "all the reasons why a loved one has not called, be brave and pick up the phone." The reason may be as simple as not wanting to "disturb the patient or caregiver." In which case, that information can then be discussed to the satisfaction of both individuals. Convey the importance of never making assumptions and always validating one another's feelings, thoughts, and behaviors. Discuss various strategies to consider in order to obtain needed support from the healthcare team [40]. Given converging scientific evidence on the interrelationships among support, coping responses, resilience, and health, you might consider sharing scientific information about the significance of support to well-being and specifically its positive effects on strengthening healing and resilient capabilities in all individuals.

In summary, the nurse should strongly consider developing a psychosocial workshop aimed at strengthening cognitive-behavioral and self-management strategies and supportive relationships for newly diagnosed patients and their family caregivers prior to the start of treatment.

Healthy Lifestyle Behaviors with a Focus on Physical Fitness, Physical Activity, Healthy Diet, and Nutrition (Review Appendix C; Part V Chap. 16)

The majority of prehabilitation programs tend to focus on physical exercise and resistance training, and increasingly on diet and nutrition in order to enhance overall fitness so that the patient may better tolerate the physical stress associated with the impending surgery. In addition to psychosocial nursing interventions, the nurse also supports the physical fitness and nutritional/dietary goals of the prehabilitation program. In collaboration with the oncology team, the nurse monitors the patient's adherence to the program at each nurse visit, identifies potential obstacles, and as relevant proposes recommendations in consultation with the oncologist, dietician, and physiotherapist. The nurse's proactive involvement in promoting healthy life style behaviors is an essential component of nursing practice. It involves providing information, education and encouragement. It becomes even more critical for newly diagnosed patients who are essentially healthy and do not necessitate the specialized diet and or nutritional supplements of an oncology dietician. Although the literature has focused on pre surgical patients with cancer, these programs are also needed for all patients facing most cancer treatments.

15.8 Nursing Implications

Physical Exercise (PE) [22]

Physical activity refers to any activity involving skeletal muscles ([22], p. 198). Exercise is regarded as (1) aerobic activity when it increases oxygen intake such as cardiovascular functioning and (2) anaerobic when it involves resistance or weight training. Measurements of physical activity combine the duration of the activity with its intensity ([22], p. 200). A frequently used measure of exercise is known as metabolic equivalents (METs) which refer to the level of intensity (i.e., sedentary, light, moderate, vigorous) of the activity in relation to the body's resting metabolic rate ([22], p. 200) One's total expenditure of energy may be assessed as the product of low-intensity activity for a long duration or high-intensity activity for a short period, with differential effects on the individual's physiology. Physical activity is also measured in terms of the physical activity ratio (PAL) defined as the overall activity level over a day.

Regular, moderately intense, daily physical activity has been heralded as a clinical imperative for cancer prevention (and other forms of chronic illness) and to increase survivability as well as to optimize resilience in patients awaiting surgery [1, 22]. There is convincing evidence that physical exercise counters obesity, unwanted weight gain and being overweight, factors which have been implicated in cancer incidence ([22], p. 200).

PE promotes psychological, physical, and metabolic strengthening through short-term repetitions that promote physiological learning as well as fitness-promoting processes [97]. Physical activity/exercise activates the stress response system for a specified length of time during which the whole body is mobilized (including cardiovascular, musculoskeletal, and metabolic, neuroendocrine, and immune systems) in order to meet physiological demands for maintaining homeostasis at a higher level, before returning to normal or reconstituted homeostatic levels [98, 99]. Repeated regularly, it leads to a higher level of overall resilience and homeostatic capability.

Recent research indicates that exercise induces cytotoxic immune cell activity, restricts inflammatory signaling pathways in myeloid immune cells, and modulates acute and chronic inflammatory responses, suggesting that exercise is likely an invaluable adjunct to cancer treatment [98, 99]. PE in both healthy individuals and those with cancer appears to lower one's cancer risk and cancer recurrence, as well as optimize resilience during active treatment, although differential effects based on gender have been noted [22, 100, 101].

How Much The optimal intensity, duration, and frequency of various physical activities to promote therapeutic outcomes for patients with various stages and phases of cancer are still unclear. However, converging evidence recommends between 130 and 150 min of moderate-intensity exercise a week or 75 min of intense exercise a week to lower one's risk of developing cancer or getting cancer again (Tables 15.2 and 15.3) ([22], p. 52; [102], p. 246). Daily moderate-intensity exercise may consist of a brisk walk, biking, or running. The duration of daily moderately intense exercise should be increased over time to 60 min (or longer) in physically fit individuals, which include cancer-free survivors. Recent studies indicate that indi-

Table 15.2 Sedentary-, light-, moderate-, and vigorous-intensity physical activities ([22], p. 200; [102])

Activity/ physiological indicators	Se Sedentary (≤1.5 METs)	Light physical activity (<3 METs)	Moderate intensity (3–5.9 METs)	Vigorous intensity (≥6 METs)
Definitions	Refers to HR, RR not raised above "resting" metabolic levels	Refers to minor increased changes to heart and breathing rates	Refers to a HR increase of an estimated 60–75% its maximum (the energy requirements usually met through *aerobic metabolism* using body stores of glycogen and then fats)	Refers to a HR estimated increase of ≥80% of its maximum capability (i.e., with energy requirements by *anaerobic metabolism* using glucose and glycogen)
Exercise/ physical activity	Sitting watching TV, working in front of computer	Casual Walking, biking <5 mph, stretching, shopping for food, preparing meals	Brisk walking, walking uphill, hiking, biking, yoga	Running, swimming, aerobic workout, fast biking (>10 mph)
			Downhill skiing, doubles tennis, golfing	Cross-country skiing, single tennis, ice/field hockey
			Maintaining the grass and gardening, house work	Digging, hauling dirt and transplanting saplings, shoveling snow

Table 15.3 Summary: physiological effects of moderate physical exercise on the whole being

- ↓es stress-activated HPA axis, SAM→ ↓ ed inflammation, ↓ed oxidative stress, ↓ing potential for cell and DNA damage [23, 103, 104]
- All PA protects against weight gain, being overweight, and obesity → linked to cancer, excluding lung cancer [22, 102]
- ↓es hormonal levels such as insulin, IGF-1, estrogens, androgens, testosterone associated with being overweight, obese, and that ↑es cell proliferation and anti-apoptosis [97]
- ↑es sensitivity to insulin (↓ing insulin resistance syndrome), ↓ing pro-inflammatory adipokines or cytokines released from adipose tissue [97]
- Strengthens immune system functioning such as ↑ing NKCA, cytotoxic T-cells, IFN-gamma (e.g., [87])

viduals undergoing anticancer treatment who also engaged in either daily light home exercise or moderate-to-vigorous exercise produced a number of clinical benefits including qualitatively less physical fatigue, improved immune functioning including cell-mediated immunity, and improved quality of sleep [4, 87, 105, 106]. Conversely *vigorous* daily prolonged exercise would be counterproductive, particularly during either the diagnostic or treatment-related phases in that it can temporarily reduce resilient immune functions and increase the risk of infection, oxidative stress, and DNA damage [87].

Nursing Goals At regular clinic visits, assess the patient's weight and waist circumference. Compared to prediagnostic levels of exercise, assess the type, frequency, duration, and intensity of exercise per week, since the diagnosis. An important goal of the diagnostic phase is to encourage patients and their caregivers to increase (to recommended levels) and continue daily physical activity throughout the pretreatment phase through survivorship. Provide emotional support (encouragement), education, and relevant information tailored to the patient's preferences regarding physical activity. This discussion may entail type of activity/exercise, time of day, frequency, and duration but also its therapeutic benefits to underscore its importance to patients diagnosed with cancer. Encourage the patient and caregiver to engage in exercise together or with a close friend or companion, which in itself is both supportive and therapeutic.

Critically, the frequency, intensity, and duration of physical activity deemed therapeutic for a patient diagnosed with cancer prior to receiving treatment will depend on the patient's current clinical status and *recommendations* by the treating physician and physiotherapist. But in principle, where prehabilitation programs may be lacking, all patients who have not lost weight and are medically deemed physically healthy should be encouraged to engage in physical activity to the best of their ability without becoming exhausted (review [22]).

Tables 15.2 and 15.3 provide information that may guide the nurse's general assessment of the individual's level of physical activity, providing a better clinical context for discussions with the oncologist and physiotherapist.

Diet (Review Part V Chap. 16)
Hippocrates' saying "Let thy food be your medicine, and medicine be thy food" manifested excellent clinical insight. Whereas "under" (i.e., inadequate)-nutrition is associated with poor immune functioning, overeating causing weight gain that exceeds the normal range for height and age, also threatens the individual's survival and increases the risk for cancer and recurrence [30]. A healthy diet comprises fruits (especially small berries with a minimum of carbohydrates), vegetables, legumes, whole grains, chicken, and fish and little to no alcohol, refined sugar, red meat, and processed food [22, 97]. Consumption of water is recommended over sugared drinks including orange juices except for an occasional indulgence. Maintaining a healthy weight, waist circumference, and BMI are recommended to lower the risk of cancer or cancer recurrence. Being overweight is associated with cancer [102].

A healthy diet is now conceptualized as a whole balanced approach in which dietary patterns across healthy food groups are preferred over a previously nutrient-centered diet [102]. A prehabilitation diet however may be supplemented, modified, or restricted as a function of the type of surgery, other medical treatments, the patient's stage and type of cancer, and clinical status (e.g., [32, 33]). If the oncology dietician has determined that a newly diagnosed patient does not require nutritional supplementation or a special diet, then with the oncologist's and dietician's agreement, encourage the adoption of an evidence-based health-promoting anticancer diet based on varying dietary patterns, which has been recommended for healthy individuals to prevent cancer and for patients in transition to survivorship to optimize physical health [22].

Health-Promoting Constituents in Foods Phytochemicals are bioactive compounds that have been discovered in plants and found to play a vital role in sustaining human life. A growing body of research suggests that an array of phytochemicals protect the human organism against disease, as well as promote physiological resilience (healing). Phytochemicals have been shown to exert immunomodulating, antioxidant, antibacterial, antiviral, and anticancer capabilities; they play a critical role in reversing pro-inflammatory pathways that cause cancer (e.g., [30]; [107], p. 79, 182; [108, 109]). These non-nutritive compounds appear to protect neuro-cellular structures including DNA from oxidative damage, lower inflammation, decrease the growth rate of some cancer cells, and enhance immunity [107]. The most well known are *the carotenoids, flavonoids* (such as the catechins, quercetin), *glucosinolates, anthocyanins, saponins,* and other polyphenols such as resveratrol and lycopene. Plant foods containing phytochemicals include red peppers, onions (cooked tomatoes, carrots, and broccoli), cabbage, brussel sprouts, apricots, apples, and sweet potatoes. Carotenoids are found in red, orange, yellow, and green plants.

The objective of healthy eating lies in healthy *eating patterns of diverse food groups* that translate into unique and overlapping biochemical constituents in order to derive optimal protective benefits from a variety of food groups [102]. Suggestions for patients and caregivers surrounding health-promoting food groups and recommended dietary patterns of consumption must be predicated on scientific evidence [22] and in collaboration with the treating oncologist and dietician.

Nurses have an important role in educating patients and caregivers and encouraging adherence to prehabilitation recommendations concerning physical exercise and diet by the oncologist, dietician, and physio-exercise therapist. This requires basic knowledge of the impact of a healthy diet and exercise on the individual's emotional, physical, and neurophysiological resilient capabilities, as well as the significance of METs as a measure of exercise, in order to be fully engaged in team discussions and recommendations. Become familiar and up to date with ACS and WCRF/AICR recommendations.

Note The biochemical properties of some foods may interact with the treatment and need to be avoided, for instance, grapefruit with some medications. Thus food groups that may interact with the chemotherapy or other treatment must be vetted before sharing or developing a healthy diet with the patient. Notwithstanding, the nurse should be knowledgeable about the principles and food types associated with a healthy diet.

15.9 Managing Consent

(Please review Part IV Chap. 12)

Final Thoughts
The overall consensus within the cancer healthcare community is that an early prehabilitation program for newly diagnosed patients improves the overall physical and psychosocial resilience of the individual and is recommended as good clinical practice (eg. [1, 2, 4]). Nurse-led psychosocial interventions aimed at strengthening overall psychosocial resilience for patients and family caregivers should be encouraged. Nurse-led workshops are especially needed in this early phase to reduce stress levels, acquire emotion-regulating coping strategies and self-management skills, enhance supportive relationships, and promote healthy lifestyle behaviors in patients and caregivers in preparatory readiness for the upcoming treatment. The content from this workshop provides important knowledge and skills to successfully confront various stressors along the treatment trajectory. Each component may be offered one on one or in group workshops—it is still unclear which delivery format is optimal and likely depends on multiple factors.

References

1. Silver JK. Cancer prehabilitation and its role in improving health outcomes and reducing health care costs. Semin Oncol Nurs. 2015;31(1):13–30. PubMed PMID: 25636392. Epub 2015/02/01. eng.
2. van Rooijen SJ, Molenaar CJL, Schep G, van Lieshout R, Beijer S, Dubbers R, et al. Making patients fit for surgery: introducing a four pillar multimodal prehabilitation program in colorectal cancer. Am J Phys Med Rehabil. 2019;98(10):888–96. PubMed PMID: 31090551. Epub 2019/05/16. eng.
3. Cohen L, Parker PA, Vence L, Savary C, Kentor D, Pettaway C, et al. Presurgical stress management improves postoperative immune function in men with prostate cancer undergoing radical prostatectomy. Psychosom Med. 2011;73(3):218–25. PubMed PMID: 21257977. Epub 2011/01/25. eng.
4. Treanor C, Kyaw T, Donnelly M. An international review and meta-analysis of prehabilitation compared to usual care for cancer patients. J Cancer Survivor Res Pract. 2018;12(1):64–73. PubMed PMID: 28900822. Epub 2017/09/14. eng.
5. Hijazi Y, Gondal U, Aziz O. A systematic review of prehabilitation programs in abdominal cancer surgery. Int J Surg. 2017;39:156–62. PubMed PMID: 28161527. Epub 2017/02/06. eng.
6. Funk R, Cisneros C, Williams RC, Kendall J, Hamann HA. What happens after distress screening? Patterns of supportive care service utilization among oncology patients identified through a systematic screening protocol. Support Care Cancer. 2016;24(7):2861–8. PubMed PMID: 26838023. Epub 2016/02/04. eng.
7. Orom H, Nelson CJ, Underwood W III, Homish DL, Kapoor DA. Factors associated with emotional distress in newly diagnosed prostate cancer patients. Psycho-Oncology. 2015;24(11):1416–22. PubMed PMID: 25631163. Epub 2015/01/30. eng.

8. Riba MB, Donovan KA, Andersen B, Braun I, Breitbart WS, Brewer BW, et al. Distress management, Version 3.2019, NCCN clinical practice guidelines in oncology. J Natl Compr Cancer Netw. 2019;17(10):1229–49. PubMed PMID: 31590149. Pubmed Central PMCID: PMC6907687. Epub 2019/10/08. eng.
9. Weisman AD, Worden JW. The existential plight in cancer: significance of the first 100 days. Int J Psychiatry Med. 1976;7(1):1–15. PubMed PMID: 1052080. Epub 1976/01/01. eng.
10. Ercolano E. Psychosocial concerns in the postoperative oncology patient. Semin Oncol Nurs. 2017;33(1):74–9. PubMed PMID: 28062332. Epub 2017/01/08. eng.
11. Janoff-Bulman R. Assumptive worlds and the stress of traumatic events: applications of the scheme construct. Soc Cogn. 1989;7:113–36.
12. Lancaster SL, Klein KR, Nadia C, Szabo L, Mogerman B. An integrated model of posttraumatic stress and growth. J Trauma Dissoc. 2015;16(4):399–418. PubMed PMID: 26011515. Epub 2015/05/27. eng.
13. Seiler A, Jenewein J. Resilience in cancer patients. Front Psychiatry. 2019;10:208. PubMed PMID: 31024362. Pubmed Central PMCID: PMC6460045. Epub 2019/04/27. eng.
14. McEwen BS. Physiology and neurobiology of stress and adaptation: central role of the brain. Physiol Rev. 2007;87(3):873–904. PubMed PMID: 17615391. Epub 2007/07/07. eng.
15. Jacobs JM, Shaffer KM, Nipp RD, Fishbein JN, MacDonald J, El-Jawahri A, et al. Distress is interdependent in patients and caregivers with newly diagnosed incurable cancers. Ann Behav Med. 2017;51(4):519–31. PubMed PMID: 28097515. Pubmed Central PMCID: PMC5513787. Epub 2017/01/18. eng.
16. Balmer C, Griffiths F, Dunn J. A 'new normal': exploring the disruption of a poor prognostic cancer diagnosis using interviews and participant-produced photographs. Health. 2015;19(5):451–72. PubMed PMID: 25323052. Epub 2014/10/18. eng.
17. Robinson S, Kissane DW, Brooker J, Burney S. A systematic review of the demoralization syndrome in individuals with progressive disease and cancer: a decade of research. J Pain Symptom Manag. 2015;49(3):595–610. PubMed PMID: 25131888. Epub 2014/08/19. eng.
18. Henoch I, Danielson E. Existential concerns among patients with cancer and interventions to meet them: an integrative literature review. Psycho-Oncology. 2009;18(3):225–36. PubMed PMID: 18792088. Epub 2008/09/16. eng.
19. Tedeschi RG, Calhoun LG. Posttraumatic growth: conceptual foundations and empirical evidence. Psychol Inq. 2004;15:1–18.
20. Fassier P, Zelek L, Partula V, Srour B, Bachmann P, Touillaud M, et al. Variations of physical activity and sedentary behavior between before and after cancer diagnosis: results from the prospective population-based NutriNet-Sante cohort. Medicine. 2016;95(40):e4629. PubMed PMID: 27749527. Pubmed Central PMCID: PMC5059029. Epub 2016/10/18. eng.
21. Foucaut AM, Berthouze SE, Touillaud M, Morelle M, Bourne-Branchu V, Kempf-Lépine AS, et al. Deterioration of physical activity level and metabolic risk factors after early-stage breast cancer diagnosis. Cancer Nurs. 2015;38(4):E1–9. PubMed PMID: 25207592. Epub 2014/09/11. eng.
22. World Cancer Research Fund AIfcr. Diet, nutrition, physical activity and cancer: a global perspective. Summary of 3rd expert report. Continuous update project expert report. 2018. https://www.wcrf.org/diet-activity-and-cancer/.
23. Kirtonia A, Sethi G, Garg M. The multifaceted role of reactive oxygen species in tumorigenesis. Cell Mol Life Sci. 2020;77(22):4459–83. PubMed PMID: 32358622. Epub 2020/05/03. eng.
24. Wang M, Zhao J, Zhang L, Wei F, Lian Y, Wu Y, et al. Role of tumor microenvironment in tumorigenesis. J Cancer. 2017;8(5):761–73. PubMed PMID: 28382138. Pubmed Central PMCID: PMC5381164. Epub 2017/04/07. eng.
25. Minnella EM, Carli F, Kassouf W. Role of prehabilitation following major uro-oncologic surgery: a narrative review. World J Urol. 2022;40:1289. PubMed PMID: 33128596. Epub 2020/11/01. eng.
26. Daniels SL, Lee MJ, George J, Kerr K, Moug S, Wilson TR, et al. Prehabilitation in elective abdominal cancer surgery in older patients: systematic review and meta-analysis. BJS Open. 2020;4(6):1022–41. PubMed PMID: 32959532. Pubmed Central PMCID: PMC7709363. Epub 2020/09/23. eng.

27. Moran J, Guinan E, McCormick P, Larkin J, Mockler D, Hussey J, et al. The ability of prehabilitation to influence postoperative outcome after intra-abdominal operation: a systematic review and meta-analysis. Surgery. 2016;160(5):1189–201. PubMed PMID: 27397681. Epub 2016/10/30. eng.
28. Ngo-Huang A, Parker NH, Bruera E, Lee RE, Simpson R, O'Connor DP, et al. Home-based exercise prehabilitation during preoperative treatment for pancreatic cancer is associated with improvement in physical function and quality of life. Integr Cancer Ther. 2019;18:1534735419894061. PubMed PMID: 31858837. Pubmed Central PMCID: PMC7050956. Epub 2019/12/21. eng.
29. Childs CE, Calder PC, Miles EA. Diet and immune function. Nutrients. 2019;11(8):1933. PubMed PMID: 31426423. Pubmed Central PMCID: PMC6723551. Epub 2019/08/21. eng.
30. Alwarawrah Y, Kiernan K, MacIver NJ. Changes in nutritional status impact immune cell metabolism and function. Front Immunol. 2018;9:1055. PubMed PMID: 29868016. Pubmed Central PMCID: PMC5968375. Epub 2018/06/06. eng.
31. Gillis C, Davies SJ, Carli F, Wischmeyer PE, Wootton SA, Jackson AA, et al. Current landscape of nutrition within prehabilitation oncology research: a scoping review. Front Nutr. 2021;8:644723. PubMed PMID: 33898499. Pubmed Central PMCID: PMC8062858. Epub 2021/04/27. eng.
32. Gillis C, Loiselle SE, Fiore JF Jr, Awasthi R, Wykes L, Liberman AS, et al. Prehabilitation with whey protein supplementation on perioperative functional exercise capacity in patients undergoing colorectal resection for cancer: a pilot double-blinded randomized placebo-controlled trial. J Acad Nutr Diet. 2016;116(5):802–12. PubMed PMID: 26208743. Epub 2015/07/26. eng.
33. Gillis C, Buhler K, Bresee L, Carli F, Gramlich L, Culos-Reed N, et al. Effects of nutritional prehabilitation, with and without exercise, on outcomes of patients who undergo colorectal surgery: a systematic review and meta-analysis. Gastroenterology. 2018;155(2):391–410 e4. PubMed PMID: 29750973. Epub 2018/05/12. eng.
34. Trépanier M, Minnella EM, Paradis T, Awasthi R, Kaneva P, Schwartzman K, et al. Improved disease-free survival after prehabilitation for colorectal cancer surgery. Ann Surg. 2019;270(3):493–501. PubMed PMID: 31318793. Epub 2019/07/19. eng.
35. Galway K, Black A, Cantwell M, Cardwell CR, Mills M, Donnelly M. Psychosocial interventions to improve quality of life and emotional wellbeing for recently diagnosed cancer patients. Cochrane Database Syst Rev. 2012;11(11):CD007064. PubMed PMID: 23152241. Pubmed Central PMCID: PMC6457819. Epub 2012/11/16. eng.
36. Jassim GA, Whitford DL, Hickey A, Carter B. Psychological interventions for women with non-metastatic breast cancer. Cochrane Database Syst Rev. 2015;5:CD008729. PubMed PMID: 26017383. Epub 2015/05/29. eng.
37. Semple C, Parahoo K, Norman A, McCaughan E, Humphris G, Mills M. Psychosocial interventions for patients with head and neck cancer. Cochrane Database Syst Rev. 2013;7:CD009441. PubMed PMID: 23857592. Epub 2013/07/17. eng.
38. Denieffe S, Gooney M. A meta-synthesis of women's symptoms experience and breast cancer. Eur J Cancer Care. 2011;20(4):424–35. PubMed PMID: 20825463. Epub 2010/09/10. eng.
39. Leventhal H, Phillips LA, Burns E. The Common-Sense Model of Self-Regulation (CSM): a dynamic framework for understanding illness self-management. J Behav Med. 2016;39(6):935–46. PubMed PMID: 27515801. Epub 2016/08/16. eng.
40. Benson H, Stuart E. The wellness book: the comprehensive guide to maintaining health and treating stress-related illness. New York, NY: Simon and Schuster; 1992.
41. Meichenbaum D. A clinical handbook for assessing and treating adults with post-traumatic stress disorder (PTSD). Waterloo, ON: Institute Press; 1994.
42. Folkman S. The case for positive emotions in the stress process. Anxiety Stress Coping. 2008;21(1):3–14. PubMed PMID: 18027121. Epub 2007/11/21. eng.
43. Folkman S, Greer S. Promoting psychological well-being in the face of serious illness: when theory, research and practice inform each other. Psycho-Oncology. 2000;9(1):11–9. PubMed PMID: 10668055. Epub 2000/02/11. eng.
44. Folkman S, Lazarus RS, Dunkel-Schetter C, DeLongis A, Gruen RJ. Dynamics of a stressful encounter: cognitive appraisal, coping, and encounter outcomes. J Pers Soc Psychol. 1986;50(5):992–1003. PubMed PMID: 3712234. Epub 1986/05/01. eng.

45. Park CL. Making sense of the meaning literature: an integrative review of meaning making and its effects on adjustment to stressful life events. Psychol Bull. 2010;136(2):257–301. PubMed PMID: 20192563. Epub 2010/03/03. eng.
46. Carver CS, Scheier MF. Dispositional optimism. Trends Cogn Sci. 2014;18(6):293–9. PubMed PMID: 24630971. Pubmed Central PMCID: PMC4061570. Epub 2014/03/19. eng.
47. Amstadter AB, Moscati A, Oxon MA, Maes HH, Myers JM, Kendler KS. Personality, cognitive/psychological traits and psychiatric resilience: a multivariate twin study. Personal Individ Differ. 2016;91:74–9. PubMed PMID: 29104336. Pubmed Central PMCID: PMC5667653. Epub 2016/03/01. eng.
48. Park CL. Meaning making in the context of disasters. J Clin Psychol. 2016;72(12):1234–46. PubMed PMID: 26900868. Epub 2016/02/24. eng.
49. Cobb S. Social support as a moderator of life stress. Psychosom Med. 1976;38(5):300–14.
50. House JS, Khan RL. Measures and concepts of social support. New York, NY: Academic Press; 1985.
51. Folkman S, Moskowitz J. Positive affect and meaning-focused coping during significant psychological stress. In: Haws MH, de Wit JBF, van den Bos K, Stroebe MS, editors. The scope of social psychology: theory and applications. New York, NY: Psychology Press; 2007. p. 193–208.
52. Park CL, Edmondson D, Fenster JR, Blank TO. Meaning making and psychological adjustment following cancer: the mediating roles of growth, life meaning, and restored just-world beliefs. J Consult Clin Psychol. 2008;76(5):863–75. PubMed PMID: 18837603. Epub 2008/10/08. eng.
53. Kissane DW. The relief of existential suffering. Arch Intern Med. 2012;172(19):1501–5. PubMed PMID: 22945389. Epub 2012/09/05. eng.
54. Creamer M, Burgess P, Pattison P. Reaction to trauma: a cognitive processing model. J Abnorm Psychol. 1992;101(3):452–9. PubMed PMID: 1500602. Epub 1992/08/01. eng.
55. Thorne S, Hislop TG, Kim-Sing C, Oglov V, Oliffe JL, Stajduhar KI. Changing communication needs and preferences across the cancer care trajectory: insights from the patient perspective. Support Care Cancer. 2014;22(4):1009–15. PubMed PMID: 24287506. Epub 2013/11/30. eng.
56. Thorne SE, Kuo M, Armstrong EA, McPherson G, Harris SR, Hislop TG. 'Being known': patients' perspectives of the dynamics of human connection in cancer care. Psycho-Oncology. 2000;14(10):887–98; discussion 99–900. PubMed PMID: 16200520. Epub 2005/10/04. eng.
57. Colloca L, Lopiano L, Lanotte M, Benedetti F. Overt versus covert treatment for pain, anxiety, and Parkinson's disease. Lancet Neurol. 2004;3(11):679–84. PubMed PMID: 15488461. Epub 2004/10/19. eng.
58. Ben-Shaanan TL, Schiller M, Azulay-Debby H, Korin B, Boshnak N, Koren T, et al. Modulation of anti-tumor immunity by the brain's reward system. Nat Commun. 2018;9(1):2723. PubMed PMID: 30006573. Pubmed Central PMCID: PMC6045610. Epub 2018/07/15. eng.
59. Dutcher JM, Creswell JD. The role of brain reward pathways in stress resilience and health. Neurosci Biobehav Rev. 2018;95:559–67. PubMed PMID: 30477985. Epub 2018/11/28. eng.
60. Colloca L, Finniss D. Nocebo effects, patient-clinician communication, and therapeutic outcomes. JAMA. 2012;307(6):567–8. PubMed PMID: 22318275. Pubmed Central PMCID: PMC6909539. Epub 2012/02/10. eng.
61. Petrie KJ, Rief W. Psychobiological mechanisms of placebo and nocebo effects: pathways to improve treatments and reduce side effects. Annu Rev Psychol. 2019;70:599–625. PubMed PMID: 30110575. Epub 2018/08/16. eng.
62. Marsland AL, Walsh C, Lockwood K, John-Henderson NA. The effects of acute psychological stress on circulating and stimulated inflammatory markers: a systematic review and meta-analysis. Brain Behav Immun. 2017;64:208–19. PubMed PMID: 28089638. Pubmed Central PMCID: PMC5553449. Epub 2017/01/17. eng.
63. Colloca L, Barsky AJ. Placebo and nocebo effects. N Engl J Med. 2020;382(6):554–61. PubMed PMID: 32023375. Epub 2020/02/06. eng.

64. Ren Y, Xu F. How patients should be counseled on adverse drug reactions: avoiding the nocebo effect. Res Soc Adm Pharm. 2018;14(7):705. PubMed PMID: 29656936. Epub 2018/04/17. eng.
65. Jacobsen J, Kvale E, Rabow M, Rinaldi S, Cohen S, Weissman D, et al. Helping patients with serious illness live well through the promotion of adaptive coping: a report from the improving outpatient palliative care (IPAL-OP) initiative. J Palliat Med. 2014;17(4):463–8. PubMed PMID: 24579823. Epub 2014/03/04. eng.
66. Jacobsen J, Brenner K, Greer JA, Jacobo M, Rosenberg L, Nipp RD, et al. When a patient is reluctant to talk about it: a dual framework to focus on living well and tolerate the possibility of dying. J Palliat Med. 2018;21(3):322–7. PubMed PMID: 28972862. Epub 2017/10/04. eng.
67. Dunkel-Schetter C, Feinstein LG, Taylor SE, Falke RL. Patterns of coping with cancer. Health Psychol. 1992;11(2):79–87. PubMed PMID: 1582383. Epub 1992/01/01. eng.
68. Carlson LE, Tamagawa R, Stephen J, Drysdale E, Zhong L, Speca M. Randomized-controlled trial of mindfulness-based cancer recovery versus supportive expressive group therapy among distressed breast cancer survivors (MINDSET): long-term follow-up results. Psycho-Oncology. 2016;25(7):750–9. PubMed PMID: 27193737. Epub 2016/05/20. eng.
69. Krok D, Telka E. The role of meaning in gastric cancer patients: relationships among meaning structures, coping, and psychological well-being. Anxiety Stress Coping. 2019;32(5):522–33. PubMed PMID: 31234657. Epub 2019/06/27. eng.
70. Kalbfleisch M, Cyr A, Gregorio N, Nyhof-Young J. Investigating coping strategies and social support among Canadian melanoma patients: a survey approach. Can Oncol Nurs J. 2015;25(1):60–72. PubMed PMID: 26642495. Epub 2015/12/09. eng.
71. Cao W, Qi X, Cai DA, Han X. Modeling posttraumatic growth among cancer patients: the roles of social support, appraisals, and adaptive coping. Psycho-Oncology. 2018;27(1):208–15. PubMed PMID: 28171681. Epub 2017/02/09. eng.
72. Bernardi L, Sleight P, Bandinelli G, Cencetti S, Fattorini L, Wdowczyc-Szulc J, et al. Effect of rosary prayer and yoga mantras on autonomic cardiovascular rhythms: comparative study. BMJ. 2001;323(7327):1446–9. PubMed PMID: 11751348. Pubmed Central PMCID: 61046.
73. Lee V, Cohen SR, Edgar L, Laizner AM, Gagnon AJ. Clarifying "meaning" in the context of cancer research: a systematic literature review. Palliat Support Care. 2004;2(3):291–303. PubMed PMID: 16594414. Epub 2006/04/06. eng.
74. Lee V, Cohen SR, Edgar L, Laizner AM, Gagnon AJ. Meaning-making and psychological adjustment to cancer: development of an intervention and pilot results. Oncol Nurs Forum. 2006;33(2):291–302. PubMed PMID: 16518445. Epub 2006/03/07. eng.
75. Frankl V. Man's search for meaning. Beacon Press, Boston 2006.
76. Coward DD, Kahn DL. Transcending breast cancer: making meaning from diagnosis and treatment. J Holist Nurs. 2005;23(3):264–83; discussion 84–6. PubMed PMID: 16049116. Epub 2005/07/29. eng.
77. Cann A, Calhoun LG, Tedeschi RG, Triplett KN, Vishnevsky T, Lindstrom CM. Assessing posttraumatic cognitive processes: the Event Related Rumination Inventory. Anxiety Stress Coping. 2011;24(2):137–56. PubMed PMID: 21082446. Epub 2010/11/18. eng.
78. Taku K, Calhoun LG, Cann A, Tedeschi RG. The role of rumination in the coexistence of distress and posttraumatic growth among bereaved Japanese university students. Death Stud. 2008;32(5):428–44. PubMed PMID: 18767236. Epub 2008/09/05. eng.
79. Kolokotroni P, Anagnostopoulos F, Tsikkinis A. Psychosocial factors related to posttraumatic growth in breast cancer survivors: a review. Women Health. 2014;54(6):569–92. PubMed PMID: 24911117. Epub 2014/06/10. eng.
80. Benson H. The relaxation response. New York, NY: HarperCollins; 2000.
81. Bhasin MK, Dusek JA, Chang BH, Joseph MG, Denninger JW, Fricchione GL, et al. Relaxation response induces temporal transcriptome changes in energy metabolism, insulin secretion and inflammatory pathways. PLoS One. 2013;8(5):e62817. PubMed PMID: 23650531. Pubmed Central PMCID: PMC3641112. Epub 2013/05/08. eng.
82. Dusek JA, Otu HH, Wohlhueter AL, Bhasin M, Zerbini LF, Joseph MG, et al. Genomic counter-stress changes induced by the relaxation response. PLoS One. 2008;3(7):e2576. PubMed PMID: 18596974. Pubmed Central PMCID: PMC2432467. Epub 2008/07/04. eng.

83. Grecucci A, Pappaianni E, Siugzdaite R, Theuninck A, Job R. Mindful emotion regulation: exploring the neurocognitive mechanisms behind mindfulness. Biomed Res Int. 2015;2015:670724. PubMed PMID: 26137490. Pubmed Central PMCID: PMC4475519. Epub 2015/07/03. eng.
84. Manuello J, Vercelli U, Nani A, Costa T, Cauda F. Mindfulness meditation and consciousness: an integrative neuroscientific perspective. Conscious Cogn. 2016;40:67–78. PubMed PMID: 26752605. Epub 2016/01/12. eng.
85. Horner JK, Piercy BS, Eure L, Woodard EK. A pilot study to evaluate mindfulness as a strategy to improve inpatient nurse and patient experiences. Appl Nurs Res. 2014;27(3):198–201. PubMed PMID: 24602399. Epub 2014/03/08. eng.
86. Carlson LE, Zelinski E, Toivonen K, Flynn M, Qureshi M, Piedalue KA, et al. Mind-body therapies in cancer: what is the latest evidence? Curr Oncol Rep. 2017;19(10):67. PubMed PMID: 28822063. Epub 2017/08/20. eng.
87. Nieman DC, Wentz LM. The compelling link between physical activity and the body's defense system. J Sport Health Sci. 2019;8(3):201–17. PubMed PMID: 31193280. Pubmed Central PMCID: PMC6523821. Epub 2019/06/14. eng.
88. Paterson C, Primeau C, Pullar I, Nabi G. Development of a prehabilitation multimodal supportive care interventions for men and their partners before radical prostatectomy for localized prostate cancer. Cancer Nurs. 2019;42(4):E47–53. PubMed PMID: 29933304. Epub 2018/06/23. eng.
89. McCorkle R, Ercolano E, Lazenby M, Schulman-Green D, Schilling LS, Lorig K, et al. Self-management: enabling and empowering patients living with cancer as a chronic illness. CA Cancer J Clin. 2011;61(1):50–62. PubMed PMID: 21205833. Pubmed Central PMCID: PMC3058905. Epub 2011/01/06. eng.
90. Bakitas MA, Tosteson TD, Li Z, Lyons KD, Hull JG, Li Z, et al. Early versus delayed initiation of concurrent palliative oncology care: patient outcomes in the ENABLE III randomized controlled trial. J Clin Oncol. 2015;33(13):1438–45. PubMed PMID: 25800768. Pubmed Central PMCID: PMC4404422. Epub 2015/03/25. eng.
91. Dionne-Odom JN, Azuero A, Lyons KD, Hull JG, Tosteson T, Li Z, et al. Benefits of early versus delayed palliative care to informal family caregivers of patients with advanced cancer: outcomes from the ENABLE III randomized controlled trial. J Clin Oncol. 2015;33(13):1446–52. PubMed PMID: 25800762. Pubmed Central PMCID: PMC4404423. Epub 2015/03/25. eng.
92. Lutgendorf S, De Geest K, Bender D, Ahmed A, Goodheart M, Dahmoush L, Zimmerman M, et al. Social influences on clinical outcomes of patients with ovarian cancer. J Clin Oncol. 2012;30(23):2885–90.
93. Lutgendorf SK, Andersen BL. Biobehavioral approaches to cancer progression and survival: mechanisms and interventions. Am Psychol. 2015;70(2):186–97. PubMed PMID: 25730724. Pubmed Central PMCID: PMC4347942. Epub 2015/03/03. eng.
94. Andersen BL, Yang HC, Farrar WB, Golden-Kreutz DM, Emery CF, Thornton LM, et al. Psychologic intervention improves survival for breast cancer patients: a randomized clinical trial. Cancer. 2008;113(12):3450–8. PubMed PMID: 19016270. Pubmed Central PMCID: PMC2661422. Epub 2008/11/19. eng.
95. House J. Work, stress and social support. Reading, MA: Addison-Wesley; 1981.
96. House JS, Landis KR, Umberson D. Social relationships and health. Science (New York, NY). 1988;241(4865):540–5. PubMed PMID: 3399889. Epub 1988/07/29. eng.
97. Latino-Martel P, Cottet V, Druesne-Pecollo N, Pierre FH, Touillaud M, Touvier M, et al. Alcoholic beverages, obesity, physical activity and other nutritional factors, and cancer risk: a review of the evidence. Crit Rev Oncol Hematol. 2016;99:308–23. PubMed PMID: 26811140. Epub 2016/01/27. eng.
98. Hojman P. Exercise protects from cancer through regulation of immune function and inflammation. Biochem Soc Trans. 2017;45(4):905–11. PubMed PMID: 28673937. Epub 2017/07/05. eng.

99. Hojman P, Gehl J, Christensen JF, Pedersen BK. Molecular mechanisms linking exercise to cancer prevention and treatment. Cell Metab. 2018;27(1):10–21. PubMed PMID: 29056514. Epub 2017/10/24. eng.
100. Nunez C, Bauman A, Egger S, Sitas F, Nair-Shalliker V. Obesity, physical activity and cancer risks: results from the cancer, lifestyle and evaluation of risk study (CLEAR). Cancer Epidemiol. 2017;47:56–63. PubMed PMID: 28126584. Epub 2017/01/28. eng.
101. Mishra SI, Scherer RW, Geigle PM, Berlanstein DR, Topaloglu O, Gotay CC, et al. Exercise interventions on health-related quality of life for cancer survivors. Cochrane Database Syst Rev. 2012;8:CD007566. PubMed PMID: 22895961. Epub 2012/08/17. eng.
102. Rock CL, Thomson C, Gansler T, Gapstur SM, McCullough ML, Patel AV, et al. American Cancer Society guideline for diet and physical activity for cancer prevention. CA Cancer J Clin. 2020;70(4):245–71. PubMed PMID: 32515498. Epub 2020/06/10. eng.
103. Aschbacher K, O'Donovan A, Wolkowitz OM, Dhabhar FS, Su Y, Epel E. Good stress, bad stress and oxidative stress: insights from anticipatory cortisol reactivity. Psychoneuroendocrinology. 2013;38(9):1698–708. PubMed PMID: 23490070. Epub 2013/03/16. eng.
104. Sillar JR, Germon ZP, DeIuliis GN, Dun MD. The role of reactive oxygen species in acute myeloid leukaemia. Int J Mol Sci. 2019;20(23):6003. PubMed PMID: 31795243. Pubmed Central PMCID: PMC6929020. Epub 2019/12/05. eng.
105. van Waart H, Stuiver MM, van Harten WH, Geleijn E, Kieffer JM, Buffart LM, et al. Effect of low-intensity physical activity and moderate- to high-intensity physical exercise during adjuvant chemotherapy on physical fitness, fatigue, and chemotherapy completion rates: results of the PACES randomized clinical trial. J Clin Oncol. 2015;33(17):1918–27. PubMed PMID: 25918291. Epub 2015/04/29. eng.
106. Hilfiker R, Meichtry A, Eicher M, Nilsson Balfe L, Knols RH, Verra ML, et al. Exercise and other non-pharmaceutical interventions for cancer-related fatigue in patients during or after cancer treatment: a systematic review incorporating an indirect-comparisons meta-analysis. Br J Sports Med. 2018;52(10):651–8. PubMed PMID: 28501804. Pubmed Central PMCID: PMC5931245. Epub 2017/05/16. eng.
107. World Cancer Research F, American Institute for Cancer R. Food, nutrition, physical activity and the prevention of cancer: a global perspective. Washington, DC: The Institute; 2007.
108. Minich DM, Brown BI. A review of dietary (phyto)nutrients for glutathione support. Nutrients. 2019;11(9):2073. PubMed PMID: 31484368. Pubmed Central PMCID: PMC6770193. Epub 2019/09/06. eng.
109. Amararathna M, Johnston MR, Rupasinghe HP. Plant polyphenols as chemopreventive agents for lung cancer. Int J Mol Sci. 2016;17(8):1352. PubMed PMID: 27548149. Pubmed Central PMCID: PMC5000748. Epub 2016/08/23. eng.

Treatment Phase 16

16.1 Introduction

This chapter covers the main concerns of patients and their caregivers during treatment, and suggests nursing approaches to enhance emotion-regulation, healing processes, and resilience during this often emotionally and physically taxing phase. The treatment itself while providing hope for most patients tends to be a source of anxiety, exacerbated by medical tests and procedures and unwelcomed side effects.

Many factors determine the optimal treatment approach for different cancers including whether it is a first-time diagnosis, the type, location, and stage of cancer; or whether it is localized, metastasized, or a cancer recurrence. Medical interventions may involve one or more of the following: surgery, chemotherapy, immunotherapy, radiation therapy, hormone therapy, monoclonal antibody, and/or other targeted therapies, including specialized ablation procedures. Some of these therapies weaken physiological resilience by temporarily killing healthy cells, causing immunosuppression, and an array of side effects [1].

The treatment phase is periodically characterized by various stressor events such as treatment modalities (e.g., surgery), illness-related symptoms, treatment-related side effects, chemoresistance, disease progression, and/or cessation of treatment. A comprehensive psychosocial nursing approach can help the patient anticipate and manage disease- and treatment-related stresses more effectively in order to protect or enhance their overall resilience.

16.2 Objectives

At the end of this chapter, you will be able to:

1. Identify typical concerns of patients and caregivers during the treatment phase
2. Describe relevant nursing approaches to manage these concerns

3. Utilize knowledge of systemic inflammation and compromised immunity to develop clinical interventions aimed at minimizing the potentially ill effects of treatment
4. Explain the interrelationships of stress, inflammatory cytokines, symptoms, and side effects caused by the disease and treatment.

Clinical Anecdote 16.1
When I was diagnosed with an aggressive, stage 4 cancer, an effective clinical protocol did not exist. Living a deliberately moment-by-moment existence was one of my coping strategies that insulated me from fearful thoughts and an active imagination.

The moment became my world. I willed myself to go through each treatment or procedure 1 min at a time, and somehow I reached the other side. That emotional resolve was enhanced by my oncologist's clinical approach. He made me feel we were an indomitable team—both fighting for the same thing—my life. He explained what I could do to make my whole being as physically and mentally healthy as possible, while he treated the disease. He recommended daily walks, the importance of eating lots of vegetables, berries, fish and chicken, and spending quality time with family and friends. My supportive family took this advice to heart, whisking me away to our favourite get-a-way for the last week of the 3-week chemotherapy cycle, when I had more energy. There. I soaked in all its magic and beauty, and fortified myself for the next round of treatment. Nothing was guaranteed but everything was possible. I felt safe, and even though I knew the odds…. I chose not to dwell on them. I focussed on hope. And interestingly, hope has been associated with a strengthened immune response [2, 3].

16.3 Definition

The treatment phase typically extends from the start to the end of medical treatment, although patients with advanced cancer may continue to receive medical therapies to keep the tumor's growth in check. Consequently, cancer has increasingly been regarded as a chronic illness.

16.4 Clinical Issues

Most patients feel extremely vulnerable and experience both symptoms and side effects. This phase is among the most emotionally distressing and uncertain for patients and caregivers [4, 5]. A lot is at stake; there is fear about whether the treatment will work, and anxiety about the potential physical "damage" caused by medical treatments. Patient and family trepidation encircles the clinical results of various tests and procedures used to monitor treatment efficacy. At some level, everyone thinks about the possibility of death.

Pivotal periods of clinical vulnerability that compromise the person's healing capability and resilience, such as the perisurgical, chemotherapeutic, and radiation periods, call out for the nurse's clinical expertise. These critical moments along the continuum require relevant psychosocial and physical nursing practices that complement the goals of oncology in order to counter immunosuppression, emotional distress, physical discomfort, and the deleterious effects of other symptoms and side effects, while striving to optimize the patient's and caregiver's resilience.

Lifestyle Health-Related Risks

An estimated 30–40% of cancers may be caused by an unhealthy lifestyle regarding nutrition, diet, physical activity, and weight, although these statistics may also be confounded by other factors such as environmental toxins, smoking, and alcohol intake [6–9]. For instance, obesity is associated with at least 12 different cancer types and is related to a number of factors including low-grade inflammation, hyperinsulinemia, and abnormalities of the insulin growth factor 1. Visceral fat is considered an endocrine organ that secretes free fatty acids and proinflammatory molecules such as leptin and adipocytokines; leptin stimulates production of IL-1, IL-6, IL-12, TNF-alpha, and cyclooxygenase, among others, contributing to the tumor microenvironment (TME) which may undermine the beneficial effects of cancer treatments [10, 11]. Evidence is mixed on whether a "healthy" lifestyle can actually be sustained among patients during treatment with chemotherapy and radiotherapy.

Diet Research data indicate that the patient's diet tends to become more inflammatory over the course of the treatment, caused in part by reduced nutritional intake, increased adiposity (obesity), and metabolic disturbances due to the treatment [12]. A prospective study of 55 women at the end of chemotherapy showed that almost 50% had consumed an inadequate diet: Both fruits and vegetables were significantly reduced; and 56% were overweight with an increased body mass index (BMI) and waist circumference, further indicating an inadequate nutritional status [13]. An estimated 49.1% of the women were shown to have reduced their intake of fruit, dark green and orange vegetables, and legumes during treatment. Their intake of macro- and micronutrients such as calcium, iron, phosphorus, magnesium, riboflavin, thiamin, vitamin B6, vitamin C, and zinc was also significantly reduced. Significantly, inadequate nutrition has been associated with immunosuppression and especially impaired T-lymphocyte cells [14]. A diet that includes moderate or greater alcohol consumption, processed foods, red meat, salt and salted foods, and beta carotene supplements not only increases the risk of cancer but a cancer recurrence [15].

In summary, an increased inflammatory index during chemotherapy highlights the importance of adopting recommended dietary and nutritional guidelines during as well as before and after treatment to ensure that all patients continue to promote their health across the continuum.

Physical activity Being physically inactive, overweight or obese, and on a diet lacking the appropriate pattern of food groups or nutrients (nutrition) constitute health-related risk factors for healthy people as well as for those already compromised by cancer and undergoing current treatment [16]. A prospective study investigated physical activity before and after a new cancer diagnosis in 942 patients [17]. Moderate-to-intense physical activity (i.e., "vigorous") was found to be significantly reduced after diagnosis, particularly in patients with skin and prostate cancers. Those patients also tended to be overweight, more sedentary, professionally inactive, and older. Other reasons included level of education, smoking, sex, stage of illness, and treatment type [17]. Given meta-analyses that have shown a dose-dependent relationship between physical activity and cancer-related mortality, patients need to be encouraged to increase their physical activity at their own rate and capability during treatment [18].

16.5 Treatment: Chemotherapy and Radiation-Related Therapy and Surgery (Review Part III Chaps. 6 and 7)

Chemotherapy, radiation therapy, brachytherapy, and surgery exacerbate systemic inflammation and temporarily suppress vital immune functions involved in anticancer surveillance. These physiological threats are on top of the patient's already distressed neurophysiology due to the physical presence of the tumor, and psychologically, the fears or concerns surrounding the treatment itself (e.g., [1]). Immunosuppressed cells include the innate natural killer cells and cell-mediated cytotoxic T lymphocyte cells that normally secrete interferon-gamma (IFN-γ), tumor necrosis factor alpha (TNF-α) and IL-17 which perform antitumor activities by identifying and eliminating nascent tumor cells (e.g. [1], p. 764).

At the same time, inflammatory cytokines *within the tumor microenvironment* (TME) facilitate the development, evasion, and spread of cancer even during treatment [1]. For instance, tumor necrosis factor-alpha (TNF-α) within the TME has been implicated in all phases of breast cancer development including tumor progression, metastases, and drug resistance [11]. TNF-α has dual roles depending on the environmental context and is not alone in this capability. To illustrate, there is a set of cell receptors known as NOTCH receptors that regulate T-cell development, maintenance, and activity. NOTCH signaling is essential for optimal T-cell-mediated immune functioning. But within the TME, NOTCH *receptors* have acquired the capability to suppress NOTCH signaling which suppresses cell-mediated immunity, enabling the tumor to avoid T-cell-mediated destruction [19]. Notch signaling within the TME has also been found to support cancer invasion, angiogenesis, tumor heterogeneity, and tumor cell dormancy within solid cancer tissues especially in epithelial cancers [20]. Moreover, cancer stem cells can alter their cell surface receptors to escape detection by anticancer immune cells as well as possess drug efflux capabilities conducive to chemoresistance [21].

This is a very simplified version of an extremely complex field of medical science involving immunodynamic responses in the face of cancer-related threats. The main point is that cell-mediated immunity is most effective in tracking down circulating and nascent tumor cells existing *outside* the TME. Temporary periods of immunosuppression associated with a cancer treatment enable the migration of cancer cells to distal regions where they tend to be embedded undetected and protected against chemotherapeutic agents, only to be activated many years later [1, 22]. These disease-related insights may be leveraged by nurses and other healthcare providers to consider clinical interventions that might counter the individual's compromised immune responses between treatments.

Moreover, systemic inflammation also gives rise to a range of symptoms and side effects associated with the cancer or treatment, as well as during cancer progression. Another question for nurses is whether it is possible through healing-promoting interventions to contain or reduce the amount and level of circulating inflammatory cytokines so that at least some relief from intense pain and suffering is possible [23].

Perisurgical Phase Review [1]

The perisurgical period, including the critical postoperative period up to the start of adjunct treatment, carries an increased risk of cancer recurrence that has been medically underestimated [23, 24]. Surgical interventions are empirically known to liberate residual tumor cells into the blood circulation which embed in distant organs serving as sites of future metastases during the postoperative period. It was previously assumed that these escaped cells could be destroyed by adjunct treatments such as chemotherapy after physical healing. But it has proven to be a more challenging problem.

Whereas cellular immunity is critical for hunting down and destroying circulating tumor cells in peripheral vessels before these rogue cells have an opportunity to seed in remote areas of the body, it appears that cell immunity is not as effective *within* the "tumor microenvironment" (TME) even in patients who are not particularly stressed [1, 23]. As previously discussed (Part III Chap. 7), tumors in the microenvironment can change their cell surface receptors (to prevent immune infiltration) as well as suppress the activity of nearby immune cells, and disrupt immune cell signaling. As a consequence, tumor cells escape detection and continue their invasive growth [23, 25].

In the treatment vacuum between the end of surgery and the start of antitumor treatment, when patients experience psychological and physical stress, natural killer cells, cytotoxic T-lymphocytes as well as IFN-γ, macrophages, and phagocytes that normally would be mobilized to eradicate residual disease after surgery are suppressed [23, 26, 27]. Postoperative patients who reported greater stress before surgery were shown to have a significant decrease in natural killer cell cytotoxic activities (NKCC) and a significant decrease in T-cell proliferative responses in peripheral vessels in keeping with an impaired immune response [24, 26]. These findings highlight the importance of enhancing cellular immunity especially in early stage postoperative patients, given the role of antitumor immune cells in tracking down residual cancer cells *circulating in peripheral blood and lymph vessels*. It underscores the value of engaging perisurgical patients in therapeutic psychosocial interventions starting in the presurgical phase aimed at reducing emotional distress in order to strengthen cell-mediated immunity.

Effects of anesthesia General anesthesia and high-dose opioids to control pain also increase the risk of cancer recurrence compared to a regional or local nerve block [27, 28]. Patients who received a combination of general and epidural anesthetics during cancer-related surgery demonstrated improved survival rates over patients who received only a general anesthetic [27, 28].

Wound healing consists of four orderly steps: clotting, inflammation, proliferation, and remodeling [29]. Inflammation depends on a healthy immune system [30]. Both acute and chronic psychological stresses are empirically known however to impair immune functioning [31], including disrupting the initial inflammation phase at the wound site, thereby prolonging wound healing [32, 33]. Specifically, the stress-activated hypothalamic–pituitary–adrenal (HPA) and sympathetic–adrenal–medullary (SAM) axes are associated with the increased flow of glucocorticoids (and other hormones) which *decrease* expression of proinflammatory TH1 cytokines such as IL-1β, IL-1α, IL-6, TNF, and IL-8 at the wound site, which are needed to start the initial inflammation process at the wound site [32, 34, 35]. The glucocorticoids serve as anti-inflammatory modulators that shift TH1 (proinflammatory) cytokines to TH2 (anti-inflammatory) cytokines, thereby inhibiting a cell-mediated immune response, which results in delayed wound healing. That TH2 anti-inflammatory shift not only slows wound healing but also suppresses cell-mediated immune functions, thereby also enabling cancer growth and metastases to proceed undetected for up to 6 weeks after surgery until chemotherapy or other anticancer treatments typically start.

The perisurgical phase provides one of the greatest opportunities for cancer to proliferate and metastasize unimpeded by treatment modalities, and further fueled by patient distress. How this phase of the treatment process is managed by healthcare providers and loved ones is thought to determine the risk of a cancer recurrence in the distant future (e.g., [27]).

Symptoms and Side Effects (Review Part III Chaps. 6 and 7)

Symptoms and side effects refer to distressing physical, biological, and emotional responses and sensations, caused by either the cancer or its treatment, respectively [36–38]. Chemotherapy is typically associated with a number of side effects such as nausea, fatigue, immunosuppression, and memory-related concerns (Also review Part V Chaps. 17 and 18). Taxanes and cyclophosphamides may cause general muscle and connective tissue aches, neuritis of the finger tips and toes, and immunosuppression. Neutrophil-inducing treatment administered to increase the number of circulating neutrophils during chemotherapy can typically induce nonspecific musculoskeletal aches, headache, and occasional bone pain (e.g., [39]).

Between 60% and 90% of patients awaiting surgery experience anxiety, worry, uncertainty, and fear of dying [40]. Typical postsurgical side effects consist of pain, fatigue, and body disfigurement. Side effects of radiation therapy may include fatigue, erythema, pruritus, shooting pain (rare), site wound, radiation pneumonitis, collapsed lung, pericardial irritation (for instance, patients with breast cancer), and immunosuppression [41]. Other common symptoms include pain, nausea, dyspnea, constipation, dry mouth, insomnia, diarrhea, fever, vomiting and/or mucositis, lymphedema, and neuritis (e.g., [36, 40, 42]). Physical symptoms and side effects need a swift medical response in order to attenuate consequential patient distress.

Symptom clusters are the external manifestations of an underlying systemic inflammation, caused by psychological and physical stress [37]. A cluster refers to "three to five concurrent symptoms that are related to one another" [36, 43]. A typical cluster consists of *depression, fatigue, and pain* and is associated with reduced physical functioning and poor quality of life in patients with advanced cancer (e.g., [44]). Another typical cluster includes *pain, sleep disturbances, and fatigue* as reported for instance by patients with acute leukemia [45–48].

The same symptom may be found in different clusters. For instance, emotional distress (anxiety, worry, uncertainty, and depression) has been shown to exacerbate fatigue and sensitivity to pain [38, 40]. Pain and fatigue are common symptoms/side effects of patients during cancer treatment. Charalambous (2019) [49] cross-sectional data of a symptom cluster in patients undergoing treatment for breast and prostate cancer revealed the interactional, direct, and indirect effects of pain, fatigue, anxiety, and depression on health-related quality of life (HRQOL). A path analysis showed that increased pain levels had significant direct effects on fatigue, anxiety, and depression. This suggested that the three symptoms co-occurred, but only *fatigue and anxiety* exerted significant direct effects on health-related quality of life, thereby serving as the key mediators of the relationship between pain and HRQOL. Similarly, the same path analysis revealed that the effect of depression on HRQOL was indirect via the mediating effects of *fatigue and anxiety*. Fatigue also was a significant mediator of the relationship between pain and HRQOL in patients with breast cancer but not prostate cancer. A clinical assessment of symptom clusters such as pain, fatigue, anxiety, and depression in patients being treated for breast or prostate cancer is a needed clinical predicate for a multimodal targeted approach to improve resilience and HRQOL.

Clinical effects The significance of these symptoms to the patient's resilience and health should not be underestimated. For instance, sleep loss has been shown to negatively impact both innate and adaptive immune functions that are critical to fighting cancer [50]. Pain, anxiety, and depression exacerbate and are exacerbated by the stress response system and the consequential inflammatory cytokine response which disrupts sleep–wake cycles and reduces cell-mediated and innate immune functions [23, 37]. Understanding these bidirectional relationships can facilitate the development of potentially effective psychosocial and/or medical interventions. More clinical research on symptom clusters based on longitudinal data of other stages and types of cancer is needed to target clinical interventions more effectively.

Body Image Impairments

Body image refers to the perceptions, thoughts, feelings, and behaviors about one's physical appearance, functions, and capabilities [51, 52]. Body image has to do with the "gap between actual and desired physical appearance, and the importance placed on appearance and physical attributes" [53, 54]. Contributing factors include sociocultural norms, interpersonal experiences, personality traits, and changes in function and appearance due to bodily impairment and disfigurement. Physical impairments create profound emotional distress in cancer patients, and their loved ones that may endure up to 5 years or longer [54]. Colostomy, head and neck surgery, limb amputations, lymphedema, mastectomy, and other impairments may adversely impact relationships with partners, friends, and family (e.g., [55–59]). For instance, family members and partners caring for colorectal patients with a stoma were found to be more depressed and anxious than caregivers of patients without a stoma [56]. Mastectomy and head and neck postsurgical patients experience the highest risk of emotional distress; head and neck patients in particular experience an abnormally high incidence of suicide, depression, substance use, relationship problems, reduced feelings of femininity or masculinity, and increased self-imposed isolation [60, 61].

In summary, the treatment phase is replete with stress-provoking challenges for the patient and caregiver. It is a phase of hope but also tremendous uncertainty and potential loss. Although the treatments aim to eliminate or contain disease progression, the residual side effects and symptoms cause emotional distress and may compromise the individual's biological and behavioral resilience. In the following section, we review the clinical research of key clinical interventions that the nurse may consider promoting healing and resilience in the patient and caregiver.

Clinical Anecdote 16.2
'When A was going through chemotherapy, she became more and more distraught at each session. A few minutes with the patient helped the nurse to understand her concerns. A had never been seriously ill in her life. She had never taken medications, not even acetaminophen for a headache. She had heard about the 'dangers' of chemotherapy to healthy cells and because she was feeling more and more tired was convinced that she was getting worse, not better. The nurse explained that (1) the effects of chemotherapy on healthy cells were temporary, that immune cells were usually able to recover between treatments. (2) The nurse also reviewed the positive goals of chemotherapy and underscored the fact that the majority of patients with A's type of cancer did very well on this treatment. The nurse used this strategy to potentially improve A's treatment expectations based on her knowledge that studies showed this strategy could enhance treatment efficacy [62]. (3) Similarly the nurse further countered the possibility of nocebo treatment side effects by emphasizing that 94% of patients did very well although at times they experienced some fatigue. (4) The nurse suggested simple exercises such as daily walks and talks with close family and friends, hand and feet massages or reflexology, and daily relaxation response practices to reduce fatigue and emotional stress,

enhance overall well being and strengthen cell mediated immune responses, based on relevant research findings (e.g. [63–68]). The nurse also provided relevant information about the resilient promoting effects of an anti cancer diet especially in promoting and protecting immune functions (in consultation with the team) [8, 69]. A acquired relevant information and the skills she needed to maintain emotional equanimity, minimize the potential for side effects, and even strengthen her resilience [62].

16.6 Psychosocial Interventions and Related Research

During treatment, the main goals of nonpharmacological psychosocial interventions are to reduce emotional stress, manage symptoms, promote emotion-regulating and self-management capabilities, enhance adaptive cognitive and behavioral coping strategies, strengthen personally supportive relationships from family as well as healthcare providers, and increase use of health-promoting lifestyle behaviors. These interventions are assessed in terms of their ability to enhance psychological adjustment, quality of life, and the reduction of an array of symptoms associated either with the disease or treatment. A number of psychosocial interventions have been identified as effective strategies for managing emotional distress and other symptoms (e.g., [70, 71]).

Perceived Support (Review Chap. 11)

Clinical research data have shown that perceived emotional support from family or significant others is critical in prolonging survival in patients with cancer [23, 72, 73]. Patients with ovarian cancer who experienced high perceived support (social attachment) showed significantly higher cell-mediated immunity, such as a higher T-cell proliferative response and the ability to successfully detect and eradicate tumor cells throughout the peripheral blood system [23, 73]. These individuals also showed higher levels of natural killer cell (NKCC) cytotoxicity *within tumor-infiltrating lymphocytes* (TIL), whereas distressed individuals lacking comparable support evidenced poorer NKCC in TILs and less TH1 (type 1 T-helper) cytokine production in all cells [74]. Tumors are generally difficult to infiltrate due to their changing cell surface markers, downregulation of immune cells within the tumor microenvironment, and their ability to disrupt immune cell signaling, which enables cancer cells to escape cell-mediated "detection" and elimination ([23], p. 190). The increased presence of natural killer cell cytotoxicity in the peripheral *and* tumor microenvironment has been attributed to patient perceptions of perceived support, especially from informal supports throughout the illness and treatment [23, 75]. However, a patient's family network has not always been shown to be supportive, and this perceived lack of support has been associated with cancer progression [76–78]. Moreover, not all patients are open to accepting nursing support, and we need to better understand these reasons [79].

A few studies investigated the effects of a supportive expressive intervention (SEI) in women in the early phase of breast cancer [75], women with a cancer recurrence [80], women with breast cancer [81], and distressed women at the end of adjuvant chemotherapy [82, 83]. The findings were inconsistent across studies and generally modest, perhaps related to the poor methodological quality of the studies [81]. The qualitative study of women who participated in a SEI intervention had mainly positive experiences. They found support within the group, felt that they had more effective coping strategies, and were more optimistic. Significantly, the most important characteristics of their "therapist" were a sense of empathy, active listening, and the promotion of coping strategies. These scientific findings underscore the importance of ongoing assessments of patient and family caregiver sources and quality of informal support which may vary over time. It calls for workshops or one-on-one interventions that cultivate the development of meaningful support between the patient and family caregiver.

Cognitive-Behavioral Interventions (CB) (Review Chaps. 5 and 9; Appendix in Chap. 9)

Cognitive-behavioral interventions are multimodal, multitargeted strategies frequently offered in one-on-one nurse-patient or caregiver sessions as well as in group workshops just prior to, immediately after and during treatment. In a Cochrane review of 28 RCTs, cognitive-behavioral interventions were related to significant improvements in quality of life, depression and anxiety (low-quality evidence), and mood (moderate-quality evidence) in patients with nonmetastatic breast cancer [84]. Similarly, an RCT of women with stage 1–3 breast cancer enrolled 4–8 weeks after surgery showed that the women assigned to the 10-week cognitive-behavioral stress management intervention compared to the 1 day psychoeducational session group showed significantly better psychosocial adaptation based on significant reductions in anxiety and cortisol levels, and higher levels of Th1 cytokine production compared to the control group following adjuvant treatment [85]. The intervention may have helped to maintain or enhance TH1 cytokines that are critical for maintaining cell-mediated immune activities against cancer cells.

A meta-analysis of 32 studies suggested that CB strategies were the most effective among psychosocial interventions to reduce depression and anxiety, and increase quality of life in women after surgery for breast cancer [86]. A three-arm randomized controlled study of men with prostate cancer who underwent a radical prostatectomy compared a stress-coping management intervention (SM) with a supportive attention intervention (SA) and a control group (see Appendix in Chap. 9 for intervention content). The perisurgical SM group showed a significant reduction in mood disturbances compared to the control group [87]. The SM group also produced significantly greater natural killer cell cytotoxicity and significantly elevated circulating inflammatory cytokines (i.e., IL-12p, IL-1B, and TNF) 48 h after surgery compared to the SA group. The results also demonstrated significant elevations of natural killer cell cytotoxicity and IL-1B compared to men in the control group. Given the increased risk of cancer progression during the perisurgical phase, the SM intervention with its clear mobilization of anticancer immune cells to track down circulating peripheral cancer cells appears to offer potentially therapeutic clinical benefits compared to the supportive attention intervention. The finding that mood was unrelated to the immune changes may be due to the fact that mood disturbances were low to start with. If so, these results suggest that psychosocial parameters cannot be completely relied on for predicting the patient's physiological parametric values.

Although marked by low-quality evidence, the findings were consistent with Antoni's landmark stress-reducing CB interventions which reported significantly enhanced cell-mediated immune activity posttreatment in patients with breast cancer [88] (Review Appendix in Chap. 9). Both Cohen's and Antoni's studies shared many of the same coping-related topics. Although more rigorously designed trials are needed to redress the moderately high risk of bias in Cohen's study, the topics in this stress management intervention are similar to other CB interventions with positive clinical outcomes, and consequently should be considered in reducing emotional distress and enhancing immune functioning in pre/postsurgical patients with cancer.

MBSR/MBCTs (Review Appendix in Chap. 9; Appendix in Chap. 13)

Mindfulness-based stress reduction and mindfulness-based cognitive therapy are multimodal, multitargeted interventions offered as workshops at different points of vulnerability along the continuum, including the treatment phase for patients with cancer. Topics may include mindfulness meditation, coping skills, strengthening family support, learning strategies to elicit needed support, improving patient–healthcare provider relationships, and discussing meaning and existential issues (e.g., [89, 90]).

In a meta-analysis of ten studies ($N = 1709$), mindfulness-based stress reduction (MBSR) and mindfulness-based cognitive therapy (MBCT) showed significant but small effect size improvements post intervention for the primary clinical outcome, health-related quality of life, and secondary outcomes of fatigue, sleep, stress, anxiety, and depression compared to usual care in women with breast cancer [91]. However, the effect size improvements did not rise to clinical significance. Similar small effect improvements in anxiety and depression were noted at 6 months, and anxiety 12 months after baseline compared to usual care. Compared to the short-term findings, later results were associated with higher heterogeneity, signifying further caution with regard to the interpretation of the findings.

In a meta-analysis of 14 RCT and non-RCT studies ($N = 1505$), MBSR showed significant improvements in cognitive functioning, fatigue, emotional well-being, anxiety, depression, stress, distress, and mindfulness compared to those with usual care in patients with breast cancer during and after treatment [92]. The effects on pain, sleep quality, and global quality of life trended toward statistical significance.

Despite the low-quality evidence, the results were generally consistent with Haller's [91] findings. One challenge to the findings of the meta-analysis was the lack of standardized programs and measures across the studies used to evaluate the overall effectiveness of the MBSR/MBCTs.

Overall, a combination of education, cognitive, and behavioral strategies and a mindfulness activity can be effective in reducing emotional distress and other symptoms while improving quality of life and well-being (Review Appendix in Chap. 9; Appendix in Chap. 13).

Self-Management Interventions (SMI) (Review Appendix A)

SMI is increasingly considered as a viable intervention for patients and family caregivers to develop self-efficacy and relevant skills in managing practical problems associated with cancer or its treatment between treatment sessions [93, 94]. In a systematic review of nine RCTs and quasiexperimental studies, a program of self-management interventions (SMI) resulted in a significant decrease in psychological distress in five of nine studies in patients undergoing treatment for diverse cancers [95]. SMI interventions consisted of education regarding problem solving, resource utilization, and action planning with a few studies also including decision making and strengthening relationships and goal setting (one study). Those studies that failed to attain a significant improvement compared to controls were patients with hematological cancers and a reliance on multimedia technologies, suggesting that the actual physical presence of healthcare providers with the patient in facilitating healing should not be underestimated. The impact of SMIs in early-to-end stage supportive care patients and family caregivers based on mainly manualized telephone sessions has generally produced mixed findings [96, 97].

Progressive Relaxation and Imagery

A systematic review of seven RCTs on progressive relaxation-guided imagery for patients with cancer on chemotherapy showed beneficial effects on mood, depression, and anxiety as well as nausea and vomiting compared to controls [98]. Three trials showed significant effects on heart rate, blood pressure, cortisol, and immunity in desired directions. Methodological quality ranged from average to very poor. Another systematic review of four RCTs and one case–control study on the effectiveness of progressive muscle relaxation showed few benefits for cancer patients on chemotherapy [99]. The quality of evidence was also poor.

An RCT of 208 patients with prostate and breast cancer on chemotherapy evaluated a 4-week intervention that combined guided imagery and progressive muscle relaxation. The intervention effectively reduced levels of fatigue and pain, and increased health-related quality of life over baseline, compared to the control group [100]. The intervention group also reported significantly less vomiting, nausea, and retching compared to controls. Significantly, the intervention group saw a significant decrease in the number of depressed individuals compared to the number of moderately depressed individuals in the control group. These findings are generally consistent with previous studies, suggesting that a combination of guided imagery and progressive muscle relaxation can be effective in managing symptoms during chemotherapy, and thus contribute to a better quality of life [100].

Massage, Foot Reflexology

Massage therapy has gained wider acceptance as a potential therapeutic to improve quality of life mainly in survivors of cancer and patients in palliative care rather than patients with tumors on active treatment, due to medical concerns about inadvertent dislocations of cancer cells from the tumor which may then embed in distal regions, for metastatic colonization (e.g., [101–103]). Findings from massage therapy tend to show significant improvements in symptom management, and even a small but significant increase in dopamine, natural killer cells, and T-lymphocytes [102, 104, 105], notwithstanding the low-quality evidence due to small samples and inadequate research designs and methodology. Rather than using massage to relieve various symptoms in patients during chemotherapy or cancer treatment, foot massage or reflexology may be a safe therapeutic alternative with promising results.

A randomized controlled study investigated the potential efficacy of two types of foot massage in patients being treated with chemoradiotherapy for colorectal cancer [106]. Sixty patients were randomized either to receive foot massage, foot reflexology, or standard care. The foot massage and reflexology groups received their respective interventions twice weekly during 5 weeks of chemoradiotherapy. The findings indicated that the classical foot massage showed significant reductions in pain levels and incidence of distension. Reflexology showed significant reductions in pain and fatigue levels, a reduction in the incidence of distension and urinary frequency, and a significant improvement in quality of life. Although both forms demonstrated clinical improvements, patients in the reflexology group appeared to do better.

A retrospective analysis of complete patient files for a 1-year program in which 28 patients receiving chemotherapy for breast cancer also received a new therapeutic combination of acupuncture and reflexology to manage chemotherapy-induced peripheral neuropathy (CIPN) [107]. Assessments were reviewed at baseline, after treatment, and periodically up to 1 year later. Sixteen of 21 (76%) patients with grade 1 and 2 neuropathy and all seven patients with grade 3 or 4 neuropathy were symptom free at 6 months (82%). By 12 months, 93% of all the patients were symptom free. These findings were compared to a systematic review and meta-analysis based on 31 studies in which 68% of patients with cancer experienced CIPN in the month after the end of treatment, and only 70% were found to be symptom free at 6 months and longer [108]. The proof-of-concept retrospective analysis suggests the need for a well-designed and powered randomized controlled trial to assess the effectiveness of a combined acupuncture-reflexology intervention during chemotherapy in order to prevent the development of CIPN or to minimize its manifestation as a consequence of anticancer treatments.

A convenient sample of hospitalized patients on chemotherapy assessed 15 patients who received reflexology foot massage by a trained nurse and 15 patients who had usual care [109]. Self-reported anxiety was assessed before, after, and 24 h later, in two separate pilot studies. The intervention produced a 7.9-point reduction on the state anxiety scale compared to usual care. A more rigorous controlled trial to evaluate the impact of massage therapy, especially its duration of effects at 24, 48, and even 60 h after the intervention, may further inform clinical practice. The findings also raise the interesting possibility that nurses might teach caregivers interested in providing reflexology to loved ones between treatments.

In summary, foot reflexology studies like massage-based studies require more rigorous and adequately powered randomized controlled trials in order to truly assess their potential short- and long-term healing and resilient capabilities in patients during anticancer treatment. Measures of the effects of reflexology on physiological parameters would also further inform our knowledge of the role of foot reflexology in cancer care.

Exercise, Weight, and Nutrition (Review Appendix C)

The WCRF/AICR [8, 68] recommends exercise and a nutritional diet to promote the health of recovering cancer patients as well as those who have never had cancer. There is growing evidence that exercise and immune-nutritional support and a healthy diet (as feasible) have positive measurable effects in patients *during* anticancer treatments.

Exercise

A Cochran review of 56 RCTs ($n = 4826$) concluded that moderate-intensity exercise for individuals with diverse cancers before, during, and following active treatment had a positive effect on health-related quality of life at 12 weeks compared to light exercise [110]. Exercise significantly improved physical role and social functioning at 12 weeks and 6 months over baseline compared to controls. It also improved the quality of sleep, anxiety, and fatigue. Exercise consisted of walking, cycling, resistance training, yoga, and/or qigong. These clinical benefits were significantly linked to mainly moderate to vigorous exercise, although the high risk of bias requires caution.

A meta-analysis based on 17 studies investigated the effect of exercise during adjuvant chemotherapy and/or radiotherapy for breast cancer on symptoms of anxiety, fatigue, depression, and quality of life [111]. Significant improvements in fatigue, depression, and quality of life compared to usual care were obtained, with effect sizes ranging from 0.2 to 0.5. The relatively low doses of exercise (less than 12 MET hours weekly) consisting of 90–120 min of moderate exercise appeared to be more effective than higher doses in improving fatigue and quality of life.

16.6 Psychosocial Interventions and Related Research

A randomized control trial assessed the effectiveness of exercise during adjuvant chemotherapy in patients with colon and breast cancer [112]. Two hundred and twenty participants were randomly assigned to the (1) low-intensity physical activity home-based program (i.e., oncomove), (2) the moderate-to-high-intensity supervised resistance and aerobic exercise program (on track), or (3) usual care. The interventions ran from the start to the end of chemotherapy. Both interventions compared to usual care significantly improved physical functioning, nausea, vomiting, and pain; and showed less decline in cardiorespiratory fitness. The OnTrack program showed significantly better outcomes for physical fatigue and muscle strength. The 6th-month follow-up showed that most gains had returned to normal. Both intervention groups also returned to work earlier than the usual controls. Whereas the supervised moderate-to-intense combined program was deemed more effective than the home-based physical activity program, the latter was deemed to be a viable alternative for those who decline to follow a more intense program during chemotherapy.

A meta-analysis of 25 RCTs ($n = 3418$) showed that exercise significantly improved physical functioning and reduced fatigue compared to controls in women during and after treatment for breast cancer [113]. The effect size differences were relatively small (physical functioning) to slightly larger (fatigue). The 6-month follow-up after chemotherapy or radiochemotherapy showed relative improvements based on even smaller effect size differences in women with breast cancer [113]. It may be noteworthy that patients who received the exercise program *after* treatment compared to *during* adjuvant treatment showed a small *but greater improvement* in physical functioning and fatigue. Notwithstanding, there may be important mediating or buffering effects of exercise during treatment, which needs to be further assessed. Five RCTs indicated that patients who received a combined aerobic and resistance training derived the greatest benefit in physical functioning; 12 RCTs demonstrated that fatigue was optimally reduced by aerobic exercise alone. Quality evidence was rated moderate to high across RCTs [113].

A meta-analysis of five RCTs ($n = 784$) showed that supervised and home-based physical exercise compared to control groups had a significant inverse effect on general fatigue (ES: -0.22) and physical fatigue (ES: -0.35) during and after treatment in four studies in which breast cancer patients received chemotherapy, radiochemotherapy, or radiochemo- and hormonal therapy [114]. Exercise had no effect on either cognitive or affective fatigue. The four supervised exercise programs that consisted of either resistance exercises ($n = 2$) or resistance/aerobic exercises ($n = 2$) had even greater inverse effects on general fatigue (-0.25) and, especially, physical fatigue (-0.39).

An RCT on the effects of exercise in patients with head and neck cancer who were undergoing chemotherapy reported significant improvements in functional capacity, quality of life as well as preventing an increase in fatigue levels [115]. Among the various physical activities favored by patients to counter fatigue during cancer treatments, relaxation exercise was ranked first followed by a combination of aerobic and resistance training [116].

A review of 45 meta-analyses, systematic reviews, and pooled analyses showed that the highest level of physical activity compared to the lowest was related to a significant reduction in the risks for esophageal adenocarcinoma and breast, bladder, colon, endometrial renal, and gastric cancers [117]. An RCT investigated the effectiveness of (1) a low-intensity physical activity home program, (2) a moderate-to-high intensity supervised aerobic exercise with resistance training, and (3) usual care during adjuvant chemotherapy in 230 patients with cancer [112]. Both the low-intensity group and moderate- to high-intensity group compared to usual care showed a significant but smaller decline in cardiorespiratory fitness ($p < 0.001$), greater physical functioning ($p \leq 0.001$) and significant improvement in pain ($p = 0.003$ and $p = 0.011$), and nausea and vomiting ($p = 0.029$ and $p = 0.031$) respectively. The *moderate-to-high intensity* physical activity demonstrated greater muscle strength ($p = 0.002$) and less physical fatigue ($p < 0.001$). All three groups returned to baseline levels on all outcome measurements at the 6-month follow-up. Both intervention groups also appeared to return to work sooner ($p = 0.012$) than the usual care group. A supervised moderate-to-intense physical exercise during chemotherapy is the optimal intervention for patients with breast cancer, although the low intensity at home option appeared to be a feasible option.

Finally, physical exercise is being explored as a possible therapeutic intervention to prevent or attenuate the chemotherapy-induced peripheral neuropathies (CIPN) caused by taxanes, platinum, or vinca alkaloids and experienced as prickly, tingling, numbness, pain, and/or cold sensations to fingers and feet. In a secondary analysis of a national phase 111 RCTs, 355 patients with cancer were randomized to (1) the chemotherapy group or (2) chemotherapy and exercise group [118]. The chemo-exercise group demonstrated an important decrease in symptoms of hot/coldness in hands or feet, and numbness and tingling compared to chemotherapy alone. Exercise appeared to decrease CIPN side effects more in male patients or patients who were older or had breast cancer. The findings suggest that moderate-to-intense exercise should be considered for patients during chemotherapy-based taxanes, vinca alkaloids, or platinum. The exercise intervention consisted of moderate-intensity, individualized home-based progressive walking and resistance training for 6 weeks.

These studies underscore the importance of physical activity during treatment for essentially healthy individuals as a function of their clinical status. Working with the physiotherapist and oncologist, the nurse plays a vital role in educating, encouraging, and supporting patients in this resilient-promoting therapy. As previously noted, studies of physical exercise have regulating effects in immune functioning vital to the body's ability to fight cancer alongside anticancer treatments [63].

Diet and Nutrition

A meta-analysis of 11 RCTs assessed the impact of (1) dietary counseling (DC), (2) high-energy oral nutritional supplements (ONS), or (3) ONS favoring protein and $n - 3$ polyunsaturated fatty acids (PUFA) aimed at regulating cancer-related metabolic changes during chemoradiation therapy [12]. There was an overall increase in body weight. Positive clinical outcomes were mainly attributed to the high protein and $n - 3$ PUFA intervention. The high protein and $n - 3$ PUFA were found to significantly decrease lean body mass loss ($N = 2$) and improve aspects of quality of life ($N = 3$). Neither the DC nor high-energy ONS exerted significant effects which may have been caused by poor adherence. Those positive findings are consistent with immunonutritional support received by surgical patients in order to regulate the inflammatory response of the perisurgical period [119]. Although the meta-analysis was predicated on a small number of underpowered studies of low-quality evidence, the results point toward potential clinical benefits of immunonutritional support that target metabolic alterations caused by the treatment or cancer [15].

Last, a small double-blind RCT randomly assigned 42 patients with cancer on chemotherapy to (1) the experimental condition in which patients received whey protein isolates with zinc and selenium every day for 12 weeks and (2) the control group that received a "maltodextrin" (i.e., carbohydrate sweetener) snack for the duration of the 12-week study [120]. The experimental group increased their levels of albumin by 2.9% and immunoglobulin G by 4.8% compared to controls at 12 weeks. The experimental group also showed a significant 11.7% increase in glutathione levels compared to the control group (6.0%). Glutathione is an anti oxidant that helps to protect cell structures from ROS -induced damage. A supplemental diet of whey protein appeared to improve immunity, glutathione levels, and nutritional status of patients undergoing chemotherapy. These studies strongly suggest that nurses work with nutritionists specialized in cancer and the oncologist to identify and treat patients at risk for inadequate nutritional requirements during chemotherapy.

Therapeutic Healing (Review Part IV Chap. 14; Appendix in Chap. 14)

Healing touch is an intentional, energy manipulating healing modality that was used in one study during chemoradiation therapy ([121], p. 2270). A randomized controlled trial of 60 women on chemoradiation for cervical cancer who received healing touch (HT) compared to relaxation training (RT) or usual care (UC) showed a minimal decrease in their natural killer cell cytotoxicity (NKCC) over the treatment span. Conversely the other two groups produced a significant decline over the same period [122]. The HT patients also experienced a significant improvement in depressed mood according to two separate measures of depression (POMS and CESD depressed mood subscale). Although the long-term clinical implications (i.e., sustainability) are unknown, the findings suggest a moderating effect of HT on depressed mood and immune functions that require further investigation based on RCTS with a double-blinded design and a sham healing group.

16.7 Family Caregivers

A meta-analysis of 29 RCTs assessed the types of psychosocial interventions that have been used to help family caregivers of patients with cancer. The identified interventions were *psychoeducation, skills training, and therapeutic counseling* based on different durations and frequency [123]. These interventions showed small-to-medium size effects that significantly reduced caregiving burden, improved coping ability, increased self-efficacy, and enhanced different facets of quality of life in caregivers of patients with early- to late-stage cancers of various types. Northouse who is a nurse recommended that clinicians implement research-based clinical interventions to enhance the quality of life of family caregivers.

In a Cochrane review of 19 trials ($n = 3725$), psychosocial interventions used to improve the quality of life, physical health, and well-being of informal caregivers did not appear to have a clinically meaningful impact on caregiver well-being, caregiver burden, depression, anxiety, physical health, and distress [124]. Patients were newly diagnosed with cancer, waiting to start treatment, on treatment, and after treatment. Clinical content included *providing information/education, coping, problem solving, and communication skills to manage symptoms or strengthen relationships,* all important components of psychosocial interventions. It is possible that the different phases of diagnosis, treatment, and survivorship, each with its corresponding clinical implications for the caregiver, likely requires a meta-analysis of each phase taken separately to reduce heterogeneity and a possible canceling out effect of various clinical outcomes

Cognitive-Behavioral Strategies CBT (Appendix in Chap. 9)

A clinical trial randomly assigned 157 Chinese informal caregivers and their loved ones with lung cancer to a CBT or an integrative mind–body spiritual intervention (I-BMS). The interventions were administered in separated groups of patients and caregivers [125]. Both the CBT and the IBMS appeared to improve caregiver psychological distress and quality of life over baseline scores, and no differences in clinical outcomes between the two interventions were found. The I-BMS intervention consisted of (1) psychoeducation, (2) qi gong and acupressure, (3) mindfulness relaxation exercises, and (4) a life review in order to enhance meaning from the caregiving experience. A 'usual care' arm is required to strengthen the design and interpretation of results. But the clinical approach suggests the value of addressing caregiver concerns separately from the patient, and also to consider tailored interventions that take into account the cultural background of individuals.

Mindfulness-Based Interventions (MB) (Review Part IV Chap. 13; Appendix in Chap. 9; Appendix in Chap. 13)

A PRISMA-guided systematic review of RCTs revealed a paucity of evidence supporting the effectiveness of MB interventions on family caregivers of patients with cancer, mainly due to the lack of well designed studies [126]. In a meta-analysis of 27 RCTS and pre/post studies of family caregivers, diverse meditative interventions appeared to effectively reduce depression, anxiety, stress, and increase self-efficacy in caregivers of individuals with dementia and other chronic illnesses including cancer (1 study) an estimated 8 weeks after starting the intervention [127]. The meditative practices included Benson's relaxation response, mindfulness meditation, and the mindfulness-based stress reduction intervention. These meditative practices may be effective for family caregivers of patients with cancer irrespective of the stage of illness. You may review the steps of the relaxation response technique in Benson and Stuart [128].

Summary

Several psychosocial interventions have been shown to reduce the severity of symptoms and side effects experienced by patients and caregivers, although in the main, the improvements are of small to medium effect sizes and of short or uncertain duration, due in part to the heterogeneity inherent in many meta-analyses. These studies nonetheless highlight the value of introducing healing- and resilient-promoting interventions during treatment including the perisurgical period for the purpose of promoting coping and self-management skills, strengthening informal supports (review Chaps. 11 and 15), and alleviating side effects and symptoms. Findings for use of foot reflexology (Chap. 14), the relaxation response technique (Chap. 13), and/or mindfulness-based stress-reducing interventions show promise as potential therapeutic interventions.

The review also highlights the importance of nurses' educating patients and caregivers to the resilient-promoting benefits of adhering to healthy lifestyle recommendations as much as possible Nurses work together with the oncologist and a *cancer*-nutritionist and physiotherapist to introduce, monitor, and/or encourage these interventions to optimize physical fitness and manage symptoms and side effects so that the body may be better enabled to fight cancer in conjunction with the medical treatment.

16.8 Nursing Approaches

Patients and caregivers may experience periodic emotional distress throughout the cancer trajectory, often triggered by transitional moments such as the start of chemotherapy/radiation therapy, the preoperative through postoperative phase, as well as by various symptoms and side effects. Systemic inflammation and immunosuppression pose a persistent potential threat to healing and long-term survival even as treatment-related efforts are directed toward eliminating and/or containing the cancer (e.g., [27, 28]). Researchers have come to realize that the patient's immune system and the developing tumor are intimately engaged in an interactive cat and mouse game that continues during the treatment phase. When the immune system is suppressed, the tumor can gain an important physiological advantage conducive to its growth and proliferative capabilities that can manifest in the future, long after the apparently successful goals of treatment have been met [1, 27].

With these considerations in mind, NCCN and other professional practice guidelines support regular assessments of (1) emotional distress (Review Part II Chap. 3) and (2) the identification of cancer- and treatment-related threats so that sources of distress may be expeditiously addressed and psychological adaptation to stress, enhanced [70, 129, 130]. Given the likelihood of periodic adverse clinical

Table 16.1 Suggested nursing goals for patients before, during, and after treatments, and caregivers as a function of the clinical status, patient preferences, and goals of treatment

1. Reduce emotional distress [31, 131, 132] (Chap. 3)
2. Manage distorted beliefs and negative expectations related to treatment [128, 133] (Chaps. 9 and 10)
3. Optimize healing processes, e.g., positive cognitive expectations [68] (Chap. 12) and wound healing
4. Manage side effects and symptoms; promote and protect immune functioning (Also Chap. 15)
5. Promote emotion-regulation [93, 134] (Chap. 9)
6. Promote self-management skills [94] (Chap. 9)
7. Promote relevant adaptive coping skills [135] (Chap. 9)
8. Strengthen supportive relationships [75, 136] (Chap. 11)
9. Support diet, nutrition and physical activity [8] (Chaps. 15–18)
10. Practice within the healing-promoting context of a quality nurse-patient (and caregiver) relationship [137] (Chap. 8)

situations along the continuum, all patients and caregivers should be beneficiaries of relevant cognitive-behavioral and support-enhancing strategies starting at diagnosis, but continuing throughout the treatment phase (Table 16.1) (e.g., [84, 85, 125]). Review the proposed nursing assessment in Chap. 15. This assessment is appropriate for patients and caregivers throughout the continuum, including treatment.

The Nurse–Patient Relationship (Review Part IV Chap. 8)

The quality of the nurse–patient–caregiver relationship serves as an invaluable, potential healing context especially during the treatment phase which is marked by tremendous uncertainty, stress, and the need for hope (Fig. 16.1). This relationship is therapeutic when a compassionate and meaningful state of connectedness between nurse and patient (with the caregiver) is established, predicated on mutual trust and hope for the best possible care and clinical outcome (e.g., [138]). That connection depends on the nurse's demonstrated scientific and technical competence, *ability to communicate effectively, that is,* to sensitively interact with and be responsive to the individual's thoughts, feelings, and behaviors [139, 140]. A sense of mutual connectedness can precipitate the downregulation of the stress response, enabling the PNS and other healing processes to restore dysregulated neurophysiological and immune pathways and functions that subsequently impact behavior, which is experienced as a sense of overall well being [23, 77, 141, 142].

16.8 Nursing Approaches

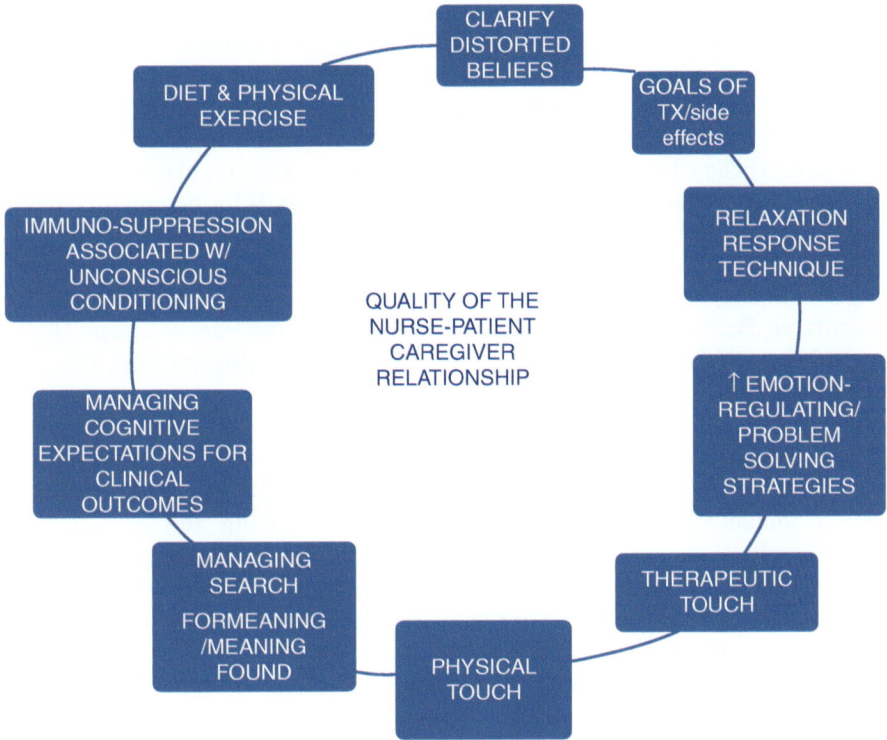

Fig. 16.1 Suggested one-on-one psychosocial discussions with patients and caregivers (Review Part IV Chaps. 8–14)

Promoting Self-Management (Problem-Solving) Capabilities
(Review Part IV Chap. 9; Appendices A and B)

The majority of patients experience some level of anxiety, but overall are sufficiently resilient to meet challenges during treatment. Most people have been effective problem solvers in their precancer lives. But the clinical context in which they now find themselves may cause some to doubt their ability to deftly manage all the big and little stresses that come their way. Promoting the patient/caregiver's knowledge and skills related to the course of the treatment and disease in *the early phase of treatment* may help both to better anticipate and handle treatment- and disease-related problems such as fatigue or pain between treatments. Facilitating problem-solving strategies consists of helping the individual to define the problem, goal, desired outcome, access relevant resources, and generate an action plan, that is the steps to achieve the desired outcome. Finally it requires evaluating the effectiveness of the executed plan of action [133, 143]. Learning to problem solve around cancer and treatment related issues can enhance their sense of self-efficacy and facilitate emotion regulation, knowing they have the capability to successfully confront the challenges they must face [93, 94, 143, 144]. Part of promoting self-management skills has to do with building a trusting relationship between nurse and patient and caregiver based on effective bidirectional communication skills [139].

Consider offering a self-management workshop for patients and especially their family caregivers *prior* to the start of any treatment in order to enhance their self-efficacy beliefs and capabilities, supported by regular bidirectional communication with the nurse (see Appendix in Chap. 9 for potential content) (e.g., [85]).

Cognitive-Behavioral Coping Approaches (Review Part IV Chaps. 9 and 10; Part IV Chap. 13; Appendix in Chap. 9; Appendix in Chap. 13; Appendix B)

Patients adjust better and are psychologically more resilient, when they adopt relevant cognitive coping strategies to manage illness- and treatment related threats and acquire pro-active problem solving self management skills (previous section) [93, 145–147]. Appendix B provides suggested cognitive promoting strategies which consist of emotion-, problem-, and meaning-oriented nursing interventions to promote resilience. Patients and caregivers may benefit from individualized coping promoting sessions (Review Appendix B) or multimodal group workshops in which cognitive-behavioral coping strategies are a key part of a broader multimodal intervention. Review Part IV (Chap. 9) and Part V (Chap. 18) on Supportive Care for suggested interventions to support patient and caregiver hope, a vital coping strategy for maintaining emotional equanimity. Some highly anxious individuals may experience intrusive ideation with avoidant behaviors. Part IV (Chap. 10) discusses strategies to reduce intrusive ideation.

Consider offering regularly scheduled (for instance monthly) nurse-led multimodal, multitargeted workshops that promote relevant cognitive-behavioral coping strategies to manage patient-identified threats and emotional distress, and strategies to enhance the quality of patient–caregiver relationships including strategies to attract and maintain needed support (See next section). Incorporate behavioral strategies such as mindful meditation or the relaxation response technique to reduce emotional distress (Review Chap. 13). Share relevant information and access to resources that facilitate better coping capabilities. Enable discussions around the process of adjusting social and family roles in response to various health-related setbacks and/or side effects or symptoms (Fig. 16.2).

Clinical research highlights the importance of enhancing resilient-promoting emotion regulating and problem-solving coping efforts especially in distressed patients and caregivers early in the disease trajectory with frequent individualized nursing support along the continuum.

16.8 Nursing Approaches

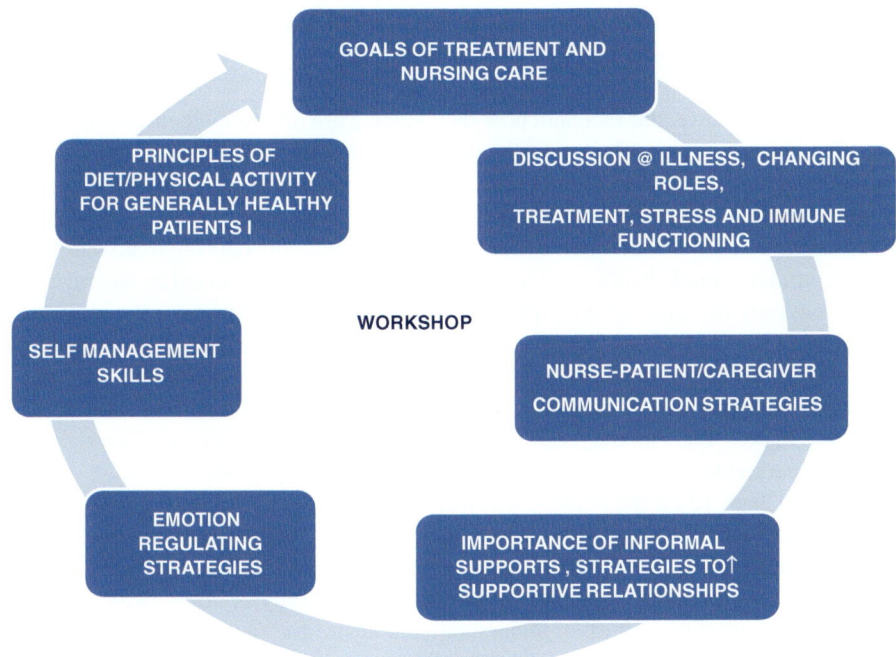

Fig. 16.2 Suggested components for a monthly workshop pretreatment (Review Part V Chap. 19)

Enhancing the Quality of Supportive Relationships (Review Part IV Chap. 11; Appendix B)

An important goal of nursing during treatment is to ensure the quality and strength of the patient's and family caregiver's supportive relationships with one another and, as needed, with family and close friends. The patients' and caregivers' perceived emotional support from loved ones has an important "buffering role" or protective function that helps to mitigate the suffering they may experience emotionally and physiologically during treatment [148]. Informal support plays a significant role in downregulating stress and its related biomarkers, and even in reducing the risk of dying of cancer [23, 136]. One of the critical functions of informal support during treatment (or any phase of the continuum) is their ability to encourage the patient to adopt relevant coping strategies to manage stress and even to facilitate a sense of meaning in life [135, 149]. The role of informal supports in either protecting or reducing the potential toxic effects of various treatments on cell-mediated immunity is strongly suggested by the findings, but more rigorous RCTs investigating the effects of supportive relationships on effective coping, meaning found, and immune responses during cancer treatment would contribute to the cancer literature and nursing practice. Chapter 11 and Appendix B offer nurse-led strategies to encourage better informal patient and caregiver supportive relationships.

Managing Positive/Negative Expectations of Treatment (Please Review Part IV Chap. 12)

What patients believe and feel, and how they behave are driven by their core beliefs, attitudes, assumptions, and previous health-related experiences [150]. These beliefs either foster healing outcomes or create obstacles to healing [151–153]. The manner in which these beliefs are managed by the nurse influences the potential for healing (the placebo effect) or for negative (nocebo) clinical outcomes during treatment [68, 154]. Comments made by the oncologist and nurse that are perceived as negative by the patient may interfere with the pharmacophysiological pathways of the intended treatment [154, 155]. Comments such as "Your cancer does not fit within the guidelines of a protocol" as opposed to "we have several options to consider," or "You *will* experience pain as opposed to you *may experience some discomfort*" may mean well, but fosters fear, anxiety, and/or an exaggerated pain response. Conversely, optimizing a treatment plan can improve treatment efficacy [156].

Review Chap. 12 on the placebo and nocebo triggers in the clinical environment that can either support the goals of treatment and healing processes, or inadvertently interfere with them. *Before starting cancer treatment*, the clinic nurse may want to review known side effects associated with the chemotherapy or other medical treatments with the patient, out of an understandable desire for caution even when consent to treat has been done. When the nurse focuses mainly on potential side effects, the unintended consequence may be to create negative expectations (doubts) surrounding the treatment that activate the biological stress response system associated with the release of inflammatory cytokines such as TNF and IL-6 among others, and suppresses PNS (healing processes) and immune functions (e.g., [157–159]).

A few helpful strategies Framing conveys the necessary clinical information within a more favorable perspective [62, 160–162]. Emphasize that *the majority* of patients who have the *same cancer as the patient* do well *rather than stating that a small number of patients suffer side effects* [68]. Remind the patient of the clinical goals of treatment in order to enhance the patient's cognitive expectations. Finally culminate the discussion by saying something to the effect of: "What is important is to let the nurse know if you feel differently than you would normally, or you have a concern or you feel good! Most of all remember that the goal of this treatment is to obtain a desired and positive clinical outcome of eliminating the cancer so that your immune capabilities are more enabled to help the treatment get rid of the cancer." Use factual information specific to the patient's treatment which can also bolster the patient's positive beliefs about the treatment. Just prior to starting the treatment (i.e., an infusion), direct the patient's attention to the drug as it starts to be administered. These simple practices can reaffirm or reactivate the patient's positive expectations (placebo) for a clinical benefit [163–165].

Conversely, negative expectations may prove more challenging to overcome. These patients are unlikely to alter their negative beliefs about the illness or treatment and in fact may reinforce their negative beliefs (i.e., known as cognitive immunization) when the clinician's information appears *nonspecific or too general*. For instance, stating that taxol is a common anticancer drug which has been "found to be effective in patients like yourself" may be too vague to be convincing enough to change their negative beliefs [68].

Helping patients make that shift toward more positive beliefs will likely necessitate greater specificity in the medical information being shared (for instance, taxol blocks cancer growth by stopping cell division and causing cancer cell death). If statistics are highly favorable, state something to the effect of "90% of patients on your protocol, and on taxol with your stage and type of cancer get better." You might also make the link between holding positive/negative beliefs and the greater likelihood of positive or negative healing outcomes by sharing the results of iconic studies in which clinical outcomes were associated with patient beliefs [68, 155, 164, 166–168].

In summary, nurse interventions involve providing information about the treatment goals within an open treatment approach that improves patient expectations which can potentially reduce symptoms and side effects, improve treatment efficacy, and perhaps improve immune functioning (e.g., [68, 156, 165, 169]). When the nurse's interventions occur within the context of a compassionate nurse–patient relationship, the placebo effect appears to be further optimized as evidenced by an RCT with patients with irritable bowel syndrome [170, 171]. These nursing interventions take very little time to do and may induce a significant therapeutic healing effect ([62], p. 206).

Promoting Immune Functioning (Review Part IV Chaps. 9, 11, 12, and 14)

Cancer- and treatment-related threats contribute to systemic inflammation, immunosuppression, and dysregulated immune signaling pathways needed for immunosurveillance [33, 172, 173]. Poor nutritional intake over the course of treatment as well as obesity and sedentary behavior are also contributing factors. Unconscious conditioning of sociophysical factors in the clinical environment during treatment is another possible cause of immunosuppression [174, 175]. The nurse's goal is to restore, protect, or minimize the decline of the patient's immune functions and in particular cell-mediated immunity during treatment via strategies empirically known to promote healing processes, immune functions, and resilience.

Part IV offers several strategies that may be considered to protect and maintain immunity during treatment. Clinical approaches to consider at regularly scheduled clinic visits:

1. Encourage physical activity during treatment in order to facilitate protein synthesis, muscle fitness and to counter immunosuppression [63, 176].
2. Introduce stress-reducing, emotion-regulating, meaning making, and problem-solving coping strategies which have been shown to improve immune cell functions [85, 88].

3. Strengthen informal supportive relationships [23, 177],
4. Encourage use of the relaxation response technique or mindful meditation [178],
5. For highly anxious individuals, consider healing touch: A small randomized controlled study of 64 patients with cervical cancer reported that natural killer cell cytotoxicity was significantly less suppressed in patients who received healing touch compared to either the relaxation group or usual care group during chemoradiation therapy [122] (review Part IV Chap. 14).
6. Last, consider the presence of unconscious conditioning during treatment which may suppress immune functioning (Review Part IV Chap. 12).

Because the clinical benefits of any one intervention above is still unclear, we need rigorously designed clinical trials to further inform the efficacy of each of these interventions. It is also possible that clear clinical benefits may depend on multi modal psycho-social interventions with unique and overlapping endpoints. A nurse-led rigorously designed RCT aimed at minimizing, protecting, or maintaining innate immune and cell-mediated immune functions in patients during treatment would inform the cancer literature with respect to the use of relevant psychosocial nursing strategies during treatment.

Unconscious Conditioning During Chemotherapy (See Part IV Chap. 12)

One nursing concern during treatment is the patient's potential for unconscious conditioning of social and physical factors within the clinical environment that may induce or maintain immunosuppression as a side effect of some types of chemotherapy (specifically, taxanes or vinca alkaloids such as doxorubicin and vincristine) [174, 179]. For example, the patient on return to the clinic and re-exposed to these factors may unconsciously reactivate previously embedded neural/humoral-immune pathways caused by the chemotherapy that result in an immunosuppressed response. Triggering social and physical factors may include repeated behaviors such as the nurse's setting up the intravenous for treatment, the clinic wall color, odors, equipment, and other recurring procedures [175].

Potential clinical clues Patients who present at the next chemotherapy still immunosuppressed may see their treatment deferred until their immune cell counts improve. If this is a frequent recurrence, assess whether the patient (1) has improved immune functioning between treatments, (2) remains immunosuppressed between treatments, (3) improves immune functioning between treatments, but manifests an immunosuppressed response on return to clinic before treatment [152].

A patient who complains of constant fatigue between treatments contrary to medical expectation may be affected by environmental factors in the home which mimic environmental conditions at the clinic, thereby adversely affecting the patient's immune recovery. For instance, the patient's home wall color may resemble the clinic wall color. But immunosuppression also may be elicited by the patient's *memories* of the clinical experience, for instance via unwanted intrusive ideation [152]. For example, a patient's blood taken on a home visit may show immune recovery between two treatments, but the blood test taken at the clinic before the upcoming treatment inexplicably shows immunosuppression; though rare, it may be indicative of unconscious immunosuppression. Knowledge of the normal chemotherapy cycle, including the expected timing of immune recovery, can be used by the nurse to determine whether salient environmental cues might be an interfering factor, adversely affecting the immune functioning of the patient.

Although unusual, suggested nursing interventions include re-emphasizing the positive goals of the chemotherapy during the *current* infusion, drawing the patient's attention to the start of the infusion, use of positive imagery at home or during the infusion, and use of deliberate rumination to dispel negative thoughts surrounding the treatment. Benson's relaxation response technique or mindful meditation has been shown to reduce emotional reactivity associated with intrusive ideation. Finally, a referral to psychology should be considered. Each of these suggestions needs to be assessed in a well-designed randomized controlled study (Review Part IV Chaps. 9, 10, and 12).

Supporting Diet, Relevant Nutrition, and Physical Activity
(Review Part V Chap. 15)

Diet and Nutrition

The WCRF/AICR [8] provides an evidenced-based recommended diet for cancer prevention and for cancer survivors. All newly diagnosed patients require a diet and nutrition assessment, preferably by the dietitian, or if agreed, by the nurse. Patients receiving anticancer treatments who are physically fit without illness- or treatment-related weight loss or other serious clinical issues and with the support of the oncologist and cancer nutritionist should be encouraged to follow the WCRF/AICR [8] diet, at least to start. These scientific-based recommendations are continuously updated on-line with the latest meta-analyses and RCTs (https://www.aicr.org/research/third-expert-report/).

At regularly scheduled clinical appointments, assess the patient's weight, pattern of dietary intake, and how they feel about adhering to a healthy diet. Look for *dietary patterns of diverse healthy foods* rather than a preference for only a few preferred items (Chap. 15). Review the recommended pattern of fruits, vegetables, legumes, and fish while discussing the patient's reasons for possibly avoiding other important food groups (Table 16.2) [8, 182]. Educate: Explain the importance of a healthy diet and its effect on proteins, physical development, and immune functioning. Patients undergoing anticancer treatments tend to progressively gain weight and eat less fruits and vegetables in their diet over time. An inadequate nutritional intake has been associated with immunosuppression. Work closely with the oncologist and nutritionist for signs of an inadequate diet and to support dietary recommendations for patients during treatment.

Table 16.2 Foods to avoid during treatment and survivorship [8, 15, 180, 181]

Processed foods (white bread, pancakes, cakes, and cookies)
Red meat
Delicatessen meats including sausages, salami, and smoked meat
Fried or barbecued foods
Salty foods and salt
Refined sugar, candy
Alcohol
Smoking
Beta carotene supplements

Immunonutrition As previously discussed, patients with cancer may reduce their nutritional intake during chemoradiotherapy which may contribute to metabolic disturbances, systemic inflammation, and immune suppression [13, 14, 183]. Various immunonutritional protocols have shown clear clinical benefits for patients on cancer treatments and patients during the perisurgical period, although some findings are mixed [12, 119]. For example, nutritional interventions fortified with protein (for collagen synthesis, wound healing) and $n - 3$ polyunsaturated fatty acids (PUFA) aimed at regulating metabolic alterations, showed significant improvements in body weight, minimizing lean body mass loss and improving some aspects of quality of life [12].

The findings strongly suggest the value of doing general nutritional assessments, such as taking the patient's weight and dietary intake to help identify patients who may not be eating properly or adhering to dietary and nutritional recommendations. (1) Explore patient thoughts and feelings regarding the recommended diet or supplements. (2) Are they well tolerated? (3) What other foods do they eat—itemize, discuss, and educate? (4) Assess for side effects especially fatigue, a sign of immunosuppression, and possible malnourishment. (5) Monitor weight, blood albumin, total protein, and ratio of albumin to globulin, which serve as indicators of a malnutrition. (6) Measure CRP as a gross measure of inflammation, and lymphocytes (%), needed to counter viruses, bacteria, and cancer cells. The nurse plays a proactive collaborative role in reviewing and promoting the appropriate diet and nutritional intake as a function of the patient's health status and the dietician's recommendation. This is all the more critical as it is impossible for the dietician to actively follow all cancer patients, in particular those who have been generally deemed healthy at the start of treatment.

Clinical Anecdote 16.3
When I was treated for cancer and even some years afterward the vast majority of oncologists and dietitians adhered to the view that unless the patient was cachectic, seriously malnourished due to the disease or treatment, patients like myself who were basically healthy during treatment, could eat almost anything so long as it was cooked. "Eat a balanced meal" was the main advice. Maybe lots of fruits and

vegetables, but carbohydrates, refined sugars, red meat, processed foods, and fried or barbecued meat and vegetables were according to the patient's taste. As one healthcare provider at the time explained to me, "These patients are not likely to recover, what they eat will not make a difference." Perhaps not. But from a whole person care perspective based on a multimodal, multitargeted approach, it also might help. And of course years later the anticancer evidence on diet and nutrition is becoming much clearer. But as a nurse one of our responsibilities is not just to educate patients and families, but to bring to the oncology team's attention, and that includes the dietician, concerns about a generally healthy patient's current diet. Complex diets may be the realm of the dietician, but every nurse should be well versed in the latest research findings produced by the WCRF/AICR [8].

Physical Activity (Review Part V Chap. 15)
Physical activity reduces the risk of developing cancer and preventing a cancer recurrence. It strengthens overall fitness prior to treatment and during survivorship (e.g., [8, 184–186]). Regular exercise appears to improve immunity and helps to regulate acute and chronic systemic inflammation, all to underscore its potential importance as an adjunct therapy during treatment [176]. However, the evidence for physical exercise during the treatment phase appears to be mixed due to the paucity of RCTs and the tendency of meta-analyses to combine exercise programs for patients during and after treatment (e.g., [187]). An integrative review of physical activity during and after adjuvant treatment in women with breast cancer indicated that a lack of information and guidance from healthcare professionals may explain in part the general paucity of physical activity programs during treatment. Facilitators to exercise were peers and also healthcare professionals who provided education and support [188].

Patients who are otherwise healthy or deemed adequately fit by the oncologist should be invited to enroll in a supervised exercise program that is increasingly referred to by oncologists as adjunct therapy. Patients who were enrolled during the diagnostic phase or the start of treatment should be encouraged to continue (e.g., [18, 111, 112]). Both moderate- and high-intensity exercise appears to improve a number of physical and psychological indicators that contribute to better overall fitness, less anxiety and fatigue, and an earlier return to work compared to chemotherapy alone [189]. One study found that a low-intensity home program also produced several clinical benefits in women undergoing chemotherapy for breast cancer who were unwilling or unable to participate in the moderate-to-intense supervised exercise program [112].

In an RCT, 143 patients received (1) a combination of diet consultations, moderate-to-intense aerobic, and resistance training, or (2) usual care during chemotherapy and radiotherapy for breast cancer [190]. The intervention compared to usual care improved fatigue, anxiety, depression, and quality of life at the end of chemotherapy, and at 26 weeks at the end of radiotherapy. In addition, body mass index and body fat showed significant reductions, and cognitive flexibility and muscle endurance improved at 26 weeks. Significant improvements in fatigue and quality of life were also reported at the 12-month follow-up, compared to usual care.

Although clinical guidelines for exercise *during* treatment were not located, Carayol's meta-analysis suggests that low doses of exercise (<12 MET hours weekly) consisting of 90–120 min weekly of moderate physical exercise were more effective than higher doses in achieving desired improvements in quality of life, fatigue, anxiety, and depression. The findings however also suggest that any physical activity is beneficial compared to inactivity [111, 112, 190]. In consultation with the oncologist and physiotherapist, all patients during treatment should be encouraged to engage in some daily exercise, such as moderately paced walking as a function of their clinical state.

Review the patient's physical activity as part of regular clinic appointments with the patient and caregiver. Review the frequency, duration, and intensity of exercise between visits, and how these vary over time and as a function of potentially interfering factors, such as the patient's state of health between treatments. Determine to what extent side effects, such as fatigue, neuralgia, and general muscular pain posttreatment, accounted for the decline in physical exercise. The nurse and patient may work together to identify periods during the day or week or between treatments when a patient usually feels "better" recognizing these moments as "opportunities" for physical activity to strengthen their overall resilience and counter fatigue or neuralgia associated with the treatment.

Facilitating Wound Healing in the Perioperative Period (Review Sect. "Body Image Impairments")

Patients may experience slow wound healing postoperatively, delaying the start of chemotherapy, and/or other anticancer treatments. Slow wound healing is associated with postoperative complications, obesity, sleep disturbances, less exercise, poor nutrition, and *ongoing psychological distress* (e.g., [29, 30, 191, 192]). Employing therapeutic strategies that can reduce stress and restore a TH-1 over TH-2 cytokine response may accelerate physical healing.

Regular exercise and a balanced nutritional diet have been shown to improve wound healing and strengthen immunity [29, 192, 193]. Meals that include fish and chicken provide protein needed to stimulate collagen synthesis and wound remodeling. Smoking and alcohol intake (which decreases angiogenesis) should be discouraged (e.g., [194]). Wound healing also has been improved by uninterrupted sleep in order to increase the secretion of growth hormone, decrease migration of monocytes, and activate macrophages (e.g., [191]) Use of a relaxation exercise accompanied by imagery, starting 3 days before surgery and continuing 7 days afterward, was shown to significantly reduce the healing time, compared to standard care [195]. There is some evidence that an emotional disclosure intervention based on writing about a trauma event showed significantly smaller "punch biopsy" wounds 14 and 21 days later compared to controls who were asked to write about "time management" [193]. Facilitating wound healing is a clinical imperative especially for postoperative individuals needing chemotherapy or radiotherapy within a timely framework.

Symptom/Side Effects

Growing evidence suggests that *interventions* that target the main symptom of a symptom cluster, that is, the one that appears to exert the greatest negative effect on physical well-being such as pain, may also attenuate the intensity of the other symptoms (for instance, anxiety and poor sleep) due to a shared underlying biological predicate [100]. A secondary analysis of data from a RCT study that investigated imagery and muscle relaxation on pain, anxiety, fatigue and depression revealed the mediating effects of various symptoms within the cluster that may eventually identify the strategic targets (ie behavioral and or physiological endpoints) of proposed clinical interventions to manage symptom clusters [49]. Currently, interventions such as exercise, at a moderate level of intensity, appears more generally to improve a number of symptoms and side effects during treatment [196].

Pain (Review Part IV Chaps. 9, 12, 13, and 14; Part V Chap. 18; Appendix A)
Cancer- and treatment-related pain, including postoperative pain, is generally undertreated [197]. A combination of pain education, medication adherence, and the acquisition of self-efficacy skills may be effective in relieving pain. Enhancing *cognitive expectations for a therapeutic benefit* for instance, in the recovery room by drawing the patient's attention to the analgesic infusion while reiterating its beneficial intent, has been shown to effectively reduce *both pain and anxiety* levels [174] (Part IV Chap. 12). As pain tends to be associated with emotional distress and/or fatigue, use of mindful meditation (MM) or the relaxation response technique (RR) may also be considered as an adjunct therapeutic option due to its ability to downregulate the stress response, reducing in principle, levels of proinflammatory cytokines associated with the sensation of pain (such as TNF and IL-6). Please review Chap. 18 on the use of acupuncture/acupressure for cancer or treatment-related pain. As an adjunct therapy, acupuncture has been found to alleviate cancer- or treatment-related pain and should be considered [198–200].

Peripheral Neuropathy
Chemotherapies including taxanes and platinum agents such as cisplatin damage nerve endings in the toes and hands, causing numbness and/or prickly and sharp, knife-like sensations that may "feel" worse at night, preventing sleep. Without an empirically effective therapeutic intervention, patients usually resort to *medications* such as Lyrica (pregabalin) with mixed results.

Hand and foot massage may improve circulation and provide temporary relief. A quasi experimental study reported that *warm foot bathing* may be more effective than foot massage in easing the symptoms of peripheral neuropathy by increasing the flow of oxygenated blood to affected areas [201]. A retrospective consecutive chart review of 30 patients with breast cancer who received a combined acupuncture and reflexology protocol (ART-N) which began an estimated 101 days after starting chemotherapy reported that 26/30 patients had a complete recovery from sensory and/or motor neuropathies by 12 months. Eight of these patients had grade 3–4 neuropathies that appeared to be successfully treated by this combined protocol [107]. Only two complained of neuropathic symptoms (grades 1 and 2) at 12 months. Two patient records lacked sufficient information to be included in the final analysis. The average number of sessions was 10.8 (range: 4–32). The protocol consisted of 1–2 weekly sessions of acupuncture (20 min) followed by reflexology (30–40 min) [107]. As a proof of concept, the finding needs to be replicated with a rigorously designed RCT, in which the protocol is administered concurrently with the start of the chemotherapy.

Kleckner and colleagues' [118] secondary analysis of an RCT of 355 cancer patients indicated that a standardized moderate-to-intense individualized 6-week, home exercise program consisting of progressive walking and resistance training during chemotherapy appeared to reduce chemotherapy-induced peripheral neuropathic (CIPN) side effects of numbness and tingling ($p = 0.06$) and hot/cold sensations of the feet and hands ($p = 0.045$). All patients suffering from foot neuropathies should be warned of an increased risk for falling and as clinically assessed referred to physiotherapy.

Fatigue (Review Appendix C)
Moderate regular exercise has been shown to be effective as a strategy for reducing treatment-associated fatigue in patients who have been medically deemed physically healthy [114, 196]. Explore the optimal time of day or within the treatment cycle when the patient generally experiences more energy. Encourage exercise for 20 min daily if possible, working up to 40–60 min, as a function of their clinical status. Even 5 min of walking or engaging in a passive range of motion exercises should be encouraged, increasing if possible, at the patient's own rate, and in consultation with the physio- or exercise-therapist.

Fatigue may also be caused by inadequate nutritional intake during chemoradiotherapy and an immunosuppressed clinical status, requiring the interventions of an onconutritionist. The nurse's role is to assess, educate, and collaborate with the oncology team to find the optimal clinical approach. This depends on a proactive nurse who is knowledgeable about the latest evidence-based WCRF/AICR [8] recommendations for a health-promoting lifestyle.

Sleep Disturbances (Review Part IV Chaps. 9 and 14; Appendix in Chap. 9; Appendix in Chap. 14)
Sleep is an important restorative healing function of the body that conserves energy and maintains homeostasis [202, 203] (see Matthews et al. [202] systematic review). Sleep disturbances have been associated with immunosuppression, delays in healing, increased pain sensitivity, poor quality of life, and poor performance on ADL, thereby posing a serious health risk to patients during chemotherapy [202, 204]. In addition to reducing environmental disturbances such as noise and unwanted light, physical exercise, slow massage, cognitive-behavioral strategies, psychoeducation, MBSR, and soft music may improve cancer- and treatment-related sleep disturbances. However, better-designed studies are needed to confirm these findings (e.g., [205–207]).

Body Image Impairments

Body image impairments due to chemotherapy, surgery, and or radiotherapy can have consequential effects on the individual's sense of self, causing intimacy problems, shame, inadequacy, avoidance, social isolation, depression, and anxiety [208–210]. The most effective clinical approaches to improve body image perceptions may depend on the type of body impairment and the main sources of distress. Research to date has tended to focus mainly on women with breast cancer [60, 211], then prostate cancer [212], and exceptionally, head and neck [61].

A number of strategies have provided some help, including a psychotherapeutic approach (CBT or MBSR), psychoeducation, brief couple sex therapy, yoga, and physical activity/exercise tailored to the type of body impairment. An early study randomly assigned 312 women with breast cancer after surgery and still on adjuvant chemotherapy to four groups: (1) education, (2) discussion, (3) combined discussion–education, and (4) control groups [213]. The education groups (1 and 3) received information to increase a sense of control over their illness and reduce feelings of uncertainty. Topics included breast cancer, nutrition, exercise, body image, nutrition, relationships and intimacy, and relaxation exercises. The education groups showed a higher sense of self-esteem, better body image, less intrusive ideation, and greater tendency to discuss their cancer with friends and family than the control group. Body image-related interventions have been offered in groups or as couples, although these therapeutic effects are generally not sustainable, and findings of effectiveness are mixed (e.g., [60, 209, 210]).

One of Lewis Smith's [60] recommendations is to offer a biophysical and psychosocial approach rather than a reductionist focus on the impairment. This is in keeping with the stress, healing and resilient-promoting model and indeed is a core value of the nursing discipline. Through a more comprehensive lens consisting of culture, values, assumptions, and beliefs about the world and the self, relationships, and social influences, body image may be considered with an aim toward incorporating a more enlightened body image into a reintegrated self.

Nursing interventions that help to dismantle patient *stereotypes* about beauty and appearance by analyzing them within the deeper context of meaningful relationships, values, and beliefs may be helpful, particularly before and after disfiguring surgical procedures [214]. Physical activity has been shown to play an important role in improving body image in some patients depending on the location and extent of physical disfigurement [209]. Disease-specific models of body image are needed to guide clinicians in their care of cancer patients with special needs such as the head and neck cancer population [53, 215, 216] or all patients with cancer and body image challenges [54]. Body image is an important component of caring for patients with cancer that starts during treatment and continues into survivorship. More qualitative studies may deepen our understanding of the distress associated with specific types of impairments, followed by controlled randomized studies to evaluate the proposed nursing interventions.

Lymphedema (LE)

This refers to "swelling of the soft interstitial tissues due to the accumulation of protein-rich fluid in extracellular spaces" ([217], p. 202). LE is caused by damage to a designated area of the body from a surgical, radiation, or chemotherapeutic procedure that causes the lymph vessels to become constricted, blocked, or disrupted so lymph fluid cannot be drained and fluid stasis occurs ([217], p. 202). Critical prognostic factors include the number of axillary nodes removed during surgery, the type of surgery, and radiation. LE is a lifelong condition that requires continuous vigilance starting in the preoperative through postsurgical phases in order to prevent, minimize, or control its swelling [218].

The pretreatment phase is the optimal time for the patient to obtain initial *information* about the early signs, potential triggers, the self-care skills, and lifelong interventions to manage lymphedema (LE) which need to be regularly implemented, and monitored after surgery or radiotherapy [219]. The International Society of Lymphology recommends preop teaching, skin care, exercise therapy, manual lymphatic drainage, compression therapy, and continuous lifelong patient vigilance throughout survivorship (e.g., [218–220]). Written guidelines that summarize the key points and offer visual representations of various skills would also be helpful for patients [218, 221]. During the treatment phase, self-care (self-management behaviors), skin care, exercise, and manual lymphatic drainage should be reinforced as lifelong behaviors of patients, ideally with the support of the family caregiver. Nurses can decrease the risk of lymphedema with *early* patient education before, during, and after anticancer treatment.

Family Caregivers (Review Part V Chap. 18)

Family caregivers of whom the majority are women tend to receive little interventional support especially during the earlier phases of the patient's cancer continuum [123, 222]. Although a clinical focus on the informal caregiver exceeds the goals of this book, it is still essential to remember that in caring for patients, the emotional, social, physical, and caregiving needs of the caregiver must be addressed. We know from several studies that the impact of cancer affects not only the patient but those he or she loves, including the informal caregiver [223]. Patients and their loved ones or partners tend to respond to cancer-related threats as "one emotional system" [224]. As Chap. 18 on Supportive care and End of Life discusses, family caregiver burden inevitably increases with disease progression and the need to care for caregivers as much as the patient becomes a clinical imperative [225].

When we care for patients and neglect the needs of the family caregiver, the result can lead to both caregiver and patient distress [226]. Informal caregivers are not only responsible for navigating the healthcare system and patient caregiving activities during treatment, but many also have their own work and family responsibilities, and suffer their own chronic illnesses, with little time for self-care activities, placing them also at serious risk health wise [227]. Caregivers may experience additional distress when they feel they cannot talk openly with the doctor or nurse about their personal concerns, the patient, or other family members. In the year following the diagnosis, caregiver health was found to deteriorate as patients improved their physical health [226]. Controlled intervention studies to enhance the self-management and coping efficacy of caregivers during treatment as they increasingly must care for their loved one is a clinical imperative of practice.

Summary

This chapter has highlighted the complex work nurses do to reduce emotional distress, manage symptoms, protect immune functioning, and enhance overall healing processes and resilient capabilities of patients and caregivers during treatment. Many nursing interventions are carried out every day in one-to-one clinical interactions with the patient and caregiver. Some may be optimally offered as part of a group workshop. Given growing evidence of the importance of strengthening immune functioning, a number of immune-promoting interventions discussed in this chapter should be evaluated in well designed studies. But given current clinical findings, these interventions should become standard nursing practice throughout the perisurgical and chemoradiotherapeutic phases of treatment.

References

1. Wang M, Zhao J, Zhang L, Wei F, Lian Y, Wu Y, et al. Role of tumor microenvironment in tumorigenesis. J Cancer. 2017;8(5):761–73. PubMed PMID: 28382138. Pubmed Central PMCID: PMC5381164. Epub 2017/04/07. eng.
2. Kim J, Han JY, Shaw B, McTavish F, Gustafson D. The roles of social support and coping strategies in predicting breast cancer patients' emotional well-being: testing mediation and moderation models. J Health Psychol. 2010;15(4):543–52. PubMed PMID: 20460411. Pubmed Central PMCID: PMC3145334. Epub 2010/05/13. eng.
3. Kim SW, Kim SY, Kim JM, Park MH, Yoon JH, Shin MG, et al. Relationship between a hopeful attitude and cellular immunity in patients with breast cancer. Gen Hosp Psychiatry. 2011;33(4):371–6. PubMed PMID: 21762834. Epub 2011/07/19. eng.
4. Rades D, Narvaez CA, Dziggel L, Tvilsted S, Kjaer TW, Schild SE, et al. Emotional problems prior to adjuvant radiation therapy for breast cancer. In Vivo. 2021;35(5):2763–70. PubMed PMID: 34410966. Pubmed Central PMCID: PMC8408699. Epub 2021/08/20. eng.
5. Yang WFZ, Lee RZY, Kuparasundram S, Tan T, Chan YH, Griva K, et al. Cancer caregivers unmet needs and emotional states across cancer treatment phases. PLoS One. 2021;16(8):e0255901. PubMed PMID: 34379667. Pubmed Central PMCID: PMC8357113. Epub 2021/08/12. eng.
6. De Almeida CV, de Camargo MR, Russo E, Amedei A. Role of diet and gut microbiota on colorectal cancer immunomodulation. World J Gastroenterol. 2019;25(2):151–62. PubMed PMID: 30670906. Pubmed Central PMCID: PMC6337022. Epub 2019/01/24. eng.
7. Childs CE, Calder PC, Miles EA. Diet and immune function. Nutrients. 2019;11(8):1933. PubMed PMID: 31426423. Pubmed Central PMCID: PMC6723551. Epub 2019/08/21. eng.
8. World Cancer Research Fund AIfcr. Diet, nutrition, physical activity and cancer: a global perspective. Summary of 3rd expert report. Continuous update project expert report. 2018. https://www.wcrf.org/diet-activity-and-cancer/.
9. Shams-White MM, Brockton NT, Mitrou P, Romaguera D, Brown S, Bender A, et al. Operationalizing the 2018 World Cancer Research Fund/American Institute for Cancer Research (WCRF/AICR) cancer prevention recommendations: a standardized scoring sys-

tem. Nutrients. 2019;11(7):1572. PubMed PMID: 31336836. Pubmed Central PMCID: PMC6682977. Epub 2019/07/25. eng.
10. Ringel AE, Drijvers JM, Baker GJ, Catozzi A, García-Cañaveras JC, Gassaway BM, et al. Obesity shapes metabolism in the tumor microenvironment to suppress anti-tumor immunity. Cell. 2020;183(7):1848–66.e26. PubMed PMID: 33301708. Pubmed Central PMCID: PMC8064125. Epub 2020/12/11. eng.
11. Cruceriu D, Baldasici O, Balacescu O, Berindan-Neagoe I. The dual role of tumor necrosis factor-alpha (TNF-α) in breast cancer: molecular insights and therapeutic approaches. Cell Oncol. 2020;43(1):1–18. PubMed PMID: 31900901. Epub 2020/01/05. eng.
12. de van der Schueren MAE, Laviano A, Blanchard H, Jourdan M, Arends J, Baracos VE. Systematic review and meta-analysis of the evidence for oral nutritional intervention on nutritional and clinical outcomes during chemo(radio)therapy: current evidence and guidance for design of future trials. Ann Oncol. 2018;29(5):1141–53. PubMed PMID: 29788170. Pubmed Central PMCID: PMC5961292. Epub 2018/05/23. eng.
13. Custódio ID, Marinho Eda C, Gontijo CA, Pereira TS, Paiva CE, Maia YC. Impact of chemotherapy on diet and nutritional status of women with breast cancer: a prospective study. PLoS One. 2016;11(6):e0157113. PubMed PMID: 27310615. Pubmed Central PMCID: PMC4911080. Epub 2016/06/17. eng.
14. Alwarawrah Y, Kiernan K, MacIver NJ. Changes in nutritional status impact immune cell metabolism and function. Front Immunol. 2018;9:1055. PubMed PMID: 29868016. Pubmed Central PMCID: PMC5968375. Epub 2018/06/06. eng.
15. De Cicco P, Catani MV, Gasperi V, Sibilano M, Quaglietta M, Savini I. Nutrition and breast cancer: a literature review on prevention, treatment and recurrence. Nutrients. 2019;11(7):1514. PubMed PMID: 31277273. Pubmed Central PMCID: PMC6682953. Epub 2019/07/07. eng.
16. Rock CL, Thomson C, Gansler T, Gapstur SM, McCullough ML, Patel AV, et al. American Cancer Society guideline for diet and physical activity for cancer prevention. CA Cancer J Clin. 2020;70(4):245–71. PubMed PMID: 32515498. Epub 2020/06/10. eng.
17. Fassier P, Zelek L, Partula V, Srour B, Bachmann P, Touillaud M, et al. Variations of physical activity and sedentary behavior between before and after cancer diagnosis: results from the prospective population-based NutriNet-Sante cohort. Medicine. 2016;95(40):e4629. PubMed PMID: 27749527. Pubmed Central PMCID: PMC5059029. Epub 2016/10/18. eng.
18. Lugo D, Pulido AL, Mihos CG, Issa O, Cusnir M, Horvath SA, et al. The effects of physical activity on cancer prevention, treatment and prognosis: a review of the literature. Complement Ther Med. 2019;44:9–13. PubMed PMID: 31126580. Epub 2019/05/28. eng.
19. Kelliher MA, Roderick JE. NOTCH Signaling in T-cell-mediated anti-tumor immunity and T-cell-based immunotherapies. Front Immunol. 2018;9:1718. PubMed PMID: 30967879. Pubmed Central PMCID: PMC6109642. Epub 2019/04/11. eng.
20. Misiorek JO, Przybyszewska-Podstawka A, Kałafut J, Paziewska B, Rolle K, Rivero-Müller A, et al. Context matters: NOTCH signatures and pathway in cancer progression and metastasis. Cells. 2021;10(1):94. PubMed PMID: 33430387. Pubmed Central PMCID: PMC7827494. Epub 2021/01/13. eng.
21. Steinbichler TB, Dudás J, Skvortsov S, Ganswindt U, Riechelmann H, Skvortsova II. Therapy resistance mediated by cancer stem cells. Semin Cancer Biol. 2018;53:156–67. PubMed PMID: 30471331. Epub 2018/11/25. eng.
22. Wang H, Unternaehrer JJ. Epithelial-mesenchymal transition and cancer stem cells: at the crossroads of differentiation and dedifferentiation. Dev Dyn. 2019;248(1):10–20. PubMed PMID: 30303578. Epub 2018/10/12. eng.
23. Lutgendorf SK, Andersen BL. Biobehavioral approaches to cancer progression and survival: mechanisms and interventions. Am Psychol. 2015;70(2):186–97. PubMed PMID: 25730724. Pubmed Central PMCID: PMC4347942. Epub 2015/03/03. eng.
24. Andersen BL, Farrar WB, Golden-Kreutz D, Kutz LA, MacCallum R, Courtney ME, et al. Stress and immune responses after surgical treatment for regional breast cancer. J Natl Cancer

Inst. 1998;90(1):30–6. PubMed PMID: 9428780. Pubmed Central PMCID: PMC2743254. Epub 1998/01/15. eng.
25. Gong XH, Wang JW, Li J, Chen XF, Sun L, Yuan ZP, et al. Physical exercise, vegetable and fruit intake and health-related quality of life in Chinese breast cancer survivors: a cross-sectional study. Qual Life Res. 2017;26(6):1541–50. PubMed PMID: 28229328. Epub 2017/02/24. eng.
26. Angka L, Khan ST, Kilgour MK, Xu R, Kennedy MA, Auer RC. Dysfunctional natural killer cells in the aftermath of cancer surgery. Int J Mol Sci. 2017;18(8):1787. PubMed PMID: 28817109. Pubmed Central PMCID: PMC5578175. Epub 2017/08/18. eng.
27. Neeman E, Ben-Eliyahu S. Surgery and stress promote cancer metastasis: new outlooks on perioperative mediating mechanisms and immune involvement. Brain Behav Immun. 2013;30(Suppl):S32–40. PubMed PMID: 22504092. Pubmed Central PMCID: PMC3423506. Epub 2012/04/17. eng.
28. Han XR, Wen X, Li YY, Fan SH, Zhang ZF, Li H, et al. Effect of different anesthetic methods on cellular immune functioning and the prognosis of patients with ovarian cancer undergoing oophorectomy. Biosci Rep. 2017;37(5):BSR20170915. PubMed PMID: 28935762. Pubmed Central PMCID: PMC5653919. Epub 2017/09/25. eng.
29. Guo S, Dipietro LA. Factors affecting wound healing. J Dent Res. 2010;89(3):219–29. PubMed PMID: 20139336. Pubmed Central PMCID: 2903966.
30. Walburn J, Vedhara K, Hankins M, Rixon L, Weinman J. Psychological stress and wound healing in humans: a systematic review and meta-analysis. J Psychosom Res. 2009;67(3):253–71. PubMed PMID: 19686881. Epub 2009/08/19. eng.
31. McEwen BS. Physiology and neurobiology of stress and adaptation: central role of the brain. Physiol Rev. 2007;87(3):873–904. PubMed PMID: 17615391. Epub 2007/07/07. eng.
32. Kiecolt-Glaser J, Marucha P, Malarkey W, Mercado A, Glaser R. Slowing of wound healing by psychological stress. Lancet. 1995;346:1–3.
33. Glaser R, Kiecolt-Glaser JK. Stress-induced immune dysfunction: implications for health. Nat Rev Immunol. 2005;5(3):243–51. PubMed PMID: 15738954.
34. Godbout JP, Glaser R. Stress-induced immune dysregulation: implications for wound healing, infectious disease and cancer. J NeuroImmune Pharmacol. 2006;1(4):421–7. PubMed PMID: 18040814. Epub 2007/11/28. eng.
35. Glaser R, Kiecolt-Glaser JK, Marucha PT, MacCallum RC, Laskowski BF, Malarkey WB. Stress-related changes in proinflammatory cytokine production in wounds. Arch Gen Psychiatry. 1999;56(5):450–6. PubMed PMID: 10232300. Epub 1999/05/08. eng.
36. Kwekkeboom KL. Cancer symptom cluster management. Semin Oncol Nurs. 2016;32(4):373–82. PubMed PMID: 27789073. Pubmed Central PMCID: PMC5143160. Epub 2016/10/30. eng.
37. Miller AH, Ancoli-Israel S, Bower JE, Capuron L, Irwin MR. Neuroendocrine-immune mechanisms of behavioral comorbidities in patients with cancer. J Clin Oncol. 2008;26(6):971–82. PubMed PMID: 18281672. Pubmed Central PMCID: PMC2770012. Epub 2008/02/19. eng.
38. Miller AH, Maletic V, Raison CL. Inflammation and its discontents: the role of cytokines in the pathophysiology of major depression. Biol Psychiatry. 2009;65(9):732–41. PubMed PMID: 19150053. Pubmed Central PMCID: PMC2680424. Epub 2009/01/20. eng.
39. Najafi S, Ansari M, Kaveh V, Haghighat S. Comparing the efficacy and side-effects of PDLASTA® (Pegfilgrastim) with PDGRASTIM® (Filgrastim) in breast cancer patients: a non-inferiority randomized clinical trial. BMC Cancer. 2021;21(1):454. PubMed PMID: 33892670. Pubmed Central PMCID: PMC8066442. Epub 2021/04/25. eng.
40. Ercolano E. Psychosocial concerns in the postoperative oncology patient. Semin Oncol Nurs. 2017;33(1):74–9. PubMed PMID: 28062332. Epub 2017/01/08. eng.
41. Hogle WP. Radiation therapy in the treatment of breast cancer. Semin Oncol Nurs. 2007;23(1):20–8. PubMed PMID: 17303513. Epub 2007/02/17. eng.

42. Nooner AK, Dwyer K, DeShea L, Yeo TP. Using relaxation and guided imagery to address pain, fatigue, and sleep disturbances: a pilot study. Clin J Oncol Nurs. 2016;20(5):547–52. PubMed PMID: 27668375. Epub 2016/09/27. eng.
43. Kwekkeboom K, Zhang Y, Campbell T, Coe CL, Costanzo E, Serlin RC, et al. Randomized controlled trial of a brief cognitive-behavioral strategies intervention for the pain, fatigue, and sleep disturbance symptom cluster in advanced cancer. Psycho-Oncology. 2018;27(12):2761–9. PubMed PMID: 30189462. Pubmed Central PMCID: PMC6279506. Epub 2018/09/07. eng.
44. Laird BJ, Scott AC, Colvin LA, McKeon AL, Murray GD, Fearon KC, et al. Pain, depression, and fatigue as a symptom cluster in advanced cancer. J Pain Symptom Manag. 2011;42(1):1–11. PubMed PMID: 21402467. Epub 2011/03/16. eng.
45. Miladinia M, Baraz S, Ramezani M, Malehi AS. The relationship between pain, fatigue, sleep disorders and quality of life in adult patients with acute leukaemia: during the first year after diagnosis. Eur J Cancer Care. 2018;27(1):e12762. PubMed PMID: 28913954. Epub 2017/09/16. eng.
46. Irwin MR. Inflammation at the intersection of behavior and somatic symptoms. Psychiatric Clin N Am. 2011;34(3):605–20. PubMed PMID: 21889682. Pubmed Central PMCID: PMC3820277. Epub 2011/09/06. eng.
47. Irwin MR. Depression and insomnia in cancer: prevalence, risk factors, and effects on cancer outcomes. Curr Psychiatry Rep. 2013;15(11):404. PubMed PMID: 24078066. Pubmed Central PMCID: PMC3836364. Epub 2013/10/01. eng.
48. Irwin MR, Carrillo C, Olmstead R. Sleep loss activates cellular markers of inflammation: sex differences. Brain Behav Immun. 2010;24(1):54–7. PubMed PMID: 19520155. Pubmed Central PMCID: 2787978.
49. Charalambous A, Giannakopoulou M, Bozas E, Paikousis L. Parallel and serial mediation analysis between pain, anxiety, depression, fatigue and nausea, vomiting and retching within a randomised controlled trial in patients with breast and prostate cancer. BMJ Open. 2019;9(1):e026809. PubMed PMID: 30679301. Pubmed Central PMCID: PMC6347855. Epub 2019/01/27. eng.
50. Irwin MR. Why sleep is important for health: a psychoneuroimmunology perspective. Annu Rev Psychol. 2015;66:143–72. PubMed PMID: 25061767. Epub 2014/07/26. eng.
51. Cash T, Pruzinsky T, editors. Body image: a handbook of theory, research, and clinica; practice. The Guilford: New York, NY; 2002.
52. Cash TF, Pruzinsky T. Future challenges for body image theory, research and clinical practice. New York, NY: The Guilford Press; 2002.
53. Fingeret MC, Hutcheson KA, Jensen K, Yuan Y, Urbauer D, Lewin JS. Associations among speech, eating, and body image concerns for surgical patients with head and neck cancer. Head Neck. 2013;35(3):354–60. PubMed PMID: 22431304. Pubmed Central PMCID: PMC4022133. Epub 2012/03/21. eng.
54. Fingeret MC, Teo I, Epner DE. Managing body image difficulties of adult cancer patients: lessons from available research. Cancer. 2014;120(5):633–41. PubMed PMID: 24895287. Pubmed Central PMCID: PMC4052456. Epub 2014/06/05. eng.
55. Smile TD, Tendulkar R, Schwarz G, Arthur D, Grobmyer S, Valente S, et al. A Review of treatment for breast cancer-related lymphedema: paradigms for clinical practice. Am J Clin Oncol. 2018;41(2):178–90. PubMed PMID: 28009597. Epub 2016/12/24. eng.
56. Cotrim H, Pereira G. Impact of colorectal cancer on patient and family: implications for care. Eur J Oncol Nurs. 2008;12(3):217–26. PubMed PMID: 18567538. Epub 2008/06/24. eng.
57. Bullen TL, Sharpe L, Lawsin C, Patel DC, Clarke S, Bokey L. Body image as a predictor of psychopathology in surgical patients with colorectal disease. J Psychosom Res. 2012;73(6):459–63. PubMed PMID: 23148815. Epub 2012/11/15. eng.
58. Taylor-Ford M, Meyerowitz BE, D'Orazio LM, Christie KM, Gross ME, Agus DB. Body image predicts quality of life in men with prostate cancer. Psycho-Oncology. 2013;22(4):756–61. PubMed PMID: 22422671. Epub 2012/03/17. eng.

59. Smith JD, Shuman AG, Riba MB. Psychosocial issues in patients with head and neck cancer: an updated review with a focus on clinical interventions. Curr Psychiatry Rep. 2017;19(9):56. PubMed PMID: 28726060. Epub 2017/07/21. eng.
60. Lewis-Smith H, Diedrichs PC, Harcourt D. A pilot study of a body image intervention for breast cancer survivors. Body Image. 2018;27:21–31. PubMed PMID: 30121489. Epub 2018/08/20. eng.
61. Davidson A, Williams J. Factors affecting quality of life in patients experiencing facial disfigurement due to surgery for head and neck cancer. Br J Nurs. 2019;28(3):180–4. PubMed PMID: 30746969. Epub 2019/02/13. eng.
62. Evers AWM, Colloca L, Blease C, Annoni M, Atlas LY, Benedetti F, et al. Implications of placebo and nocebo effects for clinical practice: expert consensus. Psychother Psychosom. 2018;87(4):204–10. PubMed PMID: 29895014. Pubmed Central PMCID: PMC6191882. Epub 2018/06/13. eng.
63. Nieman DC, Wentz LM. The compelling link between physical activity and the body's defense system. J Sport Health Sci. 2019;8(3):201–17. PubMed PMID: 31193280. Pubmed Central PMCID: PMC6523821. Epub 2019/06/14. eng.
64. Lutgendorf SK, Sood AK, Antoni MH. Host factors and cancer progression: biobehavioral signaling pathways and interventions. J Clin Oncol. 2010;28(26):4094–9. PubMed PMID: 20644093. Pubmed Central PMCID: PMC2940426. Epub 2010/07/21. eng.
65. Bhasin MK, Dusek JA, Chang BH, Joseph MG, Denninger JW, Fricchione GL, et al. Relaxation response induces temporal transcriptome changes in energy metabolism, insulin secretion and inflammatory pathways. PLoS One. 2013;8(5):e62817. PubMed PMID: 23650531. Pubmed Central PMCID: PMC3641112. Epub 2013/05/08. eng.
66. Diego MA, Field T. Moderate pressure massage elicits a parasympathetic nervous system response. Int J Neurosci. 2009;119(5):630–8. PubMed PMID: 19283590. Epub 2009/03/14. eng.
67. Henricson M, Ersson A, Määttä S, Segesten K, Berglund AL. The outcome of tactile touch on stress parameters in intensive care: a randomized controlled trial. Complement Ther Clin Pract. 2008;14(4):244–54. PubMed PMID: 18940711. Epub 2008/10/23. eng.
68. Petrie KJ, Rief W. Psychobiological mechanisms of placebo and nocebo effects: pathways to improve treatments and reduce side effects. Annu Rev Psychol. 2019;70:599–625. PubMed PMID: 30110575. Epub 2018/08/16. eng.
69. World Cancer Research F, American Institute for Cancer R. Food, nutrition, physical activity and the prevention of cancer: a global perspective. Washington, DC: The Institute; 2007.
70. Riba MB, Donovan KA, Andersen B, Braun I, Breitbart WS, Brewer BW, et al. Distress management, Version 3.2019, NCCN clinical practice guidelines in oncology. J Natl Compr Cancer Netw. 2019;17(10):1229–49. PubMed PMID: 31590149. Pubmed Central PMCID: PMC6907687. Epub 2019/10/08. eng.
71. Greenlee H, DuPont-Reyes MJ, Balneaves LG, Carlson LE, Cohen MR, Deng G, et al. Clinical practice guidelines on the evidence-based use of integrative therapies during and after breast cancer treatment. CA Cancer J Clin. 2017;67(3):194–232. PubMed PMID: 28436999. Pubmed Central PMCID: PMC5892208. Epub 2017/04/25. eng.
72. Lutgendorf SK, DeGeest K, Sung CY, Arevalo JM, Penedo F, Lucci J III, et al. Depression, social support, and beta-adrenergic transcription control in human ovarian cancer. Brain Behav Immun. 2009;23(2):176–83. PubMed PMID: 18550328. Pubmed Central PMCID: PMC2677379. Epub 2008/06/14. eng.
73. Lutgendorf SK, Sood AK, Anderson B, McGinn S, Maiseri H, Dao M, et al. Social support, psychological distress, and natural killer cell activity in ovarian cancer. J Clin Oncol. 2005;23(28):7105–13. PubMed PMID: 16192594. Epub 2005/09/30. eng.
74. Lutgendorf SK, Lamkin DM, DeGeest K, Anderson B, Dao M, McGinn S, et al. Depressed and anxious mood and T-cell cytokine expressing populations in ovarian cancer patients. Brain Behav Immun. 2008;22(6):890–900. PubMed PMID: 18276105. Pubmed Central PMCID: PMC2605940. Epub 2008/02/16. eng.

75. Brandão T, Tavares R, Schulz MS, Matos PM. Experiences of breast cancer patients and helpful aspects of supportive-expressive group therapy: a qualitative study. Eur J Cancer Care. 2019;28(5):e13078. PubMed PMID: 31038245. Epub 2019/05/01. eng.
76. Kroenke CH, Michael YL, Poole EM, Kwan ML, Nechuta S, Leas E, et al. Postdiagnosis social networks and breast cancer mortality in the After Breast Cancer Pooling Project. Cancer. 2017;123(7):1228–37. PubMed PMID: 27943274. Pubmed Central PMCID: PMC5360517. Epub 2016/12/13. eng.
77. Nausheen B, Gidron Y, Peveler R, Moss-Morris R. Social support and cancer progression: a systematic review. J Psychosom Res. 2009;67(5):403–15. PubMed PMID: 19837203. Epub 2009/10/20. eng.
78. Kroenke CH, Quesenberry C, Kwan ML, Sweeney C, Castillo A, Caan BJ. Social networks, social support, and burden in relationships, and mortality after breast cancer diagnosis in the Life After Breast Cancer Epidemiology (LACE) study. Breast Cancer Res Treat. 2013;137(1):261–71. PubMed PMID: 23143212. Pubmed Central PMCID: PMC4019377. Epub 2012/11/13. eng.
79. Zwahlen D, Tondorf T, Rothschild S, Koller MT, Rochlitz C, Kiss A. Understanding why cancer patients accept or turn down psycho-oncological support: a prospective observational study including patients' and clinicians' perspectives on communication about distress. BMC Cancer. 2017;17(1):385. PubMed PMID: 28558713. Pubmed Central PMCID: PMC5450069. Epub 2017/06/01. eng.
80. Kissane DW, Grabsch B, Clarke DM, Smith GC, Love AW, Bloch S, et al. Supportive-expressive group therapy for women with metastatic breast cancer: survival and psychosocial outcome from a randomized controlled trial. Psycho-Oncology. 2007;16(4):277–86. PubMed PMID: 17385190. Epub 2007/03/27. eng.
81. Guarino A, Polini C, Forte G, Favieri F, Boncompagni I, Casagrande M. The effectiveness of psychological treatments in women with breast cancer: a systematic review and meta-analysis. J Clin Med. 2020;9(1):209. PubMed PMID: 31940942. Pubmed Central PMCID: PMC7019270. Epub 2020/01/17. eng.
82. Park H, Oh S, Noh Y, Kim JY, Kim JH. Heart rate variability as a marker of distress and recovery: the effect of brief supportive expressive group therapy with mindfulness in cancer patients. Integr Cancer Ther. 2018;17(3):825–31. PubMed PMID: 29417836. Pubmed Central PMCID: PMC6142099. Epub 2018/02/09. eng.
83. Carlson LE, Tamagawa R, Stephen J, Drysdale E, Zhong L, Speca M. Randomized-controlled trial of mindfulness-based cancer recovery versus supportive expressive group therapy among distressed breast cancer survivors (MINDSET): long-term follow-up results. Psycho-Oncology. 2016;25(7):750–9. PubMed PMID: 27193737. Epub 2016/05/20. eng.
84. Jassim GA, Whitford DL, Hickey A, Carter B. Psychological interventions for women with non-metastatic breast cancer. Cochrane Database Syst Rev. 2015;5:CD008729. PubMed PMID: 26017383. Epub 2015/05/29. eng.
85. Antoni MH, Lechner S, Diaz A, Vargas S, Holley H, Phillips K, et al. Cognitive behavioral stress management effects on psychosocial and physiological adaptation in women undergoing treatment for breast cancer. Brain Behav Immun. 2009;23(5):580–91. PubMed PMID: 18835434. Pubmed Central PMCID: PMC2722111. Epub 2008/10/07. eng.
86. Matthews H, Grunfeld EA, Turner A. The efficacy of interventions to improve psychosocial outcomes following surgical treatment for breast cancer: a systematic review and meta-analysis. Psycho-Oncology. 2017;26(5):593–607. PubMed PMID: 27333194. Epub 2016/06/23. eng.
87. Cohen L, Parker PA, Vence L, Savary C, Kentor D, Pettaway C, et al. Presurgical stress management improves postoperative immune function in men with prostate cancer undergoing radical prostatectomy. Psychosom Med. 2011;73(3):218–25. PubMed PMID: 21257977. Epub 2011/01/25. eng.
88. Antoni MH, Lutgendorf SK, Blomberg B, Carver CS, Lechner S, Diaz A, et al. Cognitive-behavioral stress management reverses anxiety-related leukocyte transcriptional dynamics. Biol Psychiatry. 2012;71(4):366–72. PubMed PMID: 22088795. Pubmed Central PMCID: PMC3264698. Epub 2011/11/18. eng.

References

89. Carlson LE. Mindfulness-based interventions for coping with cancer. Ann N Y Acad Sci. 2016;1373(1):5–12. PubMed PMID: 26963792. Epub 2016/03/11. eng.
90. Hall DL, Luberto CM, Philpotts LL, Song R, Park ER, Yeh GY. Mind-body interventions for fear of cancer recurrence: a systematic review and meta-analysis. Psycho-Oncology. 2018;27(11):2546–58. PubMed PMID: 29744965. Pubmed Central PMCID: PMC6488231. Epub 2018/05/11. eng.
91. Haller H, Winkler MM, Klose P, Dobos G, Kümmel S, Cramer H. Mindfulness-based interventions for women with breast cancer: an updated systematic review and meta-analysis. Acta Oncol. 2017;56(12):1665–76. PubMed PMID: 28686520. Epub 2017/07/08. eng.
92. Zhang Q, Zhao H, Zheng Y. Effectiveness of mindfulness-based stress reduction (MBSR) on symptom variables and health-related quality of life in breast cancer patients-a systematic review and meta-analysis. Support Care Cancer. 2019;27(3):771–81. PubMed PMID: 30488223. Epub 2018/11/30. eng.
93. Leventhal H, Phillips LA, Burns E. The Common-Sense Model of Self-Regulation (CSM): a dynamic framework for understanding illness self-management. J Behav Med. 2016;39(6):935–46. PubMed PMID: 27515801. Epub 2016/08/16. eng.
94. McCorkle R, Ercolano E, Lazenby M, Schulman-Green D, Schilling LS, Lorig K, et al. Self-management: enabling and empowering patients living with cancer as a chronic illness. CA Cancer J Clin. 2011;61(1):50–62. PubMed PMID: 21205833. Pubmed Central PMCID: PMC3058905. Epub 2011/01/06. eng.
95. Goldberg JI, Schulman-Green D, Hernandez M, Nelson JE, Capezuti E. Self-management interventions for psychological distress in adult cancer patients: a systematic review. West J Nurs Res. 2019;41(10):1407–22. PubMed PMID: 31007160. Epub 2019/04/23. eng.
96. Bakitas MA, Tosteson TD, Li Z, Lyons KD, Hull JG, Li Z, et al. Early versus delayed initiation of concurrent palliative oncology care: patient outcomes in the ENABLE III randomized controlled trial. J Clin Oncol. 2015;33(13):1438–45. PubMed PMID: 25800768. Pubmed Central PMCID: PMC4404422. Epub 2015/03/25. eng.
97. Dionne-Odom JN, Azuero A, Lyons KD, Hull JG, Tosteson T, Li Z, et al. Benefits of early versus delayed palliative care to informal family caregivers of patients with advanced cancer: outcomes from the ENABLE III randomized controlled trial. J Clin Oncol. 2015;33(13):1446–52. PubMed PMID: 25800762. Pubmed Central PMCID: PMC4404423. Epub 2015/03/25. eng.
98. Kapogiannis A, Tsoli S, Chrousos G. Investigating the effects of the progressive muscle relaxation-guided imagery combination on patients with cancer receiving chemotherapy treatment: a systematic review of randomized controlled trials. Explore. 2018;14(2):137–43. PubMed PMID: 29506956. Epub 2018/03/07. eng.
99. Pelekasis P, Matsouka I, Koumarianou A. Progressive muscle relaxation as a supportive intervention for cancer patients undergoing chemotherapy: a systematic review. Palliat Support Care. 2017;15(4):465–73. PubMed PMID: 27890023. Epub 2016/11/29. eng.
100. Charalambous A, Giannakopoulou M, Bozas E, Marcou Y, Kitsios P, Paikousis L. Guided imagery and progressive muscle relaxation as a cluster of symptoms management intervention in patients receiving chemotherapy: a randomized control trial. PLoS One. 2016;11(6):e0156911. PubMed PMID: 27341675. Pubmed Central PMCID: PMC4920431. Epub 2016/06/25. eng.
101. Field T. Massage therapy research review. Complement Ther Clin Pract. 2016;24:19–31. PubMed PMID: 27502797. Pubmed Central PMCID: PMC5564319. Epub 2016/08/10. eng.
102. Shin ES, Seo KH, Lee SH, Jang JE, Jung YM, Kim MJ, et al. Massage with or without aromatherapy for symptom relief in people with cancer. Cochrane Database Syst Rev 2016;(6):CD009873. PubMed PMID: 27258432. Epub 2016/06/04. eng.
103. Wang T, Zhai J, Liu XL, Yao LQ, Tan JB. Massage therapy for fatigue management in breast cancer survivors: a systematic review and descriptive analysis of randomized controlled trials. Evid Based Complement Alternat Med. 2021;2021:9967574. PubMed PMID: 34603480. Pubmed Central PMCID: PMC8483909. Epub 2021/10/05. eng.

104. Hernandez-Reif M, Field T, Ironson G, Beutler J, Vera Y, Hurley J, et al. Natural killer cells and lymphocytes increase in women with breast cancer following massage therapy. Int J Neurosci. 2005;115(4):495–510. PubMed PMID: 15809216. Epub 2005/04/06. eng.
105. Hernandez-Reif M, Ironson G, Field T, Hurley J, Katz G, Diego M, et al. Breast cancer patients have improved immune and neuroendocrine functions following massage therapy. J Psychosom Res. 2004;57(1):45–52. PubMed PMID: 15256294. Epub 2004/07/17. eng.
106. Uysal N, Kutluturkan S, Ugur I. Effects of foot massage applied in two different methods on symptom control in colorectal cancer patients: randomised control trial. Int J Nurs Pract. 2017;23(3):e12532. PubMed PMID: 28176423. Epub 2017/02/09. eng.
107. Ben-Horin I, Kahan P, Ryvo L, Inbar M, Lev-Ari S, Geva R. Acupuncture and reflexology for chemotherapy-induced peripheral neuropathy in breast cancer. Integr Cancer Ther. 2017;16(3):258–62. PubMed PMID: 28150504. Pubmed Central PMCID: PMC5759933. Epub 2017/02/06. eng.
108. Seretny M, Currie GL, Sena ES, Ramnarine S, Grant R, MacLeod MR, et al. Incidence, prevalence, and predictors of chemotherapy-induced peripheral neuropathy: a systematic review and meta-analysis. Pain. 2014;155(12):2461–70. PubMed PMID: 25261162. Epub 2014/09/28. eng.
109. Quattrin R, Zanini A, Buchini S, Turello D, Annunziata MA, Vidotti C, et al. Use of reflexology foot massage to reduce anxiety in hospitalized cancer patients in chemotherapy treatment: methodology and outcomes. J Nurs Manag. 2006;14(2):96–105. PubMed PMID: 16487421. Epub 2006/02/21. eng.
110. Mishra SI, Scherer RW, Geigle PM, Berlanstein DR, Topaloglu O, Gotay CC, et al. Exercise interventions on health-related quality of life for cancer survivors. Cochrane Database Syst Rev. 2012;8:CD007566. PubMed PMID: 22895961. Epub 2012/08/17. eng.
111. Carayol M, Bernard P, Boiché J, Riou F, Mercier B, Cousson-Gélie F, et al. Psychological effect of exercise in women with breast cancer receiving adjuvant therapy: what is the optimal dose needed? Ann Oncol. 2013;24(2):291–300. PubMed PMID: 23041586. Epub 2012/10/09. eng.
112. van Waart H, Stuiver MM, van Harten WH, Geleijn E, Kieffer JM, Buffart LM, et al. Effect of low-intensity physical activity and moderate- to high-intensity physical exercise during adjuvant chemotherapy on physical fitness, fatigue, and chemotherapy completion rates: results of the PACES randomized clinical trial. J Clin Oncol. 2015;33(17):1918–27. PubMed PMID: 25918291. Epub 2015/04/29. eng.
113. Juvet LK, Thune I, Elvsaas I, Fors EA, Lundgren S, Bertheussen G, et al. The effect of exercise on fatigue and physical functioning in breast cancer patients during and after treatment and at 6 months follow-up: a meta-analysis. Breast. 2017;33:166–77. PubMed PMID: 28415013. Epub 2017/04/18. eng.
114. van Vulpen JK, Peeters PH, Velthuis MJ, van der Wall E, May AM. Effects of physical exercise during adjuvant breast cancer treatment on physical and psychosocial dimensions of cancer-related fatigue: a meta-analysis. Maturitas. 2016;85:104–11. PubMed PMID: 26857888. Epub 2016/02/10. eng.
115. Samuel SR, Maiya AG, Fernandes DJ, Guddattu V, Saxena PUP, Kurian JR, et al. Effectiveness of exercise-based rehabilitation on functional capacity and quality of life in head and neck cancer patients receiving chemo-radiotherapy. Support Care Cancer. 2019;27(10):3913–20. PubMed PMID: 30919154. Pubmed Central PMCID: PMC6728220. Epub 2019/03/29. eng.
116. Hilfiker R, Meichtry A, Eicher M, Nilsson Balfe L, Knols RH, Verra ML, et al. Exercise and other non-pharmaceutical interventions for cancer-related fatigue in patients during or after cancer treatment: a systematic review incorporating an indirect-comparisons meta-analysis. Br J Sports Med. 2018;52(10):651–8. PubMed PMID: 28501804. Pubmed Central PMCID: PMC5931245. Epub 2017/05/16. eng.
117. McTiernan A, Friedenreich CM, Katzmarzyk PT, Powell KE, Macko R, Buchner D, et al. Physical activity in cancer prevention and survival: a systematic review. Med Sci Sports Exerc.

2019;51(6):1252–61. PubMed PMID: 31095082. Pubmed Central PMCID: PMC6527123. Epub 2019/05/17. eng.
118. Kleckner IR, Kamen C, Gewandter JS, Mohile NA, Heckler CE, Culakova E, et al. Effects of exercise during chemotherapy on chemotherapy-induced peripheral neuropathy: a multicenter, randomized controlled trial. Support Care Cancer. 2018;26(4):1019–28. PubMed PMID: 29243164. Pubmed Central PMCID: PMC5823751. Epub 2017/12/16. eng.
119. Prieto I, Montemuiño S, Luna J, de Torres MV, Amaya E. The role of immunonutritional support in cancer treatment: current evidence. Clin Nutr. 2017;36(6):1457–64. PubMed PMID: 27931879. Epub 2016/12/10. eng.
120. Bumrungpert A, Pavadhgul P, Nunthanawanich P, Sirikanchanarod A, Adulbhan A. Whey protein supplementation improves nutritional status, glutathione levels, and immune function in cancer patients: a randomized, double-blind controlled trial. J Med Food. 2018;21(6):612–6. PubMed PMID: 29565716. Epub 2018/03/23. eng.
121. Armstrong K, Lanni T Jr, Anderson MM, Patricolo GE. Integrative medicine and the oncology patient: options and benefits. Support Care Cancer. 2018;26(7):2267–73. PubMed PMID: 29396594. Epub 2018/02/06. eng.
122. Lutgendorf SK, Mullen-Houser E, Russell D, Degeest K, Jacobson G, Hart L, et al. Preservation of immune function in cervical cancer patients during chemoradiation using a novel integrative approach. Brain Behav Immun. 2010;24(8):1231–40. PubMed PMID: 20600809. Pubmed Central PMCID: PMC3010350. Epub 2010/07/06. eng.
123. Northouse LL, Katapodi MC, Song L, Zhang L, Mood DW. Interventions with family caregivers of cancer patients: meta-analysis of randomized trials. CA Cancer J Clin. 2010;60(5):317–39. PubMed PMID: 20709946. Pubmed Central PMCID: PMC2946584. Epub 2010/08/17. eng.
124. Treanor CJ, Santin O, Prue G, Coleman H, Cardwell CR, O'Halloran P, et al. Psychosocial interventions for informal caregivers of people living with cancer. Cochrane Database Syst Rev. 2019;6(6):CD009912. PubMed PMID: 31204791. Pubmed Central PMCID: PMC6573123. Epub 2019/06/18. eng.
125. Xiu D, Fung YL, Lau BH, Wong DFK, Chan CHY, Ho RTH, et al. Comparing dyadic cognitive behavioral therapy (CBT) with dyadic integrative body-mind-spirit intervention (I-BMS) for Chinese family caregivers of lung cancer patients: a randomized controlled trial. Support Care Cancer. 2020;28(3):1523–33. PubMed PMID: 31280363. Epub 2019/07/08. eng.
126. Al Daken LI, Ahmad MM. The implementation of mindfulness-based interventions and educational interventions to support family caregivers of patients with cancer: a systematic review. Perspect Psychiatric Care. 2018;54(3):441–52. PubMed PMID: 29745417. Epub 2018/05/11. eng.
127. Dharmawardene M, Givens J, Wachholtz A, Makowski S, Tjia J. A systematic review and meta-analysis of meditative interventions for informal caregivers and health professionals. BMJ Support Palliat Care. 2016;6(2):160–9. PubMed PMID: 25812579. Pubmed Central PMCID: PMC4583788. Epub 2015/03/31. eng.
128. Benson H, Stuart E. The wellness book: the comprehensive guide to maintaining health and treating stress-related illness. New York, NY: Simon and Schuster; 1992.
129. Ferrell BR, Twaddle ML, Melnick A, Meier DE. National consensus project clinical practice guidelines for quality palliative care guidelines, 4th Edition. J Palliat Med. 2018;21(12):1684–9. PubMed PMID: 30179523. Epub 2018/09/05. eng.
130. Ferrell BR, Temel JS, Temin S, Alesi ER, Balboni TA, Basch EM, et al. Integration of palliative care into standard oncology care: American Society of Clinical Oncology clinical practice guideline update. J Clin Oncol. 2017;35(1):96–112. PubMed PMID: 28034065. Epub 2016/12/31. eng.
131. McEwen BS. Neurobiological and systemic effects of chronic stress. Chronic Stress. 2017;1:2470547017692328. PubMed PMID: 28856337. Pubmed Central PMCID: PMC5573220. Epub 2017/09/01. eng.

132. McEwen BS, Nasca C, Gray JD. Stress effects on neuronal structure: Hippocampus, Amygdala, and Prefrontal Cortex. Neuropsychopharmacology. 2016;41(1):3–23. PubMed PMID: 26076834. Pubmed Central PMCID: PMC4677120. Epub 2015/06/17. eng.
133. Meichenbaum D. A clinical handbook for assessing and treating adults with post-traumatic stress disorder (PTSD). Waterloo, ON: Institute Press; 1994.
134. Folkman S, Lazarus RS, Dunkel-Schetter C, DeLongis A, Gruen RJ. Dynamics of a stressful encounter: cognitive appraisal, coping, and encounter outcomes. J Pers Soc Psychol. 1986;50(5):992–1003. PubMed PMID: 3712234. Epub 1986/05/01. eng.
135. Cao W, Qi X, Cai DA, Han X. Modeling posttraumatic growth among cancer patients: the roles of social support, appraisals, and adaptive coping. Psycho-Oncology. 2018;27(1):208–15. PubMed PMID: 28171681. Epub 2017/02/09. eng.
136. Andersen BL, Thornton LM, Shapiro CL, Farrar WB, Mundy BL, Yang HC, et al. Biobehavioral, immune, and health benefits following recurrence for psychological intervention participants. Clin Cancer Res. 2010;16(12):3270–8. PubMed PMID: 20530702. Pubmed Central PMCID: PMC2910547. Epub 2010/06/10. eng.
137. Thorne SE, Kuo M, Armstrong EA, McPherson G, Harris SR, Hislop TG. 'Being known': patients' perspectives of the dynamics of human connection in cancer care. Psycho-Oncology. 2000;14(10):887–98; discussion 99-900. PubMed PMID: 16200520. Epub 2005/10/04. eng.
138. Durkin J, Jackson D, Usher K. Defining compassion in a hospital setting: consensus on the characteristics that comprise compassion from researchers in the field. Contemp Nurse. 2020;56(2):146–59.
139. Thorne S, Hislop TG, Kim-Sing C, Oglov V, Oliffe JL, Stajduhar KI. Changing communication needs and preferences across the cancer care trajectory: insights from the patient perspective. Support Care Cancer. 2014;22(4):1009–15. PubMed PMID: 24287506. Epub 2013/11/30. eng.
140. Thorne SE, Kuo M, Armstrong EA, McPherson G, Harris SR, Hislop TG. 'Being known': patients' perspectives of the dynamics of human connection in cancer care. Psycho-Oncology. 2005;14(10):887–98; discussion 99–900. PubMed PMID: 16200520. Epub 2005/10/04. eng.
141. Mikulincer M, Shaver PR. Enhancing the "Broaden and Build" cycle of attachment security in adulthood: from the laboratory to relational contexts and societal systems. Int J Environ Res Public Health. 2020;17(6):2054. PubMed PMID: 32244872. Pubmed Central PMCID: PMC7143531. Epub 2020/04/05. eng.
142. Mikulincer M, Shaver PR. Attachment orientations and emotion regulation. Curr Opin Psychol. 2019;25:6–10. PubMed PMID: 29494853. Epub 2018/03/02. eng.
143. McCorkle R, Dowd M, Ercolano E, Schulman-Green D, Williams AL, Siefert ML, et al. Effects of a nursing intervention on quality of life outcomes in post-surgical women with gynecological cancers. Psycho-Oncology. 2009;18(1):62–70. PubMed PMID: 18570223. Pubmed Central PMCID: PMC4186244. Epub 2008/06/24. eng.
144. McCorkle R, Strumpf NE, Nuamah IF, Adler DC, Cooley ME, Jepson C, et al. A specialized home care intervention improves survival among older post-surgical cancer patients. J Am Geriatr Soc. 2000;48(12):1707–13. PubMed PMID: 11129765. Epub 2000/12/29. eng.
145. Jacobsen J, Kvale E, Rabow M, Rinaldi S, Cohen S, Weissman D, et al. Helping patients with serious illness live well through the promotion of adaptive coping: a report from the improving outpatient palliative care (IPAL-OP) initiative. J Palliat Med. 2014;17(4):463–8. PubMed PMID: 24579823. Epub 2014/03/04. eng.
146. Folkman S, Moskowitz J. Positive affect and meaning-focused coping during significant psychological stress. In: Haws MH, de Wit JBF, van den Bos K, Stroebe MS, editors. The scope of social psychology: theory and applications. New York, NY: Psychology Press; 2007. p. 193–208.
147. Dunkel-Schetter C, Feinstein LG, Taylor SE, Falke RL. Patterns of coping with cancer. Health Psychol. 1992;11(2):79–87. PubMed PMID: 1582383. Epub 1992/01/01. eng.
148. Hostinar CE, Sullivan RM, Gunnar MR. Psychobiological mechanisms underlying the social buffering of the hypothalamic-pituitary-adrenocortical axis: a review of animal models and

human studies across development. Psychol Bull. 2014;140(1):256–82. PubMed PMID: 23607429. Pubmed Central PMCID: PMC3844011. Epub 2013/04/24. eng.
149. Krok D, Telka E. The role of meaning in gastric cancer patients: relationships among meaning structures, coping, and psychological well-being. Anxiety Stress Coping. 2019;32(5):522–33. PubMed PMID: 31234657. Epub 2019/06/27. eng.
150. Wright LM, Leeahey M. A guide to family assessment and intervention. 6th ed. Philadelphia, PA: FA Davis Company; 2013.
151. Benson H, Friedman R. Harnessing the power of the placebo effect and renaming it "remembered wellness". Annu Rev Med. 1996;47:193–9. PubMed PMID: 8712773.
152. Pacheco-Lopez G, Engler H, Niemi MB, Schedlowski M. Expectations and associations that heal: immunomodulatory placebo effects and its neurobiology. Brain Behav Immun. 2006;20(5):430–46. PubMed PMID: 16887325.
153. Benson H, Stark M. Timeless healing: the power and biology of belief. New York, NY: Simon & Schuster; 1997.
154. Hauser W, Hansen E, Enck P. Nocebo phenomena in medicine: their relevance in everyday clinical practice. Deutsches Arzteblatt Int. 2012;109(26):459–65. PubMed PMID: 22833756. Pubmed Central PMCID: PMC3401955. Epub 2012/07/27. eng.
155. Flaten MA, Simonsen T, Olsen H. Drug-related information generates placebo and nocebo responses that modify the drug response. Psychosom Med. 1999;61(2):250–5. PubMed PMID: 10204979. Epub 1999/04/16. eng.
156. Rief W, Shedden-Mora MC, Laferton JA, Auer C, Petrie KJ, Salzmann S, et al. Preoperative optimization of patient expectations improves long-term outcome in heart surgery patients: results of the randomized controlled PSY-HEART trial. BMC Med. 2017;15(1):4. PubMed PMID: 28069021. Pubmed Central PMCID: PMC5223324. Epub 2017/01/11. eng.
157. Marsland AL, Walsh C, Lockwood K, John-Henderson NA. The effects of acute psychological stress on circulating and stimulated inflammatory markers: a systematic review and meta-analysis. Brain Behav Immun. 2017;64:208–19. PubMed PMID: 28089638. Pubmed Central PMCID: PMC5553449. Epub 2017/01/17. eng.
158. Benedetti F, Amanzio M, Vighetti S, Asteggiano G. The biochemical and neuroendocrine bases of the hyperalgesic nocebo effect. J Neurosci. 2006;26(46):12014–22. PubMed PMID: 17108175. Pubmed Central PMCID: PMC6674855. Epub 2006/11/17. eng.
159. Dutcher JM, Creswell JD. The role of brain reward pathways in stress resilience and health. Neurosci Biobehav Rev. 2018;95:559–67. PubMed PMID: 30477985. Epub 2018/11/28. eng.
160. Faasse K, Huynh A, Pearson S, Geers AL, Helfer SG, Colagiuri B. The influence of side effect information framing on nocebo effects. Ann Behav Med. 2019;53(7):621–9. PubMed PMID: 30204841. Epub 2018/09/12. eng.
161. Faasse K, Martin LR. The power of labeling in nocebo effects. Int Rev Neurobiol. 2018;139:379–406. PubMed PMID: 30146055. Epub 2018/08/28. eng.
162. Faasse K, Parkes B, Kearney J, Petrie KJ. The influence of social modeling, gender, and empathy on treatment side effects. Ann Behav Med. 2018;52(7):560–70. PubMed PMID: 29860362. Epub 2018/06/04. eng.
163. Colloca L, Finniss D. Nocebo effects, patient-clinician communication, and therapeutic outcomes. JAMA. 2012;307(6):567–8. PubMed PMID: 22318275. Pubmed Central PMCID: PMC6909539. Epub 2012/02/10. eng.
164. Colloca L, Klinger R, Flor H, Bingel U. Placebo analgesia: psychological and neurobiological mechanisms. Pain. 2013;154(4):511–4. PubMed PMID: 23473783. Pubmed Central PMCID: PMC3626115. Epub 2013/03/12. eng.
165. Colloca L, Lopiano L, Lanotte M, Benedetti F. Overt versus covert treatment for pain, anxiety, and Parkinson's disease. Lancet Neurol. 2004;3(11):679–84. PubMed PMID: 15488461. Epub 2004/10/19. eng.
166. Bingel U, Wanigasekera V, Wiech K, Ni Mhuircheartaigh R, Lee MC, Ploner M, et al. The effect of treatment expectation on drug efficacy: imaging the analgesic benefit of the opioid remifentanil. Sci Transl Med. 2011;3(70):70ra14. PubMed PMID: 21325618. Epub 2011/02/18. eng.

167. Colloca L, Miller FG. The nocebo effect and its relevance for clinical practice. Psychosom Med. 2011;73(7):598–603. PubMed PMID: 21862825. Pubmed Central PMCID: PMC3167012. Epub 2011/08/25. eng.
168. Colloca L, Tinazzi M, Recchia S, Le Pera D, Fiaschi A, Benedetti F, et al. Learning potentiates neurophysiological and behavioral placebo analgesic responses. Pain. 2008;139(2):306–14. PubMed PMID: 18538928. Epub 2008/06/10. eng.
169. Ben-Shaanan TL, Schiller M, Azulay-Debby H, Korin B, Boshnak N, Koren T, et al. Modulation of anti-tumor immunity by the brain's reward system. Nat Commun. 2018;9(1):2723. PubMed PMID: 30006573. Pubmed Central PMCID: PMC6045610. Epub 2018/07/15. eng.
170. Kaptchuk TJ, Kelley JM, Conboy LA, Davis RB, Kerr CE, Jacobson EE, et al. Components of placebo effect: randomised controlled trial in patients with irritable bowel syndrome. BMJ. 2008;336(7651):999–1003. PubMed PMID: 18390493. Pubmed Central PMCID: PMC2364862. Epub 2008/04/09. eng.
171. Blasini M, Peiris N, Wright T, Colloca L. The role of patient-practitioner relationships in placebo and nocebo phenomena. Int Rev Neurobiol. 2018;139:211–31. PubMed PMID: 30146048. Pubmed Central PMCID: PMC6176716. Epub 2018/08/28. eng.
172. Mathew A, Doorenbos AZ, Li H, Jang MK, Park CG, Bronas UG. Allostatic load in cancer: a systematic review and mini meta-analysis. Biol Res Nurs. 2021;23(3):341–61. PubMed PMID: 33138637. Epub 2020/11/04. eng.
173. Webster Marketon JI, Glaser R. Stress hormones and immune function. Cell Immunol. 2008;252(1–2):16–26. PubMed PMID: 18279846.
174. Colloca L, Barsky AJ. Placebo and nocebo effects. N Engl J Med. 2020;382(6):554–61. PubMed PMID: 32023375. Epub 2020/02/06. eng.
175. Luckemann L, Unteroberdorster M, Kirchhof J, Schedlowski M, Hadamitzky M. Applications and limitations of behaviorally conditioned immunopharmacological responses. Neurobiol Learn Mem. 2017;142(Pt A):91–8. PubMed PMID: 28216206. Epub 2017/02/22. eng.
176. Hojman P. Exercise protects from cancer through regulation of immune function and inflammation. Biochem Soc Trans. 2017;45(4):905–11. PubMed PMID: 28673937. Epub 2017/07/05. eng.
177. Lutgendorf SK, DeGeest K, Dahmoush L, Farley D, Penedo F, Bender D, et al. Social isolation is associated with elevated tumor norepinephrine in ovarian carcinoma patients. Brain Behav Immun. 2011;25(2):250–5. PubMed PMID: 20955777. Pubmed Central PMCID: PMC3103818. Epub 2010/10/20. eng.
178. Carlson LE, Beattie TL, Giese-Davis J, Faris P, Tamagawa R, Fick LJ, et al. Mindfulness-based cancer recovery and supportive-expressive therapy maintain telomere length relative to controls in distressed breast cancer survivors. Cancer. 2015;121(3):476–84. PubMed PMID: 25367403. Epub 2014/11/05. eng.
179. Schedlowski M, Pacheco-López G. The learned immune response: Pavlov and beyond. Brain Behav Immun. 2010;24(2):176–85. PubMed PMID: 19698779. Epub 2009/08/25. eng.
180. Solans M, Romaguera D, Gracia-Lavedan E, Molinuevo A, Benavente Y, Saez M, et al. Adherence to the 2018 WCRF/AICR cancer prevention guidelines and chronic lymphocytic leukemia in the MCC-Spain study. Cancer Epidemiol. 2020;64:101629. PubMed PMID: 31756676. Epub 2019/11/23. eng.
181. Inchauspe J. Glucose revolution. New York, NY; London; Toronto, ON; Sydney, NSW; New Delhi: Simon & Schuster; 2022.
182. Latino-Martel P, Cottet V, Druesne-Pecollo N, Pierre FH, Touillaud M, Touvier M, et al. Alcoholic beverages, obesity, physical activity and other nutritional factors, and cancer risk: a review of the evidence. Crit Rev Oncol Hematol. 2016;99:308–23. PubMed PMID: 26811140. Epub 2016/01/27. eng.
183. Custódio IDD, Franco FP, Marinho EDC, Pereira TSS, Lima MTM, Molina M, et al. Prospective analysis of food consumption and nutritional status and the impact on the dietary inflammatory index in women with breast cancer during chemotherapy. Nutrients.

2019;11(11):2610. PubMed PMID: 31683752. Pubmed Central PMCID: PMC6893533. Epub 2019/11/07. eng.
184. van Rooijen SJ, Molenaar CJL, Schep G, van Lieshout R, Beijer S, Dubbers R, et al. Making patients fit for surgery: introducing a four pillar multimodal prehabilitation program in colorectal cancer. Am J Phys Med Rehabil. 2019;98(10):888–96. PubMed PMID: 31090551. Epub 2019/05/16. eng.
185. van Rooijen S, Carli F, Dalton S, Thomas G, Bojesen R, Le Guen M, et al. Multimodal prehabilitation in colorectal cancer patients to improve functional capacity and reduce postoperative complications: the first international randomized controlled trial for multimodal prehabilitation. BMC Cancer. 2019;19(1):98. PubMed PMID: 30670009. Pubmed Central PMCID: PMC6341758. Epub 2019/01/24. eng.
186. van Rooijen SJ, Engelen MA, Scheede-Bergdahl C, Carli F, Roumen RMH, Slooter GD, et al. Systematic review of exercise training in colorectal cancer patients during treatment. Scand J Med Sci Sports. 2018;28(2):360–70. PubMed PMID: 28488799. Epub 2017/05/11. eng.
187. McGettigan M, Cardwell CR, Cantwell MM, Tully MA. Physical activity interventions for disease-related physical and mental health during and following treatment in people with non-advanced colorectal cancer. Cochrane Database Syst Rev. 2020;5(5):CD012864. PubMed PMID: 32361988. Pubmed Central PMCID: PMC7196359. Epub 2020/05/04. eng.
188. Browall M, Mijwel S, Rundqvist H, Wengström Y. Physical activity during and after adjuvant treatment for breast cancer: an integrative review of women's experiences. Integr Cancer Ther. 2018;17(1):16–30. PubMed PMID: 28008778. Pubmed Central PMCID: PMC5950941. Epub 2016/12/23. eng.
189. Mijwel S, Jervaeus A, Bolam KA, Norrbom J, Bergh J, Rundqvist H, et al. High-intensity exercise during chemotherapy induces beneficial effects 12 months into breast cancer survivorship. J Cancer Surviv. 2019;13(2):244–56. PubMed PMID: 30912010. Pubmed Central PMCID: PMC6482129. Epub 2019/03/27. eng.
190. Carayol M, Ninot G, Senesse P, Bleuse JP, Gourgou S, Sancho-Garnier H, et al. Short- and long-term impact of adapted physical activity and diet counseling during adjuvant breast cancer therapy: the "APAD1" randomized controlled trial. BMC Cancer. 2019;19(1):737. PubMed PMID: 31345179. Pubmed Central PMCID: PMC6659309. Epub 2019/07/28. eng.
191. Besedovsky L, Lange T, Haack M. The sleep-immune crosstalk in health and disease. Physiol Rev. 2019;99(3):1325–80. PubMed PMID: 30920354. Pubmed Central PMCID: PMC6689741. Epub 2019/03/29. eng.
192. House SL. Psychological distress and its impact on wound healing: an integrative review. J Wound Ost Contin Nurs. 2015;42(1):38–41. PubMed PMID: 25549307. Epub 2014/12/31. eng.
193. Weinman J, Ebrecht M, Scott S, Walburn J, Dyson M. Enhanced wound healing after emotional disclosure intervention. Br J Health Psychol. 2008;13(Pt 1):95–102. PubMed PMID: 18230239. Epub 2008/01/31. eng.
194. Brown KL, Phillips TJ. Nutrition and wound healing. Clin Dermatol. 2010;28(4):432–9. PubMed PMID: 20620761. Epub 2010/07/14. eng.
195. Broadbent E, Kahokehr A, Booth RJ, Thomas J, Windsor JA, Buchanan CM, et al. A brief relaxation intervention reduces stress and improves surgical wound healing response: a randomised trial. Brain Behav Immun. 2012;26(2):212–7. PubMed PMID: 21741471. Epub 2011/07/12. eng.
196. Mishra SI, Scherer RW, Snyder C, Geigle PM, Berlanstein DR, Topaloglu O. Exercise interventions on health-related quality of life for people with cancer during active treatment. Cochrane Database Syst Rev. 2012;2012(8):CD008465. PubMed PMID: 22895974. Pubmed Central PMCID: PMC7389071. Epub 2012/08/17. eng.
197. Oldenmenger WH, Geerling JI, Mostovaya I, Vissers KCP, de Graeff A, Reyners AKL, et al. A systematic review of the effectiveness of patient-based educational interventions to improve cancer-related pain. Cancer Treat Rev. 2017;63:96–103. PubMed PMID: 29272781. Epub 2017/12/23. eng.

198. Chiu HY, Hsieh YJ, Tsai PS. Systematic review and meta-analysis of acupuncture to reduce cancer-related pain. Eur J Cancer Care. 2017;26(2):e12457. PubMed PMID: 26853524. Epub 2016/02/09. eng.
199. Birch S, Lee MS, Alraek T, Kim TH. Evidence, safety and recommendations for when to use acupuncture for treating cancer related symptoms: a narrative review. Integr Med Res. 2019;8(3):160–6. PubMed PMID: 31304088. Pubmed Central PMCID: PMC6600712. Epub 2019/07/16. eng.
200. Garcia MK, Driver L, Haddad R, Lee R, Palmer JL, Wei Q, et al. Acupuncture for treatment of uncontrolled pain in cancer patients: a pragmatic pilot study. Integr Cancer Ther. 2014;13(2):133–40. PubMed PMID: 24282103. Epub 2013/11/28. eng.
201. Park R, Park C. Comparison of foot bathing and foot massage in chemotherapy-induced peripheral neuropathy. Cancer Nurs. 2015;38(3):239–47. PubMed PMID: 25275582. Epub 2014/10/03. eng.
202. Matthews E, Carter P, Page M, Dean G, Berger A. Sleep-wake disturbance: a systematic review of evidence-based interventions for management in patients with cancer. Clin J Oncol Nurs. 2018;22(1):37–52. PubMed PMID: 29350708. Epub 2018/01/20. eng.
203. Matthews EE, Berger AM, Schmiege SJ, Cook PF, McCarthy MS, Moore CM, et al. Cognitive behavioral therapy for insomnia outcomes in women after primary breast cancer treatment: a randomized, controlled trial. Oncol Nurs Forum. 2014;41(3):241–53. PubMed PMID: 24650832. Epub 2014/03/22. eng.
204. Besedovsky L, Lange T, Born J. Sleep and immune function. Pflugers Arch. 2012;463(1):121–37. PubMed PMID: 22071480. Pubmed Central PMCID: PMC3256323. Epub 2011/11/11. eng.
205. Miladinia M, Baraz S, Shariati A, Malehi AS. Effects of slow-stroke back massage on symptom cluster in adult patients with acute leukemia: supportive care in cancer nursing. Cancer Nurs. 2017;40(1):31–8. PubMed PMID: 26925992. Epub 2016/03/02. eng.
206. DuBose JR, Hadi K. Improving inpatient environments to support patient sleep. Int J Qual Health Care. 2016;28(5):540–53. PubMed PMID: 27512130. Epub 2016/08/12. eng.
207. Lipsett A, Barrett S, Haruna F, Mustian K, O'Donovan A. The impact of exercise during adjuvant radiotherapy for breast cancer on fatigue and quality of life: a systematic review and meta-analysis. Breast. 2017;32:144–55. PubMed PMID: 28189100. Epub 2017/02/12. eng.
208. Esplen MJ, Trachtenberg L. Online interventions to address body image distress in cancer. Curr Opin Support Palliat Care. 2020;14(1):74–9. PubMed PMID: 31895065. Epub 2020/01/03. eng.
209. Duijts SF, Faber MM, Oldenburg HS, van Beurden M, Aaronson NK. Effectiveness of behavioral techniques and physical exercise on psychosocial functioning and health-related quality of life in breast cancer patients and survivors--a meta-analysis. Psycho-Oncology. 2011;20(2):115–26. PubMed PMID: 20336645. Epub 2010/03/26. eng.
210. Fang SY, Lin YC, Chen TC, Lin CY. Impact of marital coping on the relationship between body image and sexuality among breast cancer survivors. Support Care Cancer. 2015;23(9):2551–9. PubMed PMID: 25617071. Epub 2015/01/27. eng.
211. Esplen MJ, Wong J, Warner E, Toner B. Restoring Body Image After Cancer (ReBIC): results of a randomized controlled trial. J Clin Oncol. 2018;36(8):749–56. PubMed PMID: 29356610. Epub 2018/01/23. eng.
212. Langelier DM, D'Silva A, Shank J, Grant C, Bridel W, Culos-Reed SN. Exercise interventions and their effect on masculinity, body image, and personal identity in prostate cancer - a systematic qualitative review. Psycho-Oncology. 2019;28:1184. PubMed PMID: 30875710. Epub 2019/03/16. eng.
213. Helgeson VS, Cohen S, Schulz R, Yasko J. Education and peer discussion group interventions and adjustment to breast cancer. Arch Gen Psychiatry. 1999;56(4):340–7. PubMed PMID: 10197829. Epub 1999/04/10. eng.
214. Timko C, Janoff-Bulman R. Attributions, vulnerability, and psychological adjustment: the case of breast cancer. Health Psychol. 1985;4(6):521–44. PubMed PMID: 3830703. Epub 1985/01/01. eng.

References

215. Ellis MA, Sterba KR, Day TA, Marsh CH, Maurer S, Hill EG, et al. Body image disturbance in surgically treated head and neck cancer patients: a patient-centered approach. Otolaryngol Head Neck Surg. 2019;161(2):278–87. PubMed PMID: 30961419. Pubmed Central PMCID: PMC6675637. Epub 2019/04/10. eng.
216. Semple C, Parahoo K, Norman A, McCaughan E, Humphris G, Mills M. Psychosocial interventions for patients with head and neck cancer. Cochrane Database Syst Rev. 2013;7:CD009441. PubMed PMID: 23857592. Epub 2013/07/17. eng.
217. Wanchai A, Armer JM, Stewart BR, Lasinski BB. Breast cancer-related lymphedema: a literature review for clinical practice. Int J Nurs Sci. 2016;3(2):204–7.
218. McCaulley L, Smith J. Diagnosis and treatment of lymphedema in patients with breast cancer. Clin J Oncol Nurs. 2014;18(5):E97–102. PubMed PMID: 25253121. Epub 2014/09/26. eng.
219. Wilson DJ. Exercise for the patient after breast cancer surgery. Semin Oncol Nurs. 2017;33(1):98–105. PubMed PMID: 28063632. Epub 2017/07/26. eng.
220. Winkels RM, Sturgeon KM, Kallan MJ, Dean LT, Zhang Z, Evangelisti M, et al. The women in steady exercise research (WISER) survivor trial: the innovative transdisciplinary design of a randomized controlled trial of exercise and weight-loss interventions among breast cancer survivors with lymphedema. Contemp Clin Trial. 2017;61:63–72. PubMed PMID: 28739540. Pubmed Central PMCID: PMC5817634. Epub 2017/01/09. eng.
221. Dönmez AA, Kapucu S. The effectiveness of a clinical and home-based physical activity program and simple lymphatic drainage in the prevention of breast cancer-related lymphedema: a prospective randomized controlled study. Eur J Oncol Nurs. 2017;31:12–21. PubMed PMID: 29173822. Epub 2017/11/28. eng.
222. Northouse LL, Mood DW, Schafenacker A, Kalemkerian G, Zalupski M, LoRusso P, et al. Randomized clinical trial of a brief and extensive dyadic intervention for advanced cancer patients and their family caregivers. Psycho-Oncology. 2013;22(3):555–63. PubMed PMID: 22290823. Pubmed Central PMCID: PMC3387514. Epub 2012/02/01. eng.
223. Chen ML, Chu L, Chen HC. Impact of cancer patients' quality of life on that of spouse caregivers. Support Care Cancer. 2004;12(7):469–75. PubMed PMID: 15118899. Epub 2004/05/01. eng.
224. Hagedoorn M, Sanderman R, Bolks HN, Tuinstra J, Coyne JC. Distress in couples coping with cancer: a meta-analysis and critical review of role and gender effects. Psychol Bull. 2008;134(1):1–30. PubMed PMID: 18193993. Epub 2008/01/16. eng.
225. Dionne-Odom JN, Taylor R, Rocque G, Chambless C, Ramsey T, Azuero A, et al. Adapting an early palliative care intervention to family caregivers of persons with advanced cancer in the rural deep south: a qualitative formative evaluation. J Pain Symptom Manag. 2018;55(6):1519–30. PubMed PMID: 29474939. Pubmed Central PMCID: PMC5951755. Epub 2018/02/24. eng.
226. Shaffer KM, Kim Y, Carver CS. Physical and mental health trajectories of cancer patients and caregivers across the year post-diagnosis: a dyadic investigation. Psychol Health. 2016;31(6):655–74. PubMed PMID: 26680247. Pubmed Central PMCID: PMC4930392. Epub 2015/12/19. eng.
227. Kershaw T, Ellis KR, Yoon H, Schafenacker A, Katapodi M, Northouse L. The interdependence of advanced cancer patients' and their family caregivers' mental health, physical health, and self-efficacy over time. Ann Behav Med. 2015;49(6):901–11. PubMed PMID: 26489843. Pubmed Central PMCID: PMC4825326. Epub 2015/10/23. eng.

The Transition to Survivorship 17

17.1 Introduction

For most, the transition to survivorship is a positive, often transformative experience in the aftermath of cancer treatment [1–3]. For others, the transition is fraught with anxiety and trepidation [4, 5]. Survivorship is increasingly recognized as a period of great patient uncertainty and adjustment. The end of treatment may signal the elimination or containment of the disease, but it does not address the potential emotional, physical, neurophysiological, and psychosocial changes caused by having experienced a life-threatening illness, treatment, and stressful trajectory. Healthcare providers who say to their patients, "Go live your life," may be well intentioned, but to many individuals and their family caregivers, it is initially scary. It feels as if the perceived "safety" net of hospital, clinic, and the oncology team is about to dissipate, generating a whole new phase of anxiety and lack of self-efficacy with consequential implications for sustaining a health-related future. For these reasons, a nursing program that focuses on the transitional phase to survivorship by providing patients and family caregivers with the knowledge and skills to forge a healthy resilient future is integral to their future resilience and health.

17.2 Objectives

At the end of the chapter, you will be able to facilitate healing and resilience during the transition to survivor phase by:

- Addressing posttreatment fears of "professional abandonment" and providing early cues of a potential cancer recurrence.
- Promoting contextually-based self-efficacy beliefs and behaviors that enable a renewed sense of control over one's life.

- Facilitating the integration of new lifestyle behaviors through education to strengthen resilience and reduce cancer risk.
- Strengthening the quality of support of family and significant others.
- Reducing symptomatic effects of cancer and treatment such as anxiety, fatigue, sleep disruption, cognitive problems, body image, neuropathies based on relevant knowledge and therapeutic strategies.
- Providing needed information about health-related resources and early possible signs.
- Fostering a new integrated sense of self, meaning, and purpose in life.

Clinical Anecdote 17.1
The day my treatment ended, the doctor informed me that everything was fine and to "go live my life." When I asked who would be following me now, he responded, the palliative care team! Which was totally antithetical to how I had interpreted "fine." I burst into tears, my fears now cresting in a thunderous crescendo. The word, "palliative" precipitated many sleepless nights, and generated tremendous fatigue made only worse with the realization that my cognitive abilities felt different, off somehow- it was harder to retrieve words I wanted to express, and to pay attention- my working memory seemed to have been altered- I was in the midst of a perfect interactive storm of fatigue, memory problems, sleepless nights, anxiety and fear! My energy was sapped at a time when I had wanted to focus on getting back to "normal." Although with time, I found my new normal.

17.3 Definition

The definition of survivorship is still widely debated. Based on Marzorati and colleagues' [6] compilation of various conceptualizations, survivorship in this chapter refers to a life-changing process, starting at diagnosis, continuing through treatment, and extending after treatment to a cancer-free healthy life or living well with a chronic illness. The "after treatment" component of this general definition, may be said to encompass the transition phase to survivorship, which has tended to be neglected by most healthcare providers ([1, 3, 6] p. 235).

The transition phase involves the process of adapting physically, psychologically, cognitively, socially, and behaviorally to a new "normal" with its challenges and opportunities for personal and social growth and transformation, in part through the acquisition of greater self-efficacy and self-management capabilities [2, 7]. Transition to survivorship ultimately ends with the survivors' growing confidence in their health, quality of life, self-management skills, and belief in a future either healthy and cancer free or a quality of life, living with a chronic illness (e.g., [8]).

17.4 Common Patient Concerns

Patients strive to pick up the mantle of their former lives, only to discover that their life has profoundly changed in both perceptible and imperceptible ways [9]. Having been encouraged to embrace a present-oriented, day-by-day strategy during treatment, many are fearful of shifting their horizons forward toward a more hopeful future and longer-term goals (Fig. 17.1).

Feelings of Medical Abandonment (Review Part IV Chaps. 8, and 11)

Survivors are generally "unprepared" for what they may perceive as an abrupt medical discharge. Many, deemed "cancer free," now experience *feelings of* "abandonment" by the healthcare team [10]. The transition is experienced as an important loss of health-related security caused by the perceived withdrawal of the oncology team from closely monitoring the patient's health status. The oncologists and nurses had served, in the patient's mind, as saviors from the jaws of death; they were the incontrovertible experts in their treatment, clinical surveillance, and compassionate care.

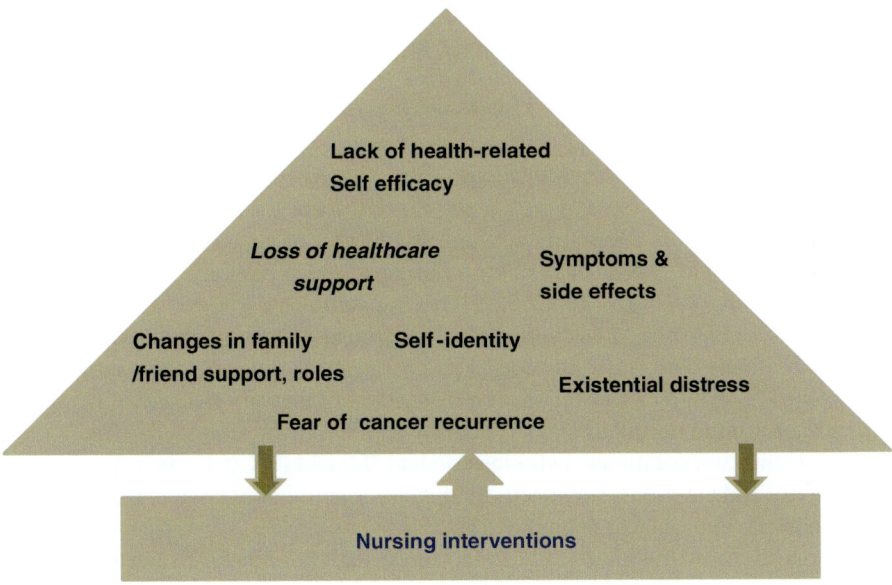

Fig. 17.1 Patient and family caregiver concerns transitioning to survivorship

Survivors may now find they have to fend for themselves, with inadequate or no guidelines on how to live a healthy life, prevent a cancer recurrence, identify future clinical signs of cancer, manage persistent side effects and symptoms, or have regular access to a healthcare practitioner who *knows them* (e.g., [9, 11, 12]). Posttreatment concerns, if left unaddressed, can impede their ability to restore (heal) resilient capabilities, promote health potential, and their ability to forge into their future with confidence [7].

These issues continue to resonate among most new survivors, with the literature revealing only a paucity of posttreatment programs to support individuals and family caregivers in their transition to a healthy future life (e.g., [13]). The empirically known stress-related adverse effects on the whole person's resilience and healing capabilities underscore the importance of offering a transition-to-survivorship workshop for patients and their family caregivers, addressing an important gap in meeting the adaptive health-related needs of survivors and their caregivers ([14], e.g., [15]).

An Altered Self-Identity

Many survivors have been psychologically and physically changed—*they feel* they are no longer the same resilient and capable person as before; they may perceive the world and themselves in it differently, with less confidence, greater vulnerability, less sense of personal control, and uncertainty. Always looming in the back of their mind is the question of how to protect themselves against a recurrence (e.g., [16–18]).

Fear of a Cancer Recurrence (FCR)

One-third of survivors are highly anxious and fearful of a cancer recurrence [14]. FCR refers to "fear, worry or concern relating to the possibility that cancer will come back or progress" ([4] p. 3265, [5]). FCR is unrelated to the individual's cancer prognosis [19]. Individuals with stage 1 may be as distressed about the possibility as individuals with stage 4 cancer. Yet, prolonged feelings of fear can increase the potential risk of a cancer recurrence by sustaining the very cascade of neuroendocrinal and immune inflammatory pathways (previously discussed) which *suppress* TH1 anticancer immune cytokines such as $IL2$ and $IFN-\gamma$, innate natural killer cell activity and cytotoxic T-cell activity that are scientifically known to hunt down and eliminate rogue cancer cells [20, 21].

Factors associated with a fear of recurrence include a lack of relevant health-related information, dissatisfaction with their health professionals, and a personal history in which loved ones have died of cancer. Other factors involve new or persistent physical symptoms, stage of cancer, treatment type, low optimism, fewer significant relationships, low quality of life, distrust of one's own body, and death anxiety [19, 22]. For many, cancer has been the Trojan horse that hijacked their physical self, growing and proliferating before making its presence known [23].

This realization causes many survivors to profoundly distrust their body, even when the nurse has given them a list of clinical signs that warrant a timely return to the clinic such as indefatigable fatigue, an unremitting cough, a constant cold, inexplicable or rapid weight loss, new persistent headaches, loss of appetite, constant diarrhea, or persistent new body aches, pain or sensations, and/or shortness of breath.

Changes in Family Support (Review Part IV Chap. 11)

Supportive relationships generally undergo changes posttreatment [24]. Family caregivers understandably desire to resume their own daily life and responsibilities, yet may also experience conflicting emotions due to the reduced time now available for their loved one [25]. Conversely, new survivors may experience feelings of guilt at having disrupted the lives of loved ones, but also anxiety about the potential loss of previously received support, at a time when they are experiencing new feelings of vulnerability [25].

Whereas some survivors may be relieved, feeling that their loved ones have become overly involved in their daily life, others may experience anticipatory feelings of loneliness in the wake of changes in the nature of their relationships with other family members and close friends. Subjective feelings of abandonment from loved ones may play into the survivors' sense of helplessness and loneliness which are associated with poor resilience and an increased risk of cancer recurrence [26, 27]. The loss of a significant source of meaningful support was found to be associated with depression in cancer patients, as well as an increased risk of morbidity and mortality [27–29].

Enduring Symptoms and Side Effects of Treatment or Cancer (Review Chaps. 6 and 7)

Individuals may experience various symptoms and side effects such as poor stamina, fatigue, sleep disturbances, memory problems, neuritis, pain, depression, sexual dysfunction, body image disfigurement, and anxiety for months into survivorship that impede their return to activities of daily living and even a return to work as assessed in survivors of breast cancer and other cancers [8, 30, 31]. Up to 66% of breast cancer patients, for example, experience cancer-related fatigue, 46% experience problems concentrating, and up to 49% suffer muscular/joint pain after treatment (e.g., [32, 33]).

Studies have found that the threat-induced anxiety of a cancer diagnosis persists throughout the treatment phase and into survivorship [34]. Other clinical research has focused on a symptom cluster frequently manifested in survivors consisting of fatigue, sleep disturbances, and pain [35, 36]. These symptoms and side effects have been attributed to the residual effects of radiation, chemotherapy, and surgical procedures, possible residual effects of the tumor, emotional distress, and other related host factors [37–41]. Activated proinflammatory cytokines released by the immune system appear to give rise to fatigue, depression, anxiety, and difficulty sleeping [42, 43]. But the anxiety and depressive mood may also be attributed to other factors including fear of a cancer recurrence [5].

Additional side effects may include neuropathies, cognitive, and body image impairments (such as lymphedema). Body image changes can negatively impact intimacy, sexuality and by extension quality of life [44–47]. Undertreated symptoms constitute a "symptom burden" that not only aggravates emotional distress but contributes to allostatic load which increases the individual's risk of future illness, including cancer. As a consequence, these side effects and symptoms must be clinically addressed [48].

Insomnia In the cancer population, insomnia is two to three times greater than in the general population, for instance in an estimated 6-% of breast cancer survivors with an estimated prevalence of 40% (e.g., [49]). Insomnia refers to the inability to fall asleep, stay asleep, or fall back to sleep. It may be associated with pain, depressive symptoms, fatigue, poor quality of life, increased risk of a cancer recurrence, and shortened life [50]. Whereas sedation typically is used to manage insomnia, sedatives are also associated with unwanted side effects such as ongoing sleep, drowsiness, memory problems, and/or performance difficulties [51].

Cancer-related fatigue (CRF) An estimated 25–30% of patients who are cancer free at the end of treatment experience cancer-related fatigue persisting up to 10 years into survivorship [38, 52]. CRF is one of the most prevalent and distressing symptoms caused by the cancer and its treatment, but also by other related psychosocial, behavioral as well as biological factors [38, 53]. CRF's definition, based on Cella's conceptualization, refers to "the subjective state of overwhelming and sustained exhaustion and decreased capacity for physical and mental work that is not relieved by rest" ([53] p. 2, [54]). CRF undermines the individual's ability for normal work, social relationships, activities of daily living, and a quality life after treatment [55]. Cancer-related fatigue also may be exacerbated by a lack of instrumental or emotional support. CRF is associated with typical cancer-related symptoms such as depression, sleep disturbances, emotional distress, and pain [41, 53, 56].

Cancer-related fatigue is associated with a dysregulated HPA axis, inadequate PNS healing-related functions, disruptions in circadian rhythm, and significantly the presence of proinflammatory cytokines released by the immune system in response to the cancer and its treatments [41, 56]. Various studies have shown a specific relationship between cancer-related fatigue and increased levels of inflammatory C-reactive protein (CRP), tumor necrosis factor (TNF), and possibly interleukin 6 (IL-6) [38, 53]. A genomic study that focused on cancer-related fatigue in survivors showed increased gene expression of proinflammatory cytokines and Nuclear Factor Kappa B (NF_KB) (an inflammatory transcription factor). The elevated cytokines and transcription factors were also associated with reduced gene expression of glucocorticoids, suggesting some impairment in normal glucocorticoid activity ([53] p. 5). Longitudinal studies are needed across phases in the cancer trajectory including survivorship to determine the relationships among transcription factors, other cytokines, glucocorticoid activity and fatigue.

One hypothesis is that fatigue levels may be improved by downregulating proinflammatory cytokines and the proinflammatory transcription factor, NFKB. Restoring the balance between pro- and anti-inflammatory cytokines (TH1/TH2 relationship) may also reduce symptoms induced by an inflammatory environment. However, nutritional deficiencies, physical inactivity, and a higher body mass index have also been shown to account for fatigue and need to be investigated as part of an overall assessment and clinical action plan [38, 53, 56]. The majority of studies are still based on patients with breast cancer. Further studies are needed in underrepresented cancer populations.

In summary, symptoms are not unusual among survivors of cancer, although research in this area has underrepresented the diverse cancer population. Notwithstanding, persistent symptoms reduce the survivors' ability to heal and achieve a present and future quality of life. Significantly, the prolonged manifestation of symptoms also poses a long-term threat to the individual's survivability by maintaining an inflammatory environment in which residual cancer cells, unimpeded by cell-mediated immune cells, may continue to circulate and embed in various organs for later metastatic colonization.

Cognitive impairment An estimated 80% of cancer survivors experience some form of cognitive difficulty which tends to go untreated [57, 58]. It is a common side effect of treatment (surgery, chemotherapy, and radiation therapy), although personal and social factors such as loneliness, distress, anxiety, and depression are likely contributing factors [59, 60]. *Posthoc* analyses of baseline data from a randomized controlled study that investigated the effectiveness of an intervention to improve cognitive difficulty in survivors of early stage breast cancer revealed significant contributing factors [61]. Cognitive difficulties were related to fatigue and stress along with other demographic and medical factors including the number of chemotherapy cycles that had been completed [61]. Persistent cognitive problems in survivorship may lead to a lack of confidence and self-efficacy particularly within work- and social-related functions [62]. Cognitive capability (as well as body image) is an integral component of one's self-concept, self-image, or self-identity.

Self-image is the way in which individuals "see" themselves not only physically, but in terms of their self-concept (self-identity), which includes roles (functions), responsibilities, competencies, and relationships. These attributes of the person's self-concept shape an individual's values, beliefs, and attitudes about the self in relation to the world and contribute to one's sense of purpose and meaning in life [63, 64]. Physical changes to body image may alter beliefs about the self, negatively impacting personal relationships, the ability to return to work, social and occupational functioning, and for some daily activities (Review Part V, Chap. 16).

Lifestyle Behaviors (Review Part V Chap. 16)

A healthy lifestyle refers to all behaviors that promote resilience and health by maintaining a dietary pattern of healthy food and nutrition, daily physical exercise, a normal weight, a good night's sleep, as well as engaging in stress-reducing strategies (Table 17.1) (e.g., [65]). Survivors have been shown to gain weight, increase their body mass index (BMI), and gain abdominal adiposity during treatment while also manifesting immunosuppression and an increased inflammatory profile according to clinical research based mainly in breast cancer [66–68]. Yet, the evidence is strong that a healthy lifestyle is essential not only for cancer prevention but also to reduce the risk of a cancer recurrence, and to improve quality of life in survivors of cancer (e.g., [69]). The Canadian National Breast Screening Study ($N = 49,613$), which followed women for a mean of 16.6 years, showed that adherence to the American Cancer Society (ACS) Guidelines was effective in producing a 31% reduction in breast cancer risk compared to those who only adhered to one guideline or none [70]. Adherence to 6 or 7 of the WCRF/AICR guidelines showed a 31% reduction in breast cancer risk, strongly underscoring the importance of providing health-related information and guidance to new survivors to enhance their adoption of health behaviors, not only in survivors of breast cancer, but head and neck, liver, prostate, colorectal, gastric, and other forms of cancers [71–73].

However, most survivors of any cancer are unsure where to obtain health-promoting information, resulting in uncertainty and misconceptions of what constitutes a healthy lifestyle [74, 75]. A qualitative study revealed that some survivors were unclear about the role of diet in a cancer recurrence [74]. Even when survivors of breast and endometrial cancers were aware of the importance of health-promoting behaviors, persistent symptoms interfered with their making health-promoting behavioral changes [75–77]. A cross-sectional study of 315 survivors of breast cancer reported that fatigue was the most frequently cited "barrier" to making healthy food choices (72.1%) and in engaging in physical activity (65.7%) [76]. Cited barriers to eating healthily or being physically active included stress (69.5%) and treatment-related changes such as loss of appetite, taste, and a desire for unhealthy

Table 17.1 Definitions from diet, nutrition, physical activity, and cancer: Global perspective: A summary of the Third Expert Report ([65] p. 16)

Healthy behaviors	Definition
Nutrition	"The processes of ingestion, digestion, absorption, transportation, assimilation and excretion used by the whole organism specifically its cells, tissues, organs in order to acquire energy and nutrients to function normally and have a normal structure" (p. 16)
Diet	"Food that consists of needed nutrients and energy for life-sustaining biochemical reactions" (p. 16)
Physical activity	"Movement of skeletal muscle that includes exercises, manual labor, standing, walking, housework, and fidgeting" (p. 16)

foods which negatively impacted eating healthily (31.4–48.6%). Experiencing pain or discomfort (53.7%) also thwarted physical activity [76]. Other studies have mentioned emotions and bowel irregularities as a function of the treatment or cancer site, neuropathies, and lymphedema as limiting factors [75]. A recent cross-sectional study (n = 66) obtained similar findings, reporting that only 7.6% of cancer survivors had met NCCN's (2016) six health behavior guidelines [78]. For these reasons, new survivors require education regarding how they may promote their health and overcome or effectively manage side effects and symptoms, and in so doing, facilitate their ability to take back control over their resilient capabilities and health.

17.5 Clinical Research: Psychosocial Interventions

The main goal of survivorship-promoting interventions is to strengthen overall resilience and health by (a) promoting healthy lifestyle behaviors, (b) reducing emotional distress, (c) effectively managing side effects/symptoms, (d) promoting self-efficacy through self-management and emotion-regulating skills, and (e) providing psychosocial support, psychoeducation, and medically-relevant information to newly transitioning survivors of cancer and their family caregivers. Systematic reviews, meta-analyses, RCTs, and a few one-arm clinical studies have provided evidence of various psychosocial interventions that address survivor and/or caregiver concerns, and can inform the nurse's practice.

Cognitive-Behavioral (CB) Strategies (Review Appendix in Part IV Chap. 9 and Appendix B)

Cognitive-behavioral interventions appear to be effective in reducing a number of symptoms such as insomnia, depression, stress, fear of a cancer recurrence, social disruption, as well as improving quality of life and mood in survivors of mainly breast cancer, but also prostate and colorectal cancer [14, 79–81]. In a meta-analysis of 14 RCTs (N = 1363), compared to controls, the CB interventions showed significant medium to large effect size reductions in insomnia at the postintervention assessment with prolonged effects up to at least 12 months across studies [82]. The intervention was shown to be effective for improving insomnia and enhancing quality of sleep in individuals with breast cancer.

An RCT compared the effectiveness of 8 weeks of either acupuncture or CB interventions to reduce insomnia in 160 cancer survivors [51]. Findings indicated that both significantly reduced the severity of insomnia over baseline with significant improvements observed over 20 weeks, based on clinically meaningful change values of −8.31 for acupuncture and −10.91 for the CB strategies. Notwithstanding, a significant mean difference still favored the CB intervention over acupuncture.

The cognitive-behavioral intervention showed significantly better *overall sleep quality, faster sleep onset, reduced waking after sleep onset, and improved sleep efficiency*. Acupuncture was found to effectively increase total sleep time over

CBT-I. Both interventions significantly reduced *fatigue, the use of sedatives, and improved mood and quality of life* posttreatment. Although baseline pain was generally low, acupuncture was found to be more effective than CBT in reducing *pain intensity* posttreatment. The multimodal CB intervention consisted of sleep hygiene, coping strategies, education, cognitive restructuring, stimulus control, i.e., learning to associate one's bed with sleep by getting out of bed 15–20 min after failing to fall asleep, in order to do something relaxing before returning to bed, and repeating the process. The third component referred to shortening the time spent in bed in order to optimize the potential for falling and remaining asleep [51].

An RCT of an internet-delivered CBT based on 114 cancer survivors showed a significant moderate effect reduction in *fears of a cancer recurrence* and an even greater effect size improvement in quality of life postintervention compared to usual care [83]. Significant and large effect size reductions in *anxiety and depressive symptoms* and *general distress* strongly suggested that the internet may be an acceptable mode for implementing this intervention.

A few randomized controlled trials have also investigated the efficacy of cognitive-behavioral stress reduction (CBSR) interventions in new survivors of cancer, with significant clinical outcomes (e.g., [79, 81, 84]). One hundred and ninety-nine early stage, nonmetastatic women with breast cancer postsurgery were randomly assigned to either a 10-week group CBSR intervention or a control group [79]. The intervention a significantly improved several clinical outcomes, including social interactions, recreational activities, positive affect, emotional well-being, finding benefit, lifestyle behaviors, and feeling more relaxed for up to 12 months after the intervention. The CBSR components included stress-reducing activities such as imagery and relaxation exercises, discussions of social support resources, effective coping responses to cancer, and treatment-related topics. The CBSR group also addressed negative beliefs and encouraged participants to engage in more positive reappraisals, greater expression of positive emotions, and learned skills in conflict resolution.

These studies strongly suggest that cognitive-behavioral strategies are effective in reducing a number of side effects and symptoms including fears about a cancer recurrence using face-to-face individual and group as well as teleinternet modes of delivery. The findings indicate that a workshop based on a multi-modal CB approach would make an important clinical contribution to the overall health and quality of life of new survivors.

Mind–Body Stress Reduction (MBSR) and Mindfulness-Based Cancer Recovery (MBCR) (Review Appendix in Part IV Chap. 13)

MBSR/MBCR are multimodal interventions organized around mindful meditation that typically incorporates CB strategies, relaxation, and psychoeducation. In randomized controlled trials, both MBSR and MBCR have been associated with significant improvements in anxiety, depression, fatigue, perceived stress, quality of life, emotional well-being, fear of a cancer recurrence, and cognitive confusion in survivors of breast and prostate cancer compared to a waitlist usual care or supportive expressive intervention (SET) [85–89].

A meta-analysis of 29 RCTs with 3274 patients with cancer and survivors investigated the effectiveness of MBSR compared to controls on psychological and physical health outcomes [90]. The MBSR interventions produced a small-to-medium effect reduction in psychological distress at the end of the treatment as well as at follow-up. Small-to-medium effect size improvements of secondary clinical outcomes were also reported for anxiety, fear of a cancer recurrence, depression, fatigue, sleep disturbances, and pain [90]. The potential effectiveness of this intervention to improve the lives of survivors who continue to experience cancer- or treatment-related symptoms is compelling. Future studies that identify the optimal components of an effective MBSR on targeted clinical outcomes would further inform clinical practice.

In an RCT of breast cancer survivors, participants randomly assigned to the MBCR intervention ($n = 134$) reported significant increases in emotional and affective support, spirituality, meaning in life, and posttraumatic growth compared to participants in the supportive expressive intervention (SET) ($n = 118$) who achieved similar outcomes albeit at lower levels [91]. Women in the MBCR group also reported significant reductions in tension, fatigue, cognitive confusion, and anxiety compared to the SET group. In this study the MBCR program was specifically *tailored* to the needs of cancer survivors [91].

Finally, an RCT randomly assigned *healthy* participants (n-42) either to a meditation or control group. The meditation intervention compared to the control group produced significant improvements in attention, working memory, and recognition memory as well as reductions in anxiety and negative mood states, suggesting its potential viability as an adjunct therapy for posttreatment-related cognitive difficulties [92]. The meditation intervention completed 13 min of daily meditation for 8 weeks. Although the small study was underpowered, the findings strongly suggest the need to replicate this study in survivors with a rigorously designed and powered RCT. The cognitive and emotional improvements after 8 weeks of meditating only 13 min every day have important clinical implications for patients, caregivers, and nurses.

Future RCTs might also evaluate the effectiveness of MBCR or MBSR interventions on normalizing the parametric values of proinflammatory cytokines caused by the cancer, its treatment, and symptoms, with a particular focus on enhancing cell-mediated immunity. This clinical research may further inform nursing practice, given the critical role of anticancer immune surveillance in tracking down and eliminating roving cancer cells. Specific markers might include glucocorticoid levels, NOR, IL-2, and/or IFN-γ in conjunctions with behavioral (e.g., anxiety or distress) as observed by other effective resilient-promoting clinical interventions [93, 94]. IL-2 increases natural killer cells and provides immunologic surveillance of cancer cells, while IFN-γ inhibits the growth of specific tumor cells. Both are typically suppressed in emotionally distressed individuals, which have been increasingly acknowledged in new survivors [94]. Because of the likelihood of residual cancer cells even at the end of treatment, the need for a multitargeted intervention that restores immune parameters to their normal range of values as soon as possible during the transition phase to survivorship should be a clinical goal of practice.

Massage and Foot Reflexology (Review Part V Chap. 20; Review Appendix in Chap. 14)

A small number of studies have assessed the effectiveness of massage and foot reflexology in survivors and caregivers. An early phase single-blinded RCT of survivors of breast cancer ($n = 66$) assessed a 6-week Swedish massage intervention with moderately applied pressure compared to either the light touch control or the wait list control group [95]. The Swedish massage with applied moderate pressure was significantly more effective in reducing fatigue, compared to the other two groups [95].

Although applied moderate massage may alleviate cancer-related fatigue temporarily in survivors, the effects of massage on residual cancer cells pose, in my opinion, a justifiable caution. The question of the amount of time that needs to transpire before engaging in a body massage during survivorship must be asked, and clinical guidelines developed before a clinical recommendation for full body massage in the transition period to survivorship is feasible.

A double-blind placebo-controlled RCT of 66 informal caregivers of cancer showed that foot reflexology had a significant positive effect in reducing anxiety and improving sleep compared to the placebo control [96]. The finding suggests that foot reflexology is a safe and effective strategy that nurses might recommend to symptomatic informal caregivers and survivors during the transition to survivorship. Findings from a well designed and sufficiently powered RCT of the potential effects of foot massage on immune functioning of cancer survivors would make an important contribution to their health and potential survivability.

Self-Management Interventions (SMI) (Review Part V, Chap. 16; Appendix A)

SMIs are increasingly recommended to facilitate the transition to survivorship. They offer relevant knowledge and skills that survivors and caregivers can use to more effectively manage persistent physical and psychological symptoms SMIs may address changes in role functioning, specific information on healthy lifestyle behaviors, problem-solving approaches to manage health -related concerns (eg persistent side effects and symptoms). SMI workshops include how to collaborate and maintain relationships with healthcare providers [10].

In a systematic review of 12 studies and meta-analysis of 9 RCTs consisting of 2804 adult cancer survivors, SMI interventions that were compared to usual care, an attention control group, or a waitlist group showed a significant medium effect size improvement in health-related quality of life and a large effect size reduction in fatigue levels that trended toward statistical significance [97]. The effects of the SMI on anxiety, depression, and self-efficacy were not significant posttreatment, although long-term SMI showed a relatively small albeit significant increased effect in self-efficacy. SMI content was generally delivered by web or the internet and/or combined with face-to-face interventions. These trials tended to evaluate interventions aimed at emotional distress, symptom and uncertainty management, empowerment and coping skills, exercise, and diet. Substantial heterogeneity limits interpretation of the findings. More research on the optimal mode of delivery, content, and number of sessions is needed in light of other SMI findings with mixed results for instance in caregivers and patients in the palliative cancer population (e.g., [98–100]).

A recent systematic review of 41 mostly randomized-controlled trials evaluating the effectiveness of SMIs was mostly based on survivors of breast cancer [101]. Less than half the studies were organized around a theoretical framework, and the psychoeducational interventions varied in design with variable therapeutic effects. Risk of bias could not be fully assessed, and it was unclear the extent to which survivor needs were assessed prior to the development of the SMI across the studies.

A feasibility study of 79 survivors of breast cancer in transition to survivorship suggested that a one session intervention on survivorship care planning was significantly effective in increasing self-reported health, decreasing social role limitations, and improving self-efficacy compared to usual care [12]. Guided by the chronic care model, the survivor-centered session helped to establish priorities and goals, highlighted resources for problem solving, and encouraged the development of a plan for improving their health. Although the duration of effects was unknown, the study underscores the value of offering a posttreatment SMI intervention to facilitate the individual's transition to survivorship. To date, the majority of RCTs evaluating the efficacy of SMIs are for patients with advanced cancer in supportive care and their caregivers [97, 102].

Health-Related Education (Review Appendices A and B)

Education is a large component of the nurse's psychosocial interventions. A three-wave repeated measures experimental design compared the effectiveness of two psychosocial interventions: an interpersonal counseling intervention (TIP-C) and a health education attention condition (HEAC) intervention on quality of life in 71 survivors of prostate cancer and 70 partners [103]. The TIP-C intervention focused on mood/affect management, emotional expression, interpersonal communication, social support, and cancer information. The HEAC consisted of written materials about prostate cancer, the diagnosis and treatment, and health topics such as nutrition during cancer, exercise to reduce fatigue, health resources, and quitting smoking. Both interventions were telephone-delivered.

The survivors in the HEAC group showed significant improvements in depression, negative affect, fatigue, stress, and spiritual well-being compared to survivors on the TIP-C counseling group. Partners in the HEAC group showed significant improvements in depression, fatigue, family support, social well-being, and spiritual well-being compared to those in the TIP-C condition. The importance of relevant cancer- and treatment-related information, ways to strengthen health as well as address the unmet needs of survivors and their partners must be an essential component of any survivor-based intervention. The lack of relevant information interferes with the ability to obtain needed resources, make relevant health-related decisions, and modulate emotional distress.

Health-Promoting Lifestyle Interventions (Review Appendix C)

At every phase along the disease and treatment outcome, the importance of promoting healthy lifestyle behaviors is critical to the individual's survivability. Convergent evidence indicates that a healthy lifestyle is associated with a better prognosis, survival, and health-related quality of life [65]. It is all the more important in the transition to survivorship. A prospective within group study from a multisite RCT of 227 breast cancer survivors investigated the effects of a healthy 12-month lifestyle program which consisted of a Mediterranean diet, brisk walking every day, and daily Vitamin D [104]. Significant improvements in health-related quality of life compared to baseline measures were reported in global health status, physical functioning, and role and social functioning. Significant positive effects were also found for well-being, body image, and future outlook with significant reductions in fatigue, nausea and vomiting, dyspnea, constipation, systemic side effects, sexual functioning, and breast-related symptoms. Finally, BMI was shown to be negatively related to global health status, and serum 25(OH) D levels negatively associated with breast-related symptoms. At baseline, only 16% of participants were still on treatment. Almost half the participants started the program less than 8 months after surgery ($n = 105$, 46.3%) and 53% 8 months or more after surgery ($n = 122$), suggesting that introducing a healthy lifestyle during but especially after treatment for stage 1 to stage 3 breast cancer has significant positive effects on HRQOL in survivorship. Similar programs should be evaluated in other under represented cancer populations during the transition to survivorship.

Nutrition and Diet

An essential component of a healthy lifestyle has to do with a varied dietary pattern of healthy foods. Meta-analyses of 83 RCTs and observational (cohort and case control) studies ($N = 2,130,753$) showed that *people without cancer* who adhered to a Mediterranean diet (MedD) had a significantly lower risk of overall cancer mortality compared to those in the MedD group with the lowest adherence [73]. The significantly lower risk was for colorectal cancer, breast cancer, gastric cancer, liver cancer, head and neck cancer, and prostate cancer. Notwithstanding, the findings of the cancer survivor group with the highest adherence to a MedD diet was not shown to be associated with either cancer mortality or a cancer recurrence. However the MedD was defined differently across the studies. Moreover the quality of the research designs, the size and composition of the samples (including cancer type, age and gender) in the 4 studies based on survivors, could not be assessed. Factors shown to impact risk of cancer mortality and a cancer recurrence are age, gender, and alcohol consumption [73]. The moderate consumption of alcohol which is an integral part of the MEDd raises health-related concerns for survivors as well as healthy populations [65, 73, 105]. Conversely a systematic review and meta analysis with 1,670,179 participants which evaluated *diet quality* defined by validated indexes, such as the Healthy Eating index (and others), the findings showed that a high quality diet was significantly and inversely related to all cancer mortality and cancer mortality in cancer survivors [71].

Pooled analyses from Schwingshackl's 2017 study showed that fruits, vegetables, and whole grains were most protective for *healthy participants*: specifically, fruit intake significantly reduced cancer risk, as did vegetable and whole grain consumption. Dairy trended toward a reduced cancer risk, whereas meat consumption trended toward an increased cancer risk [73]. The worldwide compilation of meta-analyses suggests that prostate cancer carries a slight increased risk in relation to dairy products [65].

Similarly an analysis of relationships between 10 selected nutritional factors and the risk of cancer based on 108 meta-analyses, 20 pooled analyses, 4 intervention RCTs, and 1 postintervention study showed that the factors that increased risk of cancer were alcohol, being overweight and obese, consumption of red and processed meat, salt and salted foods, and consumption of beta carotene supplements [69]. Factors that reduced the cancer risk were physical activity, daily consumption of fruits and vegetables, dietary fiber, and breastfeeding. Dairy products were found to reduce cancer risk with the possible exception of prostate cancer ([106] p. 38). Overall evidence indicates the importance of (a) maintaining a balanced and varied diet, (b) significantly reducing alcohol intake, (c) maintaining a physically active lifestyle, and (d) a healthy weight, which are all consistent with recent findings from the WCRR/AICR Third Expert Report on diet, nutrition, physical activity, and cancer which is recommended for healthy persons as well as cancer survivors (2018).

A meta-analysis of 117 cohort studies ($n = 209,597$) assessed the relationship between food intake and *dietary patterns*, and overall mortality in survivors of cancer [107]. Greater consumption of vegetables and fish was inversely related to overall mortality; higher alcohol intake was associated with overall mortality. Adherence to the highest category of a quality diet was inversely related to overall mortality. Similarly, adhering to the highest category of a healthy *dietary pattern* was inversely related to overall mortality. Conversely, a western dietary pattern was significantly related to an increased risk of mortality [107]. A healthy diet based on dietary patterns of intake underscores the importance of encouraging patients to adopt a healthier diet and pattern of intake, with long-term clinical benefits. Investing in healthy lifestyle behaviors also enables survivors to restore a sense of personal control over their health. In summary, diet plays an important role in preventing cancer.

Exercise/Physical Activity

In a meta-analysis of 20 studies ($N = 1223$), exercise was significantly more effective than either usual care or usual lifestyle exercise interventions in improving cardiopulmonary fitness based on a significant increase in $VO_{2\,peak}$, decreased fasting insulin levels, and lowered insulin resistance in survivors of colorectal cancer [108]. An impaired $VO_{2\,peak}$ during treatment and survivorship has been associated with a greater symptom burden and higher cancer-related mortality [108]. At least 150 min/week of aerobic exercise, which varied in intensity across studies, significantly improved $VO_{2\,peak}$ and cardiopulmonary fitness in cancer survivors. Exercise also decreased the intercellular adhesion molecule (sICAM-1), which is normally overexpressed in cancer and associated with angiogenesis and with suppressing immune recognition of tumor cells [108] (Review Part III Chaps. 6 and 7).

A recent review of the relationship between moderate to intense *daily* physical activity of less than 60 minutes and the immune system indicated that regular exercise appeared to regulate and likely strengthen the immune response [109]. A number of restorative (healing) health-promoting immune changes included: (a) reduced levels of inflammatory cytokines, (b) increased T-lymphocyte cell proliferation, (c) increased neutrophil phagocyte functioning, and (d) increased natural killer cell activities ([109] p. 212). Regular exercise has a resilient-promoting, strengthening effect on the immune response that enhances its functional efficacy over time, i.e., regular exercise exerts a training function on resilient promoting physical, biological, and, specifically, immune processes.

A Cochrane review of 40 trials ($n = 3694$) based on survivors of diverse cancers showed that exercise compared to usual care had a significant positive effect on global *quality of life* at 12 weeks and at 6 months [110]. Survivor concerns also significantly improved between the 12-week and 6-month follow-up as did *body image/self-esteem* using the Rosenberg scale at 12 weeks and between the 12-week and 6-month follow-up. Other significant improvements included *emotional well-being at 12 weeks, sexuality at 6 months, sleep disturbances at 12 weeks, social functioning* at 12 weeks and 6 months, *anxiety* at 12 weeks, *fatigue a*t 12 weeks and between 12 weeks and 6 months, and *pain* at 12 weeks compared to usual care data [110]. Another meta-analysis based on exercise corroborated its effectiveness in reducing fatigue [111].

A Cochrane review of 23 studies (1372 participants) involving people with cancer and survivors of breast, prostate, colorectal, and lung cancer investigated the strategies used to encourage people living with cancer and survivors to engage in daily exercise. Thirteen of these studies were based on a moderate-intensity exercise program (150 min per week) or resistance training (a minimum of two days per week) [112]. Eight of the 13 studies demonstrated a 75% adherence or higher to exercise programs based on specified guidelines, and all involved some level of supervision. Setting goals, use of graded physical activity, and instructions were thought to facilitate use of exercise. Further research is needed to understand how to motivate survivors to adopt exercise as a health behavior that has substantial positive effects on psychological and physical well-being, symptom management, and the immune system. In the main, the studies produced low-quality evidence due to methodological issues.

Summary RCTs assessing the effectiveness of therapeutic interventions in cancer care are disproportionately based on individuals who have had breast cancer. Clinical therapeutic interventions specifically designed for survivors of various cancer types at every stage of the disease are needed. As Carlson's study findings [87] suggest, clinical content (topics) must be tailored to the specific medical, emotional, social, and behavioral concerns of the intended beneficiaries of the intervention. The transition to survivorship is still in its early phases of scientific evidence. More rigorous trials are needed in order to produce meta-analyses based on studies with low heterogeneity and risk of bias.

17.6 Proposed Nursing Approaches (See Part IV, Chaps. 8–14; Part V Chap. 16)

The transition phase from "patient" to survivor is the optimal time for nurses to provide patients and families with the support, knowledge, and skills they require to walk with confidence into their future. The main goal is to facilitate their successful transition to a resilient-promoting and healthy reintegrated life. The majority of posttreatment survivors are highly motivated to take a proactive role in their health but have been largely discouraged by the lack of programs available (e.g., [15]).

Nursing goals include (a) Reducing fears of a cancer recurrence or expressions of existential/emotional distress, (b) providing self-management interventions to increase self-efficacy beliefs and problem-solving capabilities around survivor-identified medical and health-related concerns, such as dealing with residual or persistent treatment- or cancer-related symptoms, and (c) promoting a healthy lifestyle with respect to physical exercise, diet, and weight. Through a nursing assessment, the presence of distorted beliefs and dysfunctional coping behaviors need to be identified and addressed (Chaps. 9 and 10). In the final analysis, a tailored multimodal intervention within a supportive nurse-patient/caregiver relationship is most likely to optimize the survivor's and caregiver's capabilities and strengths to face their future with confidence. Establishing regular workshops on transitioning to survivorship may be an effective means for addressing the main concerns of patients and family caregivers in combination with follow-up individualized clinical visits, as assessed.

Maintain a Sense of Connectedness between Nurse and Individual and Family (Part IV, Chap. 8)

An important nursing objective is to maintain a supportive relationship during the transition phase with the patient and family caregiver. The transition to a new normal life may entail adjustments in the nature of their supportive relationships with family and friends who tend to resume personal and work-related responsibilities and social activities [113–115]. Establish regular follow-ups during this phase, enabling individuals to feel that they are still connected to their healthcare team and the nurse, in particular, as they acquire relevant cognitive and behavioral coping strategies and self-management capabilities. The nurse's presence, reassurance, relevant responses, and health-related suggestions for the new survivor and family member can reduce feelings of anxiety and provide the needed impetus to embrace their survivorship. Both one-on-one interactions and nurse-led workshops may be effective psychosocial interventions [9, 12].

Promote Self-Management Capabilities (Review Content in Part IV Chap. 9; Review Appendix A)

Individuals with various chronic conditions, including cancer, who are highly motivated to acquire self-management capabilities have reported improved health outcomes and quality of life compared to less motivated patients [9, 12, 116]. The goals of self-management programs are to increase self-efficacy and problem-solving capabilities for dealing with current and future health-related issues emanating from the disease or treatment in order to promote the individual's sense of personal control over her or his health (e.g., [117, 118]). Common components of SMI are described in Chap. 9. The key to a successful SMI workshop is to first do an assessment of the intended group's concerns and needs and develop a tailored SMI to effectively address them.

Fear of a Cancer Recurrence (Part IV, Chap. 10)

Fear of a cancer recurrence has been shown to trigger a readiness to develop self-management capabilities [9, 12]. Perhaps the key to overcoming this fear is gaining relevant information that provides a sense of personal control and self efficacy regarding how to reduce the risk of a cancer recurrence and enables early recognition of salient cues that signal a need to return to clinic in a timely manner. Another key aspect is providing relevant strategies to control one's intrusive ideation as well as to reduce anxiety. Addressing fears of a cancer recurrence may be optimally managed by a multimodal approach. Tomei and colleagues (2020) designed a randomized controlled pilot study to assess the effects of a 6-week *cognitive existential psychological intervention* specifically designed to address survivors' fear of a cancer recurrence. Individuals were asked to imagine the situation that evoked fear, which was then accompanied by discussions of existential concerns, relaxation exercises, and use of cognitive restructuring (Review Part IV Chap. 9). Survivors' fears of a cancer recurrence, uncertainty about the illness, the need to seek reassurances, and the use of cognitive avoidance were significantly reduced. The intervention group also manifested more positive reappraisals and improved quality of life compared to controls. An RCT based on a rigorous design with a larger sample could provide evidence of the effectiveness of this intervention in helping survivors. *Other strategies to consider as part of the intervention include introducing CB strategies and* mindful meditation of the relaxation response technique [119, 120].

Nursing interventions also must include sharing relevant information regarding a healthy lifestyle (i.e., moderately intense physical activity, maintaining an appropriate weight, reducing/abstaining from alcohol, and following guidelines for an appropriate diet, e.g., Healthy Eating index). Because a healthy lifestyle has been shown to significantly reduce the risk of a cancer recurrence, survivors may be especially motivated to live a healthy life and in so doing gain some mastery over their fears [71, 73]. It is incumbent upon the nurse to develop an educational program that includes a take away pamphlet with relevant *and practical information for maintaining a healthy diet and regular exercise as well as strategies to reduce emotional distress*. Refer survivors as well to the websites for the WCRF/AICR and its CUP updates [65].

The Quality and Quantity of Informal Support (See Part IV, Chaps. 10 and 11)

The transition phase is an opportunity for the family caregiver (or significant other) and the new survivor to clarify mutual expectations, feelings, and thoughts about the nature of their personal relationship as both transition to survivorship. Subsequent to an assessment, the cancer-free individual and the family may be helped to navigate these changes in their relationship.

Discussions should be facilitated about meaningful supportive relationships within the family now that the threat of cancer has subsided. Suggestions include engaging the survivor and loved one in a discussion of things they have learned about the meaning of family support through the cancer experience. The patient and his or her supportive network should be encouraged to share their thoughts and feelings surrounding the illness and treatment, what the whole experience has meant emotionally to each person, what they have learned from that experience, and from one another, and perhaps the toll it has taken on each person [121]. This may involve enabling survivor and caregiver the opportunity to clarify misunderstandings and concerns around the cancer-related experience as well as possible changes in the nature of their supportive relationship in the future.

Sharing the behaviors that have enhanced or fortified one another's emotional well-being can be mutually therapeutic and validating. And while the nature of support may change now that the survivor has completed treatment, the lessons learned from this life-threatening experience and the strengths (knowledge, skills, and presence) both patient and family have gleaned from this experience are worth articulating to underscore the importance of supportive relationships as the resilient-promoting predicate for a meaningful and healthy life [21, 28, 121]. Link these lessons learned and explore ways that these mutually supportive relationships may continue to be expressed perhaps differently as they move into survivorship.

New normal relationships Facilitate survivor and family discussions involving how the survivor and family imagine their daily life moving forward while continuing to demonstrate caring and supportive behaviors toward one another in ways that are commensurate with their new reality. Encourage discussions of what would constitute supportive behaviors in this new phase of life. Engage the family and patient in developing new strategies for ensuring the survivor feels connected and cared for as he/she transitions to a more independent life. Encourage adaptive coping strategies such as planning new opportunities to enjoy one another's company as two healthy, independent, resilient-promoting loved ones. Encourage both survivor and family to identify supportive behaviors that are personally meaningful, such as making daily telephone calls, going for walks together, meditating together, helping with groceries, sharing healthy recipes, a movie, and so on (e.g., [122, 123]).

Supportive relationships are sources of meaning throughout our lives, and a discussion of the significance of supportive relationships can serve as a reminder to both of the invaluable contribution of meaningful relationships in the quality of one's life. Consider doing an updated review of the research literature on support and survivorship, and develop your own workshop on support in the transition to survivorship.

Managing Symptoms and Side Effects of Treatment and the Cancer (See Part V, Chap. 16)

Review potential links among symptoms in terms of timing, sequencing, triggers, intensity, duration and cluster presentation. A nursing assessment includes an exploration of aberrant patient beliefs about cancer and/or its treatment that may have persisted into survivorship and inadvertently have triggered the manifestation of symptoms [124]. The presence of concurring symptoms (clusters) generally indicates a persistent underlying inflammatory environment [35, 36, 43, 125].

Survivors and family caregivers require relevant information/education about the likely significance of clustered symptoms as well as suggested interventions and a plan of action (that is, acquiring self-management, problem-solving actions developed with the nurse) to manage the cluster [101]. Increased physical activity has been shown to significantly reduce anxiety in breast cancer survivors; physical activity also appears to reduce fatigue, depression, and sleep disturbances in survivors of other cancers [126]. The mindfulness-based stress reduction program for survivors of breast cancer has been shown to be an effective intervention for managing symptom clusters, specifically anxiety, depression, perceived stress, as well as fatigue, sleep problems, and drowsiness, and improvements have been sustained 6–12 weeks afterward [127] (review Appendix A and Appendix in Chap. 13)

Other effective emotion-regulating strategies include the relaxation response technique, cognitive-behavioral stress reduction interventions, and various cognitive-behavioral strategies (Part IV, Chap. 9) [39, 40, 79, 91, 127]. Cognitive strategies, such as reappraisal, problem solving, use of distraction, and ways to seek, obtain and maintain needed support, are among the nonpharmacological strategies that have been shown to reduce anxiety, fear, and depressed mood (e.g., [10, 93, 128]) (Part IV Chap. 9).

These interventions may be most effective by incorporating three interrelated components: The first is to educate the individual on the relationships among most symptoms, emotional distress, and their underlying inflammatory environment. Second, share evidentiary information regarding the general effectiveness of the proposed interventions in reducing systemic inflammation and enhancing biological resilience and psychological well-being. Third, review the critical steps of a given intervention, encourage daily practice, provide a hand out sheet or audio recording to facilitate home practice, and incorporate an evaluation follow-up with the nurse.

Specific Side Effects (Review Part III, Chaps. 6 and 7)
Some side effects of treatment can be more challenging to overcome. Typically, these include fatigue and cognitive problems with recall and memory (as well as an altered body image, lymphedema, and neuropathies). Each has its own individualized concerns and worries that must be addressed in order to alleviate the survivor's distress. Body impairment, lymphedema, and neuropathies require clinical interventions during treatment as well as in survivorship, and for these reasons, they are discussed in Part V Chap. 16.

Cancer-Related Fatigue Although medical researchers have identified pharmacological antagonists to counter the presence of persistent proinflammatory markers associated with fatigue after treatment, many survivors prefer to first try nonpharmacological interventions. When fatigue is part of a symptom cluster, the relaxation response and mindful meditation have been shown to improve fatigue as well as the intensity of the related symptoms by downregulating the stress response, and presumably reducing corresponding cytokines [127, 129]. *Both modalities* have been found to help people deal with *the uncontrolled ideation* that can impede sleep and contribute to feelings of fatigue [124]. Daily moderately intense physical exercise also has been shown to alleviate symptoms of fatigue, possibly due to the recently reported normalizing effects of exercise on the immune system which would include restoring the TH1/TH2 homeostatic balance [109, 130].

Yoga, psychoeducation, acupuncture, and cognitive-behavioral strategies also appear to be effective in reducing fatigue (e.g., [38, 124, 131, 132]). A randomized-controlled study using a crossover wait list design investigated the effectiveness of a CB intervention organized around six factors thought to perpetuate the subjective experience of fatigue ([131] p. 4483): (a) inadequate coping responses to the cancer experience, (b) distorted cognitions related to fatigue, (c) irregular sleep–wake pattern, (d) dysregulated activity, (e) inadequate support, and (f) negative social interactions. A manual was developed for each factor to enhance a standardized clinical approach. A survivor assessment determined the number of factors to be included in a tailored intervention. The survivors in the intervention showed a significant improvement in the severity of their fatigue and also a significant increase in functional capabilities compared to the wait list condition [131]. This is a nice example of a fairly well-described intervention that nurses with advanced degrees might wish to learn more about. A more rigorous clinical research design using a control group and blinding would further inform the effectiveness of this well-described intervention.

Cognitive Difficulties Although pharmacological agents can help patients with cancer-related cognitive changes, medication may also cause side effects. A combined approach that includes nonpharmacological interventions may be more effective. Three nonpharmacological interventions have had a significant positive effect on cognitive difficulties following treatment. In order of significance, they were: (a) a meditation/mindfulness program aimed at reducing stress which also included learning to strengthen attentiveness and cognitive-behavioral coping approaches; (b) a combination of cognitive training and exercise; and (c) a combination of cognitive training, cognitive rehabilitation, and exercise [133]. An interdisciplinary approach may be most effective, depending on the individual's degree of cognitive difficulties. Nurses can play a role by encouraging individuals to adopt stress-reducing exercises such as taking daily brisk walks, daily practice of the meditation/relaxation response techniques, as well as helping individuals to develop strategies for remembering tasks or functions.

Finding Meaning in the New Normal Life (See Part IV Chap. 10; Part V Chap. 18; Appendix B)

Life is fragile and extremely precious to the survivor, compelling some to question how they truly want to spend the rest of their life. Individuals may struggle to "know" themselves and to conceptualize a recognizable self-identity following a life-threatening experience which may have left physical as well as psychic scars. This may lead to self-reflection and a quest for renewed meaning and purpose. The end of treatment offers the chance to take stock of a life already lived and discover paths toward creating a personally coherent life moving into the future, fraught as it is with uncertainty. This quest for a new reintegrated self may also be triggered by the need to restore oneself at the helm of one's life, making the decisions about healthcare needs but also setting personal goals guided by reprioritized or reasserted values and beliefs about oneself in relation to the world and others. In other words, determining how to live a life they were uncertain, they still would have in the future. The meaning a person ascribes to the cancer, treatment, and survivorship predicts how well he or she will adapt and thus enable the possibility of a meaningful life [134–137].

A small but growing number of studies indicates that finding meaning in life is associated with psychological well-being and even longer survivability [135, 138–140]. Moreover, intervention studies aimed at improving a sense of meaning in life, such as van der Spek's meaning-centered intervention, was associated with significant improvements in personal meaning, purpose in life, and significant reductions in depression, anxiety, hopelessness, and distress [141]. One effective one-on-one meaning-making intervention was developed by a nurse, Dr. Virginia Lee (2006). It is easy to administer in a clinic or at home. As a manualized intervention, the effectiveness of this meaning-making intervention depends on the expertise of the nurse leading the intervention. A training workshop for nurses in cancer care that incorporated the theoretical underpinnings of meaning making, the clinical evidence and a training phase to develop the nurse's clinical expertise, would provide a useful skill to help patients and caregivers across the trajectory as well as into survivorship [142–144]. Another effective intervention for new survivors might be a life review to help provide a more hopeful future within the context of their past and present experiences [1, 145].

17.6 Proposed Nursing Approaches

Promoting a Healthy Lifestyle (Review Part V, Chaps. 15 and 16 Sections on Healthy Lifestyle Behaviors, Physical Activity, Diet) (Tables 17.2, 17.3 and 17.4)

Survivors of diverse cancers may be physically compromised by an inadequate diet and physical inactivity during treatment resulting in an increased inflammatory index that can predispose individuals to an increased risk of health-related problems, including a cancer recurrence [67, 146]. A healthy lifestyle has been strongly

Table 17.2 Recommendations from the Third Expert Reports on Diet, Nutrition, physical activity, and cancer [65]

Lifestyle-related factors	Recommendations	Rationale
1. Maintain a healthy weight (p. 48)	Maintain your normal weight throughout life	(a) Strong evidence that increased body fat causes many cancers, even within the normal range for weight!
2. Maintain regular physical activity (p. 50)	Maintain daily moderate-to-intense physical activity (a) This requires 45–60 min of moderate–intensity exercise each day: Cycling, walking, gardening, swimming, dancing	(a) Strong evidence that physical activity is protective against many cancers (b) Protects against weight gain
3. A diet replete with whole grains, vegetables, fruit, beans, and lentils (p. 53)	Diet should include 30 g at a minimum of fiber such as (a) Whole grains—Brown rice, wheat, barley, rye and oats (b) Red, green, white yellow, purple orange fruit (c) Nonstarchy vegetables—Green leafy vegetables, eggplant, broccoli, chick peas, bok choy (d) Eat at least 5 helpings or 400 g of various nonstarchy vegetables and fruit everyday	(a) Strong evidence that eating whole grains protects again colorectal cancer, and trends toward protective effects for other cancers (b) Dietary fiber protects against weight gain, overweight, obesity, and colorectal cancer (c) Greater body fat causes diverse cancers (d) Some evidence that fruits and vegetables may decrease risk of many cancers, weight gain, and obesity
4. Limit eating processed foods, high in fat, starch or sugars; also fast foods, prepared meals, snacks, bakery foods, candy, which are associated with excess energy intake (p. 56)	Diet may include nuts high in fat, oils of plant	(a) Strong evidence that fast foods are energy dense and are associated with weight gain, obesity (b) A western diet associated with too much free sugar, meat, fat— Also causes weight gain, obesity, and likely increases risk of cancer (c) Glycemic load, i.e., an increase in blood glucose and insulin after food intake has been associated with endometrial cancer (d) Greater body adiposity causes many cancers

Table 17.3 Recommendations from the Third Expert Reports on Diet, Nutrition, physical activity, and cancer

Lifestyle related factors	Recommendations	Rationale
5. Limit intake of red and processed meat (p. 58)	(a) Restrict intake of red meat to only about 3 portions per week (b) Eat little to NO processed meat (c) Red meat in recommended doses is good source of zinc, iron, protein, and vitamin B 12 (d) Meat-free diets may obtain protein from mix of whole grains (cereals) and pulses (legumes), i.e., beans and lentils (e) Iron from lentils, spinach, soybeans, dark chocolate, and oysters	(a) Strong evidence that red meat and processed meat can cause colorectal cancer (b) Processed meat contains high levels of salt, and methods used produce carcinogens
6. Limit intake of sugar sweetened drinks (p. 60)	(a) Do not drink sugar sweetened drinks (b) Drink water or unsweetened drinks such as tea or coffee without added sugar (c) Coffee and tea have caffeine: Maximum daily intake of caffeine (according to European food safety authority) is 4 brewed cups (d) Fruit juices in large quantities even with no added sugar cause weight gain, and intake should be restricted (e) No strong evidence that artificially sweetened drink with minimal energy (e.g., diet soda) cause cancer	(a) Strong evidence that sugared drinks provide energy without reducing appetite leading to weight gain and obesity in adults and kids made worse by low levels of physical activity (b) Overweight or obese caused by excess of energy intake relative to energy expenditure (c) Great body fat causes many cancers (d) Fatness also causes type 2 diabetes and CVD
7. Limit alcohol intake (p. 62)	(a) Alcohol intake should not exceed national guidelines (b) Children must not drink alcohol (c) Pregnant women must not drink alcohol (d) See alcoholic drinks (wcrf.org/cancer-prevention-recommendations)	(a) Strong evidence that alcohol causes many cancers (b) There is no threshold below which alcohol intake does not contribute to a risk of some cancers (c) Although drinking alcohol (at least two drinks per day) seems to be protective against kidney cancer, it does not counter the significant risk of developing all other kinds of cancers (d) Alcohol drinks of ALL types increase the risk of cancer

17.6 Proposed Nursing Approaches

Table 17.4 Recommendations from the Third Expert Reports on Diet, Nutrition, physical activity, and cancer

Lifestyle related factors	Recommendations	Rationale
8. Do not use supplements for cancer prevention (p. 62)	(a) Meet nutritional needs through diet, not dietary supplements (b) Take supplements only recommended by a qualified health professional for health or developmental considerations such as pregnancy	There is strong evidence that: (a) Taking high-dose beta carotene supplements causes cancer in current and former smokers (b) Trials of other high-dose supplements have produced inconsistent findings on cancer risk based on observational studies (c) Prescribed by a medical professional, supplements may be needed for specific nutrient insufficiencies, such as dietary anemia that may require iron or folic acid supplementation; others in northern climates may need vitamin D
9. Mothers without cancer breastfeed their baby if they can (p. 66)	(a) This recommendation in keeping with WHO that babies should be breast fed exclusively for 6 months, and then up to 2 years or beyond alongside appropriate diet for the growing baby	(a) Strong evidence that breast feeding protects mother against breast cancer, and lowers risk for type 2 diabetes (b) Children who were breast fed are protected against excess weight gain, obesity (c) Excess body fatness in childhood is associated with earlier menarche in girls and increases risk of several cancers (d) Breastfeeding protects the development of the baby's immune system, and protects against infections in infancy and childhood diseases

(continued)

Table 17.4 (continued)

Lifestyle related factors	Recommendations	Rationale
10. After a cancer diagnosis follow WCRF/AICR CUP 2018 recommendations (p. 68)	(a) All cancer survivors should receive guidance on nutrition and physical activity from health professionals (b) Unless medically contra indicated, all cancer survivors should follow cancer prevention recommendations starting right after the acute stage of the treatment (c) People diagnosed with cancer should see a trained health professional to advise them on these lifestyle behaviors (d) Patients undergoing treatment may have special nutritional needs, those who are posttreatment, and in palliative stage who are losing weight may require special nutritional interventions	(a) Growing consensus of the important role of diet, nutrition, physical activity and body fatness in improving cancer survival (b) For breast cancer survivors: persuasive evidence that nutritional factors, especially low body fatness and physical activity enhance survival and future risk of breast cancer (c) Research on the effects of diet, physical activity, and obesity is growing in other forms of cancer

recommended for cancer survivors in order to lower the risk of a cancer recurrence [65]. Key components of a healthy life style include a good night's sleep, daily physical activity preferably at moderate- to- intense levels of physical activity (and for no more than 60 minutes per session at intense levels), resistance training, a varied diet of fruit, dark and leafy vegetables, whole grains, fish and minimal alcohol while maintaining a healthy weight (e.g., [69, 109, 147]).

Diet The importance of a diversified healthy diet cannot be emphasized enough. For instance, a multicentered trial of survivors of breast cancer who showed a higher adherence to a Mediterranean diet compared to those who were rated as lower adherents had significantly better scores on physical functioning, sleep, symptomatic pain, and overall well-being [148]. The WCRF/AICR's ([65], pp. 38) latest global research evidence on cancer prevention and survivorship have also reported that dairy products were not associated with an increased risk of cancer, including for postmenopausal breast cancer or premenopausal breast cancer, or prostate cancer, contrary to earlier evidence. Dairy products showed a "probable decrease" in cancer risk for colorectal cancer.

Bioactive phytonutrients in various plant foods that have been scientifically shown to have antioxidant, anti-inflammatory, immunomodulating as well as antimicrobial effects in laboratory experiments (e.g., [149, 150] p. 182) include flavonoids, carotenoids, glucosinolates, isoflavones, terpenes, and saponins, among others. Although not designated as essential nutrients for maintaining life, numerous studies and meta-analyses strongly suggest that phytonutrients exert beneficial effects on maintaining or promoting health by preventing some diseases, including cancer or its recurrence (chemoprevention). Different phytochemicals are present in fruits, vegetables, legumes, herbs, and teas, which explain why, for instance, fruits and vegetables are so important to a healthy, diversified diet. A healthy dietary pattern of eating improves physical and cognitive function by providing the necessary nutrients and metabolic requirements to maintain homeostasis, development, healing, and resilient processes that sustain overall health [151–153].

Encourage adherence to a healthy and nutritious diet and to maintaining a healthy weight offering a guideline that summarizes your discussions. Prior to meeting with a survivor and caregiver, consult with the oncologist and dietician to ensure that the WCRF/AICR's guidelines are appropriate given the clinical status of the survivor at the end of treatment.

Physical activity has been shown to significantly improve physical fitness, function, strength, and quality of life in mostly survivors of breast and prostate cancers [154, 155]. Physical activity in survivors of breast cancer was associated with a significantly lower risk of all-cause mortality, death from breast cancer, and a nonsignificant lower risk of a cancer recurrence (e.g., [154]). Similarly, physical activity of survivors of prostate cancer showed significant improvements in fatigue, fitness, function, and overall quality of life. More research based on survivors with other cancer sites is needed.

Become familiar with general guidelines for moderate activity and consult with the oncology team with respect to the intensity, frequency, and duration of daily activity to promote overall fitness and health in each survivor, depending on their clinical status. A consultation with the exercise physiologist should result in a guideline for each survivor to follow at home. A nurse plays a huge role in educating survivors and loved ones with respect to explaining the biological as well as behavioral benefits of a healthy diet and exercise on weight, critical anticancer immune cell functions, physical fitness, emotion regulation, and cognitive thinking. Moreover, a healthy lifestyle facilitates the normalization of TH1/TH2 cytokines which, when dysregulated, have been implicated in a number of side effects and symptoms. The amount of information provided and at what level is a function of the survivor's and caregiver's education and preferences. In addition to encouraging a healthy diet and exercise, encourage the patient and family to help one another integrate these new lifestyle behaviors into their daily life by planning and preparing meals together, sharing recipes, and by engaging in regular physical activity together.

Final Thoughts

The transition to survivorship is filled with hope but also fraught with anxiety that can undermine the survivor's resilience and health potential. It requires a thoughtful nursing approach which is optimally supported by a combination of one-on-one nursing interventions and/or a posttreatment nurse-led survivorship workshop. Armed with what we know now about the effects of support, coping, meaning-making strategies, and healthy lifestyle behaviors throughout, the whole person incorporating these therapeutic modalities into a workshop for survivors and/or caregivers in transition should constitute a clinical imperative.

References

1. Denlinger CS, Sanft T, Baker KS, Broderick G, Demark-Wahnefried W, Friedman DL, et al. Survivorship, version 2.2018, NCCN clinical practice guidelines in oncology. J Natl Compr Canc Netw. 2018;16(10):1216–47; PubMed PMID: 30323092. Pubmed Central PMCID: PMC6438378. Epub 2018/10/17. eng.
2. Skeath P, Norris S, Katheria V, White J, Baker K, Handel D, et al. The nature of life-transforming changes among cancer survivors. Qual Health Res. 2013;23(9):1155–67; Epub 2013/07/19. eng.
3. Denlinger CS, Sanft T, Moslehi JJ, Overholser L, Armenian S, Baker KS, et al. NCCN guidelines insights: survivorship, version 2.2020. J Natl Compr Canc Netw. 2020;18(8):1016–23; PubMed PMID: 32755975. Pubmed Central PMCID: PMC7785060. Epub 2020/08/07. eng.
4. Lebel S, Ozakinci G, Humphris G, Mutsaers B, Thewes B, Prins J, et al. From normal response to clinical problem: definition and clinical features of fear of cancer recurrence. Support Care Cancer. 2016;24(8):3265–8; PubMed PMID: 27169703. Epub 2016/05/14. eng.
5. Lebel S, Ozakinci G, Humphris G, Thewes B, Prins J, Dinkel A, et al. Current state and future prospects of research on fear of cancer recurrence. Psychooncology. 2017;26(4):424–7; PubMed PMID: 26891602. Epub 2016/02/20. eng.
6. Marzorati C, Riva S, Pravettoni G. Who is a cancer survivor? A systematic review of published definitions. J Cancer Educ. 2017;32(2):228–37; PubMed PMID: 26854084. Epub 2016/02/09. eng.
7. Wood SK. Transition to cancer survivorship: a concept analysis. ANS Adv Nurs Sci. 2018;41(2):145–60; PubMed PMID: 29059066. Epub 2017/10/24. eng.
8. Fitch MI. Transition to survivorship: can there be improvement? Curr Opin Support Palliat Care. 2018;12(1):74–9; PubMed PMID: 29176332. Epub 2017/11/28. eng.
9. Kvale EA, Meneses K, Demark-Wahnefried W, Bakitas M, Ritchie C. Formative research in the development of a care transition intervention in breast cancer survivors. Eur J Oncol Nurs. 2015;19(4):329–35; PubMed PMID: 25726359. Epub 2015/03/03. eng.
10. McCorkle R, Ercolano E, Lazenby M, Schulman-Green D, Schilling LS, Lorig K, et al. Self-management: enabling and empowering patients living with cancer as a chronic illness. CA Cancer J Clin. 2011;61(1):50–62; PubMed PMID: 21205833. Pubmed Central PMCID: PMC3058905. Epub 2011/01/06. eng.
11. Meade E, McIlfatrick S, Groarke AM, Butler E, Dowling M. Survivorship care for postmenopausal breast cancer patients in Ireland: what do women want? Eur J Oncol Nurs. 2017;28:69–76; PubMed PMID: 28478858. Epub 2017/05/10. eng.
12. Kvale EA, Huang CS, Meneses KM, Demark-Wahnefried W, Bae S, Azuero CB, et al. Patient-centered support in the survivorship care transition: outcomes from the patient-owned survivorship care plan intervention. Cancer. 2016;122(20):3232–42; PubMed PMID: 27387096. Epub 2016/07/09. eng.

13. Reb A, Ruel N, Fakih M, Lai L, Salgia R, Ferrell B, et al. Empowering survivors after colorectal and lung cancer treatment: pilot study of a self-management survivorship care planning intervention. Eur J Oncol Nurs. 2017;29:125–34; PubMed PMID: 28720259. Pubmed Central PMCID: PMC5539921. Epub 2017/07/20. eng.
14. van de Wal M, Thewes B, Gielissen M, Speckens A, Prins J. Efficacy of blended cognitive behavior therapy for high fear of recurrence in breast, prostate, and colorectal cancer survivors: the SWORD study, a randomized controlled trial. J Clin Oncol Off J Am Soc Clin Oncol. 2017;35(19):2173–83; PubMed PMID: 28471726. Epub 2017/05/05. eng.
15. Mazanec SR, Sattar A, Delaney CP, Daly BJ. Activation for health management in colorectal cancer survivors and their family caregivers. West J Nurs Res. 2016;38(3):325–44; PubMed PMID: 26385501. Epub 2015/09/20. eng.
16. Duijts SF, Faber MM, Oldenburg HS, van Beurden M, Aaronson NK. Effectiveness of behavioral techniques and physical exercise on psychosocial functioning and health-related quality of life in breast cancer patients and survivors--a meta-analysis. Psychooncology 2011;20(2):115-126; PubMed PMID: 20336645. Epub 2010/03/26. eng.
17. Duijts SF, van der Beek AJ, Boelhouwer IG, Schagen SB. Cancer-related cognitive impairment and patients' ability to work: a current perspective. Curr Opin Support Palliat Care. 2017;11(1):19–23; PubMed PMID: 27898512. Epub 2016/11/30. eng.
18. Vehling S, Philipp R. Existential distress and meaning-focused interventions in cancer survivorship. Curr Opin Support Palliat Care. 2018;12(1):46–51; PubMed PMID: 29251694. Epub 2017/12/19. eng.
19. Butow P, Sharpe L, Thewes B, Turner J, Gilchrist J, Beith J. Fear of cancer recurrence: a practical guide for clinicians. Oncology (Williston Park). 2018;32(1):32–8; PubMed PMID: 29447419. Epub 2018/02/16. eng.
20. Wang M, Zhao J, Zhang L, Wei F, Lian Y, Wu Y, et al. Role of tumor microenvironment in tumorigenesis. J Cancer. 2017;8(5):761–73; PubMed PMID: 28382138. Pubmed Central PMCID: PMC5381164. Epub 2017/04/07. eng.
21. Lutgendorf SK, Andersen BL. Biobehavioral approaches to cancer progression and survival: mechanisms and interventions. Am Psychol. 2015;70(2):186–97; PubMed PMID: 25730724. Pubmed Central PMCID: PMC4347942. Epub 2015/03/03. eng.
22. Simard S, Thewes B, Humphris G, Dixon M, Hayden C, Mireskandari S, et al. Fear of cancer recurrence in adult cancer survivors: a systematic review of quantitative studies. J Cancer Surviv. 2013;7(3):300–22; PubMed PMID: 23475398. Epub 2013/03/12. eng.
23. Holmberg C. No one sees the fear: becoming diseased before becoming ill--being diagnosed with breast cancer. Cancer Nurs. 2014;37(3):175–83; PubMed PMID: 23448954. Epub 2013/03/02. eng.
24. Fong AJ, Scarapicchia TMF, McDonough MH, Wrosch C, Sabiston CM. Changes in social support predict emotional well-being in breast cancer survivors. Psychooncology. 2017;26(5):664–71; PubMed PMID: 26818101. Epub 2016/01/29. eng.
25. Dorros SM, Segrin C, Badger TA. Cancer survivors' and partners' key concerns and quality of life. Psychol Health. 2017;32(11):1407–27; PubMed PMID: 29047300. Epub 2017/10/20. eng.
26. McGinty HL, Small BJ, Laronga C, Jacobsen PB. Predictors and patterns of fear of cancer recurrence in breast cancer survivors. Health Psychol. 2016;35(1):1–9; PubMed PMID: 26030308. Epub 2015/06/02. eng.
27. Lutgendorf SK, DeGeest K, Dahmoush L, Farley D, Penedo F, Bender D, et al. Social isolation is associated with elevated tumor norepinephrine in ovarian carcinoma patients. Brain Behav Immun. 2011;25(2):250–5; PubMed PMID: 20955777. Pubmed Central PMCID: PMC3103818. Epub 2010/10/20. eng.
28. Lutgendorf S, De Geest K, Bender D, Ahmed A, Goodheart M, Dahmoush L, Zimmerman M, et al. Social influences on clinical outcomes of patients with ovarian cancer. J Clin Oncol. 2012;30(23):2885–90.

29. Lutgendorf SK, Sood AK, Anderson B, McGinn S, Maiseri H, Dao M, et al. Social support, psychological distress, and natural killer cell activity in ovarian cancer. J Clin Oncol Off J Am Soc Clin Oncol. 2005;23(28):7105–13; PubMed PMID: 16192594. Epub 2005/09/30. eng.
30. Carreira H, Williams R, Müller M, Harewood R, Stanway S, Bhaskaran K. Associations between breast cancer survivorship and adverse mental health outcomes: a systematic review. J Natl Cancer Inst. 2018;110(12):1311–27; PubMed PMID: 30403799. Pubmed Central PMCID: PMC6292797. Epub 2018/11/08. eng.
31. Yi JC, Syrjala KL. Anxiety and depression in cancer survivors. Med Clin North Am. 2017;101(6):1099–113; PubMed PMID: 28992857. Pubmed Central PMCID: PMC5915316. Epub 2017/10/11. eng.
32. Schmid-Büchi S, Halfens RJ, Dassen T, van den Borne B. Psychosocial problems and needs of posttreatment patients with breast cancer and their relatives. Eur J Oncol Nurs. 2011;15(3):260–6; PubMed PMID: 20089447. Epub 2010/01/22. eng.
33. Joly F, Lange M, Dos Santos M, Vaz-Luis I, Di Meglio A. Long-term fatigue and cognitive disorders in breast cancer survivors. Cancers (Basel). 2019;11(12):1896; PubMed PMID: 31795208. Pubmed Central PMCID: PMC6966680. Epub 2019/12/05. eng.
34. Berry-Stoelzle MA, Mark AC, Kim P, Daly JM. Anxiety-related issues in cancer survivorship. J Patient Cent Res Rev. 2020;7(1):31–8; PubMed PMID: 32002445. Pubmed Central PMCID: PMC6988709. Epub 2020/02/01. eng.
35. Kwekkeboom KL. Cancer symptom cluster management. Semin Oncol Nurs. 2016;32(4):373–82; PubMed PMID: 27789073. Pubmed Central PMCID: PMC5143160. Epub 2016/10/30. eng.
36. Kwekkeboom K, Zhang Y, Campbell T, Coe CL, Costanzo E, Serlin RC, et al. Randomized controlled trial of a brief cognitive-behavioral strategies intervention for the pain, fatigue, and sleep disturbance symptom cluster in advanced cancer. Psychooncology. 2018;27(12):2761–9; PubMed PMID: 30189462. Pubmed Central PMCID: PMC6279506. Epub 2018/09/07. eng.
37. Blomberg BB, Alvarez JP, Diaz A, Romero MG, Lechner SC, Carver CS, et al. Psychosocial adaptation and cellular immunity in breast cancer patients in the weeks after surgery: an exploratory study. J Psychosom Res. 2009;67(5):369–76; PubMed PMID: 19837199. Pubmed Central PMCID: PMC2764537. Epub 2009/10/20. eng.
38. Bower JE. Cancer-related fatigue--mechanisms, risk factors, and treatments. Nat Rev Clin Oncol. 2014;11(10):597–609; PubMed PMID: 25113839. Pubmed Central PMCID: PMC4664449. Epub 2014/08/13. eng.
39. Miller AH, Ancoli-Israel S, Bower JE, Capuron L, Irwin MR. Neuroendocrine-immune mechanisms of behavioral comorbidities in patients with cancer. J Clin Oncol Off J Am Soc Clin Oncol. 2008;26(6):971–82; PubMed PMID: 18281672. Pubmed Central PMCID: PMC2770012. Epub 2008/02/19. eng.
40. Miller AH, Maletic V, Raison CL. Inflammation and its discontents: the role of cytokines in the pathophysiology of major depression. Biol Psychiatry. 2009;65(9):732–41; PubMed PMID: 19150053. Pubmed Central PMCID: PMC2680424. Epub 2009/01/20. eng.
41. Levkovich I, Cohen M, Pollack S, Drumea K, Fried G. Cancer-related fatigue and depression in breast cancer patients postchemotherapy: different associations with optimism and stress appraisals. Palliat Support Care. 2015;13(5):1141–51; PubMed PMID: 25201115. Epub 2014/09/10. eng.
42. Dantzer R, Kelley KW. Twenty years of research on cytokine-induced sickness behavior. Brain Behav Immun. 2007;21(2):153–60; PubMed PMID: 17088043. Pubmed Central PMCID: PMC1850954. Epub 2006/11/08. eng.
43. Dantzer R, O'Connor JC, Freund GG, Johnson RW, Kelley KW. From inflammation to sickness and depression: when the immune system subjugates the brain. Nat Rev Neurosci. 2008;9(1):46–56; PubMed PMID: 18073775. Pubmed Central PMCID: PMC2919277. Epub 2007/12/13. eng.
44. Reese JB, Handorf E, Haythornthwaite JA. Sexual quality of life, body image distress, and psychosocial outcomes in colorectal cancer: a longitudinal study. Support Care Cancer.

2018;26(10):3431–40; PubMed PMID: 29679138. Pubmed Central PMCID: PMC6474341. Epub 2018/04/22. eng.
45. Lewis-Smith H, Diedrichs PC, Harcourt D. A pilot study of a body image intervention for breast cancer survivors. Body Image. 2018;27:21–31; PubMed PMID: 30121489. Epub 2018/08/20. eng.
46. Jonsdottir JI, Jonsdottir H, Klinke ME. A systematic review of characteristics of couple-based intervention studies addressing sexuality following cancer. J Adv Nurs. 2018;74(4):760–73; PubMed PMID: 28986928. Epub 2017/10/08. eng.
47. Frick MA, Vachani CC, Hampshire MK, Bach C, Arnold-Korzeniowski K, Metz JM, et al. Survivorship after treatment of pancreatic cancer: insights via an internet-based survivorship care plan tool. J Gastrointest Oncol. 2017;8(5):890–6; PubMed PMID: 29184694. Pubmed Central PMCID: PMC5674255. Epub 2017/12/01. eng.
48. Deshields TL, Penalba V, Liu J, Avery J. Comparing the symptom experience of cancer patients and non-cancer patients. Support Care Cancer. 2017;25(4):1103–9; PubMed PMID: 27966024. Epub 2016/12/15. eng.
49. Leysen L, Lahousse A, Nijs J, Adriaenssens N, Mairesse O, Ivakhnov S, et al. Prevalence and risk factors of sleep disturbances in breast cancersurvivors: systematic review and meta-analyses. Support Care Cancer. 2019;27(12):4401–33; PubMed PMID: 31346744. Epub 2019/07/28. eng.
50. Zachariae R, Amidi A, Damholdt MF, Clausen CDR, Dahlgaard J, Lord H, et al. Internet-delivered cognitive-behavioral therapy for insomnia in breast cancer survivors: a randomized controlled trial. J Natl Cancer Inst. 2018;110(8):880–7; PubMed PMID: 29471478. Pubmed Central PMCID: PMC6093474. Epub 2018/02/23. eng.
51. Garland SN, Xie SX, DuHamel K, Bao T, Li Q, Barg FK, et al. Acupuncture versus cognitive behavioral therapy for insomnia in cancer survivors: a randomized clinical trial. J Natl Cancer Inst. 2019;111(12):1323–31; PubMed PMID: 31081899. Pubmed Central PMCID: PMC6910189. Epub 2019/05/14. eng.
52. Bower JE, Ganz PA, Desmond KA, Bernaards C, Rowland JH, Meyerowitz BE, et al. Fatigue in long-term breast carcinoma survivors: a longitudinal investigation. Cancer. 2006;106(4):751–8; PubMed PMID: 16400678. Epub 2006/01/10. eng.
53. Bower JE, Lamkin DM. Inflammation and cancer-related fatigue: mechanisms, contributing factors, and treatment implications. Brain Behav Immun. 2013;30 Suppl(0):S48–57; PubMed PMID: 22776268. Pubmed Central PMCID: PMC3978020. Epub 2012/07/11. eng.
54. Cella D, Peterman A, Passik S, Jacobsen P, Breitbart W. Progress toward guidelines for the management of fatigue. Oncology (Williston Park). 1998;12(11A):369–77; PubMed PMID: 10028520. Epub 1999/02/24. eng.
55. Bower JE, Ganz PA, Desmond KA, Rowland JH, Meyerowitz BE, Belin TR. Fatigue in breast cancer survivors: occurrence, correlates, and impact on quality of life. J Clin Oncol. 2000;18(4):743–53; PubMed PMID: 10673515. Epub 2000/02/16. eng.
56. Seiler A, Klaas V, Troster G, Fagundes CP. eHealth and mHealth interventions in the treatment of fatigued cancer survivors: a systematic review and meta-analysis. Psychooncology. 2017;26(9):1239–53; PubMed PMID: 28665554. Epub 2017/07/01. eng.
57. Hardy SJ, Krull KR, Wefel JS, Janelsins M. Cognitive changes in cancer survivors. Am Soc Clin Oncol Educ Book. 2018;38:795–806; PubMed PMID: 30231372. Epub 2018/09/21. eng.
58. Vannorsdall TD. Cognitive changes related to cancer therapy. Med Clin North Am. 2017;101(6):1115–34; PubMed PMID: 28992858. Epub 2017/10/11. eng.
59. Jaremka LM, Peng J, Bornstein R, Alfano CM, Andridge RR, Povoski SP, et al. Cognitive problems among breast cancer survivors: loneliness enhances risk. Psychooncology. 2014;23(12):1356–64; PubMed PMID: 24729533. Pubmed Central PMCID: PMC4194180. Epub 2014/04/15. eng.
60. Klaver KM, Duijts SFA, Engelhardt EG, Geusgens CAV, Aarts MJB, Ponds R, et al. Cancer-related cognitive problems at work: experiences of survivors and professionals. J Cancer Surviv. 2020;14(2):168–78; PubMed PMID: 31768861. Pubmed Central PMCID: PMC7182611. Epub 2019/11/27. eng.

61. Gutenkunst SL, Vardy JL, Dhillon HM, Bell ML. Correlates of cognitive impairment in adult cancer survivors who have received chemotherapy and report cognitive problems. Support Care Cancer. 2021;29(3):1377–86; PubMed PMID: 32666213. Epub 2020/07/16. eng.
62. Li M, Caeyenberghs K. Longitudinal assessment of chemotherapy-induced changes in brain and cognitive functioning: a systematic review. Neurosci Biobehav Rev. 2018;92:304–17; PubMed PMID: 29791867. Epub 2018/05/24. eng.
63. Ownsworth T, Chambers S, Hawkes A, Walker DG, Shum D. Making sense of brain tumour: a qualitative investigation of personal and social processes of adjustment. Neuropsychol Rehabil. 2011;21(1):117–37. PubMed PMID: 21154113. Epub 2010/12/15. eng.
64. Ownsworth T, Nash K. Existential well-being and meaning making in the context of primary brain tumor: conceptualization and implications for intervention. Front Oncol. 2015;5:96; PubMed PMID: 25964883. Pubmed Central PMCID: PMC4410611. Epub 2015/05/13. eng.
65. World Cancer Research Fund AIfcr. Diet, nutrition, physical activity and cancer: a global perspective. Summary of 3rd expert report. Continuous update project expert report. dietandcancerreport.org; 2018.
66. Carayol M, Ninot G, Senesse P, Bleuse JP, Gourgou S, Sancho-Garnier H, et al. Short- and long-term impact of adapted physical activity and diet counseling during adjuvant breast cancer therapy: the "APAD1" randomized controlled trial. BMC Cancer. 2019;19(1):737; PubMed PMID: 31345179. Pubmed Central PMCID: PMC6659309. Epub 2019/07/28. eng.
67. Custódio ID, Marinho Eda C, Gontijo CA, Pereira TS, Paiva CE, Maia YC. Impact of chemotherapy on diet and nutritional status of women with breast cancer: a prospective study. PLoS One. 2016;11(6):e0157113; PubMed PMID: 27310615. Pubmed Central PMCID: PMC4911080. Epub 2016/06/17. eng.
68. Custódio IDD, Franco FP, Marinho EDC, Pereira TSS, Lima MTM, Molina M, et al. Prospective analysis of food consumption and nutritional status and the impact on the dietary inflammatory index in women with breast cancer during chemotherapy. Nutrients. 2019;11(11):2610; PubMed PMID: 31683752. Pubmed Central PMCID: PMC6893533. Epub 2019/11/07. eng.
69. Latino-Martel P, Cottet V, Druesne-Pecollo N, Pierre FH, Touillaud M, Touvier M, et al. Alcoholic beverages, obesity, physical activity and other nutritional factors, and cancer risk: a review of the evidence. Crit Rev Oncol Hematol. 2016;99:308–23; PubMed PMID: 26811140. Epub 2016/01/27. eng.
70. Catsburg C, Miller AB, Rohan TE. Adherence to cancer prevention guidelines and risk of breast cancer. Int J Cancer. 2014;135(10):2444–52; PubMed PMID: 24723234. Epub 2014/04/12. eng.
71. Schwingshackl L, Bogensberger B, Hoffmann G. Diet quality as assessed by the healthy eating index, alternate healthy eating index, dietary approaches to stop hypertension score, and health outcomes: an updated systematic review and meta-analysis of cohort studies. J Acad Nutr Diet. 2018;118(1):74–100.e11; PubMed PMID: 29111090. Epub 2017/11/08. eng.
72. Van Blarigan EL, Meyerhardt JA. Role of physical activity and diet after colorectal cancer diagnosis. J Clin Oncol. 2015;33(16):1825–34; PubMed PMID: 25918293. Pubmed Central PMCID: PMC4438267 online at www.jco.org. Author contributions are found at the end of this article. Epub 2015/04/29. eng.
73. Schwingshackl L, Schwedhelm C, Galbete C, Hoffmann G. Adherence to Mediterranean diet and risk of cancer: an updated systematic review and meta-analysis. Nutrients. 2017;9(10):1063; PubMed PMID: 28954418. Pubmed Central PMCID: PMC5691680. Epub 2017/09/29. eng.
74. Beeken RJ, Williams K, Wardle J, Croker H. "What about diet?" A qualitative study of cancer survivors' views on diet and cancer and their sources of information. Eur J Cancer Care. 2016;25(5):774–83; PubMed PMID: 27349812. Pubmed Central PMCID: PMC4995727. Epub 2016/06/29. eng.
75. Koutoukidis DA, Beeken RJ, Lopes S, Knobf MT, Lanceley A. Attitudes, challenges and needs about diet and physical activity in endometrial cancer survivors: a qualitative study. Eur J Cancer Care. 2017;26(6).; PubMed PMID: 27324208. Epub 2016/06/22. eng.

76. Keaver L, McGough AM, Du M, Chang W, Chomitz V, Allen JD, et al. Self-reported changes and perceived barriers to healthy eating and physical activity among global breast cancer survivors: results from an exploratory online novel survey. J Acad Nutr Diet. 2021;121(2):233–41. e8; PubMed PMID: 33109503. Epub 2020/10/29. eng.
77. Koutoukidis DA, Knobf MT, Lanceley A. Obesity, diet, physical activity, and health-related quality of life in endometrial cancer survivors. Nutr Rev. 2015;73(6):399–408; PubMed PMID: 26011914. Pubmed Central PMCID: PMC4477700. Epub 2015/05/27. eng.
78. Hyland KA, Jacobs JM, Lennes IT, Pirl WF, Park ER. Are cancer survivors following the national comprehensive cancer network health behavior guidelines? An assessment of patients attending a cancer survivorship clinic. J Psychosoc Oncol. 2018;36(1):64–81; PubMed PMID: 29303476. Pubmed Central PMCID: PMC6536303. Epub 2018/01/06. eng.
79. Antoni MH, Lechner SC, Kazi A, Wimberly SR, Sifre T, Urcuyo KR, et al. How stress management improves quality of life after treatment for breast cancer. J Consult Clin Psychol. 2006;74(6):1143–52; PubMed PMID: 17154743. Epub 2006/12/13. eng.
80. Herschbach P, Book K, Dinkel A, Berg P, Waadt S, Duran G, et al. Evaluation of two group therapies to reduce fear of progression in cancer patients. Support Care Cancer. 2010;18(4):471–9; PubMed PMID: 19865833. Epub 2009/10/30. eng.
81. Peoples AR, Garland SN, Pigeon WR, Perlis ML, Wolf JR, Heffner KL, et al. Cognitive behavioral therapy for insomnia reduces depression in cancer survivors. J Clin Sleep Med. 2019;15(1):129–37; PubMed PMID: 30621831. Pubmed Central PMCID: PMC6329536. Epub 2019/01/10. eng.
82. Ma Y, Hall DL, Ngo LH, Liu Q, Bain PA, Yeh GY. Efficacy of cognitive behavioral therapy for insomnia in breast cancer: a meta-analysis. Sleep Med Rev. 2021;55:101376; PubMed PMID: 32987319. Epub 2020/09/29. eng.
83. Murphy MJ, Newby JM, Butow P, Loughnan SA, Joubert AE, Kirsten L, et al. Randomised controlled trial of internet-delivered cognitive behaviour therapy for clinical depression and/or anxiety in cancer survivors (iCanADAPT early). Psychooncology. 2020;29(1):76–85; PubMed PMID: 31659822. Epub 2019/10/30. eng.
84. Stagl JM, Bouchard LC, Lechner SC, Blomberg BB, Gudenkauf LM, Jutagir DR, et al. Long-term psychological benefits of cognitive-behavioral stress management for women with breast cancer: 11-year follow-up of a randomized controlled trial. Cancer. 2015;121(11):1873–81; PubMed PMID: 25809235. Pubmed Central PMCID: PMC4441540. Epub 2015/03/27. eng.
85. Nissen ER, O'Connor M, Kaldo V, Højris I, Borre M, Zachariae R, et al. Internet-delivered mindfulness-based cognitive therapy for anxiety and depression in cancer survivors: a randomized controlled trial. Psycho-Oncology. 2020;29(1):68–75; PubMed PMID: 31600414. Pubmed Central PMCID: PMC7004073. Epub 2019/10/11. eng.
86. Bower JE, Crosswell AD, Stanton AL, Crespi CM, Winston D, Arevalo J, et al. Mindfulness meditation for younger breast cancer survivors: a randomized controlled trial. Cancer. 2015;121(8):1231–40; PubMed PMID: 25537522. Pubmed Central PMCID: PMC4393338. Epub 2014/12/30. eng.
87. Carlson LE. Distress management through mind-body therapies in oncology. J Natl Cancer Inst Monogr. 2017;2017(52). PubMed PMID: 29140490. Epub 2017/11/16. eng.
88. Lengacher CA, Reich RR, Paterson CL, Ramesar S, Park JY, Alinat C, et al. Examination of broad symptom improvement resulting from mindfulness-based stress reduction in breast cancer survivors: a randomized controlled trial. J Clin Oncol. 2016;34(24):2827–34; PubMed PMID: 27247219. Pubmed Central PMCID: PMC5012660 online at www.jco.org. Author contributions are found at the end of this article. Epub 2016/06/02. eng.
89. Reich RR, Lengacher CA, Klein TW, Newton C, Shivers S, Ramesar S, et al. A randomized controlled trial of the effects of mindfulness-based stress reduction (MBSR[BC]) on levels of inflammatory biomarkers among recovering breast cancer survivors. Biol Res Nurs. 2017;19(4):456–64; PubMed PMID: 28460534. Pubmed Central PMCID: PMC5942506. Epub 2017/05/04. eng.
90. Cillessen L, Johannsen M, Speckens AEM, Zachariae R. Mindfulness-based interventions for psychological and physical health outcomes in cancer patients and survivors: a

systematic review and meta-analysis of randomized controlled trials. Psychooncology. 2019;28(12):2257–69; PubMed PMID: 31464026. Pubmed Central PMCID: PMC6916350. Epub 2019/08/30. eng.
91. Carlson LE, Tamagawa R, Stephen J, Drysdale E, Zhong L, Speca M. Randomized-controlled trial of mindfulness-based cancer recovery versus supportive expressive group therapy among distressed breast cancer survivors (MINDSET): long-term follow-up results. Psychooncology. 2016;25(7):750–9; PubMed PMID: 27193737. Epub 2016/05/20. eng.
92. Basso JC, McHale A, Ende V, Oberlin DJ, Suzuki WA. Brief, daily meditation enhances attention, memory, mood, and emotional regulation in non-experienced meditators. Behav Brain Res. 2019;356:208–20; PubMed PMID: 30153464. Epub 2018/08/29. eng.
93. Antoni MH, Lutgendorf SK, Blomberg B, Carver CS, Lechner S, Diaz A, et al. Cognitive-behavioral stress management reverses anxiety-related leukocyte transcriptional dynamics. Biol Psychiatry. 2012;71(4):366–72; PubMed PMID: 22088795. Pubmed Central PMCID: PMC3264698. Epub 2011/11/18. eng.
94. Fava GA, McEwen BS, Guidi J, Gostoli S, Offidani E, Sonino N. Clinical characterization of allostatic overload. Psychoneuroendocrinology. 2019;108:94–101; PubMed PMID: 31252304. Epub 2019/06/30. eng.
95. Kinkead B, Schettler PJ, Larson ER, Carroll D, Sharenko M, Nettles J, et al. Massage therapy decreases cancer-related fatigue: results from a randomized early phase trial. Cancer. 2018;124(3):546–54; PubMed PMID: 29044466. Pubmed Central PMCID: PMC5780237. Epub 2017/10/19. eng.
96. Toygar İ, Yeşilbalkan ÖU, Malseven YG, Sönmez E. Effect of reflexology on anxiety and sleep of informal cancer caregiver: randomized controlled trial. Complement Ther Clin Pract. 2020;39:101143; PubMed PMID: 32379631. Epub 2020/05/08. eng.
97. Kim SH, Kim K, Mayer DK. Self-management intervention for adult cancer survivors after treatment: a systematic review and meta-analysis. Oncol Nurs Forum. 2017;44(6):719–28; PubMed PMID: 29052663. Epub 2017/10/21. eng.
98. Dionne-Odom JN, Azuero A, Lyons KD, Hull JG, Tosteson T, Li Z, et al. Benefits of early versus delayed palliative care to informal family caregivers of patients with advanced cancer: outcomes from the ENABLE III randomized controlled trial. J Clin Oncol Off J Am Soc Clin Oncol. 2015;33(13):1446–52; PubMed PMID: 25800762. Pubmed Central PMCID: PMC4404423. Epub 2015/03/25. eng.
99. Bakitas MA, Tosteson TD, Li Z, Lyons KD, Hull JG, Li Z, et al. Early versus delayed initiation of concurrent palliative oncology care: patient outcomes in the ENABLE III randomized controlled trial. J Clin Oncol. 2015;33(13):1438–45; PubMed PMID: 25800768. Pubmed Central PMCID: PMC4404422 online at www.jco.org. Author contributions are found at the end of this article. Epub 2015/03/25. eng.
100. Dionne-Odom JN, Taylor R, Rocque G, Chambless C, Ramsey T, Azuero A, et al. Adapting an early palliative care intervention to family caregivers of persons with advanced cancer in the rural deep south: a qualitative formative evaluation. J Pain Symptom Manag. 2018;55(6):1519–30; PubMed PMID: 29474939. Pubmed Central PMCID: PMC5951755. Epub 2018/02/24. eng.
101. Cuthbert CA, Farragher JF, Hemmelgarn BR, Ding Q, McKinnon GP, Cheung WY. Self-management interventions for cancer survivors: a systematic review and evaluation of intervention content and theories. Psychooncology. 2019;28(11):2119–40; PubMed PMID: 31475766. Epub 2019/09/03. eng.
102. Kavalieratos D, Corbelli J, Zhang D, Dionne-Odom JN, Ernecoff NC, Hanmer J, et al. Association between palliative care and patient and caregiver outcomes: a systematic review and meta-analysis. JAMA. 2016;316(20):2104–14; PubMed PMID: 27893131. Pubmed Central PMCID: PMC5226373. Epub 2016/11/29. eng.
103. Badger TA, Segrin C, Figueredo AJ, Harrington J, Sheppard K, Passalacqua S, et al. Psychosocial interventions to improve quality of life in prostate cancer survivors and their intimate or family partners. Qual Life Res Int J Qual Life Asp Treat Care Rehab.

2011;20(6):833–44; PubMed PMID: 21170682. Pubmed Central PMCID: PMC3117079. Epub 2010/12/21. eng.
104. Montagnese C, Porciello G, Vitale S, Palumbo E, Crispo A, Grimaldi M, et al. Quality of life in women diagnosed with breast cancer after a 12-month treatment of lifestyle modifications. Nutrients. 2021;13:1–15; PubMed PMID: 33396551. Pubmed Central PMCID: PMC7824271. Epub 2021/01/06. eng.
105. (CUP) WCRFICup. Cancer prevention and survival. London: WCRF; 2017.
106. World Cancer Research Fund/AICR. Diet, nutrition, physical activity and cancer: a global perspective. Summary of 3rd expert report. Continuous update project expert report. dietandcancerreport.org; 2018.
107. Schwedhelm C, Boeing H, Hoffmann G, Aleksandrova K, Schwingshackl L. Effect of diet on mortality and cancer recurrence among cancer survivors: a systematic review and meta-analysis of cohort studies. Nutr Rev. 2016;74(12):737–48; PubMed PMID: 27864535. Pubmed Central PMCID: PMC5181206. Epub 2016/11/20. eng.
108. Gao R, Yu T, Liu L, Bi J, Zhao H, Tao Y, et al. Exercise intervention for post-treatment colorectal cancer survivors: a systematic review and meta-analysis. J Cancer Surviv. 2020;14(6):878–93. PubMed PMID: 32533468. Epub 2020/06/14. eng.
109. Nieman DC, Wentz LM. The compelling link between physical activity and the body's defense system. J Sport Health Sci. 2019;8(3):201–17; PubMed PMID: 31193280. Pubmed Central PMCID: PMC6523821. Epub 2019/06/14. eng.
110. Mishra SI, Scherer RW, Geigle PM, Berlanstein DR, Topaloglu O, Gotay CC, et al. Exercise interventions on health-related quality of life for cancer survivors. Cochrane Database Syst Rev. 2012;8:CD007566; PubMed PMID: 22895961. Epub 2012/08/17. eng.
111. Hilfiker R, Meichtry A, Eicher M, Nilsson Balfe L, Knols RH, Verra ML, et al. Exercise and other non-pharmaceutical interventions for cancer-related fatigue in patients during or after cancer treatment: a systematic review incorporating an indirect-comparisons meta-analysis. Br J Sports Med. 2018;52(10):651–8; PubMed PMID: 28501804. Pubmed Central PMCID: PMC5931245. Epub 2017/05/16. eng.
112. Turner RR, Steed L, Quirk H, Greasley RU, Saxton JM, Taylor SJ, et al. Interventions for promoting habitual exercise in people living with and beyond cancer. Cochrane Database Syst Rev. 2018;9(9):CD010192; PubMed PMID: 30229557. Pubmed Central PMCID: PMC6513653 known John Saxton: None known Stephanie Taylor: None known Derek Rosario: None known Mohamed Thaha: None known Liam Bourke: received honoraria for lecturing from Sanofi and Astellas and research funding from the NIHR and CRUK. Epub 2018/09/20. eng.
113. Merluzzi TV, Philip EJ, Yang M, Heitzmann CA. Matching of received social support with need for support in adjusting to cancer and cancer survivorship. Psychooncology. 2016;25(6):684–90; PubMed PMID: 26126444. Pubmed Central PMCID: PMC4960824. Epub 2015/07/02. eng.
114. Foster C, Breckons M, Cotterell P, Barbosa D, Calman L, Corner J, et al. Cancer survivors' self-efficacy to self-manage in the year following primary treatment. J Cancer Surviv. 2015;9(1):11–9; PubMed PMID: 25028218. Pubmed Central PMCID: PMC4341005. Epub 2014/07/17. eng.
115. Merluzzi TV, Serpentini S, Philip EJ, Yang M, Salamanca-Balen N, Heitzmann Ruhf CA, et al. Social relationship coping efficacy: a new construct in understanding social support and close personal relationships in persons with cancer. Psychooncology. 2019;28(1):85–91; PubMed PMID: 30303251. Epub 2018/10/12. eng.
116. Jerofke T, Weiss M, Yakusheva O. Patient perceptions of patient-empowering nurse behaviours, patient activation and functional health status in postsurgical patients with life-threatening long-term illnesses. J Adv Nurs. 2014;70(6):1310–22; PubMed PMID: 24847530.
117. Tomei C, Lebel S, Maheu C, Lefebvre M, Harris C. Examining the preliminary efficacy of an intervention for fear of cancer recurrence in female cancer survivors: a randomized controlled clinical trial pilot study. Support Care Cancer. 2018;26(8):2751–62; PubMed PMID: 29500582. Epub 2018/03/04. eng.

118. Lashbrook MP, Valery PC, Knott V, Kirshbaum MN, Bernardes CM. Coping strategies used by breast, prostate, and colorectal cancer survivors: a literature review. Cancer Nurs. 2018;41(5):E23–39; PubMed PMID: 28723724. Epub 2017/07/21. eng.
119. Lengacher CA, Reich RR, Ramesar S, Alinat CB, Moscoso M, Cousin L, et al. Feasibility of the mobile mindfulness-based stress reduction for breast cancer (mMBSR(BC)) program for symptom improvement among breast cancer survivors. Psychooncology. 2018;27(2):524–31; PubMed PMID: 28665541. Epub 2017/07/01. eng.
120. Hall DL, Luberto CM, Philpotts LL, Song R, Park ER, Yeh GY. Mind-body interventions for fear of cancer recurrence: a systematic review and meta-analysis. Psychooncology. 2018;27(11):2546–58; PubMed PMID: 29744965. Pubmed Central PMCID: PMC6488231. Epub 2018/05/11. eng.
121. Haugland T, Wahl AK, Hofoss D, DeVon HA. Association between general self-efficacy, social support, cancer-related stress and physical health-related quality of life: a path model study in patients with neuroendocrine tumors. Health Qual Life Outcomes. 2016;14:11; PubMed PMID: 26787226. Pubmed Central PMCID: PMC4717553. Epub 2016/01/21. eng.
122. Uchino BN. Social support and health: a review of physiological processes potentially underlying links to disease outcomes. J Behav Med. 2006;29(4):377–87; PubMed PMID: 16758315. Epub 2006/06/08. eng.
123. Uchino BN, Bowen K, Carlisle M, Birmingham W. Psychological pathways linking social support to health outcomes: a visit with the "ghosts" of research past, present, and future. Soc Sci Med. 2012;74(7):949–57; PubMed PMID: 22326104. Pubmed Central PMCID: PMC3298603. Epub 2012/02/14. eng.
124. Desautels C, Trudel-Fitzgerald C, Ruel S, Ivers H, Savard J. Do cancer-related beliefs influence the severity, incidence, and persistence of psychological symptoms? Cancer Nurs. 2017;40(4):E50–E8; PubMed PMID: 27398794. Epub 2016/07/12. eng.
125. Dantzer R, Capuron L, Irwin MR, Miller AH, Ollat H, Perry VH, et al. Identification and treatment of symptoms associated with inflammation in medically ill patients. Psychoneuroendocrinology. 2008;33(1):18–29; PubMed PMID: 18061362. Pubmed Central PMCID: 2234599.
126. Mishra SI, Scherer RW, Snyder C, Geigle PM, Berlanstein DR, Topaloglu O. Exercise interventions on health-related quality of life for people with cancer during active treatment. Cochrane Database Syst Rev. 2012;2012(8):CD008465; PubMed PMID: 22895974. Pubmed Central PMCID: PMC7389071. Epub 2012/08/17. eng.
127. Reich RR, Lengacher CA, Alinat CB, Kip KE, Paterson C, Ramesar S, et al. Mindfulness-based stress reduction in post-treatment breast cancer patients: immediate and sustained effects across multiple symptom clusters. J Pain Symptom Manag. 2017;53(1):85–95; PubMed PMID: 27720794. Epub 2016/10/11. eng.
128. Jassim GA, Whitford DL, Hickey A, Carter B. Psychological interventions for women with non-metastatic breast cancer. Cochrane Database Syst Rev. 2015;5:CD008729; PubMed PMID: 26017383. Epub 2015/05/29. eng.
129. Benson H, Stuart E. The wellness book: the comprehensive guide to maintaining health and treating stress-related illness. New York: Simon and Schuster; 1992.
130. Thong MSY, van Noorden CJF, Steindorf K, Arndt V. Cancer-related fatigue: causes and current treatment options. Curr Treat Options in Oncol. 2020;21(2):17; PubMed PMID: 32025928. Pubmed Central PMCID: PMC8660748. Epub 2020/02/07. eng.
131. Gielissen MF, Verhagen S, Witjes F, Bleijenberg G. Effects of cognitive behavior therapy in severely fatigued disease-free cancer patients compared with patients waiting for cognitive behavior therapy: a randomized controlled trial. J Clin Oncol. 2006;24(30):4882–7; PubMed PMID: 17050873. Epub 2006/10/20. eng.
132. McCusker J, Yaffe M, Faria R, Lambert S, Li M, Poirier-Bisson J, et al. Phase II trial of a depression self-care intervention for adult cancer survivors. Eur J Cancer Care. 2017;6; PubMed PMID: 28984000. Epub 2017/10/07. eng.

References

133. Zeng Y, Dong J, Huang M, Zhang JE, Zhang X, Xie M, et al. Nonpharmacological interventions for cancer-related cognitive impairment in adult cancer patients: a network meta-analysis. Int J Nurs Stud. 2020;104:103514; PubMed PMID: 32004776. Epub 2020/02/01. eng.
134. Leventhal H, Phillips LA, Burns E. The common-sense model of self-regulation (CSM): a dynamic framework for understanding illness self-management. J Behav Med. 2016;39(6):935–46; PubMed PMID: 27515801. Epub 2016/08/16. eng.
135. Windsor TD, Curtis RG, Luszcz MA. Sense of purpose as a psychological resource for aging well. Dev Psychol. 2015;51(7):975–86; PubMed PMID: 26010384. Epub 2015/05/27. eng.
136. Mosher CE, Winger JG, Hanna N, Jalal SI, Einhorn LH, Birdas TJ, et al. Randomized pilot trial of a telephone symptom management intervention for symptomatic lung cancer patients and their family caregivers. J Pain Symptom Manag. 2016;52(4):469–82; PubMed PMID: 27401514. Pubmed Central PMCID: PMC5075493. Epub 2016/10/25. eng.
137. Winger JG, Adams RN, Mosher CE. Relations of meaning in life and sense of coherence to distress in cancer patients: a meta-analysis. Psychooncology. 2016;25(1):2–10; PubMed PMID: 25787699. Pubmed Central PMCID: PMC4575247. Epub 2015/03/20. eng.
138. Boyle PA, Buchman AS, Bennett DA. Purpose in life is associated with a reduced risk of incident disability among community-dwelling older persons. Am J Geriatr Psychiatry. 2010;18(12):1093–102; PubMed PMID: 20808115. Pubmed Central PMCID: PMC2992099. Epub 2010/09/03. eng.
139. Boyle PA, Barnes LL, Buchman AS, Bennett DA. Purpose in life is associated with mortality among community-dwelling older persons. Psychosom Med. 2009;71(5):574–9; PubMed PMID: 19414613. Pubmed Central PMCID: PMC2740716. Epub 2009/05/06. eng.
140. Steptoe A, Deaton A, Stone AA. Subjective wellbeing, health, and ageing. Lancet. 2015;385(9968):640–8; PubMed PMID: 25468152. Pubmed Central PMCID: PMC4339610. Epub 2014/12/04. eng.
141. van der Spek N, Vos J, van Uden-Kraan CF, Breitbart W, Cuijpers P, Holtmaat K, et al. Efficacy of meaning-centered group psychotherapy for cancer survivors: a randomized controlled trial. Psychol Med. 2017;47(11):1990–2001; PubMed PMID: 28374663. Pubmed Central PMCID: PMC5501751. Epub 2017/04/05. eng.
142. Lee V, Cohen SR, Edgar L, Laizner AM, Gagnon AJ. Meaning-making and psychological adjustment to cancer: development of an intervention and pilot results. Oncol Nurs Forum. 2006;33(2):291–302; PubMed PMID: 16518445. Epub 2006/03/07. eng.
143. Lee V. The existential plight of cancer: meaning making as a concrete approach to the intangible search for meaning. Support Care Cancer. 2008;16(7):779–85; PubMed PMID: 18197427. Epub 2008/01/17. eng.
144. Lee V, Cohen SR, Edgar L, Laizner AM, Gagnon AJ. Clarifying "meaning" in the context of cancer research: a systematic literature review. Palliat Support Care. 2004;2(3):291–303; PubMed PMID: 16594414. Epub 2006/04/06. eng.
145. Haber D. Life review: implementation, theory, research, and therapy. Int J Aging Hum Dev. 2006;63(2):153–71; PubMed PMID: 17137032. Epub 2006/12/02. eng.
146. de van der Schueren MAE, Laviano A, Blanchard H, Jourdan M, Arends J, Baracos VE. Systematic review and meta-analysis of the evidence for oral nutritional intervention on nutritional and clinical outcomes during chemo(radio)therapy: current evidence and guidance for design of future trials. Ann Oncol. 2018;29(5):1141–53; PubMed PMID: 29788170. Pubmed Central PMCID: PMC5961292. Epub 2018/05/23. eng.
147. McEwen BS, Karatsoreos IN. Sleep deprivation and circadian disruption: stress, allostasis, and allostatic load. Sleep Med Clin. 2015;10(1):1–10; PubMed PMID: 26055668. Epub 2015/06/10. eng.
148. Porciello G, Montagnese C, Crispo A, Grimaldi M, Libra M, Vitale S, et al. Mediterranean diet and quality of life in women treated for breast cancer: a baseline analysis of DEDiCa multicentre trial. PLoS One. 2020;15(10):e0239803; PubMed PMID: 33031478. Pubmed Central PMCID: PMC7544033 following competing interests: LSAA is a founding member of the International Carbohydrate Quality Consortium (ICQC) and has received honoraria from the Nutrition Foundation of Italy (NFI), research grants from LILT (a non-profit orga-

nization for the fight against cancer) and in-kind research support from Abiogen Pharma, the Almond Board of California (USA), Barilla (Italy), Consorzio Mandorle di Avola (Italy), DietaDoc (Italy), Ello Frutta (Italy), Panificio Giacomo Luongo (Italy), Perrotta (Italy), Roberto Alimentare (Italy), SunRice (Australia). However, no funding that she has received has been involved in the current project. GLB reports personal fees from Janssen-Cilag, personal fees from Boehringer Ingelheim, personal fees from Roche, non-financial support from Bristol-Myers Squibb, non-financial support from AstraZeneca/MedImmune, non-financial support from Pierre Fabre, non-financial support from Ipsen, outside the submitted work. DG has received speaking and/or consulting fees from Abiogen Pharma, Amgen, Eli-Lilly, Janssen-Cilag, Merck and Mundipharma. MP has received research support from Amgen. GR has received research grants from the Barilla Company to his University Department and is member of the scientific advisory boards of the foundation "Barilla Center for Food and Nutrition" and of "Nutrition Foundation of Italy". DJAJ has received research grants from Saskatchewan & Alberta Pulse Growers Associations, the Agricultural Bioproducts Innovation Program through the Pulse Research Network, the Advanced Foods and Material Network, Loblaw Companies Ltd., Unilever Canada and Netherlands, Barilla, the Almond Board of California, Agriculture and Agri-food Canada, Pulse Canada, Kellogg's Company, Canada, Quaker Oats, Canada, Procter & Gamble Technical Centre Ltd., Bayer Consumer Care, Springfield, NJ, Pepsi/Quaker, International Nut & Dried Fruit (INC), Soy Foods Association of North America, the Coca-Cola Company (investigator initiated, unrestricted grant), Solae, Haine Celestial, the Sanitarium Company, Orafti, the International Tree Nut Council Nutrition Research and Education Foundation, the Peanut Institute, Soy Nutrition Institute (SNI), the Canola and Flax Councils of Canada, the Calorie Control Council, the Canadian Institutes of Health Research (CIHR), the Canada Foundation for Innovation (CFI)and the Ontario Research Fund (ORF). He has received in-kind supplies for trials as a research support from the Almond board of California, Walnut Council of California, American Peanut Council, Barilla, Unilever, Unico, Primo, Loblaw Companies, Quaker (Pepsico), Pristine Gourmet, Bunge Limited, Kellogg Canada, WhiteWave Foods. He has been on the speaker's panel, served on the scientific advisory board and/or received travel support and/or honoraria from the Almond Board of California, Canadian Agriculture Policy Institute, Loblaw Companies Ltd, the Griffin Hospital (for the development of the NuVal scoring system), the Coca-Cola Company, EPICURE, Danone, Diet Quality Photo Navigation (DQPN), Better Therapeutics (FareWell), Verywell, True Health Initiative (THI), Heali AI Corp, Institute of Food Technologists (IFT), Soy Nutrition Institute (SNI), Herbalife Nutrition Institute (HNI), Saskatchewan & Alberta Pulse Growers Associations, Sanitarium Company, Orafti, the American Peanut Council, the International Tree Nut Council Nutrition Research and Education Foundation, the Peanut Institute, Herbalife International, Pacific Health Laboratories, Nutritional Fundamentals for Health (NFH), Barilla, Metagenics, Bayer Consumer Care, Unilever Canada and Netherlands, Solae, Kellogg, Quaker Oats, Procter & Gamble, Abbott Laboratories, Dean Foods, the California Strawberry Commission, Haine Celestial, PepsiCo, the Alpro Foundation, Pioneer Hi-Bred International, DuPont Nutrition and Health, Spherix Consulting and WhiteWave Foods, the Advanced Foods and Material Network, the Canola and Flax Councils of Canada, Agri-Culture and Agri-Food Canada, the Canadian Agri-Food Policy Institute, Pulse Canada, the Soy Foods Association of North America, the Nutrition Foundation of Italy (NFI), Nutra-Source Diagnostics, the McDougall Program, the Toronto Knowledge Translation Group (St. Michael's Hospital), the Canadian College of Naturopathic Medicine, The Hospital for Sick Children, the Canadian Nutrition Society (CNS), the American Society of Nutrition (ASN), Arizona State University, Paolo Sorbini Foundation and the Institute of Nutrition, Metabolism and Diabetes. He received an honorarium from the United States Department of Agriculture to present the 2013 W.O. Atwater Memorial Lecture. He received the 2013 Award for Excellence in Research from the International Nut and Dried Fruit Council. He received funding and travel support from the Canadian Society of Endocrinology and Metabolism to produce mini cases for the Canadian Diabetes Association (CDA). He is a member of the International Carbohydrate

Quality Consortium (ICQC). His wife, Alexandra L Jenkins, is a director and partner of INQUIS Clinical Research for the Food Industry, his 2 daughters, Wendy Jenkins and Amy Jenkins, have published a vegetarian book that promotes the use of the foods described here, The Portfolio Diet for Cardiovascular Risk Reduction (Academic Press/Elsevier 2020 ISBN:978-0-12-810510-8) and his sister, Caroline Brydson, received funding through a grant from the St. Michael's Hospital Foundation to develop a cookbook for one of his studies. He has had close contact with the food industry to produce plant based diets. However, no funding that he has received has been involved in the current project. All other authors declare no competing interests. This does not alter our adherence to PLOS ONE policies on sharing data and materials. Epub 2020/10/09. eng.
149. Gupta C, Prakash D. Phytonutrients as therapeutic agents. J Complement Integr Med. 2014;11(3):151–69; PubMed PMID: 25051278. Epub 2014/07/23. eng.
150. World Cancer Research Fund, American Institute for Cancer Research. Food, nutrition, physical activity and the prevention of cancer: a global perspective. Washington, DC: American Institute for Cancer Research; 2007.
151. Coro DG, Hutchinson AD, Banks S, Coates AM. Diet and cognitive function in cancer survivors with cancer-related cognitive impairment: a qualitative study. Eur J Cancer Care. 2020;29(6):e13303; PubMed PMID: 32875677. Epub 2020/09/03. eng.
152. Coro D, Hutchinson A, Dahlenburg S, Banks S, Coates A. The relationship between diet and cognitive function in adult cancer survivors: a systematic review. J Cancer Surviv. 2019;13(5):773–91; PubMed PMID: 31399855. Epub 2019/08/11. eng.
153. McGrattan AM, McGuinness B, McKinley MC, Kee F, Passmore P, Woodside JV, et al. Diet and inflammation in cognitive ageing and Alzheimer's disease. Curr Nutr Rep. 2019;8(2):53–65; PubMed PMID: 30949921. Pubmed Central PMCID: PMC6486891. Epub 2019/04/06. eng.
154. Spei ME, Samoli E, Bravi F, La Vecchia C, Bamia C, Benetou V. Physical activity in breast cancer survivors: a systematic review and meta-analysis on overall and breast cancer survival. Breast. 2019;44:144–52; PubMed PMID: 30780085. Epub 2019/02/20. eng.
155. Bourke L, Smith D, Steed L, Hooper R, Carter A, Catto J, et al. Exercise for men with prostate cancer: a systematic review and meta-analysis. Eur Urol. 2016;69(4):693–703; PubMed PMID: 26632144. Epub 2015/12/04. eng.

Supportive Care and End of Life 18

> Hope" is the thing with feathers
> That perches in the soul
> And sings the tune without the words
> And never stops - at all."
>
> Emily Dickinson

18.1 Introduction

Supportive cancer care is the last phase in a continuous journey of the nurse, patient, and caregiver which starts at diagnosis through to the end of life, and just afterward, with the patient's funeral which may include serving as a source of support in the early phase of caregiver and family mourning. It is a continuity-of-nursing care perspective that enables the patient and family to feel secure in the knowledge that the nurse knows them well as whole individuals, promoting their healing and resilient capabilities. Some patients and family caregivers with early stage disease may be fortunate to step off the cancer trajectory indefinitely. Some patients with stage 1 to stage 3 cancers and deemed "treatable" at diagnosis, nevertheless arrive in the terminal phase. And others, diagnosed with stage 4 advanced cancer, make incredible recoveries. All patients and their caregivers regardless of the type of cancer or stage throughout the continuum should be encouraged to participate in comprehensive multimodal, multitargeted, and tailored psychosocial nursing interventions to promote quality of life, wellness, acceptance, and comfort according to their clinical status. The content of these interventions may vary as a function of the main concerns and clinical state of the patient. This is so, especially, for patients in the nonactive treatment phase of supportive care services.

18.2 Objectives

At the end of this chapter, you will have knowledge of:

- Palliative/supportive care interventions for patients with advanced/terminal disease, and their family caregiver
- Clinical criteria considered in the cessation of active treatment
- Patient and family caregiver concerns during the immediate cessation of treatment phase
- Patient and caregiver concerns during the terminal phase
- Empirically known psychosocial nursing interventions

Clinical Anecdote 18.1
Each person deals with this ultimate rite of passage in his or her own way, in his or her own time. Some appear to face the unfathomable with purposeful acquiescence. 'I am now ready to explore what awaits me beyond the boundaries of a life well lived.'

Others, despite the odds, fight for every day they can rob death of its final reckoning. People have their beliefs: a life fulfilled but wanting more or a life incomplete with goals unrealized. Others are gripped by an overwhelming fear of the unknown, and of being 'alone' even in death. In the end, most people find comfort when they are surrounded by love and understanding and an ability to die on their own terms.

18.3 Definition

A medical trend in oncology refers to any patient with advanced disease as "palliative" starting at diagnosis even when active treatment is given [1]. This chapter focuses on the supportive care phase starting mainly with the end of active treatment usually associated with disease progression. Palliative care or supportive care continues until the death of the patient, and extends into the mourning period of the grieving caregiver and family [2].

Disease progression is typically accompanied by a more intensified symptom burden which generally includes greater pain, physical discomfort, and psychological suffering in patients. Family caregivers experience feelings of growing helplessness and distress with the realization that their loved one's life is drawing to a close [2]. During this phase of illness, both family and the patient need one another, and the support of a compassionate and tailored nursing approach. In keeping with the stress, healing and resilience nursing model, the philosophy, goals and interventions of whole person care are consistent across the patient continuum. The model is aimed at all patients with cancer and family caregivers regardless of the stage or phase of the illness, shaped only by the changing health-related needs of the patient and family caregiver.

Table 18.1 Suggested criteria for transfer to supportive care services [3–5]

Major criteria	Of 36 other "minor" criteria identified:
Severe physical symptoms such as uncontrolled pain and severe fatigue	Hypercalcemia
Severe emotional symptoms	Bone and/or liver metastases
Disease recurrence and/or cancer progression uncontrolled by active treatment	Malignant ascites
Emergency visits related to clinical status	Moderate physical symptoms (4–6 on 10-point scale)
Rapid deterioration of physical status	Moderate emotional symptoms (4–6 on 10-point scale)
Patient requests transfer	Inadequate support
Multiorgan failure (very late)	Decision-making or care planning needs
Brain/leptomeningeal metastases within 3 months of diagnosis of advanced disease	
Request for hastened death	
Advanced bone and/or liver metastases	

18.4 Cessation of Treatment

NCCN Guidelines on palliative/supportive care suggest that the process of transitioning to supportive care services occurs when active treatment no longer is a viable option by the oncology treatment team (Table 18.1) [6]. Cancer progression and/or severe and unacceptable side effects preclude further treatment. Subsequently, supportive care becomes the main therapeutic option for patients and family [6–8]. Notwithstanding, the timing of palliative care referrals has been problematic, for example, only 28% of patients with advanced ovarian cancer used palliative care referrals, and 38% transferred to palliative care within only 30 days of death [9, 10]. Because of negative connotations associated with the term "palliative," these services are increasingly known as *supportive care* which tends to result in earlier, more successful referrals [9, 11, 12]. Both patients and family caregivers remain the main unit of nursing care. Following the patient's death, the family continues to be supported through the bereavement phase [6].

18.5 Transition to Supportive Care Services

Marsella [13] has identified characteristics of the transition phase that contribute to patient and family distress at the end of active treatment.

Nature of Transition and Lack of Information

The transition phase involves *changes* in the goals of care, in patient and family roles, the composition and roles of the healthcare team, and frequently the location of care. Patients and families may be confused about the goals of *active* versus *palliative chemotherapy*, and the nature of a cure versus palliation [12, 14]. They need the opportunity to discuss their feelings of impending loss, sadness, fear, helplessness, and fear of abandonment associated with the transfer to a new team [6, 13].

During the transition (if not sooner), the patient and caregiver are introduced to the supportive care physician and nurse, and learn about the various healthcare services and resources, the in-hospital supportive care unit, hospice, and home care [15, 16]. Because patients with cancer may deteriorate unexpectedly, the time needed to fulfill the patient's and family's stated goals and wishes for realizing an optimal end of life may be challenging, and depends in part on the patient's and family's readiness to make decisions and take action. Miscommunications during transition can lead to complicated and conflicted feelings and adverse beliefs about the loved one's quality of care which often emerges only after his or her death [12].

Timing

The optimal time to introduce supportive care services has become a notable topic in the supportive care literature due to clinical observations that many patients are transferred too late or are reluctant at first to transfer in order to fully benefit from supportive care services [4, 17, 18]. Recent studies suggest that earlier rather than later access to supportive care services may provide greater quality of life for patients with advanced disease and their caregivers, although meta-analyses report only small effect size improvements over usual care, especially regarding the health-related outcomes of caregivers [17, 19]. Patients who received 8.5 *months* or more of supportive care were less likely to receive chemotherapy and more likely to experience a better quality of life. Those with more than 8 *weeks* of palliative care had more than a three-fold chance of dying at home, received more opioid medication, and experienced fewer emergency room visits [17]. Early supportive care (more than 3 months before death) for patients with end-stage disease was associated with an improved symptom burden, better quality of life, and a decrease in aggressive chemotherapy and resuscitative efforts [20, 21]. Notwithstanding there also appeared to be differential results according to the type of terminal cancer, for instance, lung cancer versus gastrointestinal cancer [21]. Conversely, caregiver outcomes were mixed, and their health-related issues remained a clinical concern (e.g., [22, 23]).

Clinical Anecdote 18.2
Mr R and his wife knew that Mr R's advanced cancer and obvious physical decline meant that they had to come to terms with his approaching death. For the first time in 60 years they would have to go their separate ways until 'reunited' in the afterlife. This realization was particularly hard for Mrs R to accept. But in those final weeks, at the couple's insistence, what made it more bearable was that Mr R was cared for in a medical rather than palliative care unit. It represented hope over hopelessness.

18.6 Patient Concerns, Distress, and Symptom Burden

Many patients still die without an opportunity for psychological healing, personal growth, inner peace, and acceptance. This may be due to many factors, including the lack of advanced practice clinical nurses who possess specialized knowledge, psychosocial strategies, and expert skills of communication needed to create a healing environment for patients and loved ones [2, 24–27].

Patients seek relief from the intensified symptoms of progressive disease, and relief from existential suffering (e.g., [28]). Most seek love, presence, and support from family and friends, and an evidentiary conviction that the nurse and oncologist will be readily accessible to ensure physical and emotional comfort, technical and medical expertise, and an engaged and compassionate presence. Many want information about what to expect clinically as the disease advances, and how to manage various symptoms, especially at home. Some will seek and find solace in religion or the spiritual [29]. All seek an oncologist and nurse who can promote their quality of life for as long as possible, suggest effective coping strategies, facilitate their last wishes in a timely manner, and enable, for as long as possible, physical comfort and cognitive clarity in the presence of loved ones.

Emotional Distress and Existential Suffering (Review Part IV Chap. 10)

Terminating active treatment may ignite feelings of extreme emotional distress, confusion, fear and uncertainty about the goals of medical and nursing care in relation to their chances of survival (e.g., [30]). The transition to supportive care signals a clear message that one's life is drawing to a close, which may trigger a crisis of existential distress [31–33]. Existential suffering occurs when a severe threat calls into question "fundamental expectations about security, interrelatedness with justness, controllability, certainty and hope for a long life" [34, p. 2526]. It refers to a state of powerlessness, meaninglessness, death anxiety, and futility in the face of a threat, such as the existential threat of nonexistence and/or beliefs in one's impending mortality, which can have profound disruptive effects on self-identity (e.g., [34]). Existential distress can be characterized by spiritual distress, hopelessness, and demoralization, and is associated with a perceived loss of control, physical suffering, profound loneliness, anticipatory grief, regrets, and/or embitterment about an unfulfilled life [35–37]. It may be exacerbated when patients perceive a lack of emotional support from significant others, feel they are a burden to loved ones, perceive a lack of adequate communication with the supportive care team and for some, experience a heightened awareness of aloneness, borne of the realization that in irrefutable ways their life is on a path distinct from their loved ones [38]. These thoughts and feelings may come into acute focus when the patient and family experience new caregivers at the end of life—people who no longer *know* them [39].

Symptom Burden

A high symptom burden can contribute to a demoralized state of existential suffering [31, 38]. As cancer progresses, the individual's symptom burden intensifies. Regardless of cancer type, an estimated 38–64% of patients endure severe-to-difficult to control pain in the end of life phase which may present as part of a symptom cluster with depression and fatigue [40]. Pain continues to be undertreated in an estimated one third of patients with advanced cancer [41, 42]. In addition to pain, patients generally suffer anxiety, chronic fatigue, cachexia, nausea and vomiting, constipation, and/or breathlessness [43, 44]. Constipation is a common symptom frequently related to increased opioid intake and/or an abdominal blockage [2]. There is compelling evidence that delays in identifying patients who need palliative care lead to poor quality of life and can even negatively impact interventions to effectively manage symptoms and provide optimal physical comfort [2].

18.7 Family Caregiver Concerns

Caregiver burden refers to the extent to which the individual feels that their emotional, physical, social, and/or financial health has been compromised as a consequence of caring for the patient [45]. Family caregivers tend to be older and female. They also tend to feel they have insufficient knowledge and skills to manage the medical, personal and family-related concerns of their loved one [46–49]. Caregivers are involved in daily management of progressively worsening patient symptoms, they monitor the patient's emotional and physical health, and provide various supportive functions for the patient, day in and day out. Given *corroborated evidence of the reciprocal* emotional relationship between patient and family caregiver, the patient's poor prognosis, advancing disease and increased symptom burden significantly contribute not only to the patient's but family caregiver's distress [50–52]. Family caregivers may experience even greater emotional distress, depression and anxiety than their loved one as they bear witness to the deteriorating signs of disease progression and impending death, which are only reinforced when supportive care services are perceived as failing to meet patient and caregiver needs [47, 53, 54].

A systematic review of ten studies revealed that the pain experienced by patients with advanced cancer who were cared for at home, was influenced by the carer's distress related to care giving responsibilities, knowledge of pain management, distress experienced by both patient and caregiver, and the extent to which pain ratings between patient and caregiver were concordant or divergent [55]. An unreasonable caregiving burden carried by an increasingly distressed carer, may be associated with ineffective pain management, contributing to the patient's suffering [53, 56]. Family caregivers who looked after their loved one at home with the support of a palliative outreach program revealed the need for healthcare assistance to address *their own feelings* of losing control, anger toward the patient, and a desire to leave care to someone else [53].

Compounding their caregiving-distress, family caregivers have little time to exercise, attend to other family responsibilities, engage in social activities, or care for their own health-related needs [48, 57]. More than half are at risk health-wise due to lack of sleep, fatigue, and often their own neglected chronic illnesses (e.g., [45, 58]). This cumulative stress is also manifested by negative effects on their physical health, immune function, and financial well-being [59].

The cumulative evidence points toward family caregivers who require greater clinical support for patient care which only amplifies in the terminal phase [54, 60, 61]. As death encroaches, caregivers may find care giving itself too emotionally and physically draining [45]. Many caregivers may be hesitant to ask for help.

18.8 Clinical Benefits of Early Integrated Oncology-Supportive Care Services

The idea of integrating supportive care with oncology care in ambulatory clinic settings for patients with *advanced disease* has received widespread oncologic support [62]. In this model of care, *integrated oncology and supportive* care teams work in tandem to provide comprehensive care across ambulatory settings, community, family settings, and in-patient palliative care units (e.g., [22]). Starting in the diagnostic phase, the supportive care team manages symptoms and side effects and addresses coping-related issues in the clinic, whereas the oncology team "treats the disease" in patients with *advanced cancer*. Both teams frequently include more than one advanced clinical nurse although the goals of nursing care from a *medical perspective* may differ. The medical philosophy of the oncology and supportive care approach is to enable relationships to be established over time between the patients with advanced disease (and their family caregivers), and the supportive care team, in principle, enabling a more seamless transition to supportive care [62, 63].

Although this clinical approach to patients with advanced disease is gaining widespread acceptance, care still must be taken not to directly assign advanced patients to a supportive care team even as the patient receives active treatment, without taking serious and full measure of the sensibilities, philosophy and preferences of the patient and caregiver. The majority of patients presenting with Stage 3 disease are likely to recover completely or live well with a chronic illness, and may balk at being assigned at diagnosis, to the supportive care team even as they continue active treatment [11]. They may balk at being assigned to a supportive care nurse rather than a nurse on the treatment team when they perceive themselves as healthy and their emotional reactivity as normal, given the diagnosis. It also must be acknowledged that an ever increasing proportion of stage 4 patients are prolonging their survivability thanks to the latest pharmacotherapeutics. However well intentioned, the majority of patients with stage 3–4 disease who may eventually qualify for "palliative" supportive care services may not be so amenable in the diagnostic phase [17]. To assume otherwise may be to intensify the patient's emotional distress, amplifying the biological stress response system with its corresponding suppression of immune functions, including innate immune and cell mediated immune activities needed for cancer surveillance and elimination [64].

Extreme clinical sensitivity must be exercised when individuals *with advanced disease* are designated supportive care patients at diagnosis. The goal of transitioning to supportive care at any phase of advanced disease requires tremendous professional sensitivity and depends in large part on the patient's clinical status, how they feel physically and how the information is conveyed [65]. Patient expectations refer to "specific cognitions about the likelihood of future events" [65, p. 602]. Patients tend to hold specific expectations about their illness, the efficacy of the treatment, the side effects and even their ability to modulate clinical outcomes. Bundle all these expectations together and it reflects something about the patient's hopes.

Clinical Anecdote 18.3 (Review Hope Chap. 9)
Mr M was an extremely intelligent and highly successful self-made man who provided a luxurious lifestyle for himself, his wife and teenage daughter. At 47 he showed no signs of slowing down. But at the urging of his wife Mr M went for a check up because of a dry cough and shortness-of-breath that had increased over the previous few months. It came as a profound shock to be told he had advanced nonoperable cancer. Although he received anti-cancer treatment, he clearly 'remembered' being told that he had 'about 11 months to live' and should 'get his affairs in order'. After that, the patient quickly went downhill. According to his family, he simply gave up, became depressed and without hope. He essentially succumbed to that prognosis, dying exactly 11 months later.

This clinical anecdote illustrates how a health professional's attitudes and behaviors, even when well intentioned, may suppress the patient's hope regarding his treatment and possibly hasten death. Hope helps patients manage health-related threats and uncertainty, even when having hope appears to be unrealistic. It provides an emotional buffer while the patient comes to terms with his life threatening clinical reality [66]. To challenge the patient's "unrealistic" expectations is to potentially plummet the patient into the morass of hopelessness (Review Part IV, Chap. 9). Clinical research shows that a sense of hopelessness is a key property of demoralization and is associated with depression, and a desire for a hastened death in individuals with cancer and progressive disease [34, 67, 68]. A sense of hopelessness also is associated with suppressed cell mediated immunity as also evidenced by patients with breast cancer [69, 70]. By dashing the patient's cognitive expectations about treatment, the patient's doctor may have eradicated any patient hope regarding his future, and unwittingly may even have hastened his death.

It is not that the patients' beliefs per se can "save" an individual from cancer's life-threatening reality. But a body of clinical research strongly suggests that having hope even as a palliative patient tends to improve the deleterious effects of symptoms including depression and anxiety, improve cell mediated immune functions, and enhance quality of life and posttraumatic growth [71, 72]. Providing patients with a positive upbeat description of how the team plans to *optimize his or her wellness f*or as long as possible, *may support the patient's hope* in the early palliative phase giving the family and patient metaphorical space to come to terms with the consequential implications of ending treatment [1, 20, 21, 73]. Providing in a general way the research findings of prolonged survival for instance, from Temel's study of supportive care patients with advanced lung cancer [1, 21]. Highlighting the value of mutually supportive patient-family caregiver relationships on immunity may help to attenuate the initial distress of becoming a 'supportive care' patient. [74–76]. (Other psychosocial strategies will be discussed in the Nursing approaches section).

18.9   RCTs: Psychosocial Interventions

Supportive care services usually take place in supportive care hospital units, ambulatory oncology clinics and in the community (home or hospice care). According to different models of care, the focus of psychosocial interventions may be the patient, the patient–caregiver dyad, and/or the family caregiver.

Patient-Focused Studies (Appendix A)

Integrated supportive care may refer to the care received by patients with advanced disease who are on active treatment at diagnosis with supportive care providing psychosocial and symptom-related interventions. When treatment is no longer viable, the patient continues with the supportive care team. In a meta-analysis of 43 RCTs ($N = 12{,}731$) compared to usual care, palliative care interventions effectively improved *quality of life* and decreased *symptom burden* in patients with advanced disease at the 1- to 3 month-follow-up [77]. When only five trials with low risk of bias were analyzed, the supportive care effect size on the patient's *quality of life* was reduced but remained significant compared to usual care. No significant improvement in either symptom burden or length of survival was found. Palliative care was associated with improvements in patient *satisfaction, advance care planning*, and less use of *health care resources* consistent with a self-management model of care [77]. The sample consisted of patients with advanced cancer (69.7%) and heart failure (32.5%) who were cared for in ambulatory care, home based, and in hospital. Because of substantial heterogeneity across trials, the results need to be interpreted with caution.

Conversely, in a meta-analysis of eight randomized controlled and two cluster-randomized trials, an integrated supportive/oncology care intervention significantly improved quality of life and symptom burden in patients, compared to usual care [78]. When trials with greater homogeneity were analyzed ($I^2 = 0\%$), the supportive care component appeared to significantly decrease all-cause mortality [78]. The patients received active treatment while also being cared for by supportive care services for physical and psychological symptoms and side effects.

In a landmark RCT of 151 newly diagnosed patients with metastatic nonsmall cell lung cancer, the early *integrated palliative*/oncology care intervention starting after diagnosis was significantly more effective in improving quality of life compared to usual care. (It begs the question: how was "usual" care defined?) Moreover, fewer patients in the intervention than usual care group reported symptoms of depression. Although fewer patients in the intervention than usual care group experienced aggressive end-of-life care, the early supportive care group still showed a longer median survival of 11.6 months compared to 8.9 months [1]. There were also fewer ER visits and hospitalizations compared to usual care. Interventions involved discussions with the patient about the illness, treatment goals; information guiding treatment decisions, advance care planning, patient care-related preferences, symptom management, learning effective coping strategies, spiritual coping, managing moods, redirecting hope; establishing a "rapport" with patient and caregiver; conducting a life review, facilitating caregiver referrals to meet their special health-related needs [21] (Appendix A). Advanced practice nursing care of patients with cancer across *all stages* of the disease should provide similar a whole person approach drawing on relevant psychosocial interventions.

Another RCT of newly diagnosed incurable lung cancer and/or colorectal GI cancer ($N = 350$) based on the same early integrated-palliative/oncological care intervention compared to usual care revealed differential effects according to cancer type [21]. Patients with lung cancer demonstrated significant improvements in quality of life and depression at 12 and 24 weeks over baseline scores whereas patients in the usual care group deteriorated. Conversely, patients with GI cancer in both the early integrated palliative care intervention and usual care group showed improvements in QOL and mood only at 12 weeks. However, those in the palliative care intervention were more apt to discuss their wishes with healthcare providers compared to the *usual care group* when they realized they were in the terminal phase (30.2% versus 14.5% $P = 0.004$) [21].

The importance of tailoring interventions to the specific needs of patients with different forms of cancer may be underscored by the differential results of patients with lung versus GI cancer. The GI patients appeared to have greater clinical care demands, greater complexity of treatment necessitating longer hospitalizations, although other clinical studies with heterogeneous cancer populations have reported no differences in clinical benefit across patients with different types of cancer, including those with GI cancer [79]. Temel's two studies highlight the importance of patient-centered interventions that include both symptom management and promoting effective coping strategies. Significantly helping patients *to redirect their hope toward more realistic goals* was a vital component of facilitating coping capabilities. Sharing the prognosis and the disease trajectory with patients helped them to make more informed clinical decisions and advanced care planning.

In a nurse-led controlled trial, the effects of an *early* integrated palliative care intervention (ENABLE 11) based on a self-management model showed effective improvements in quality of life with a significant reduction in depressed mood in patients with incurable cancer living in a rural community, compared to patients who received usual care [79]. However, symptom intensity did not improve significantly more than the usual care group. Patients had *advanced* gastro intestinal, lung, genitourinary, and breast cancers. When this integrative palliative care intervention was replicated to assess its effects based on *an early* versus *delayed* implementation, there were no differences in terms of quality of life, symptom impact and mood [80]. But the early start intervention was associated with a 15% increase in survival at 1 year, consistent with Temel's [1] study findings. "Early" referred to patients who started the palliative care intervention within 30 to 60 days of an advanced cancer diagnosis, cancer recurrence or disease progression, whereas a *delayed* integrative palliative care intervention started 3 months later. The fact that symptom intensity did not improve suggests that patients either had difficulty assessing prodromal signs and determining the optimal time to intervene with adequate medication, or lacked the confidence to self-medicate to the level required for relief. It is possible that patients in the terminal phase (with their caregiver) are too distressed by the disease progression and the patient's physical deterioration to effectively assume this aspect of self-management.

A systematic review investigated the types of psycho social interventions which appeared to promote patient well-being, quality of life, and meaning in life [81, 82]. Six clinical interventions were identified: cognitive-behavioral strategies, life review, dignity, narrative, meaning-making, counseling, education, music, and writing, among others. The meaning-making intervention appeared to be most effective in promoting quality of life and meaning in patients with advanced cancer.

These RCTs highlight the clinical imperative *of providing all patients* with cancer a comprehensive whole person approach to their care which includes the provision of psychosocial nursing interventions aimed at reducing emotional distress and promoting healing and resilient capabilities starting at diagnosis.

Focus on Patient and Caregiver Dyads

In principle, supportive care services that involve both the patient and the family caregiver are thought to promote a better overall illness experience, such as better symptom management, an enhanced quality of life and effective treatment planning [83]. However, most controlled trials that assessed the effectiveness of clinical interventions which were conjointly given to patients and caregivers resulted in clinical benefits that were mostly experienced by the patient [77]. Given the well documented presence of depression, anxiety and other symptoms experienced by caregivers of patients with advanced and terminal disease, Kavalieratos' findings lend credence to the suggestion that the real *focus* of many dyadic interventions is on patient rather than caregiver concerns (e.g., [45]).

Temel's [21] early integrated palliative care intervention (reported in the previous section) specifically targeted patients with advanced lung and GI cancers, although family caregivers were welcomed. When the caregiver data were analyzed, the intervention nevertheless significantly improved caregiver distress and depression, but not anxiety [46]. This improvement may have been more related to the reduction in the patient's distress than to any intervention aimed at addressing the family caregiver's unique needs (e.g., [50]).

A nurse-led three-arm RCT ($N = 302$ dyads) randomly assigned patients with advanced stage III and IV cancer and their caregivers to (1) a *brief dyadic intervention* (2 home visits plus 1 phone session) or (2) *an extended dyadic intervention* (4 home visits plus 2 telephone sessions) or (3) *usual care* [49]. The intent of the home-based, patient–caregiver centered, case management intervention was to help patients with advanced cancer and their caregivers manage the disease and symptoms. Significant improvements in dyads' coping capabilities, self-efficacy and social quality of life, and in caregivers' emotional quality of life were observed. Most effects were seen only 3 months after baseline. Brief and extensive dyadic interventions showed significant but not sustainable benefits for both patient and caregiver. It is possible that the lack of sustainable effects had to do with the patients' cancer progression and the commensurate increase in caregiver burden, suggesting the need for greater and more tailored interventions including a significant proactive increase in the nurse and team's support to patients and caregivers. It is the only study along with Temel's clinical trial [1] that was located, which highlighted the value of supporting hope as a coping strategy in patients and caregivers.

Focus on the Family Caregiver

Family caregivers experience emotional distress at levels similar to their loved ones, attributed in part to shared emotional reactions between patients and caregivers [51]. Only a few studies have investigated the effects of clinical interventions specifically designed for caregivers of palliative patients [22, 57, 84]. A meta-analysis of 29 RCTs investigated the main interventions provided to family caregivers of patients with cancer and their effects on caregiver outcomes. P*sychoeducational, skills training, and therapeutic counseling were identified* [48] (Appendix A). The majority of these interventions were delivered to patients and caregivers together (62.9%) and one third were administered only to caregivers (37.5%), but all were varied in duration and frequency. These interventions had small to medium effects which significantly decreased caregiver burden, increased caregiver's ability to cope, improved self-efficacy and increased aspects of quality of life posttreatment. The caregivers' clinical benefits might be explained in part by the fact that most interventions were delivered face-to-face (68.6%), and only one-fifth of the interventions were by telephone. But significantly the interventions addressed topics of concern to both caregivers and patients.

A systematic review of 11 RCTs and quasi-experimental studies examined the effects of supportive care interventions that supported family caregivers caring for patients at home [84]. Eight studies focused only on caregivers whereas three were centered on the patient–caregiver as the unit of care. *Education ($k = 3$), psychosocial ($k = 2$), and psychoeducational ($k = 6$) interventions* had a statistically significant effect in reducing psychological distress and the burden of care giving, and in improving perceived self-efficacy, competence in care giving and quality of life. Several interventions included *information about nutrition, symptom management and self-care,* although the descriptions of the interventions across the studies varied. Significantly, the review highlighted the lack of clinical interventions aimed at the caregiver's *physical health*, which is of concern given the empirically known progressive risk of poor physical health among caregivers due to caregiver burden [84].

A 6-session telehealth intervention (ENABLE 111) was specifically designed to address the concerns of caregivers of patients with advanced disease living in rural communities [22]. The RCT randomly assigned 122 caregivers to receive either the early or delayed intervention. Patients were newly diagnosed with recurrent or progressive metastatic cancer and cared for by family caregivers at home. The early intervention for caregivers started shortly after randomization; the delayed intervention started 3 months after randomization. Key components of the caregiver's self-management intervention included: the acquisition of problem-solving skills, self-care capabilities such as learning about a healthy diet, exercise and relaxation. It also included ways to collaborate with the nurse on managing patient symptoms, preventing crises and enhancing timely referrals to palliative care.

Family caregivers who received the *early intervention* experienced significantly less depression 3 months later compared to baseline scores [22, 23]. Following the patient's death these caregivers also experienced significantly less depression and less stress related to caregiving compared to caregivers in the delayed intervention group. However, no differences in quality of life, perceived burden, and stress between the two caregiver groups before the patient died were observed. Persistent caregiver burden highlights the need to find better solutions to address caregiver burden. Dionne-Odom's findings underscore the value of assigning a separate nurse each for the caregiver and for the patient in order to encourage the open expression of feelings and thoughts, and to address the unique needs of caregivers.

It is possible that both the patient and caregiver experience emotional needs (distress, fear) which cannot be adequately met via a mainly telehealth intervention. Following the patient's death, one-on-one semistructured interviews with the caregivers highlighted their preferences for a more flexible intervention format which would also include face-to-face sessions with the nurse in order to establish a better working relationship [57]. In qualitative interviews, the family caregivers conveyed their preference for person-centered communications that responded to their unique as well as shared needs with the patient. Significantly they preferred healthcare providers who treated them as whole individuals, rather than just as caregivers and patients [85].

There may be something else at play: the recent push toward patient and especially caregiver self-management capabilities may become an unfair burden on caregivers as the patient's disease reaches its terminal phase. Telehealth communications may facilitate the patient's wish to die at home when health care resources are scarce. But this does not lend itself to a natural healing environment in which caregivers may experience the timely and compassionate human assistance that may only be possible when the nurse is physically present in the home, and can fully address the care needs of the caregiver and patient. Because the end of life phase is emotionally distressing, it often leads to existential distress and questions about the meaning of life, which is generally not taken into account in a self-management model of practice [34]. Addressing existential distress along with effective symptom management are two essential components of compassionate nursing care.

To Summarize

Supportive care services may center on the patient, the dyadic patient–caregiver and the caregiver with varying therapeutic effects. The growing emphasis on self-management interventions particularly for caregivers caring for their loved ones at home, require regular and careful assessments, greater nursing support and more uniquely targeted, face-to-face interventions in the clinic or at home [57]. There is a healthcare imperative to develop tailored clinical interventions that meet the unique health-related needs of caregivers as well as palliative patients. One of the challenges of providing whole person care to patients and caregivers in the terminal phase, especially at home, is determining the frequency of face-to-face nursing visits required to effectively address caregiver and patient concerns, and to convey a sense of emotional security that comes with feeling truly cared for.

18.10 Nursing Approaches (Review Part IV Chaps. 8–14; Also, Part III, Chaps. 6 and 7; Appendix in Chaps. 9, 10, 11, 13, and 14, Appendices A–C)

According to Clinical Oncology Practice Guidelines, key palliative care practices include: establishing a working relationship with the patient and caregiver, assessing the patient's and caregiver's understanding of the illness and its prognosis, clarifying treatment goals, facilitating their participation in medical decision making, and coordinating care needs with other healthcare providers [8]. Notwithstanding, a multimodal, comprehensive approach must go beyond patient and caregiver understanding of the disease, "illness" related tasks and caregiver functions to embrace psychosocial interventions that address the behavioral as well as biological adaptive needs of the whole person [85]. Clinical research shows that patients with advanced disease may live well, and even longer if they *possess* emotion-regulating, cognitive-behavioral coping skills, meaningful support from loved ones, succeed in finding meaning and purpose in their life that corresponds with their clinical reality, and embrace a relevant diet and regular physical activity at one's own rate, *starting in the earlier rather than later* phases of the cancer trajectory (e.g., [79, 80]).

These therapeutic skills and informal supports are of therapeutic benefit to caregivers as well. As the burden of caregiving increases, their physical and emotional health is also at risk (e.g., [22, 48]) (Review Part IV Chap. 11). The purpose of this section is to focus mainly on managing emotion regulating cognitive-behavioral strategies, meaning-making strategies to reduce existential distress/suffering, and psychosocial strategies empirically known to reduce the intensity of symptoms that become progressively challenging to treat as the cancer progresses toward the terminal phase.

Quality of the Nurse–Patient/Family Relationship (Review Part IV Chap. 8; Appendix B)

Effective nursing care is anchored by the quality of the nurse–patient/caregiver relationship (Review Part IV Chap. 8). An enduring relationship over the course of the illness through the mourning phase enables the family and patient to feel known and their needs and concerns as whole individuals acknowledged and validated, which in itself is therapeutic (e.g., [85]). Establishing an authentic relationship involves meeting the physical, emotional, social, spiritual, medical, health-related and resilient-promoting needs of patients and caregivers with sensitivity and competence. The relationship is fostered by a compassionate and collaborative nursing approach, the nurse's ability to be fully present, drawing on effective communication skills that balance honesty with hope [27, 86]. Within this nurturing and secure context, the patient and family caregiver are more likely to share their thoughts and feelings, and experience a sense of security amidst great medical uncertainty and portending loss.

A healing-promoting relationship however depends on regularly scheduled clinic, unit or home visits to foster a sense of connectedness and mutual understanding. Regular appointments provide opportunities to *know* the patient and family caregiver and *to be known*. They enable the nurse to ascertain and respond to changing fears, emotional distress, and worries; and to facilitate realizable patient and caregiver goals. These nurse–patient and caregiver visits carve out healing opportunities characterized by active listening, providing comfort, hope and encouragement. Regular patient visits facilitate the possibility of engaging in resilient-promoting cognitive-behavioral strategies to reduce emotional distress and manage symptoms and side effects, clarify palliative goals and engage in advanced care planning within a safe and supportive environment.

Cognitive-Behavioral Emotion-Regulating Coping Strategies (Review Part IV Chaps. 9 and 10; Appendix B)

Nursing goals will change with disease progression. In the earlier phases of supportive care, goals strive to maintain overall wellness, quality of life, and activities of daily living for as long as possible. Psychologically adjusted patients and caregivers may experience rational worries and fears during the earlier supportive care phase which may be alleviated by providing relevant information, and engaging the patient and caregiver in tailored cognitive-behavioral coping strategies, redirecting fears about the future toward the meaningful possibilities in the present. Remind the patient and caregiver that the nurse and oncologist are working toward the same shared goals as the patient in promoting *optimal wellness* [73]. Encourage the use of Benson's relaxation response technique to reduce the intensity of disturbing thoughts which interfere with the possibility of living a better quality life.

Daily coping efforts usually include emotion-focused coping such as use of distraction, meaning-focused coping such as reappraisal as well as problem-focused behaviors [87].

Many patients and caregivers in the terminal phase suffer intensified anxiety, accompanied by negative thoughts that are profoundly distressing. Frequently anxiety escalates in tandem with worsening symptoms such as cachexia, pain, shortness of breath, or fatigue. A pilot study of a brief cognitive intervention to reduce anxiety in patients in the end stage of life randomly assigned 40 patients to either the intervention or the wait list condition [88]. The intervention produced a significant large effect size reduction in anxiety over the wait list condition based on the Hamilton Anxiety Rating Scale with an adjusted mean group difference of −5.51. The study suggests that a tailored brief cognitive-behavioral intervention may be an effective strategy to consider in alleviating anxiety. A multimodal module may include the following components as relevant (Review [88]):

1. Goal setting and education about anxiety, emotional distress or other symptoms.
2. Introduce Benson's relaxation response technique training and include education about the stress response system. The RR technique has been used to reduce the intensity of anxiety, distress, other symptoms (Review Part IV, Chap. 13).
3. Assess symptoms such as breathlessness to determine precipitating factors (i.e., emotional distress, disease progression or as a side effect of anticancer treatment) and suggest strategies, (i.e., learning forward in a seated position to breathe, breathing with pursed lips, slowing respirations and elongating expiration phase rather than taking deep breaths).
4. Use deep relaxation techniques and imagery to relax all muscles and to promote distraction.
5. Use active listening and as relevant, engage in discussions of the spiritual to help manage cancer-related fears such as fear of dying, loneliness and leaving loved ones behind. Treat distorted beliefs by providing relevant information and facts; use cognitive restructuring strategies and breaking down exaggerated beliefs or generalizations into manageable parts; encourage a present-oriented perspective (Review Part IV Chaps. 9 and 10). Facilitate the ability to differentiate realistic worries from unrealistic ones. (See encouraging supportive relationships, below)
6. Problem solving strategies to manage practical health related concerns. Acceptance of the terminal illness will occur at the patient's and caregiver's own pace, or not at all (Chap. 9). Greer's intervention recommends setting short-term goals with the patient and prioritizing quality of life (over length). The patient may come to realize the clinical reality due to his own perceived clinical deterioration, without necessarily acknowledging openly his or her impending death.
7. Planning and pacing oneself become more important as patients enter the terminal phase. This may involve assessing the patient's stamina throughout a typical day, the daily routine and its expenditure of energy. Review patient goals and facilitate priority goals: For example, work with the patient and the caregiver to leverage identified times during the day when more energy is available, enabling

a preferred activity. Build in opportunities to conserve energy by taking rests as well. For instance T. knew she had less and less energy to enjoy each day, but she was determined to continue her participation in a community choir where she also enjoyed the company of good friends. So each Monday, she carefully parsed her energy and incorporated a long afternoon nap which enabled her to attend choir for a few weeks more, and even a rock concert.

Regularly assess patient and caregiver distress and worries (as well as potential sources of distress) that may have arisen between nurse visits [30]. Actively listen to individual concerns. This may necessitate meeting separately with the caregiver and patient so that each individual may air their distress and concerns openly and in confidence, which in itself relieves anxiety if only temporarily.

More Cognitive Strategies (Review Part IV, Chaps. 8, 9, and 10)

These are invaluable cognitive coping strategies that can stand alone within a clinic visit or be incorporated within a more comprehensive multimodal, multitargeted nursing intervention.

Validate Patient Strategies That Work Ask the patient to describe what he or she is doing to cope with his or her worries/concerns. Jacobsen [73] suggests validating patient or caregiver strategies that seem to work. For instance, the patient might recount that she unusually contacted a close friend to go to the museum and the next day invited him for supper. The nurse might ask "What did you think of that strategy?" "How did it make you *feel*?" "Did it help? In what ways?" "Would you *consider doing this again?*" The patient might explain that these social encounters served as *needed distractions* from worries about the illness. The nurse could validate the emotion-focused coping behavior *by offering a commendation and reinforcing the strategy as a good one* for achieving "a little time out" and for obtaining needed support.

Encourage Positive Emotions (PE) Happiness or joy is a subjective, fluctuating, and resilient-promoting emotion that has its theoretical predicate in stress-coping [89] and emotion-regulation theories (Table 18.2) [91–93]. Waugh [92] posits that PE is involved in three different ways to regulate emotions. First, positive reappraisal regulates emotions by enhancing PE, even in the presence of negative emotions (NE). For instance this may be achieved by simply asking the patient or caregiver to share any event since the last clinic visit that made their hearts sing. Positive memories, self-affirmations and finding benefit are all strategies that enhance PE which mediate the relationship between emotion regulation and negative emotions [92]. An unexpected positive event such as a personal achievement or visit from a favorite relative or friend induces an unexpected positive emotion that moderates the relationship of emotion regulation on both PE and NE. For

Table 18.2 Encouraging positive emotions [73, 89, 90] (Review Part IV Chap. 9)

Ways to activate positive emotions	Examples
1. Help patients find some benefit in stressful situations "the silver lining in the cloud"	Explore/suggest walking with a friend, going on a bike ride, swim, spending more time with a grandchild, family and friends, reading a great book, going to a hockey game, painting, visiting a favorite place
2. Optimize a positive experience or memory by asking patient to share it with you, and then someone else: Each time elicits pleasure from the retelling	Invite the patient to share such a memory
3. Help patients change a negative view of a situation for a more positive or at least neutral reappraisal	1. When you are anxious, try changing the *meaning* of the source of stress, so you feel better. For instance, when the doctor suggested that you get all ducks in order, he was suggesting that as mortal beings we hope for the best but always prepare for any eventuality—Which is part of our human condition! 2. When you are anxious, try redirecting your mind to something positive that you can control in the present on this day rather than focusing on a future no one can control, for instance, spending time with a loved one. Try to redirect your mind to the present moment
4. Socialize with significant others induces positive emotions associated with meaningful experiences, and enhances vagal tone (emotional equanimity) and well-being	Organize outings with loved ones
5. Help patient identify what is most meaningful in his life	For example, spend time with loving relationships, going to church every day, listen to favorite music
6. Suggest and accompany patient/caregiver in relaxation response technique	When you focus on your breath, it is harder to perseverate on negative thoughts. Let's try together.
7. Increase patient opportunities for religious/spiritual experiences that enhance positive emotions (see Puchalski, p. 131 for interview questions)	Conduct a spiritual history; Start with "Do you consider yourself spiritual or religious?" [90, p. 131]
8. Focus on the present, not too much the future	When we focus on the future we miss all the possibilities that exist in the, moment or the day

instance, a surprise birthday party for the patient can trigger positive emotions that strengthen emotion regulation which also can serve as a buffer against negative emotion.

Depending on its source, positive emotions provide temporary relief from distress, may buffer against negative emotions and help to restore (heal) an individual's physiological, psychological, social coping resources by down regulating stress induced biological and behavioral stress response systems [89, 91, 94, 95]. Although positive emotions may co-occur with negative emotions in extremely stressful situations such as living with terminal cancer, they are directly and independently related to subjective well-being [96]. Positive emotions predispose a person to feel that life is meaningful, and may serve as an impetus for finding meaning within the context of the stressful situation [97, 98]. Finding something meaningful in each day can also make the person's heart sing even as the negative emotions associated with impending death threaten to overwhelm the patient [99]. PE strengthens resilience and the ability to live well with cancer.

Infuse the Ordinary with Meaning The patient's ability to adhere to a familiar daily routine provides order, purpose and/or meaning to daily life [89, 100–102]. A daily routine provides all humans with a sense of predictability or security, albeit a false one, which we all use to obscure the reality of our fragile existence. The nurse may leverage that knowledge by encouraging the patient and family to find meaning and purpose in everyday activities in their present life. This can be achieved by the nurse "infusing ordinary events with positive meanings" [89]. For instance, a nurse and patient might review the patient's usual day, let's say, of phone calls with family or friends, food shopping, reading a great book, taking a nap. The nurse might explore the effects of each activity on the patient's thoughts and feelings. And the nurse might further share something to the effect of, "when you just focus on the day, there are many ordinary events that can make the heart sing. Can you think of other events in your life that also make you feel content?" Of course patients may also say that these things no longer fill their heart, which would open a different equally salient conversation. For instance it might lead the nurse to try some cognitive restructuring in which connections between feelings, thoughts and behaviors are made to highlight to the patient, that by changing our thoughts to something more positive we can automatically improve our emotions (Review Part IV, Chap. 9). Persistent depression, however, may lead the nurse to suggest a referral to the physician for possible medication.

Distraction Encourage the use of this typical emotion-focused coping strategy, that was referred to in an earlier section. For example, "When I start to feel anxious, I go to the movie channel and watch anything to take my mind off my thoughts." *Normalize* these coping behaviors as strategies typically used by most people because they work! Ask if there are other symptoms that may be alleviated by distraction.

Support Hope (Review Part IV, Chap. 9) *Hope* is a dynamic, context driven coping strategy replete with meanings that vary from one individual to another [66, p. 907]. Hope is an essential coping strategy for all patients living with a life threatening cancer and family caregivers [1, 73, 103]. Hope takes on even greater significance when active treatment is terminated and patients must confront impending death. It is not unusual for patients to toggle between moments of clinical realism and hope, underscoring the personal struggle to come to terms with their approaching death while retaining the right to hope as a temporary coping effort to keep that reality at bay [103]. Healthcare providers unwittingly dash hope when they believe in "telling it like it is" failing to assess whether their patient is ready to receive such devastating news. Patients generally know when there is little hope, but it is sometimes easier to accept when it is not stated out loud *by others*. Dashing hope in favor of "calling a spade a spade" is tantamount to sinking a ship before it has had the opportunity to mend itself in a safe harbor before having to face life's ultimate act. Jacobsen [103] draws on a dual clinical framework in which the patient is encouraged to focus on living well even as the "possibility of dying is acknowledged" with references such as "making the most of each day," "doing things that make your heart sing." For instance one strategy Jacobsen uses is to support the patient's *hope* by saying, "I share your *wish* and let's keep you feeling well for as long as possible," a supportive intervention within a realistic framework. It is a gentle and sensitive approach that enables the patient and family caregiver to gradually re align their hopes to reality, on their own terms, not ours.

Support a Sense of the Spiritual and/or a Religion Many individuals find deep solace in a higher order of spiritual connectedness. It may involve the spiritual or formalized religion, the natural world or other modalities (music, art, literature, sports) through which the individual may transcend his or her corporeal being, and attain deep feelings of peace, comfort and meaning at the end of life [29, 104–106]. Being spiritual or having religious faith is associated with a particular set of beliefs, values, traditions, cognitions, feelings (emotional experiences) and behavioral practices that connect the person's being to something greater than or beyond the self [107, 108]. Spiritual well-being tends to reduce depression and emotional distress at the end of life, and enables acceptance [32, 109].

Nurses may be therapeutic when conversations lead to religious or spiritual sources of comfort (e.g., [110]). Sometimes doing a spiritual history facilitates the patient's and caregiver's ability to express their thoughts and feelings about the role of spirituality and religion in their life. A spiritual history focuses on deeply experienced beliefs and feelings belonging to the patient's inner world of core beliefs, existential meanings about life and death, feelings of despair or gratitude, and connections that in the process of sharing these beliefs with the nurse, re affirm or bestow greater meaning and acceptance. Review [90, p. 131] for the interview questions. Carrying out a spiritual history is a therapeutic intervention in itself.

Alleviate Existential Suffering (Review Part IV Chap. 10, Appendix B) Patients and caregivers may experience existential distress. Existential distress occurs when the individual is preoccupied by life and death issues and possibly overcome by a sense of meaninglessness. Existential distress arises when a gap occurs between the individual's global and situational meanings [33, 111]. It may escalate when patients perceive a lack of emotional support from significant others, feel they are a burden to loved ones, and experience a heightened awareness of aloneness or fear of approaching death [38].

Psychological healing can occur anytime, but it usually involves a process of reflection about the self in relation to the world, relationships and/or a higher order (Review Chap. 10, Table 10.3). Invite the patient's narrative within the broad context of past and current life experiences such as through a life review, which has been shown to provide a source of comfort and acceptance. Facilitating a patient narrative can help individuals' reorder life's priorities and find emotional solace in *accepting* death as an integral part of life. Self-reflection through narratives can lead to acceptance through realizing a life well lived or even a life with mistakes that may still be redeemed, by passing hard earned lessons on to loved ones, or reaching out to make "amends." With the nurse's assistance, an individual may learn not to be so hard on him-/herself in reflections—we are all part of the human condition.

Two narratives often led by nurses consist of the life review and the meaning-making intervention. The nurse may invite the patient or caregiver to engage in either a *life review or a meaning-making* intervention in order to enhance the ability to come to terms with their life's circumstance, and through this dynamic process find psychological well-being and maybe even acceptance [112–114]. As has been described in Chap. 10, advanced practice nurses need to acquire the skills of implementing these manualized interventions from clinical experts through university workshops and courses with clinical practicums, as is the case in medicine when a new therapeutic enters the medical field of clinical practice.

Behavioral Coping Strategies (See Part IV Chap. 13; Appendix in Chaps. 9 and 13, Appendices A and B) Progressive relaxation techniques have been incorporated into cognitive-behavioral stress management interventions to reduce anxiety and to down regulate the stress response system (e.g., [115, 116]). Other behavioral strategies that have achieved significant clinical benefits include Benson's relaxation response technique, mindful meditation, and yoga [117–120]. The mindfulness strategies may be effective in reducing the intensity of intrusive ideation that perpetuates emotional distress. Because these techniques also appear to reduce stress-activated pro inflammatory cytokines associated with some symptoms, the intensity of other symptoms also may improve. Ngamkham and colleagues' [121] meta-analysis of mindful interventions identified three studies with a low risk of bias which showed that mindful meditation (MM) significantly reduced pain, anxiety, stress, depression and intrusive ideation in patients with cancer [122–125].

Strengthening Supportive Relationships (Review Part IV Chap. 11)

Perceived support from family and friends has been associated with adaptive coping and *longer survival* in patients with cancer (e.g., [1, 126, 127]). One possible explanation is that informal perceived support has been significantly related to higher natural killer cell cytotoxicity *with in* tumor-infiltrating lymphocytes, for instance in patients with ovarian cancer [128]. Conversely poor perceived support or social isolation has been associated with elevated inflammatory cytokines including concentrations of intra tumor norepinephrine, scientifically known to drive tumor growth [75, 129]. Even the expression of genes associated with transcription RNA within the tumor cells of individuals with ovarian cancer differ between those individuals with perceived support, and those without [129]. Thus promoting the patient's and caregiver's relationships with loved ones and each other is a critical goal throughout the cancer trajectory in attenuating disease progression [130].

Nurture *emotional*, informational and instrumental support between patient and family caregiver, and the family throughout the palliative phase [131, 132]. Regularly check in with the patient and family caregiver separately as well as together to assess *the fit* between the support each needs and the support they receive from significant others, including healthcare workers. As needed, facilitate basic communication skills among family members by proposing strategies such as starting a conversation with "I feel" rather than making accusatory statements such as "You never listen" [133, pp. 249–265].

The nurse also facilitates patient–caregiver mutual support by encouraging the patient and caregiver to talk about the patient's approaching passing [131]. A nationwide survey of 678 mourners in Japan found that 76% of those surveyed had discussions with their loved ones before death, and appeared to experience less depression or "complicated" grief after their loved one's death than those who did not. This survey would be worthwhile repeating to ascertain the feasibility of developing a subsequent end of life supportive intervention for caregivers who are reluctant to talk to their loved ones about death.

Help the family or close friend overcome potential fears of death that may impede their ability to be present for their dying loved one. Some family members may need the nurse's support in experiencing this ultimate milestone of the lifespan. Explore what would be the worst thing that could happen if their loved one died in their presence and to close their eyes and imagine it. Then ask, what would be the best thing to happen, and imagine it. Ask: How did you feel imagining being there for your loved one? Encourage perspective taking, asking the family member to imagine being the person dying, if needed. Suggest simple gestures, such as holding the patient's hand which reassures the patient that he is not alone. Often this is more than enough to convey love and support to the dying patient. Many years ago, a much beloved aunt was dying at home from cancer. And her best friend could not find the strength to go to her bedside. She was afraid to cry "too much," and lost an invaluable opportunity to share precious last moments with a dear friend, irretrievable moments that would have given both such comfort, and it was something she regretted the rest of her life. Other suggestions may be found in Part IV Chap. 11.

Symptom Management (Review Part V Chap. 16; Part IV Chaps. 9, 12, 13 and 14; Part III Chaps. 6 and 7)

One of the most challenging aspects of caring for patients in the last 6 to 12 months of life is symptom management. The nursing goal is to maintain the patient's quality life for as long as possible, provide optimal comfort and enable cognitive acuity in order to facilitate meaningful gatherings with family and friends [6, 134]. A second critical goal is to reassess and discuss face to face the extent to which distressed family caregivers caring for their loved ones at home are comfortable in "self-management-related activities" such as assessing clinical signs and administrating narcotics and other medications at the appropriate dose [23, 57]. Patients often experience a cluster of symptoms that become overwhelming for the caregiver to manage.

Symptom clusters are the outer manifestation of dysregulated inflammatory processes exacerbated by distress, disease progression, and types of treatment/palliation (e.g., [135–138]). Increased symptom intensity exacerbates interrelated psychological and physical suffering [31, 41]. Providing psychosocial support, physical comfort, active listening, therapeutic use of touch, and reassurance can contribute to the patient's emotional equanimity which becomes an exponential part of the nurse's psychosocial care of the patient and family caregiver. Psychosocial interventions must work in tandem with pharmacological, palliative treatment and other complementary therapeutics.

Pain (e.g., Cognitive-Behavioral Strategies, Mindful Meditation, Relaxation Response Technique, Leveraging Cognitive Expectations, and Acupuncture)

Pain is undertreated in an estimated 64–66% of cancer patients with advanced metastatic and end-stage disease [41, 139]. Even when opioids are administered, pain has been found to persist in a certain proportion of patients [42]. An estimated 62–86% of patients dying of cancer take progressively higher doses of opioids which cause drowsiness and a haze-like consciousness which interfere with the patient's and family's ability to share precious time together in a more mutually satisfying way [17].

Pain Assessment

The NCCN Guidelines recommends using a 10-point numerical scale ranging from 1: no pain to 10: severe pain. Or a measure of pain intensity may be effective: 1–3: mild; 4–7: moderate; and 8–10: severe [140]. Assess the quality of the pain, specifically: somatic (aching, stabbing or pressure like pain), visceral (gnawing, cramping), neuropathic (burning, tingling or shooting). Assess duration, frequency, intensity of pain and location, and whether the pain has changed in character. Is it new or progressively worse or the same. Explore the etiology of the pain: precipitating factors, "relief-related" factors (and level of relief on the 10-point scale), related symptoms (e.g., anxiety, depression, nausea, constipation). Determine a pattern of pain in the preceding week, an analgesic history and perceived results. Explore the frequency and character of break through pain in relation to the medication's duration of effects. Assess for previous experiences with pain, cultural or personal attitudes to pain and use of medication; *presence of existential suffering or emotional distress* tends to exacerbate perceptions of pain acuity.

Nursing Goals
To alleviate the physical pain associated mainly with advanced disease and palliative treatment, such as, palliative chemotherapy or surgery involves optimizing the patient's physical comfort, physical and cognitive functionality, and safety. This involves ensuring the optimal dosing of narcotic medications and mobilizing other therapeutic modalities to work in tandem to control the intensity of pain and its break through manifestations between administered doses.

Nursing Approaches
NCCN guidelines recommend the use of integrative therapies to complement medical treatments [140]. As previously discussed in Part IV, mindful meditation, cognitive coping strategies and the relaxation response technique may be effective in reducing pain intensity by downregulating stress-related biomarkers associated with various symptoms including pain. Mindfulness based stress reduction, leveraging cognitive expectations for clinical treatment benefits, and cognitive-behavioral strategies may be suitable as complementary therapies with opioids in the earlier phases of end of life care. This also may have the added clinical benefit of reducing the opioid dose and protecting the patient's cognitive alertness [140–142]. There is some evidence that pain and anxiety may be alleviated also by leveraging the patient's clinical expectation for a treatment benefit may even improve treatment efficacy, and should be implemented (See below) [143, 144].

Symptom Cluster Moderate-to-severe, cancer-related pain *frequently co-occurs within a symptom* cluster typically consisting of emotional distress, fatigue and sleep disturbances (e.g., [136, 139, 145]). Treating pain as part of a symptom cluster can often improve or alleviate co-occurring symptoms or side effects [146, 147]. For instance, a randomized controlled trial investigated the effectiveness of a cognitive-behavioral intervention on a symptom cluster in 208 patients with breast and prostate cancers receiving chemotherapy [146, pp. 4–5]. Patients were randomly assigned either to the 4 week *cognitive-behavioral intervention* or to usual care. The intervention group showed significant reductions in fatigue and pain levels compared to the usual care group. Within group analysis demonstrated significant decreases in both pain and fatigue, with a significant increase over baseline measures in health-related quality of life. Other improvements included a reduction in anxiety, depression and nausea. Conversely the usual care group showed an increase in both fatigue and pain at 4 weeks with a corresponding decrease in health related quality of life compared to baseline scores.

The intervention consisted of 4 weekly supervised sessions of *breathing exercises, progressive muscle relaxation and guided imagery, accompanied by soft music* followed by daily unsupervised sessions [146, pp. 4–6]. This multimodal intervention may be well suited for patients with advanced disease experiencing intensified pain levels, with or without related symptoms, as part of a comprehensive approach to pain management.

Barriers to effective pain control include poor patient-nurse communications, poor understanding by caregivers of pain management in terms of dosing and duration of pain relief, quality and intensity of continuous and/or breakthrough pain, typical side effects of sedation including cognitive impairments, inadequate medication and lack of adherence to the medication.

Dyspnea Review [148] Mindfulness Techniques, Music Therapy, Breathing Retraining, Relaxation, Acupressure, and Acupuncture

One of the most difficult symptoms for any patient to bear is dyspnea or shortness of breath. An estimated 10–70% of patients with advanced cancer have been reported to experience refractory dyspnea [148, 149]. The American Thoracic Society defines dyspnea as "the subjective experience of breathing discomfort that consists of qualitatively distinct sensations that vary in intensity" [150, p. 436] Dyspnea or air hunger increases in intensity over the last few weeks of life. Dyspnea in patients with advanced cancer may be the consequential effects of advanced disease, chemotherapy, surgery or irradiation as well as emotional distress or anxiety, and other chronic illness such as heart failure or chronic obstructive pulmonary disease [148]. The main medical treatment for patients with advanced, terminally ill cancer are opioids such as morphine, increasingly, as an integrative part of a more multimodal approach that has been shown to increase clinical effectiveness over opioids alone.

Nursing Assessment

Dyspnea should be assessed each time the nurse is with the patient. A suggested validated measure is the Multidimensional Dyspnea Profile (MDP), with each item being rated on a 10-point visual analogue scale [151, p. 509]: (1) An overall assessment of discomfort 0–10 (2) effort in terms of muscle work, air hunger, tightness, mental effort and type of breathing such as fast and/or shallow (3) intensity of emotional factors such as anger, anxiety, depression, fear, frustration. In addition assess for triggers and functional ability and changes. For instance is breathlessness present at rest (a poor prognosis), running up a flight of stairs or walking. If this marks a change, note the length of time, whether it is the same or worse. What helps to relieve the discomfort according to the patient.

Nursing Goals

The main goals of care are to promote more regular breathing, physical comfort and relieve the emotional distress and anxiety associated with dyspnea or shortness of breath.

Nursing Approaches

The main clinical interventions for patients with advanced, terminally ill cancer are opioids such as morphine, as an integrative part of a more multimodal approach that has been shown to increase clinical effectiveness over opioids alone [148]. Psychosocial interventions such as mindful meditation, relaxation strategies, psychoeducation and use of music can help to reduce the emotional distress and anxiety associated with shortness of breath [148, 152–154].

Well known behavioral strategies to improve dyspnea also include specialized breathing exercises, breathing retraining to promote ventilation, resistance breathing or pursed lips breathing, diaphragmatic breathing, sitting slightly forward, pacing the breath (e.g.., [155, 156]). A multisite RCT evaluated an 8-week combined breathing retraining and psychosocial intervention for 144 patients with cancer-related dyspnea [155]. The intervention group showed a significant improvement over the control group with respect to dyspnea, anxiety and self-perceived control over dyspnea. The patients had small or nonsmall cell lung cancer, mesothelioma or lung metastasis. Learning workshops should be regularly conducted to ensure clinical expertise in using *all* these effective behavioral strategies to improve the physical comfort and breathing capability of patients in the terminal phase.

Other Nonpharmacological Interventions for Symptom Management (also Review Chaps. 9, 12, and 14)

Acupuncture, Auricular Acupuncture, and Acupressure [157]

Acupuncture has suffered from scientific skepticism in some circles of western medicine due to a paucity of rigorously designed clinical trials, leading to scientific claims that acupuncture is the result of a placebo effect [158] (Please review Part IV, Chap. 12). Acupuncture is included in this chapter due to growing evidence that acupuncture and acupressure appear to improve shortness of breath and cancer pain in patients in the terminal phase, often in combination with other nonpharmacological interventions (e.g., [148, 157, 159, 160]).

Dyspnea Acupuncture and even acupressure appear to improve *dyspnea* alone or in conjunction with opioids, according to a number of clinical studies (e.g., [161, 162]). A phase 11, clinical trial randomly assigned 173 patients to receive (1) acupuncture only (2) morphine only, or (3) both morphine and acupuncture [163]. Although no significant differences between the three groups were found at 4 h, dyspnea as measured by a visual analogue scale improved in 74% of patients who received acupuncture alone; 60% who received only morphine; and 66% who had both morphine and acupuncture. Acupuncture appeared to also relieve anxiety and increase a state of relaxation which may have been a critical factor in alleviating dyspnea. Future studies based on a combined multimodal strategy of morphine and acupuncture could further inform therapeutic strategies for dyspnea.

A systematic review and meta-analysis of 12 studies investigated the effectiveness of acupuncture and acupressure on dyspnea in 597 patients with malignant and nonmalignant disease that included 190 patients with advanced cancer [159]. Evidence from six studies suggested that 3 weeks of acupuncture compared to sham acupuncture significantly reduced the severity of breathlessness. However, these studies had a high risk of bias and considerable heterogeneity so that findings must be considered with caution.

Pain Acupuncture has been similarly incorporated into therapeutic strategies for managing cancer-related pain. A recent meta-analysis that evaluated the effects of acupuncture based on 36 studies (n = 2213) and samples ranging between 21 and 215 participants, reported differential and significant effects on cancer-related pain, malignancy-related pain, and surgical-related pain [160]. Acupuncture significantly reduced malignancy-related and surgically-related pain but not radiation or chemotherapy-related pain (see Appendix in Chap. 14). This meta-analysis has provided the strongest evidence yet of the differential effects of acupuncture on pain as a function of the cause of pain.

Acupuncture in conjunction with standard medical treatment for cancer-related pain has been shown to be effective in reducing the amount of prescribed opioids [164]. In a pragmatic, single-arm pilot study that assessed uncontrollable cancer-related pain in 41 patients who received ten sessions of acupuncture, significant improvements over baseline measures in pain severity, pain interference, and patient satisfaction were reported. When combined with prescribed opioids or nonopioid analgesics, it led to a *reduction in medication* use in 34% of patients over the course of the study [164]. Although 44% of patients did not alter their medication dosages, they still reported a significant reduction in pain severity and pain interference. Patients who want acupuncture may be psychologically predisposed to its therapeutic effects, and if so, as previously reviewed in Chap. 12 this cognitive expectation may trigger physiological pathways associated with pain relief [143].

One hypothesis is that Aß fibers in the skin that are stimulated by the needle points, reduce painful stimuli. Another hypothesis implicates the release of ß-endorphins and/or other substances in the brain and spinal cord as a consequence of needle stimulation at different Meridien points. As acupuncture does no harm, it should be considered, and may be effective for major postsurgical pain and malignant types of uncontrollable pain in some individuals. However, acupuncture, similar to massage and foot reflexology, suffers from a short duration of effects, although in combination with pharmacological agents may actually improve consistent pain relief in patients with advanced cancer. Carefully timed acupuncture may minimize the potential for breakthrough pain in patients taking opioids.

Reflexology and Massage Therapy (Pain, Anxiety, Depression) (See Part V Chap. 16; Part IV Chap. 14)
A meta-analysis of 12 controlled studies ($N = 559$) suggested that massage and reflexology significantly reduced cancer-related pain, treatment-related pain and especially surgically-related pain compared to usual care although the size effects were small (e.g., [165]). Reflexology compared to progressive relaxation was also

shown to be more effective in *reducing anxiety and depression* and enhancing mental health after 6 weeks, although these effects were not sustainable. Both interventions consisted of 6, 30-min weekly sessions, perhaps suggesting the need for more frequent sessions each week to increase the dosing efficacy [166]. Other meta-analyses have highlighted the lack of sustainability as well as the generally poor methodological quality of the studies [134, 167]. It is possible that reflexology and massage are effective in reducing anxiety which then alleviates the intensity of physical pain.

Therapeutic Touch (TT) or Reiki (R) (Anxiety, Intrusive Ideation, Physical Discomfort) (See Appendix in Chap. 14; Part IV Chap. 14)
This therapeutic intervention may be useful to consider when patients are in such physical pain and suffering that they cannot bear to be physically touched or moved. Recent clinical and immune findings suggest that we need to reconsider its potential contribution to healing under certain conditions [123, 168]. Reiki and therapeutic touch like acupuncture have been pilloried within the health care sciences due to their poorly understood theoretical underpinnings, and mostly poorly designed studies. Yet anecdotally, healing touch, increasingly supported by better designed studies, appears to improve clinical outcomes, although the mechanism of action is still unclear (Chap. 14).

Enhance Cognitive Expectations Open Treatment Approach
Above and beyond the possible clinical benefits associated with the therapeutic strategies discussed above, consider informing the patient each time a pharmacological agent is *being* administered and its intended therapeutic effects. Doing so has been shown to optimize pharmacodynamic efficacy, especially analgesics and anxiolytics [143, 144] See Part IV Chap. 12). By extension, also describe the intended therapeutic benefits of nonpharmacological therapies as they are administered.

Health Education (Review Part V Chap. 16; Appendix C)

Diet and Nutrition Given the unpredictability of advancing disease and the patient's changing clinical status, the nurse works closely with the oncology dietician who must provide regular dietary counseling and determine nutritional requirements (e.g., [169, 170]). Patients in the earlier phases of supportive care may still enjoy food. The nurse's role is to mainly monitor the patient's adjustment to the dietician's recommended dietary or nutritional intake, identify patient issues, encourage the patient and the caregiver to follow the suggested recommendations and provide relevant information. This is a team effort in which patient assessments are shared among the oncologist, nurse, dietitian and physiotherapist in order to optimize the patient's well-being. As cancer progresses, appetite may be very poor and cachexia may become a medical concern.

Physical Activity Similarly, the nurse works closely with the oncologist and oncology physiotherapist with respect to the recommended type, frequency, duration and intensity of physical activity which will also change over time. Patients in the earlier phases of supportive care should be encouraged to incorporate daily activity or exercise into their routine. Encourage the caregiver to accompany the patient given the important health promoting effects for both. Moderate to intense activity is empirically known to strengthen physical fitness and functional capability and to normalize immune functioning and improve cell-mediated immunity [171]. But daily walking as a low intensity activity is also therapeutic. The intensity, frequency and duration should be determined by the oncologist and exercise physiologist with the patient (Review Part IV Chap. 12; Part V, Chaps. 16 and 17). The nurse's role is to prolong quality of life for as long as possible through education and encouragement, collaborating with the patient and caregiver to identify potential obstacles to exercise and proactively to help to find appropriate solutions.

Self-Management Interventions (Review Part IV Chap. 9; Appendices A and B)

In principle the nursing goal is to enhance overall wellness and a sense of self-efficacy among patients and caregivers through a collaborative initiative with the nurse that promotes solutions to practical problems, mainly arising from the patient's disease and treatment, such as learning to manage symptoms between clinic visits and use relevant health related resources [172]. As previously mentioned, topics such as advance care planning, leaving a legacy, making a will, writing a letter to loved ones, strategies for effective participation in medical decision making and utilization of health resources are typically addressed (Appendix A). Provide a handout of health-related resources to review with the patient and caregiver such as information about the in-patient palliative care unit, hospice care, funeral homes or at home care. Consider the patient's and caregiver's level of health literacy, including their comfort level in assessing and acting upon symptoms, and other aspects of physical care, especially as the patient enters the terminal phase [173].

Patient and caregiver self-management knowledge and skills *should be introduced as early as* possible in the supportive care phase while the patient is still feeling generally well and has psychologically adjusted to palliative care; even so, results still are mixed [1, 21, 57]. An important component of self-management is to include a discussion on healthy lifestyle behaviors for the informal caregiver given the empirically known health-related risks associated with caregiving [2].

18.11 Unique Needs of Caregivers [22, 57] (Review Part IV; Appendix A)

Family caregivers may experience progressively greater emotional distress and a heavier caregiver burden as cancer advances and their loved one deteriorates [45]. Added to these concerns, healthcare provider support may be inadequate with many caregivers lacking clinical knowledge and skills to adequately manage various symptoms in the terminal phase [45, 174]. With increasing complexity of patient care and growing intensity of a patient's symptoms, the caregiver's understandable distress also threatens their own physical and emotional health. Caregivers caring for their loved ones at home need the nurse's emotional support and understanding should they decide against further hands-on involvement in the patient's physical care, and in particular the management of symptom relief. Some may need to distance themselves from the difficult emotional and physical care-giving responsibilities, although others may seek greater personal input into clinical decisions [53].

A systematic review of caregivers caring for loved ones at home identified three nursing interventions that may help caregivers through the palliative care phase: (a) Psychosocial education, (b) strengthening caregiver self-efficacy beliefs and coping skills, and (c) therapeutic counseling [84]. Conversely, a Cochrane review of 19 clinical trials reported that psychosocial interventions for the caregiver had no long lasting effects on caregiver distress, anxiety or depression [19]. Other RCTs that assessed the efficacy of self-management interventions on caregiver well-being have produced mixed results [22, 48]. More tailored face-to-face nurse support may be a clinical imperative for some caregivers caring for loved ones at home especially in the final weeks before death. As disease approaches the terminal phase family caregivers may no longer be willing or able to assume the major burden of patient care. As caregiver distress mounts, the ability to critically assess patient signs of symptomatic distress decreases, as evidenced by numerous research findings of the inverse relationship between a stress-induced prefrontal cortex and highly activated amygdala [94]

Mindfulness Strategies Systematic reviews have assessed the efficacy of mindful meditation (MM) for *family caregivers* of loved ones with cancer [175, 176]. The results suggest that MM may exert potential therapeutic effects on the family caregiver by alleviating depression, stress, and anxiety as well as improving overall well-being, with and without an educational component. Given health risks of caregivers, and interdependent effects between caregivers and patients, implementing effective strategies to meet the psychosocial needs of caregivers is a clinical imperative. As part of this therapeutic initiative the nurse and team need to follow caregivers as regularly as patients during the advanced stages of the illness.

Health-Related Needs The nurse's care must consider the health of the caregiver with respect to weight, diet, nutrition, and exercise during this particularly stressful phase. Encouraging a healthy diet and exercise are an integral part of nursing's legacy that must be restored and tailored to the needs of caregivers, throughout the cancer trajectory, including the terminal phase [177].

Clinical Anecdote 18.4
Most communities have their own way of grieving. Some hold a wake, others who follow the Jewish faith sit shiva, still others as I experienced in a remote northern community lead a procession of mourners through the village to their loved one's final resting place. Most nurses in cancer care who work closely with patients and caregivers understand that death, loss and mourning constitute an essential grieving phase within the nurse-family caregiver relationship, and by extension the family. Nurses understand the extent to which family healing may be facilitated by the presence of the nurse at the funeral, and afterward during the customary mourning rituals in which the whole family participates. As needed, the nurse may continue to check up on the family caregiver until both are ready to say goodbye. In so doing, the nurse who has known the patient and caregiver throughout the highs and lows of the illness journey may help to mitigate the family's last concerns, fears and even guilt.

Bereavement

Few studies have focused on the bereavement phase. There is a need for healthcare providers to prepare family caregivers for the passing of their loved one, and to visit with the family during their bereavement as an integral part of facilitating healing (e.g., [45, 61]). Bereavement outreach is defined as "contact from the clinical team that occurs immediately after death and continues until several months later" [56]. In response to a bereavement survey, families suggested that straightforward communications about the patient's prognosis, compassionate care, competency and reaching out to the family after death were key factors that helped the family during bereavement. These contact communications included letters and calls from the doctor and the nurse, attending the patient's funeral, receiving relevant literature, as well as attending a bereavement support group.

Family caregivers have identified at least three preferred forms of communication with health care providers [56]: First, a compassionate connection with the family by conveying empathy, understanding, and by providing needed clinical guidance and comfort. Second, effective communication skills that provide truthful information about the prognosis, the clinical implications associated with the changing clinical status of the loved one, and *what to expect* at the end of life. Third, regular contact during bereavement in order to help the family cope with their loss. Above all, treat family caregivers as whole individuals with their own unique beliefs, expectations and needs [85]. Regularly setting aside time to be fully present, actively listening, and providing needed information, reassurances, and support, including respecting the family's choices, are clinical imperatives. Caregiver anxiety and fatigue may be temporarily lifted when the caregiver feels that the nurse has validated their feelings and their efforts to do their best for their loved one during the illness.

Final Thoughts

This chapter covers the early, middle and terminal stages of the supportive care trajectory. In the early and middle phases of disease progression, nursing goals include promoting physical and emotional wellness and healthy activities of daily living for as long as possible. It involves helping to tailor patient and caregiver expectations to changing clinical circumstances and encouraging the meaningfulness of living fully in the moment rather than focusing on a longer life. The terminal phase is increasingly enveloped by the intensity, complexity, and scope of symptoms and side effects associated with the patient's cancer type and areas of general metastases. It may include intensified fatigue, pain, emotional distress, shortness of breath, severe headaches and seizures, overall discomfort as well as other disease-related problems such as cancer related blockages. In addition to the nurses' psychosocial interventions, acupuncture, massage, music, and even therapeutic touch may provide therapeutic relief, and nurses should be aware of these therapeutic benefits in order to advocate for their use as adjunct therapies.

A recurring theme of myriad research papers is the growing widespread clinical recognition that nurses and doctors must improve their clinical expertise with respect to communication skills, which is the predicate for all clinical interactions with patients and family caregivers. This should be made possible through university or hospital-based clinical courses/workshops or programs that include supervised clinical practicums with clinical experts (e.g., [22, 23, 178, 179]). Clinical trials that have investigated the effectiveness of clinical interventions delivered by nurses who were specially "trained" generally achieved the goals of the clinical research. But unless those effective interventions are then taught to a wider circle of clinical nurses who are the daily custodians of cancer care, those evidence based skills are essentially lost to the nursing profession in the drift of time. Patients and caregivers expect clinical expertise from nurses who accompany them on the difficult and challenging cancer trajectory. They expect this clinical expertise within the context of a connected and compassionate nurse–patient and caregiver relationship.

References

1. Temel JS, Greer JA, Muzikansky A, Gallagher ER, Admane S, Jackson VA, et al. Early palliative care for patients with metastatic non-small-cell lung cancer. N Engl J Med. 2010;363(8):733–42. PubMed PMID: 20818875. Epub 2010/09/08. eng.
2. Cotogni P, Saini A, De Luca A. In-hospital palliative care: should we need to reconsider what role hospitals should have in patients with end-stage disease or advanced cancer? J Clin Med. 2018;7(18):1–9.

3. George N, Phillips E, Zaurova M, Song C, Lamba S, Grudzen C. Palliative care screening and assessment in the emergency department: a systematic review. J Pain Symptom Manag. 2016;51(1):108–19 e2. PubMed PMID: 26335763. Epub 2015/09/04. eng.
4. Hui D, Anderson L, Tang M, Park M, Liu D, Bruera E. Examination of referral criteria for outpatient palliative care among patients with advanced cancer. Support Care Cancer. 2020;28(1):295–301. PubMed PMID: 31044305. Pubmed Central PMCID: PMC6824973. Epub 2019/05/03. eng.
5. Hui D, Meng YC, Bruera S, Geng Y, Hutchins R, Mori M, et al. Referral criteria for outpatient palliative cancer care: a systematic review. Oncologist. 2016;21(7):895–901. PubMed PMID: 27185614. Pubmed Central PMCID: PMC4943399. Epub 2016/05/18. eng.
6. Dans M, Smith T, Back A, Baker JN, Bauman JR, Beck AC, et al. NCCN guidelines insights: palliative care, version 2.2017. J Natl Compr Canc Netw. 2017;15(8):989–97. PubMed PMID: 28784860. Epub 2017/08/09. eng.
7. Ferrell BR, Temel JS, Temin S, Smith TJ. Integration of palliative care into standard oncology care: ASCO clinical practice guideline update summary. J Oncol Pract. 2017;13(2):119–21. PubMed PMID: 28972832. Epub 2017/10/04. eng.
8. Ferrell BR, Twaddle ML, Melnick A, Meier DE. National consensus project clinical practice guidelines for quality palliative care guidelines, 4th edition. J Palliat Med. 2018;21(12):1684–9. PubMed PMID: 30179523. Epub 2018/09/05. eng.
9. Mo L, Urbauer DL, Bruera E, Hui D. Recommendations for palliative and hospice care in NCCN guidelines for treatment of cancer. Oncologist. 2021;26(1):77–83. PubMed PMID: 32915490. Pubmed Central PMCID: PMC7794182. Epub 2020/09/12. eng.
10. Nitecki R, Diver EJ, Kamdar MM, Boruta DM 2nd, Del Carmen MC, Clark RM, et al. Patterns of palliative care referral in ovarian cancer: a single institution 5 year retrospective analysis. Gynecol Oncol. 2018;148(3):521–6. PubMed PMID: 29395315. Epub 2018/02/06. eng.
11. Zimmermann C, Swami N, Krzyzanowska M, Leighl N, Rydall A, Rodin G, et al. Perceptions of palliative care among patients with advanced cancer and their caregivers. CMAJ. 2016;188(10):E217–E27. PubMed PMID: 27091801. Pubmed Central PMCID: PMC4938707. Epub 2016/04/20. eng.
12. Davis MP, Bruera E, Morganstern D. Early integration of palliative and supportive care in the cancer continuum: challenges and opportunities. Am Soc Clin Oncol Educ Book. 2013:144–50. PubMed PMID: 23714482. Epub 2013/05/30. eng.
13. Marsella A. Exploring the literature surrounding the transition into palliative care: a scoping review. Int J Palliat Nurs. 2009;15(4):186–9. PubMed PMID: 19430414. Epub 2009/05/12. eng.
14. Canzona MR, Love D, Barrett R, Henley J, Bridges S, Koontz A, et al. "Operating in the dark": nurses' attempts to help patients and families manage the transition from oncology to comfort care. J Clin Nurs. 2018;27(21–22):4158–67. PubMed PMID: 29968315. Epub 2018/07/04. eng.
15. Gardiner C, Ingleton C, Gott M, Ryan T. Exploring the transition from curative care to palliative care: a systematic review of the literature. BMJ Support Palliat Care. 2011;1(1):56–63. PubMed PMID: 24653051. Epub 2011/06/01. eng.
16. Gardiner C, Ingleton C, Gott M, Ryan T. Exploring the transition from curative care to palliative care: a systematic review of the literature. BMJ Support Palliat Care. 2015;5(4):335–42. PubMed PMID: 26586682. Epub 2015/11/21. eng.
17. Ziegler LE, Craigs CL, West RM, Carder P, Hurlow A, Millares-Martin P, et al. Is palliative care support associated with better quality end-of-life care indicators for patients with advanced cancer? A retrospective cohort study. BMJ Open. 2018;8(1):e018284. PubMed PMID: 29386222. Pubmed Central PMCID: PMC5829853. Epub 2018/02/02. eng.
18. Hui D, Mori M, Watanabe SM, Caraceni A, Strasser F, Saarto T, et al. Referral criteria for outpatient specialty palliative cancer care: an international consensus. Lancet Oncol. 2016;17(12):e552–e9. PubMed PMID: 27924753. Epub 2016/12/08. eng.

19. Treanor CJ, Santin O, Prue G, Coleman H, Cardwell CR, O'Halloran P, et al. Psychosocial interventions for informal caregivers of people living with cancer. Cochrane Database Syst Rev. 2019;6(6):CD009912. PubMed PMID: 31204791. Pubmed Central PMCID: PMC6573123. Epub 2019/06/18. eng.
20. Temel JS, Greer JA, Admane S, Gallagher ER, Jackson VA, Lynch TJ, et al. Longitudinal perceptions of prognosis and goals of therapy in patients with metastatic non-small-cell lung cancer: results of a randomized study of early palliative care. J Clin Oncol Off J Am Soc Clin Oncol. 2011;29(17):2319–26. PubMed PMID: 21555700. Epub 2011/05/11. eng.
21. Temel JS, Greer JA, El-Jawahri A, Pirl WF, Park ER, Jackson VA, et al. Effects of early integrated palliative care in patients with lung and gi cancer: a randomized clinical trial. J Clin Oncol Off J Am Soc Clin Oncol. 2017;35(8):834–41. PubMed PMID: 28029308. Pubmed Central PMCID: PMC5455686. Epub 2016/12/29. eng.
22. Dionne-Odom JN, Azuero A, Lyons KD, Hull JG, Tosteson T, Li Z, et al. Benefits of early versus delayed palliative care to informal family caregivers of patients with advanced cancer: outcomes from the ENABLE III randomized controlled trial. J Clin Oncol Off J Am Soc Clin Oncol. 2015;33(13):1446–52. PubMed PMID: 25800762. Pubmed Central PMCID: PMC4404423 online at www.jco.org. Author contributions are found at the end of this article. Epub 2015/03/25. eng.
23. Dionne-Odom JN, Azuero A, Lyons KD, Hull JG, Prescott AT, Tosteson T, et al. Family caregiver depressive symptom and grief outcomes from the ENABLE III randomized controlled trial. J Pain Symptom Manag. 2016;52(3):378–85. PubMed PMID: 27265814. Pubmed Central PMCID: PMC5023481. Epub 2016/06/07. eng.
24. Banerjee SC, Manna R, Coyle N, Penn S, Gallegos TE, Zaider T, et al. The implementation and evaluation of a communication skills training program for oncology nurses. Transl Behav Med. 2017;7(3):615–23. PubMed PMID: 28211000. Pubmed Central PMCID: PMC5645276. Epub 2017/02/18. eng.
25. Wittenberg E, Reb A, Kanter E. Communicating with patients and families around difficult topics in cancer care using the COMFORT communication curriculum. Semin Oncol Nurs. 2018;34(3):264–73. PubMed PMID: 30100368. Pubmed Central PMCID: PMC6156926. Epub 2018/08/14. eng.
26. Blanch-Hartigan D. An effective training to increase accurate recognition of patient emotion cues. Patient Educ Couns. 2012;89:274–80.
27. Thorne S, Hislop TG, Kim-Sing C, Oglov V, Oliffe JL, Stajduhar KI. Changing communication needs and preferences across the cancer care trajectory: insights from the patient perspective. Support Care Cancer. 2014;22(4):1009–15. PubMed PMID: 24287506. Epub 2013/11/30. eng.
28. Park CL. Meaning making in the context of disasters. J Clin Psychol. 2016;72(12):1234–46. PubMed PMID: 26900868. Epub 2016/02/24. eng.
29. Park CL, Sherman AC, Jim HS, Salsman JM. Religion/spirituality and health in the context of cancer: cross-domain integration, unresolved issues, and future directions. Cancer. 2015;121(21):3789–94. PubMed PMID: 26258608. Pubmed Central PMCID: PMC4618033. Epub 2015/08/11. eng.
30. Riba MB, Donovan KA, Andersen B, Braun I, Breitbart WS, Brewer BW, et al. Distress management, version 3.2019, NCCN clinical practice guidelines in oncology. J Natl Compr Canc Netw. 2019;17(10):1229–49. PubMed PMID: 31590149. Pubmed Central PMCID: PMC6907687. Epub 2019/10/08. eng.
31. An E, Lo C, Hales S, Zimmermann C, Rodin G. Demoralization and death anxiety in advanced cancer. Psycho-Oncology. 2018;27(11):2566–72. PubMed PMID: 30053317. Epub 2018/07/28. eng.
32. Jim HS, Pustejovsky JE, Park CL, Danhauer SC, Sherman AC, Fitchett G, et al. Religion, spirituality, and physical health in cancer patients: a meta-analysis. Cancer. 2015;121(21):3760–8. PubMed PMID: 26258868. Pubmed Central PMCID: PMC4618080. Epub 2015/08/11. eng.
33. Park CL, Pustejovsky JE, Trevino K, Sherman AC, Esposito C, Berendsen M, et al. Effects of psychosocial interventions on meaning and purpose in adults with cancer: a systematic

review and meta-analysis. Cancer. 2019;125(14):2383–93. PubMed PMID: 31034600. Pubmed Central PMCID: PMC6602826. Epub 2019/04/30. eng.
34. Vehling S, Kissane DW. Existential distress in cancer: alleviating suffering from fundamental loss and change. Psycho-Oncology. 2018;27(11):2525–30. PubMed PMID: 30307088. Epub 2018/10/12. eng.
35. Vehling S, Kamphausen A, Oechsle K, Hroch S, Bokemeyer C, Mehnert A. The preference to discuss expected survival is associated with loss of meaning and purpose in terminally Ill cancer patients. J Palliat Med. 2015;18(11):970–6. PubMed PMID: 26288027. Epub 2015/08/20. eng.
36. Masterson MP, Slivjak E, Jankauskaite G, Breitbart W, Pessin H, Schofield E, et al. Beyond the bucket list: unfinished and business among advanced cancer patients. Psycho-Oncology. 2018;27(11):2573–80. PubMed PMID: 29947443. Pubmed Central PMCID: PMC6219918. Epub 2018/06/28. eng.
37. Breitbart W, Pessin H, Rosenfeld B, Applebaum AJ, Lichtenthal WG, Li Y, et al. Individual meaning-centered psychotherapy for the treatment of psychological and existential distress: a randomized controlled trial in patients with advanced cancer. Cancer. 2018;124(15):3231–9. PubMed PMID: 29757459. Pubmed Central PMCID: PMC6097940. Epub 2018/05/15. eng.
38. Dalal S, Bruera E. End-of-life care matters: palliative cancer care results in better care and lower costs. Oncologist. 2017;22(4):361–8. PubMed PMID: 28314840. Pubmed Central PMCID: PMC5388382. Epub 2017/03/21. eng.
39. Thorne SE, Kuo M, Armstrong EA, McPherson G, Harris SR, Hislop TG. 'Being known': patients' perspectives of the dynamics of human connection in cancer care. Psycho-Oncology. 2000;14(10):887–98; discussion 99–900. PubMed PMID: 16200520. Epub 2005/10/04. eng.
40. van den Beuken-van Everdingen MH, Hochstenbach LM, Joosten EA, Tjan-Heijnen VC, Janssen DJ. Update on prevalence of pain in patients with cancer: systematic review and meta-analysis. J Pain Symptom Manag. 2016;51(6):1070–90.e9. PubMed PMID: 27112310. Epub 2016/04/27. eng.
41. Scarborough BM, Smith CB. Optimal pain management for patients with cancer in the modern era. CA Cancer J Clin. 2018;68(3):182–96. PubMed PMID: 29603142. Pubmed Central PMCID: PMC5980731. Epub 2018/04/01. eng.
42. Greco MT, Roberto A, Corli O, Deandrea S, Bandieri E, Cavuto S, et al. Quality of cancer pain management: an update of a systematic review of undertreatment of patients with cancer. J Clin Oncol Off J Am Soc Clin Oncol. 2014;32(36):4149–54. PubMed PMID: 25403222. Epub 2014/11/19. eng.
43. Henson LA, Maddocks M, Evans C, Davidson M, Hicks S, Higginson IJ. Palliative care and the management of common distressing symptoms in advanced cancer: pain, breathlessness, nausea and vomiting, and fatigue. J Clin Oncol Off J Am Soc Clin Oncol. 2020;38(9):905–14. PubMed PMID: 32023162. Pubmed Central PMCID: PMC7082153. Epub 2020/02/06. eng.
44. Cotogni P, Saini A, De Luca A. In-hospital palliative care: should we need to reconsider what role hospitals should have in patients with end-stage disease or advanced cancer? J Clin Med. 2018;7(2):18. PubMed PMID: 29385757. Pubmed Central PMCID: PMC5852434. Epub 2018/02/02. eng.
45. Alam S, Hannon B, Zimmermann C. Palliative care for family caregivers. J Clin Oncol Off J Am Soc Clin Oncol. 2020;38(9):926–36. PubMed PMID: 32023152. Epub 2020/02/06. eng.
46. El-Jawahri A, Greer JA, Pirl WF, Park ER, Jackson VA, Back AL, et al. Effects of early integrated palliative care on caregivers of patients with lung and gastrointestinal cancer: a randomized clinical trial. Oncologist. 2017;22(12):1528–34. PubMed PMID: 28894017. Pubmed Central PMCID: PMC5728034. Epub 2017/09/13. eng.
47. Northouse LL, Katapodi MC, Schafenacker AM, Weiss D. The impact of caregiving on the psychological Well-being of family caregivers and cancer patients. Semin Oncol Nurs. 2012;28(4):236–45. PubMed PMID: 23107181. Epub 2012/10/31. eng.
48. Northouse LL, Katapodi MC, Song L, Zhang L, Mood DW. Interventions with family caregivers of cancer patients: meta-analysis of randomized trials. CA Cancer J Clin.

2010;60(5):317–39. PubMed PMID: 20709946. Pubmed Central PMCID: PMC2946584. Epub 2010/08/17. eng.
49. Northouse LL, Mood DW, Schafenacker A, Kalemkerian G, Zalupski M, LoRusso P, et al. Randomized clinical trial of a brief and extensive dyadic intervention for advanced cancer patients and their family caregivers. Psycho-Oncology. 2013;22(3):555–63. PubMed PMID: 22290823. Pubmed Central PMCID: PMC3387514. Epub 2012/02/01. eng.
50. Krug K, Miksch A, Peters-Klimm F, Engeser P, Szecsenyi J. Correlation between patient quality of life in palliative care and burden of their family caregivers: a prospective observational cohort study. BMC Palliat Care. 2016;15:4. PubMed PMID: 26767785. Pubmed Central PMCID: PMC4714452. Epub 2016/01/16. eng.
51. Hodges LJ, Humphris GM, Macfarlane G. A meta-analytic investigation of the relationship between the psychological distress of cancer patients and their carers. Soc Sci Med. 2005;60(1):1–12. PubMed PMID: 15482862. Epub 2004/10/16. eng.
52. Duimering A, Turner J, Chu K, Huang F, Severin D, Ghosh S, et al. Informal caregiver quality of life in a palliative oncology population. Support Care Cancer. 2020;28(4):1695–702. PubMed PMID: 31292753. Epub 2019/07/12. eng.
53. Naoki Y, Matsuda Y, Maeda I, Kamino H, Kozaki Y, Tokoro A, et al. Association between family satisfaction and caregiver burden in cancer patients receiving outreach palliative care at home. Palliat Support Care. 2018;16(3):260–8. PubMed PMID: 28462749. Epub 2017/05/04. eng.
54. Hudson PL, Trauer T, Lobb E, Zordan R, Williams A, Quinn K, et al. Supporting family caregivers of hospitalised palliative care patients: a psychoeducational group intervention. BMJ Support Palliat Care. 2012;2(2):115–20. PubMed PMID: 24654051. Epub 2012/06/01. eng.
55. Smyth JA, Dempster M, Warwick I, Wilkinson P, McCorry NK. A systematic review of the patient- and carer-related factors affecting the experience of pain for advanced cancer patients cared for at home. J Pain Symptom Manag. 2018;55(2):496–507. PubMed PMID: 28843458. Epub 2017/08/28. eng.
56. Morris SE, Nayak MM, Block SD. Insights from bereaved family members about end-of-life care and bereavement. J Palliat Med. 2020;23(8):1030–7. PubMed PMID: 32040370. Epub 2020/02/11. eng.
57. Dionne-Odom JN, Taylor R, Rocque G, Chambless C, Ramsey T, Azuero A, et al. Adapting an early palliative care intervention to family caregivers of persons with advanced cancer in the rural deep south: a qualitative formative evaluation. J Pain Symptom Manag. 2018;55(6):1519–30. PubMed PMID: 29474939. Pubmed Central PMCID: PMC5951755. Epub 2018/02/24. eng.
58. Haley WE, LaMonde LA, Han B, Burton AM, Schonwetter R. Predictors of depression and life satisfaction among spousal caregivers in hospice: application of a stress process model. J Palliat Med. 2003;6(2):215–24. PubMed PMID: 12854938. Epub 2003/07/12. eng.
59. Northouse L, Williams AL, Given B, McCorkle R. Psychosocial care for family caregivers of patients with cancer. J Clin Oncol Off J Am Soc Clin Oncol. 2012;30(11):1227–34. PubMed PMID: 22412124. Epub 2012/03/14. eng.
60. Hudson P, Trauer T, Kelly B, O'Connor M, Thomas K, Summers M, et al. Reducing the psychological distress of family caregivers of home-based palliative care patients: short-term effects from a randomised controlled trial. Psycho-Oncology. 2013;22(9):1987–93. PubMed PMID: 23335153. Epub 2013/01/22. eng.
61. Hudson P, Trauer T, Kelly B, O'Connor M, Thomas K, Zordan R, et al. Reducing the psychological distress of family caregivers of home based palliative care patients: longer term effects from a randomised controlled trial. Psycho-Oncology. 2015;24(1):19–24. PubMed PMID: 25044819. Pubmed Central PMCID: PMC4309500. Epub 2014/07/22. eng.
62. Hoerger M, Greer JA, Jackson VA, Park ER, Pirl WF, El-Jawahri A, et al. Defining the elements of early palliative care that are associated with patient-reported outcomes and the delivery of end-of-life care. J Clin Oncol Off J Am Soc Clin Oncol. 2018;36(11):1096–102. PubMed PMID: 29474102. Pubmed Central PMCID: PMC5891131. Epub 2018/02/24. eng.
63. Ferrell BR, Temel JS, Temin S, Alesi ER, Balboni TA, Basch EM, et al. Integration of palliative care into standard oncology care: American Society of Clinical Oncology clini-

cal practice guideline update. J Clin Oncol Off J Am Soc Clin Oncol. 2017;35(1):96–112. PubMed PMID: 28034065. Epub 2016/12/31. eng.
64. Wang M, Zhao J, Zhang L, Wei F, Lian Y, Wu Y, et al. Role of tumor microenvironment in tumorigenesis. J Cancer. 2017;8(5):761–73. PubMed PMID: 28382138. Pubmed Central PMCID: PMC5381164. Epub 2017/04/07. eng.
65. Petrie KJ, Rief W. Psychobiological mechanisms of placebo and nocebo effects: pathways to improve treatments and reduce side effects. Annu Rev Psychol. 2019;70:599–625. PubMed PMID: 30110575. Epub 2018/08/16. eng.
66. Folkman S. Stress, coping and hope. Psycho-Oncology. 2010;19:901–8.
67. Hultgren BA, Turrisi R, Mallett KA, Ackerman S, Robinson JK. Influence of quality of relationship between patient with melanoma and partner on partner-assisted skin examination education: a randomized clinical trial. JAMA Dermatol. 2016;152(2):184–90. PubMed PMID: 26422745. Pubmed Central PMCID: PMC4890560. Epub 2015/10/01. eng.
68. Robinson S, Kissane DW, Brooker J, Burney S. A systematic review of the demoralization syndrome in individuals with progressive disease and cancer: a decade of research. J Pain Symptom Manag. 2015;49(3):595–610. PubMed PMID: 25131888. Epub 2014/08/19. eng.
69. Mathew A, Doorenbos AZ, Li H, Jang MK, Park CG, Bronas UG. Allostatic load in cancer: a systematic review and mini meta-analysis. Biol Res Nurs. 2021;23(3):341–61. PubMed PMID: 33138637. Epub 2020/11/04. eng.
70. Mathews HL, Konley T, Kosik KL, Krukowski K, Eddy J, Albuquerque K, et al. Epigenetic patterns associated with the immune dysregulation that accompanies psychosocial distress. Brain Behav Immun. 2011;25(5):830–9. PubMed PMID: 21146603. Pubmed Central PMCID: PMC3079772. Epub 2010/12/15. eng.
71. Leong Abdullah MFI, Hami R, Appalanaido GK, Azman N, Mohd Shariff N, Md Sharif SS. Diagnosis of cancer is not a death sentence: examining posttraumatic growth and its associated factors in cancer patients. J Psychosoc Oncol. 2019;1:1–16. PubMed PMID: 30821660. Epub 2019/03/02. eng.
72. Steffen LE, Cheavens JS, Vowles KE, Gabbard J, Nguyen H, Gan GN, et al. Hope-related goal cognitions and daily experiences of fatigue, pain, and functional concern among lung cancer patients. Support Care Cancer. 2020;28(2):827–35. PubMed PMID: 31152302. Pubmed Central PMCID: PMC6885110. Epub 2019/06/04. eng.
73. Jacobsen J, Kvale E, Rabow M, Rinaldi S, Cohen S, Weissman D, et al. Helping patients with serious illness live well through the promotion of adaptive coping: a report from the improving outpatient palliative care (IPAL-OP) initiative. J Palliat Med. 2014;17(4):463–8. PubMed PMID: 24579823. Epub 2014/03/04. eng.
74. Lutgendorf S, De Geest K, Bender D, Ahmed A, Goodheart M, Dahmoush L, Zimmerman M, et al. Social influences on clinical outcomes of patients with ovarian cancer. J Clin Oncol. 2012;30(23):2885–90.
75. Lutgendorf SK, DeGeest K, Dahmoush L, Farley D, Penedo F, Bender D, et al. Social isolation is associated with elevated tumor norepinephrine in ovarian carcinoma patients. Brain Behav Immun. 2011;25(2):250–5. PubMed PMID: 20955777. Pubmed Central PMCID: PMC3103818. Epub 2010/10/20. eng.
76. Lutgendorf SK, Sood AK, Antoni MH. Host factors and cancer progression: biobehavioral signaling pathways and interventions. J Clin Oncol Off J Am Soc Clin Oncol. 2010;28(26):4094–9. PubMed PMID: 20644093. Pubmed Central PMCID: PMC2940426. Epub 2010/07/21. eng.
77. Kavalieratos D, Corbelli J, Zhang D, Dionne-Odom JN, Ernecoff NC, Hanmer J, et al. Association between palliative care and patient and caregiver outcomes: a systematic review and meta-analysis. JAMA. 2016;316(20):2104–14. PubMed PMID: 27893131. Pubmed Central PMCID: PMC5226373. Epub 2016/11/29. eng.
78. Fulton JJ, LeBlanc TW, Cutson TM, Porter Starr KN, Kamal A, Ramos K, et al. Integrated outpatient palliative care for patients with advanced cancer: a systematic review and meta-analysis. Palliat Med. 2019;33(2):123–34. PubMed PMID: 30488781. Pubmed Central PMCID: PMC7069657. Epub 2018/11/30. eng.

79. Bakitas M, Lyons KD, Hegel MT, Balan S, Brokaw FC, Seville J, et al. Effects of a palliative care intervention on clinical outcomes in patients with advanced cancer: the project ENABLE II randomized controlled trial. JAMA. 2009;302(7):741–9. PubMed PMID: 19690306. Pubmed Central PMCID: PMC3657724. Epub 2009/08/20. eng.
80. Bakitas MA, Tosteson TD, Li Z, Lyons KD, Hull JG, Li Z, et al. Early versus delayed initiation of concurrent palliative oncology care: patient outcomes in the ENABLE III randomized controlled trial. J Clin Oncol Off J Am Soc Clin Oncol. 2015;33(13):1438–45. PubMed PMID: 25800768. Pubmed Central PMCID: PMC4404422. Epub 2015/03/25. eng.
81. Teo I, Baid D, Ozdemir S, Malhotra C, Singh R, Harding R, et al. Family caregivers of advanced cancer patients: self-perceived competency and meaning-making. BMJ Support Palliat Care. 2020;10(4):435–42. PubMed PMID: 31806656. Epub 2019/12/07. eng.
82. Teo I, Krishnan A, Lee GL. Psychosocial interventions for advanced cancer patients: a systematic review. Psycho-Oncology. 2019;28(7):1394–407. PubMed PMID: 31077475. Epub 2019/05/12. eng.
83. Greer JA, Jackson VA, Meier DE, Temel JS. Early integration of palliative care services with standard oncology care for patients with advanced cancer. CA Cancer J Clin. 2013;63(5):349–63. PubMed PMID: 23856954. Epub 2013/07/17. eng.
84. Ahn S, Romo RD, Campbell CL. A systematic review of interventions for family caregivers who care for patients with advanced cancer at home. Patient Educ Couns. 2020;103(8):1518–30. PubMed PMID: 32201172. Pubmed Central PMCID: PMC7311285. Epub 2020/03/24. eng.
85. Washington KT, Craig KW, Parker Oliver D, Ruggeri JS, Brunk SR, Goldstein AK, et al. Family caregivers' perspectives on communication with cancer care providers. J Psychosoc Oncol. 2019;37(6):777–90. PubMed PMID: 31204604. Pubmed Central PMCID: PMC7350905. Epub 2019/06/18. eng.
86. Harrington KJ, Affronti ML, Schneider SM, Razzak AR, Smith TJ. Improving attitudes and perceptions about end-of-life nursing on a hospital-based palliative care unit. J Hosp Palliat Nurs. 2019;21(4):272–9. PubMed PMID: 30893285. Epub 2019/03/21. eng.
87. Dunkel-Schetter C, Feinstein LG, Taylor SE, Falke RL. Patterns of coping with cancer. Health Psychol. 1992;11(2):79–87. PubMed PMID: 1582383. Epub 1992/01/01. eng.
88. Greer JA, Traeger L, Bemis H, Solis J, Hendriksen ES, Park ER, et al. A pilot randomized controlled trial of brief cognitive-behavioral therapy for anxiety in patients with terminal cancer. Oncologist. 2012;17(10):1337–45. PubMed PMID: 22688670. Pubmed Central PMCID: PMC3481900 indicated no financial relationships. Section Editors: Eduardo Bruera: None; Russell K. Portenoy: Arsenal Medical Inc., Pfizer, Grupo Ferrer, Transcript Pharma, Xenon (C/A); Allergan, Ameritox, Boston Scientific, Covidien Mallinckrodt Inc., Endo Pharmaceuticals, Forest Labs, K-Pax Pharmaceuticals, Medtronics, Otsuka Pharma, ProStrakan, Purdue Pharma, Salix, St. Jude Medical (RF) Reviewer "A": None Reviewer "B": None. Epub 2012/06/13. eng.
89. Folkman S. The case for positive emotions in the stress process. Anxiety Stress Coping. 2008;21(1):3–14. PubMed PMID: 18027121. Epub 2007/11/21. eng.
90. Puchalski C, Romer AL. Taking a spiritual history allows clinicians to understand patients more fully. J Palliat Med. 2000;3(1):129–37. PubMed PMID: 15859737. Epub 2005/04/30. eng.
91. Gross JJ. Emotion regulation: current status and future prospects. Psychol Inq. 2015;26:1–26.
92. Waugh CE. The roles of positive emotion in the regulation of emotional responses to negative events. Emotion (Washington, DC). 2020;20(1):54–8. PubMed PMID: 31961178. Epub 2020/01/22. eng.
93. Seiler A, Jenewein J. Resilience in cancer patients. Front Psych. 2019;10:208. PubMed PMID: 31024362. Pubmed Central PMCID: PMC6460045. Epub 2019/04/27. eng.
94. McEwen BS. Physiology and neurobiology of stress and adaptation: central role of the brain. Physiol Rev. 2007;87(3):873–904. PubMed PMID: 17615391. Epub 2007/07/07. eng.
95. Gross JJ, John OP. Individual differences in two emotion regulation processes: implications for affect, relationships, and well-being. J Pers Soc Psychol. 2003;85(2):348–62. PubMed PMID: 12916575. Epub 2003/08/15. eng.

96. Kuppens P, Realo A, Diener E. The role of positive and negative emotions in life satisfaction judgment across nations. J Pers Soc Psychol. 2008;95(1):66–75. PubMed PMID: 18605852. Epub 2008/07/09. eng.
97. King LA, Hicks JA, Krull JL, Del Gaiso AK. Positive affect and the experience of meaning in life. J Pers Soc Psychol. 2006;90(1):179–96. PubMed PMID: 16448317. Epub 2006/02/02. eng.
98. Tugade MM, Fredrickson BL. Resilient individuals use positive emotions to bounce back from negative emotional experiences. J Pers Soc Psychol. 2004;86(2):320–33. PubMed PMID: 14769087. Pubmed Central PMCID: PMC3132556. Epub 2004/02/11. eng.
99. Sevan Schreiber D. Not the last good bye: on life, death, healing and cancer. Melbourne, London: Scribe; 2011.
100. Salander P. "Spirituality" hardly facilitates our understanding of existential distress-but "everyday life" might. Psycho-Oncology. 2018;27(11):2654–6. PubMed PMID: 29843191. Epub 2018/05/31. eng.
101. Park C, Folkman S. Meaning in the context of stress and coping. Rev Gen Psychol. 1997;1:115–44.
102. Folkman S. Positive psychological states and coping with severe stress. Soc Sci Med. 1997;45(8):1207–21. PubMed PMID: 9381234. Epub 1997/09/25. eng.
103. Jacobsen J, Brenner K, Greer JA, Jacobo M, Rosenberg L, Nipp RD, et al. When a patient is reluctant to talk about it: a dual framework to focus on living well and tolerate the possibility of dying. J Palliat Med. 2018;21(3):322–7. PubMed PMID: 28972862. Epub 2017/10/04. eng.
104. Li Y, Xing X, Shi X, Yan P, Chen Y, Li M, et al. The effectiveness of music therapy for patients with cancer: a systematic review and meta-analysis. J Adv Nurs. 2020;76(5):1111–23. PubMed PMID: 32017183. Epub 2020/02/06. eng.
105. Mount BM, Boston PH, Cohen SR. Healing connections: on moving from suffering to a sense of Well-being. J Pain Symptom Manag. 2007;33(4):372–88. PubMed PMID: 17397699. Epub 2007/04/03. eng.
106. Sherman AC, Merluzzi TV, Pustejovsky JE, Park CL, George L, Fitchett G, et al. A meta-analytic review of religious or spiritual involvement and social health among cancer patients. Cancer. 2015;121(21):3779–88. PubMed PMID: 26258730. Pubmed Central PMCID: PMC4618183. Epub 2015/08/11. eng.
107. Salsman JM, Fitchett G, Merluzzi TV, Sherman AC, Park CL. Religion, spirituality, and health outcomes in cancer: a case for a meta-analytic investigation. Cancer. 2015;121(21):3754–9. PubMed PMID: 26258400. Epub 2015/08/11. Eng.
108. Puchalski CM, Vitillo R, Hull SK, Reller N. Improving the spiritual dimension of whole person care: reaching national and international consensus. J Palliat Med. 2014;17(6):642–56. PubMed PMID: 24842136. Pubmed Central PMCID: PMC4038982. Epub 2014/05/21. eng.
109. Bernard M, Strasser F, Gamondi C, Braunschweig G, Forster M, Kaspers-Elekes K, et al. Relationship between spirituality, meaning in life, psychological distress, wish for hastened death, and their influence on quality of life in palliative care patients. J Pain Symptom Manag. 2017;54(4):514–22. PubMed PMID: 28716616. Epub 2017/07/19. eng.
110. Puchalski C, Ferrell B, Virani R, Otis-Green S, Baird P, Bull J, et al. Improving the quality of spiritual care as a dimension of palliative care: the report of the Consensus Conference. J Palliat Med. 2009;12(10):885–904. PubMed PMID: 19807235. Epub 2009/10/08. eng.
111. Park CL. Making sense of the meaning literature: an integrative review of meaning making and its effects on adjustment to stressful life events. Psychol Bull. 2010;136(2):257–301. PubMed PMID: 20192563. Epub 2010/03/03. eng.
112. Lee V, Cohen SR, Edgar L, Laizner AM, Gagnon AJ. Meaning-making and psychological adjustment to cancer: development of an intervention and pilot results. Oncol Nurs Forum. 2006;33(2):291–302. PubMed PMID: 16518445. Epub 2006/03/07. eng.
113. Lee V, Robin Cohen S, Edgar L, Laizner AM, Gagnon AJ. Meaning-making intervention during breast or colorectal cancer treatment improves self-esteem, optimism, and self-efficacy. Soc Sci Med. 2006;62(12):3133–45. PubMed PMID: 16413644. Epub 2006/01/18. eng.

114. Zhang X, Xiao H, Chen Y. Effects of life review on mental health and Well-being among cancer patients: a systematic review. Int J Nurs Stud. 2017;74:138–48. PubMed PMID: 28692880. Epub 2017/07/12. eng.
115. Andersen BL, Thornton LM, Shapiro CL, Farrar WB, Mundy BL, Yang HC, et al. Biobehavioral, immune, and health benefits following recurrence for psychological intervention participants. Clin Cancer Res. 2010;16(12):3270–8. PubMed PMID: 20530702. Pubmed Central PMCID: PMC2910547. Epub 2010/06/10. eng.
116. Antoni MH, Lechner S, Diaz A, Vargas S, Holley H, Phillips K, et al. Cognitive behavioral stress management effects on psychosocial and physiological adaptation in women undergoing treatment for breast cancer. Brain Behav Immun. 2009;23(5):580–91. PubMed PMID: 18835434. Pubmed Central PMCID: PMC2722111. Epub 2008/10/07. eng.
117. Carlson LE. Distress management through mind-body therapies in oncology. J Natl Cancer Inst Monogr. 2017;2017(52). PubMed PMID: 29140490. Epub 2017/11/16. eng.
118. Dusek JA, Otu HH, Wohlhueter AL, Bhasin M, Zerbini LF, Joseph MG, et al. Genomic counter-stress changes induced by the relaxation response. PLoS One. 2008;3(7):e2576. PubMed PMID: 18596974. Pubmed Central PMCID: PMC2432467. Epub 2008/07/04. eng.
119. Bhasin MK, Dusek JA, Chang BH, Joseph MG, Denninger JW, Fricchione GL, et al. Relaxation response induces temporal transcriptome changes in energy metabolism, insulin secretion and inflammatory pathways. PLoS One. 2013;8(5):e62817. PubMed PMID: 23650531. Pubmed Central PMCID: PMC3641112. Epub 2013/05/08. eng.
120. Carlson LE, Beattie TL, Giese-Davis J, Faris P, Tamagawa R, Fick LJ, et al. Mindfulness-based cancer recovery and supportive-expressive therapy maintain telomere length relative to controls in distressed breast cancer survivors. Cancer. 2015;121(3):476–84. PubMed PMID: 25367403. Epub 2014/11/05. eng.
121. Ngamkham S, Holden JE, Smith EL. A systematic review: mindfulness intervention for cancer-related pain. Asia Pac J Oncol Nurs. 2019;6(2):161–9. PubMed PMID: 30931361. Pubmed Central PMCID: PMC6371675. Epub 2019/04/02. eng.
122. Lengacher CA, Reich RR, Paterson CL, Ramesar S, Park JY, Alinat C, et al. Examination of broad symptom improvement resulting from mindfulness-based stress reduction in breast cancer survivors: a randomized controlled trial. J Clin Oncol Off J Am Soc Clin Oncol. 2016;34(24):2827–34. PubMed PMID: 27247219. Pubmed Central PMCID: PMC5012660 online at www.jco.org. Author contributions are found at the end of this article. Epub 2016/06/02. eng.
123. Reeve K, Black PA, Huang J. Examining the impact of a Healing Touch intervention to reduce posttraumatic stress disorder symptoms in combat veterans. Psychol Trauma Theory Res Pract Policy. 2020;12(8):897–903. PubMed PMID: 33346680. Epub 2020/12/22. eng.
124. Bower JE, Crosswell AD, Stanton AL, Crespi CM, Winston D, Arevalo J, et al. Mindfulness meditation for younger breast cancer survivors: a randomized controlled trial. Cancer. 2015;121(8):1231–40. PubMed PMID: 25537522. Pubmed Central PMCID: PMC4393338. Epub 2014/12/30. eng.
125. Johns SA, Brown LF, Beck-Coon K, Talib TL, Monahan PO, Giesler RB, et al. Randomized controlled pilot trial of mindfulness-based stress reduction compared to psychoeducational support for persistently fatigued breast and colorectal cancer survivors. Support Care Cancer. 2016;24(10):4085–96. PubMed PMID: 27189614. Pubmed Central PMCID: PMC5221754. Epub 2016/05/18. eng.
126. Cao W, Qi X, Cai DA, Han X. Modeling posttraumatic growth among cancer patients: the roles of social support, appraisals, and adaptive coping. Psycho-Oncology. 2018;27(1):208–15. PubMed PMID: 28171681. Epub 2017/02/09. eng.
127. Andersen BL, Yang HC, Farrar WB, Golden-Kreutz DM, Emery CF, Thornton LM, et al. Psychologic intervention improves survival for breast cancer patients: a randomized clinical trial. Cancer. 2008;113(12):3450–8. PubMed PMID: 19016270. Pubmed Central PMCID: PMC2661422. Epub 2008/11/19. eng.

128. Lutgendorf SK, Sood AK, Anderson B, McGinn S, Maiseri H, Dao M, et al. Social support, psychological distress, and natural killer cell activity in ovarian cancer. J Clin Oncol Off J Am Soc Clin Oncol. 2005;23(28):7105–13. PubMed PMID: 16192594. Epub 2005/09/30. eng.
129. Lutgendorf SK, DeGeest K, Sung CY, Arevalo JM, Penedo F, Lucci J 3rd, et al. Depression, social support, and beta-adrenergic transcription control in human ovarian cancer. Brain Behav Immun. 2009;23(2):176–83. PubMed PMID: 18550328. Pubmed Central PMCID: PMC2677379. Epub 2008/06/14. eng.
130. Lutgendorf SK, Andersen BL. Biobehavioral approaches to cancer progression and survival: mechanisms and interventions. Am Psychol. 2015;70(2):186–97. PubMed PMID: 25730724. Pubmed Central PMCID: PMC4347942. Epub 2015/03/03. eng.
131. Mori M, Yoshida S, Shiozaki M, Morita T, Baba M, Aoyama M, et al. "What I did for my loved one is more important than whether we talked about death": a nationwide survey of bereaved family members. J Palliat Med. 2018;21(3):335–41. PubMed PMID: 29154690. Epub 2017/11/21. eng.
132. Koffman J, Morgan M, Edmonds P, Speck P, Higginson IJ. 'The greatest thing in the world is the family': the meaning of social support among black Caribbean and white British patients living with advanced cancer. Psycho-Oncology. 2012;21(4):400–8. PubMed PMID: 21259379. Epub 2011/01/25. eng.
133. Benson H, Stuart E. The wellness book: the comprehensive guide to maintaining health and treating stress-related illness. New York: Simon and Schuster; 1992.
134. Zeng YS, Wang C, Ward KE, Hume AL. Complementary and alternative medicine in hospice and palliative care: a systematic review. J Pain Symptom Manag. 2018;56(5):781–94.e4. PubMed PMID: 30076965. Epub 2018/08/05. eng.
135. Wood LJ, Weymann K. Inflammation and neural signaling: etiologic mechanisms of the cancer treatment-related symptom cluster. Curr Opin Support Palliat Care. 2013;7(1):54–9. PubMed PMID: 23314015. Epub 2013/01/15. eng.
136. Kwekkeboom KL. Cancer symptom cluster management. Semin Oncol Nurs. 2016;32(4):373–82. PubMed PMID: 27789073. Pubmed Central PMCID: PMC5143160. Epub 2016/10/30. eng.
137. Kirtonia A, Sethi G, Garg M. The multifaceted role of reactive oxygen species in tumorigenesis. Cell Mol Life Sci. 2020;77(22):4459–83. PubMed PMID: 32358622. Epub 2020/05/03. eng.
138. Sillar JR, Germon ZP, DeIuliis GN, Dun MD. The role of reactive oxygen species in acute myeloid leukaemia. Int J Mol Sci. 2019;20(23):6003. PubMed PMID: 31795243. Pubmed Central PMCID: PMC6929020. Epub 2019/12/05. eng.
139. Kwekkeboom K, Zhang Y, Campbell T, Coe CL, Costanzo E, Serlin RC, et al. Randomized controlled trial of a brief cognitive-behavioral strategies intervention for the pain, fatigue, and sleep disturbance symptom cluster in advanced cancer. Psycho-Oncology. 2018;27(12):2761–9. PubMed PMID: 30189462. Pubmed Central PMCID: PMC6279506. Epub 2018/09/07. eng.
140. Swarm RA, Paice JA, Anghelescu DL, Are M, Bruce JY, Buga S, et al. Adult cancer pain, version 3.2019, NCCN clinical practice guidelines in oncology. J Natl Compr Canc Netw. 2019;17(8):977–1007. PubMed PMID: 31390582. Epub 2019/08/08. eng.
141. Rouleau CR, Garland SN, Carlson LE. The impact of mindfulness-based interventions on symptom burden, positive psychological outcomes, and biomarkers in cancer patients. Cancer Manag Res. 2015;7:121–31. PubMed PMID: 26064068. Pubmed Central PMCID: PMC4457221. Epub 2015/06/13. eng.
142. Dhingra L, Ahmed E, Shin J, Scharaga E, Magun M. Cognitive effects and sedation. Pain Med (Malden, MA). 2015;16(Suppl 1):S37–43. PubMed PMID: 26461075. Epub 2015/10/16. eng.
143. Colloca L, Barsky AJ. Placebo and nocebo effects. N Engl J Med. 2020;382(6):554–61. PubMed PMID: 32023375. Epub 2020/02/06. eng.
144. Colloca L, Lopiano L, Lanotte M, Benedetti F. Overt versus covert treatment for pain, anxiety, and Parkinson's disease. Lancet Neurol. 2004;3(11):679–84. PubMed PMID: 15488461. Epub 2004/10/19. eng.

145. Kwekkeboom KL, Cherwin CH, Lee JW, Wanta B. Mind-body treatments for the pain-fatigue-sleep disturbance symptom cluster in persons with cancer. J Pain Symptom Manag. 2010;39(1):126–38. PubMed PMID: 19900778. Pubmed Central PMCID: PMC3084527. Epub 2009/11/11. eng.
146. Charalambous A, Giannakopoulou M, Bozas E, Marcou Y, Kitsios P, Paikousis L. Guided imagery and progressive muscle relaxation as a cluster of symptoms management intervention in patients receiving chemotherapy: a randomized control trial. PLoS One. 2016;11(6):e0156911. PubMed PMID: 27341675. Pubmed Central PMCID: PMC4920431. Epub 2016/06/25. eng.
147. Charalambous A, Giannakopoulou M, Bozas E, Paikousis L. A randomized controlled trial for the effectiveness of progressive muscle relaxation and guided imagery as anxiety reducing interventions in breast and prostate cancer patients undergoing chemotherapy. Evid Based Complement Alternat Med. 2015;2015:270876. PubMed PMID: 26347018. Pubmed Central PMCID: PMC4545275. Epub 2015/09/09. eng.
148. Zemel RA. Pharmacologic and non-pharmacologic dyspnea management in advanced cancer patients. Am J Hosp Palliat Care. 2021;39(7):847–55. PubMed PMID: 34510917. Epub 2021/09/14. eng.
149. Hui D, Bohlke K, Bao T, Campbell TC, Coyne PJ, Currow DC, et al. Management of dyspnea in advanced cancer: ASCO guideline. J Clin Oncol Off J Am Soc Clin Oncol. 2021;39(12):1389–411. PubMed PMID: 33617290. Epub 2021/02/23. eng.
150. Parshall MB, Schwartzstein RM, Adams L, Banzett RB, Manning HL, Bourbeau J, et al. An official American Thoracic Society statement: update on the mechanisms, assessment, and management of dyspnea. Am J Respir Crit Care Med. 2012;185(4):435–52. PubMed PMID: 22336677. Pubmed Central PMCID: PMC5448624. Epub 2012/02/18. eng.
151. Stevens JP, Sheridan AR, Bernstein HB, Baker K, Lansing RW, Schwartzstein RM, et al. A multidimensional profile of dyspnea in hospitalized patients. Chest. 2019;156(3):507–17. PubMed PMID: 31128117. Pubmed Central PMCID: PMC7090324. Epub 2019/05/28. eng.
152. Ergin E, Sagkal Midilli T, Baysal E. The effect of music on dyspnea severity, anxiety, and hemodynamic parameters in patients with dyspnea. J Hosp Palliat Nurs. 2018;20(1):81–7. PubMed PMID: 30063618. Epub 2018/08/01. eng.
153. Gallagher LM, Lagman R, Rybicki L. Outcomes of music therapy interventions on symptom management in palliative medicine patients. Am J Hosp Palliat Care. 2018;35(2):250–7. PubMed PMID: 28274132. Epub 2017/03/10. eng.
154. Gallagher LM, Lagman R, Bates D, Edsall M, Eden P, Janaitis J, et al. Perceptions of family members of palliative medicine and hospice patients who experienced music therapy. Support Care Cancer. 2017;25(6):1769–78. PubMed PMID: 28105524. Epub 2017/01/21. eng.
155. Yates P, Hardy J, Clavarino A, Fong KM, Mitchell G, Skerman H, et al. A randomized controlled trial of a non-pharmacological intervention for cancer-related dyspnea. Front Oncol. 2020;10:591610. PubMed PMID: 33335858. Pubmed Central PMCID: PMC7737519. Epub 2020/12/19. eng.
156. Molassiotis A, Charalambous A, Taylor P, Stamataki Z, Summers Y. The effect of resistance inspiratory muscle training in the management of breathlessness in patients with thoracic malignancies: a feasibility randomised trial. Support Care Cancer. 2015;23(6):1637–45. PubMed PMID: 25417042. Epub 2014/11/25. eng.
157. Birch S, Lee MS, Alraek T, Kim TH. Evidence, safety and recommendations for when to use acupuncture for treating cancer related symptoms: a narrative review. Integrat Med Res. 2019;8(3):160–6. PubMed PMID: 31304088. Pubmed Central PMCID: PMC6600712. Epub 2019/07/16. eng.
158. McGeeney BE. Acupuncture is all placebo and here is why. Headache. 2015;55(3):465–9. PubMed PMID: 25660556. Epub 2015/02/11. eng.
159. von Trott P, Oei SL, Ramsenthaler C. Acupuncture for breathlessness in advanced diseases: a systematic review and meta-analysis. J Pain Symptom Manag. 2020;59(2):327–38 e3. PubMed PMID: 31539602. Epub 2019/09/21. eng.

160. Chiu HY, Hsieh YJ, Tsai PS. Systematic review and meta-analysis of acupuncture to reduce cancer-related pain. Eur J Cancer Care. 2017;26(2). PubMed PMID: 26853524. Epub 2016/02/09. eng.
161. Bauml J, Haas A, Simone CB 2nd, Li SQ, Cohen RB, Langer CJ, et al. Acupuncture for dyspnea in lung cancer: results of a feasibility trial. Integr Cancer Ther. 2016;15(3):326–32. PubMed PMID: 27114385. Pubmed Central PMCID: PMC5739187. Epub 2016/04/27. eng.
162. Doğan N, Taşcı S. The effects of acupressure on quality of life and dyspnea in lung cancer: a randomized, controlled trial. Altern Ther Health Med. 2020;26(1):49–56. PubMed PMID: 31221935. Epub 2019/06/22. eng.
163. Minchom A, Punwani R, Filshie J, Bhosle J, Nimako K, Myerson J, et al. A randomised study comparing the effectiveness of acupuncture or morphine versus the combination for the relief of dyspnoea in patients with advanced non-small cell lung cancer and mesothelioma. Eur J Cancer (Oxford, Engl: 1990). 2016;61:102–10. PubMed PMID: 27156228. Epub 2016/05/09. eng.
164. Garcia MK, Driver L, Haddad R, Lee R, Palmer JL, Wei Q, et al. Acupuncture for treatment of uncontrolled pain in cancer patients: a pragmatic pilot study. Integr Cancer Ther. 2014;13(2):133–40. PubMed PMID: 24282103. Epub 2013/11/28. eng.
165. Lee SH, Kim JY, Yeo S, Kim SH, Lim S. Meta-analysis of massage therapy on cancer pain. Integr Cancer Ther. 2015;14(4):297–304. PubMed PMID: 25784669. Epub 2015/03/19. eng.
166. Mantoudi A, Parpa E, Tsilika E, Batistaki C, Nikoloudi M, Kouloulias V, et al. Complementary therapies for patients with cancer: reflexology and relaxation in integrative palliative care. A randomized controlled comparative study. J Altern Complement Med. 2020;26(9):792–8. PubMed PMID: 32924560. Epub 2020/09/15. eng.
167. Shin ES, Seo KH, Lee SH, Jang JE, Jung YM, Kim MJ, et al. Massage with or without aromatherapy for symptom relief in people with cancer. Cochrane Database Syst Rev. 2016;(6):CD009873. PubMed PMID: 27258432. Epub 2016/06/04. eng.
168. Lutgendorf SK, Mullen-Houser E, Russell D, Degeest K, Jacobson G, Hart L, et al. Preservation of immune function in cervical cancer patients during chemoradiation using a novel integrative approach. Brain Behav Immun. 2010;24(8):1231–40. PubMed PMID: 20600809. Pubmed Central PMCID: PMC3010350. Epub 2010/07/06. eng.
169. de van der Schueren MAE, Laviano A, Blanchard H, Jourdan M, Arends J, Baracos VE. Systematic review and meta-analysis of the evidence for oral nutritional intervention on nutritional and clinical outcomes during chemo(radio)therapy: current evidence and guidance for design of future trials. Ann Oncol. 2018;29(5):1141–53. PubMed PMID: 29788170. Pubmed Central PMCID: PMC5961292. Epub 2018/05/23. eng.
170. Argilés JM, López-Soriano FJ, Busquets S. Mechanisms and treatment of cancer cachexia. Nutr Metab Cardiovasc Dis. 2013;23(Suppl 1):S19–24. PubMed PMID: 22749678. Epub 2012/07/04. eng.
171. Nieman DC, Wentz LM. The compelling link between physical activity and the body's defense system. J Sport Health Sci. 2019;8(3):201–17. PubMed PMID: 31193280. Pubmed Central PMCID: PMC6523821. Epub 2019/06/14. eng.
172. Leventhal H, Phillips LA, Burns E. The Common-Sense Model of Self-Regulation (CSM): a dynamic framework for understanding illness self-management. J Behav Med. 2016;39(6):935–46. PubMed PMID: 27515801. Epub 2016/08/16. eng.
173. Parker Oliver D, Washington K, Demiris G, Wallace A, Propst MR, Uraizee AM, Craig K, et al. Shared decision making in home hospice nursing visits: a qualitative study. J Pain Symptom Manag. 2018;55(3):922–9.
174. Mehta A, Chan LS, Cohen SR. Flying blind: sources of distress for family caregivers of palliative cancer patients managing pain at home. J Psychosoc Oncol. 2014;32(1):94–111. PubMed PMID: 24428253. Epub 2014/01/17. eng.
175. Al Daken LI, Ahmad MM. The implementation of mindfulness-based interventions and educational interventions to support family caregivers of patients with cancer: a systematic review. Perspect Psychiatr Care. 2018;54(3):441–52. PubMed PMID: 29745417. Epub 2018/05/11. eng.

176. Li G, Yuan H, Zhang W. The effects of mindfulness-based stress reduction for family caregivers: systematic review. Arch Psychiatr Nurs. 2016;30(2):292–9. PubMed PMID: 26992885. Epub 2016/03/20. eng.
177. World Cancer Research Fund AIfcr. Diet, nutrition, physical activity and cancer: a global perspective. Summary of 3rd expert report. Continuous update project expert report. dietandcancerreport.org; 2018.
178. Moore PM, Rivera S, Bravo-Soto GA, Olivares C, Lawrie TA. Communication skills training for healthcare professionals working with people who have cancer. Cochrane Database Syst Rev. 2018;7(7):CD003751. PubMed PMID: 30039853. Pubmed Central PMCID: PMC6513291 known. Camila Olivares: none known. Theresa A Lawrie: none known. Epub 2018/07/25. eng.
179. Schram AW, Hougham GW, Meltzer DO, Ruhnke GW. Palliative care in critical care settings: a systematic review of communication-based competencies essential for patient and family satisfaction. Am J Hosp Palliat Care. 2017;34(9):887–95. PubMed PMID: 27582376. Epub 2016/09/02. eng.

Is It Feasible 19

19.1 Introduction

The stress, healing and resilience nursing model of whole person care is designed to promote multimodal, multitargeted psychosocial nursing interventions to enhance healing and resilience in patients and their informal caregivers. Each psychosocial approach described in this book falls within the purview of the nursing profession with demonstrated clinical benefits for patients and their family caregiver.

Is a model relevant? The nursing model provides the goals of practice and the theoretical and empirical predicate that justify the psychosocial interventions to promote healing and resilience in patients and caregivers. Moreover, it provides a patient-centered, theoretical, and scientific context to advance clinical, research, and educational practice. Adopting the model promotes the nurses' purposeful acquisition of relevant scientific knowledge and related psychosocial clinical skills needed to facilitate healing and resilient capabilities, enhance health, and promote quality of life of the whole person with cancer with the family caregiver. It provides a substantive base for clinical researchers to carry out qualitative, cross sectional, longitudinal, and randomized controlled studies that may deepen knowledge of the model's substantive base. It facilitates the development and evaluation of relevant psychosocial interventions aimed at promoting the biological and psychological processes of healing and resilience in order to advance the nursing care of the whole patient with cancer and their caregivers across the stages of illness and the transition to survivorship (e.g., [1–6]).

Is it justifiable The model's goals, desired clinical outcomes and core content of stress, healing, resilience (coping) and health are consistent with the goals and values of the nursing discipline. Of equal import, it allows nurses to speak the same substantive "language" among their colleagues for the clinical benefit of patients and their caregivers. And it enables clinic nurses and the nursing leadership to defend, justify and explain Nursing's goals, objectives and substantive areas of professional practice to other health care professionals and hospital administrators.

Clinic nurses have relevant insights into the thoughts, feelings and behaviors of patients and caregivers due to their daily interactions with patients and loved ones, yet often feel inadequate due to the lack of a substantive body of knowledge denoting the whole person as well as related clinical expertise to intervene beyond active listening. Because most patients who have cancer view themselves as basically healthy, they seek help from health care providers who know them best, that is nurses, who understand their anxieties and fears as normal reactions to a traumatic situation, rather than as emotions to be pathologized. Patients and caregivers expect compassionate and connected nurses who listen to their concerns and use their psychosocial skills to facilitate the patient's and caregiver's adjustment to their clinical reality. The patient-centered stress, healing and resilience model highlights the importance of the nurse's compassion, connection, communication, competence in promoting patient and caregiver resilience. This essential therapeutic relationship serves as the key context for the nurse's interventions with patients and caregivers (e.g., [7, 8]). The nursing goal of promoting the healing and resilience of the whole person also complements and supports the medical goal of treating the disease in order to eliminate it or live well with it as a chronic illness. Treatment efficacy in relation to health outcomes may be mediated by strengthened healing and resilient capabilities of the whole person, which are critical objectives of the nursing profession (Review Part IV).

Is it feasible? To act to the full scope and extent of our profession not only depends on the nurse's professional capabilities but the professional support received by nursing and medical colleagues and the administrative leadership mainly in hospitals where evidence-based nursing has experienced the greatest challenge. Is this model feasible? Absolutely for advanced practice nurse practitioners who are able to work to the full extent and scope of their profession. They typically work in remote communities, urban community clinics, or in their own individual or group practices. It is also feasible for advanced practice nurses who work in hospital clinics alongside their medical colleagues in which the goals of nursing and medicine are mutually recognized to advance the health of individuals and their families. It is also most feasible within university nursing programs in which students are exposed to its theoretical tenets and psychosocial interventions. In addition, university programs expose future nurses to research methods and critical analytic skills, the essential "tools" of evidence-based practice. Adopting a model is a professionally-driven process that may progress at differential rates across university and clinical settings, but progress it must.

This chapter examines the factors that may impede the use of a conceptual model of practice in hospital settings, and particularly on hospital units. It offers strategies that may be considered to overcome resistance. But it also lays out the many psychosocial nursing interventions that are simple to incorporate into practice, and take very little time, yet hold the potential to make a significant clinical benefit.

19.2 Nursing Objectives

At the end of the chapter you will be able to:

1. Gain knowledge of the facilitators of a healing and resilient model of whole person practice.
2. Identify barriers to adopting a model.
3. Consider strategies to overcome these barriers in practice.
4. Identify a range of nursing interventions that take little to more time to implement.

19.3 Definitions

Professional practice refers to evidence-based practice guided by the values of its discipline within which a relevant conceptual model of practice delineates the goals, objectives and predicted outcomes based on critical interrelated concepts that serve as the predicate for purposeful research, education, clinical and administrative practice [9, 10].

19.4 Barriers to Evidence-Based Nursing Practice

Evidence-based practice has been shown to improve the health outcomes of patients, increase nursing satisfaction and enhance the quality of the nurse–patient relationship, the cornerstone of optimal care (Table 19.1) [15, 16]. Yet, decades after the stated clinical imperative of evidence-based practice was first articulated in the health science literature, barriers to professional practice have endured.

Table 19.1 Barriers to professional nursing practice

1. Work-related stress [11]
2. Lack of time [7, 12]
3. Lack of organizational flexibility to promote evidence-based learning, quality time with patients and families [13, 14]
4. Practice emphasized tasks over psychosocial person-centered care
5. Lack of clarity among nurses' regarding the key attributes of a nurse patient therapeutic relationship [7]
6. Lack of psychosocial evidence based nursing in clinical units—insufficient scientific knowledge and clinical intervention skills of the whole person in the care of individuals in clinical setting [13]
7. Lack of effective communication skills [8, 13]
8. Absence of nursing leadership [12, 15]
9. Problems with team collaboration [12]
10. Lack of specialized nurses or advanced practice nurses on hospital units [12]

Peer-Reviewed Research Versus Clinical Nursing Journals

Evidence based findings unsurprisingly are mainly published in peer-reviewed research journals, and not clinical journals where articles may consist of best practices, nursing guidelines, the latest procedures and tellingly education based articles proposing strategies for improving the evidence based *skills of clinic nurses* in order to knowledgeably access and interpret clinical research findings.

Despite the wealth of relevant scientific knowledge now available to clinical nurses, most clinic nurses lack the methodological skills to translate research findings from peer-reviewed journals into their clinical practice. As a result the practice of nursing as a health profession has been on a fool's errand, with consequential effects on patient care, and the ability of the profession to practice according to the values, goals and theoretical perspectives delineated by its discipline [10, 16, 17]. This chasm between patient-centered evidence-based research published in research journals and the nurse's practice has enabled hospital nursing units to be dominated by a medical paradigm that has also relegated the nursing profession toward its customary reliance on mainly procedural knowledge and skills. Advanced practice nurses guided by a whole person model of healing and resilience driven by essential methodological skills to incorporate relevant research findings into their practice are clinical imperatives of comprehensive hospital nursing care.

A Paucity of Patient-Centered Conceptual Practice Models

In the last several years, academic interest in conceptual nursing models has waned. Evidence-based findings may be interpreted by a theory, but use of a conceptual model reflective of the nursing discipline tailored to a particular patient population such as cancer or a chronic illness appears to be lacking (e.g., [18–20]). A conceptual nursing model in which the focus of practice is the whole person immediately calls for an integrated understanding of the biology and behavior of the person as the scientific substrate for a biopsychosocial nursing approach. From that deeper understanding of the biology and psychology of the whole person, relevant psychosocial interventions that target specific biomarkers as well as behavioral indicators may be justifiably considered. A conceptual model lays out a coherent and interrelated theoretical context that enables a more meaningful evidence-based practice. Without an integrated understanding of nursing's domain of practice, it is clinically impossible for the nurse to purposefully assess and comprehensively care for the whole person with cancer and their family caregiver.

To drive home the point, a scoping review of nursing psychotherapeutic interventions was carried out to address the unmet *psychological needs of patients* with cancer who were not part of supportive care services [21]. Of 86 studies, only 14 stated that these interventions were led by a nurse. The most frequent nursing interventions involved dignity therapy, a life review and supportive expressive therapies. The researchers concluded that nursing research needs to focus more on assessing the effectiveness of nurse-led psychosocial interventions to promote the well-being of patients with advanced cancer. Certainly, studies have evaluated the effectiveness of self-management, meaning-making, and cognitive-behavioral coping interventions which are easy to implement at the bedside or in a clinic (e.g., [22–27]). Yet, these evidence-based interventions have not been widely appropriated by advanced practice nurses in their care of patients and caregivers. A conceptual nursing model of practice, adopted by a nursing unit with advanced practice nurses would provide the needed professional rationale to purposefully develop the nurses' theoretical predicate and corresponding evidence to guide practice including the adoption of relevant psychosocial interventions?

Because the medical model prevails in hospitals, Nursing tends to be distinguished mainly by a series of medically-dominated tasks: procedures, techniques, treatment-related infusions, medications and dressings—all related to the care of different aspects of the person's illness, but still unrelated to the health of the whole person. A conceptual model would facilitate a more comprehensive, scientific understanding of interrelationships among a set of relevant variables of the whole biopsychosocial person that would also justify the use of appropriate psychosocial interventions.

Definitions of Evidence-Based Practice

The most enduring definition of evidence-based practice in the Nursing literature is still Sackett's definition ([28], p. 3): "… the practice of the best evidence-based 'medicine' means integrating individual clinical expertise with a critical appraisal of the best available external clinical evidence from systematic research" [28, 29]. This definition does not delineate the goals, objectives and knowledge base (of nursing) that would direct practice to relevant research findings. It may be an appropriate definition for a medical model of disease in which clinical concerns relate to the diagnosis, prognosis, therapy and other clinical and healthcare issues serving as the predicate for medical evidence-based learning ([28], p. 4). Although the principle appears to function well for a disease-focused practice, it is arguably too narrow in scope for nursing's whole person perspective, which until relatively recently also lacked conceptual clarity, accounting in part for the paucity of "evidence-based" nursing content beyond the acquisition of procedural knowledge. Notwithstanding the growing number of nurse scholars (e.g., [30–32]), one only has to do a review of nursing's clinical literature to realize that for a significant proportion of clinicians, evidence-based practice tends to be operationalized in terms of (1) *process* (e.g., tracking down evidence based on a clinical question as opposed to a nursing model that delineates the scope of the discipline's practice), (2) *the nurse's attitudes* (e.g., "evidence-based practice is fundamental to professional practice"), and (3) acquisition of *knowledge* refers to the *methodological process of retrieving* research and critical analysis. The findings highlight that nurses value the framework for professional practice but are still hindered by the lack of basic methodological skills and conceptual knowledge upon which to develop academic practice [16, 33]. The difference in definitions of evidence-based practice across settings has to do with the aspirational goals of academic practice on the one hand and the reality of clinical and educational preparedness of most nurses working on hospital units and clinics.

Work-Related Stress

Caring for patients with cancer and their loved ones is an emotionally draining and exceedingly stressful experience for nurses due to the life-threatening and serious nature of the disease and its emotional impact on the patient and loved ones (Table 19.2) [11]. This stress-related clinical care can exert a heavy toll on the nurse's own biological and psychological resilience, eventually resulting in exhausted nurses who are unable to bring their *whole* self, their whole presence to the therapeutic relationship with the patient and family caregiver (e.g., [37]).

Every day clinical demands compound the nurses' work-related stresses (e.g., staff shortages, heavy workload, unsatisfactory nurse–patient interactions due to a lack of time, inadequate scientific knowledge and clinical skills) which may fuel a professional crisis of meaning that gives way to feelings of apathy, and an insidious lack of compassion and connectedness with the patient [36, 39–41]. Depression, depersonalization, emotional exhaustion marked by a poor sense of personal accomplishment are clear signs of burnout and have been reported in an estimated third of nurses caring for patients with cancer [37, 38].

Conversely, interventions that foster healthcare provider resilience, emotional well-being and capacity for emotional engagement are associated with better quality patient outcomes. Nursing units with regular "in-service" journal club and preceptor programs have been found to decrease burnout and staff turnover (e.g., [11]). The reality of chronic stress only highlights the importance of addressing the professional concerns and emotional distresses of nurses as much as the clinical needs of patients and caregivers [37].

Table 19.2 Causes of chronic stress in nurses (e.g., [14, 34, 35])

Potential causes include:
1. Inability to practice according to academic qualifications, and goals and objectives of the profession [7, 14].
2. Feeling powerless or helpless [14, 15].
3. Competing work demands [14].
4. Lack of time for psychosocial concerns of patient and family [7].
5. Lack of collaboration and support among the nurses on a team [14].
6. Inadequate knowledge and skills to meet psychosocial needs of patients and family caregivers [13, 14].
7. Nurse shortages on units [36].
8. A clinical environment that fails to promote or support evidence based practice [11, 15].
Impact of chronic work place stress on the nurse [37, 38]
1. Emotional disconnect with patient care, lack of empathy negatively impacting patient care [36, 38].
2. Sense of numbness to others [38].
3. Lack of a meaningful practice and poor job satisfaction, poor self-worth [38].

19.4 Barriers to Evidence-Based Nursing Practice

Clinical Anecdote 19.1
Two Masters prepared nurses whom I had the privilege to mentor as part of their university clinical rotations, asked to see me. Both were gifted graduate student nurses working in an oncology clinic. In separate meetings and in different years, each explained that their academic preparation at the university exceeded the clinical realities of nursing practice in university hospitals where both worked. Although each could "see" exactly how their patients could benefit from their academic preparation, they were frustrated and felt unfulfilled at work. One of these students stated she had already applied to a 3 year medical program where she hoped to become a family doctor, and was apologizing to me for leaving Nursing! The other student expressed complete frustration that her day was spent giving intravenous medications and other procedures on a busy unit that was chronically short staffed. As a new graduate she had the temerity to try and discuss alternative ways of working together so that the nurses could spend more quality time talking to the patients who were extremely ill. She was rebuffed and actually shunned by her nurse colleagues. She too left, taking her life and career into her own hands, landing a stimulating job in the private sector where she was valued for her clinical capabilities.

The Quality of the Nurse-Patient Relationship

At the core of nursing practice lies the quality of the nurse–patient relationship [42] (Part IV Chap. 8). This relationship has been described as a therapeutic alliance or therapeutic engagement with the patient and family that has been shown to have a small but significant effect on the health outcomes of patients and families, although more rigorously designed research is needed (e.g., [43]). Although the therapeutic nurse–patient relationship is highly esteemed as a core value of nursing practice, it has generally not been reflected in the practices of most nurses in most hospital units and clinics (e.g., [34, 44]).

Studies of oncology nurses' practice have revealed patient dissatisfaction with the quality of communication and psychosocial interventions with their nurses [36]. Many patients seek shared decision making in which their treatments and options are explained, so they may more knowledgeably participate in clinical decisions [45]. Meaningful time set aside for such quality interactions with patients and caregivers has been impeded by the increased complexity of care, staff shortages, a lack of specialized nurses, the number of unrelated administrative activities assumed by advanced practice nurses and the lack of flexibility within the nursing schedule to ensure quality time between nurses and their patients and caregivers [13, 34, 41].

A multisite feasibility study in which "time" was carved out of the day from Monday to Friday for a minimum of 5 h/week so that the nurse could have protected time for therapeutic interventions with the patient, was perceived to be a success by the nurses on a psychiatric unit [7]. But the results showed nonsignificant patient outcomes (on measures of perceived quality of the nurse's interactions with the patient, and on anxiety and depressive mood). Similarly the nurse's stress only minimally improved. The lack of significant patient outcomes raises the issue of the nurses' clinical expertise in competently addressing the patients' concerns.

A Lack of Scientific Knowledge and Psychosocial Skills Among Clinical Nurses

Nurses caring for patients with cancer and their families in palliative care have reported a lack of evidence-based information, education and access to *relevant educational* databases [37]. Nonspecialist nurses caring for palliative end of life patients and caregivers have reported being ill-equipped to adequately care for patients and family during the terminal phase of cancer due to a lack of relevant knowledge and clinical skills which contributed to a perceived lack of autonomy in clinical decision making [41]. Although most nurses appear to value evidence based practice, a descriptive survey in the United States identified a number of obstacles to evidence-based care including resistance from nurse colleagues, managers and nurse leaders, with more receptive responses from nurses with Master's (non Master's degrees), as well as nurses' working at Magnet versus non-Magnet hospitals [15]. Melnyk (2012) [15] argued for Nursing's leadership and educators to provide relevant academic preparation, greater access to needed information and the time to actually utilize clinical skills in their practice, a call that has been repeated over the years (e.g., [12, 15]).

To strengthen evidence-based practice and job satisfaction, different strategies have been employed. A secondary analysis of nursing data from 282 hospitals found that nurses who were provided active "in service" and preceptors in oncology units were less likely to report burnout, and more likely to stay in their positions [11]. A multisite quality improvement strategy for oncology nurses, oncologists, and psychologists was implemented in 28 medical cancer centers in Italy [13]. The intervention consisted of (1) 2- to 3-day communication courses for nurses and oncologists, (2) a patient prompt list of questions to ask their oncologist that had to be given to every new patient, (3) the *use of specialist nurses* for patient care, (4) screening patients for psychological distress as well as social needs, and (5) all patients and families were given the opportunity to visit a library with internet access within the hospital with a nurse present to discuss any cancer-related issues [13]. These interventions were derived from Clinical Practice Guidelines for psychosocial care of adults with cancer [46]. The project team held four to six problem-solving visits to each center to help them identify obstacles and to find solutions. Up to 85% of the clinicians adhered to each recommendation, indicating the feasibility of mounting such an intervention.

By depending exclusively on clinical guidelines for improving psychosocial practice, nursing remains process driven unless the nurses' practice has been anchored within the broader purview of a model articulated by goals and objectives, and concepts relevant to professional practice. Clinical guidelines are more likely to be sustainable when they are meaningfully situated within the larger delineated parameter of the nurse's clinical practice shaped by the goals, expected outcomes, content and skills that are consistent with the goals and theoretical perspectives of the Nursing discipline. A model of practice serves to 'embed' the selected clinical guidelines within *a scientific nursing context that provides a deeper more meaningful rationale for integrating the guidelines into one's practice.* Notwithstanding, the 2–3 day communication workshops were a critical component of the intervention described above. Communication skills must be regarded as the first essential requisite toward developing skilled psychosocial nursing strategies.

In summary The first part of this chapter identifies some of the compelling arguments why academic nursing practice has been so difficult to implement particularly in the hospital setting. It is against this backdrop that suggestions for introducing a conceptual model on an in hospital unit are made. In perusing these suggestions, pick and choose whatever meets your clinical and professional needs. These suggestions will have done their work if they stimulate the team to proactively generate a more comprehensive nursing approach guided by the practice model. Progress at your own rate, first selecting what may be most easily integrated into your clinical practice as you move forward. It may not be realistic to incorporate the whole of the model, but just its essence, by learning about its goals and objectives and interrelationships among the concepts of stress, healing and resilience, and cancer. You might decide to read a relevant research article in stress, healing, or resilience and share what you have learned with colleagues. Chapter 2 which describes the key concepts of the model, is a good place to start. Part IV (Chaps. 8–14) describes seven relevant clinical interventions consistent with the goals of the model, and Part V on Nursing approaches also includes lifestyle behaviors associated with each phase of the cancer trajectory. Many are easy enough to implement and can have a significant positive effect on the well-being and quality of life of your patients and caregivers (review Chaps. 3–7).

19.5 Toward Academic Practice

Although a magnet hospital may be the optimal "cultural" environment for adopting the stress, healing and resilience practice model, it is absolutely feasible to adopt its vision and key conceptual elements as the goal directed basis for practice in any motivated clinical setting (Fig. 19.1).

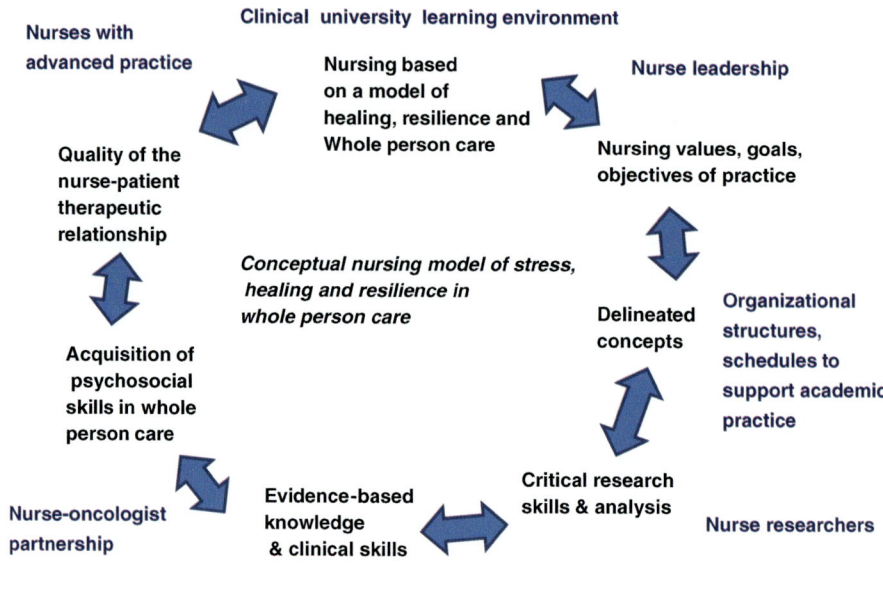

Fig. 19.1 Professional nursing practice

The Nursing Leadership

Leadership may be conceived as the "ability to influence employees" attitudes and beliefs by guiding and motivating them to achieve organizational goals, and "is … essential for a successful and efficient organisation" [47]. Transformational leadership refers to a set of skills and knowledge that includes: effective communication skills, a clear vision of practice, an ability to collaborate and motivate the nursing team, provide purposeful intellectual stimulation that advances practice, treats each staff member with respect and with the awareness of individual needs/concerns [47]. It also entails the ability to transform individual goals of practice into a shared purpose within the larger framework of the working organization or conceptual nursing model of the nursing unit. This may be accomplished in part via an ability to "market" the need for professional nursing practice throughout the multilayers of the working organization, by highlighting both patient and professional benefits of the proposed changes [47]. Another related leadership style is known as resonant leadership in which leaders are effective in self-regulating their emotions while able to be highly in tune with the emotions of the staff nurses [48]. These leaders are effective in developing highly engaged individuals capable of growing to potential within an inclusive and collaborative team.

A nurse leader with an advanced nursing degree (PhD or Master's at a minimum) and the qualities of a transformational and resonant leader is likely to succeed in navigating the nursing team around minefields, toward professional practice. A nurse leader must possess advanced academic qualifications in order to be viewed by the hospital administration, medical leadership and medical colleagues as equal partners in the pursuit of optimal quality care and treatment of the whole person. An advanced degree can facilitate collaboration with university partners in developing relevant courses and clinical stages for *both* nurses and students. It is incumbent upon the nurse leader to justify the implementation of a conceptual model at all relevant levels of the hospital and university and community organizations. These leaders must not only possess advanced nursing knowledge and skills but invest in personally learning about the scientific evidence associated with the key concepts and psychosocial strategies of the model alongside their nursing team through staff discussions, workshops, journal club and courses.

Implementing the Model

There are many ways to start the process. This is just a suggestion to get the discussion started.

1. Discuss definitions of professional nursing practice. Describe together its key elements, what professional practice brings to the quality of patient care, the nurse-patient relationship, and nursing satisfaction. Conversely discuss the potential obstacles to realizing professional nursing on the unit.
2. Introduce the model as a strategy toward adopting evidence-based practice. Identify the focus of nursing care as the whole person. Describe the attributes of person-centered or whole person care. Clarify why techniques and procedures are essential but ancillary components of psychosocial nursing of the whole person. Discuss strategies to enhance the psychosocial skills needed to effectively promote the health and well-being of the whole person, especially given that nurses spend more time with, and potentially know the patient better than any other healthcare profession.
3. If everyone is on board, suggest that the nursing leader and team begin to examine each of the key concepts, goals and objectives, and why this model is well suited to promoting the quality of life, well being and overall health of the whole person with cancer, and family caregiver (Review Chap. 2). It might be subsequently helpful to review each chapter of this book *together* as a way to progressively become familiar with the concepts and the psychosocial interventions in the model. Staff input, concerns, and proposed ideas must be an integral part of these discussions. Flexibility is key, and if your group discussions take you in another direction that leads to professional practice that's perfect.

All change is challenging. No doubt the team will ask pragmatic questions the unit strategy nurses for deepening their knowledge and skills related to the model; how will the hospital facilitate their learning, and how will the unit gain the support of the hospital administration and medical leadership, including the oncology team and other healthcare providers. Some of those considerations are addressed in the subsequent sections. The important thing to remember is that it is a process; the only important measure being evidence of the progressive acquisition of scientific knowledge (e.g., Chaps. 1–7 and psychosocial skills for nursing the whole person with cancer (e.g., Chaps. 8–14). One suggestion is to make a list of staff and manager ordered priorities, developed altogether.

Team Values

Creating an evidence-based environment depends on clarifying shared values, priorities and articulating a shared vision of practice. Shared values include: the importance of professional self-actualization and evidence-based practice predicated on scientific knowledge and skills (for instance, the stress, healing and resilience of the *whole* person and family *within the* nurse–patient therapeutic relationship). Shared values also consist of mutual respect, competence, compassion, and shared accountability within a nursing network of open communication and collaboration. Supportive communications include active listening, validating one another's capabilities, committing to professional learning, helping colleagues to manage stressful clinical situations in ways that reduce stress by engaging in problem-solving behaviors that empower, energize, and validate the team's and therefore the individual's sense of personal worth and potential for self-actualization.

It is the *bonds of colleagueship* within which the goals and objectives of practice evolve, where clinical decision making arising from the needs of the clinical context, are made. These bonds can alleviate the psychological and physiological effects of stress among colleagues when embedded within a supportive network [49–51]. When nurses feel that they are part of a supportive team, toxic psychological and physiological stress levels may be reduced and opportunities for personal and team growth become possible [52, 53].

Critical Analytic Research Skills

Evidence-based practice ultimately depends on the acquisition of critical analytic skills including the skills for accessing and critiquing research articles, systematic reviews, meta analyses and clinical guidelines [29, 54]. Clinically the ability to critique research articles is essential to bridge the gap between research and clinical practice, and for cultivating a scientific culture of up-to-date scientific evidence that informs and is informed by the delineated concepts in the model. Thus, the acquisition of critical analytic skills of clinical nurses needs to be a clinical imperative so that all nurses can meaningfully interpret the research literature. All clinic nurses need to know how to review relevant research studies to enhance scientific knowledge and clinical skills; Translating research findings into practice must be encouraged and promoted as the standard of practice. The main concepts of stress, healing and resilience in the model can serve as a purposeful predicate for the unit's first objective of gaining knowledge about the steps involved in scientific inquiry while also developing their scientific knowledge of relevant concepts. Of course this process must be facilitated by research experts from an affiliated university nursing program who can orient the staff to basic methods of inquiry and the significance of typical statistics used to evaluate controlled trials.

Introduce the acquisition of basic research skills through workshops, university courses, and regularly held journal club drawing on clinical research studies from the delineated concepts of the model and clinical concerns from the nurses' practice. The Iowa Model of evidence based practice may provide a useful guide for critiquing relevant research articles and relating the articles to other findings and theory [55]. On-line learning combined with face-to-face group learning has also been shown to be effective [56].

Clinical Skills

The clinical research literature strongly recommends that nurses acquire greater clinical expertise in providing psychosocial interventions to foster quality of life and well being in people with cancer across the continuum through university programs, courses or hospital workshops that provide *clinical practicums* and on the unit mentorship led by clinical nurse experts (e.g., [32, 41]). Essential psychosocial interventions includ: a primer in communication skills as the basis for other targeted psychosocial interventions. The nursing model specifically identifies a number of psychosocial interventions that have been empirically shown to promote resilience and health: meaning-making and cognitive-behavioral strategies, strategies to promote cognitive expectations and reduce nocebo effects during treatment, cognitive-behavioral stress management, self-management interventions, the relaxation response technique, and recommended healthy lifestyle behaviors across phases of the cancer and survivorship trajectory. Each intervention should be studied in terms of its theoretical tenets, and empirical findings. Nurses also need clinical practicums to develop clinical expertise using these interventions [8, 57].

Suggestions include:

(1) Review the psychosocial interventions in Part IV. Discuss the nursing strategies in terms of the goals of whole person care, the latest research findings (through weekly journal clubs), and the clinical contexts and scenarios where these might be effective strategies for implementation. Determine as a team which clinical skills could be strengthened by attending workshops on site, doing internships, role playing and or taking relevant university clinical courses and practicums. Loosely categorize skills according to the length of time each intervention generally takes to implement effectively in respective clinical contexts (see below). Time may initially factor into your prioritization of clinical learning. The proposed psychosocial interventions described in Part IV may be divided into three time sensitive categories: Effective nursing interventions that take between: 1 and 10 min; 30 and 40 min; greater than 40 min.

The 1- to 10-min Nursing Interventions (Table 19.3)

Many clinical strategies take only a few minutes to implement but can make a huge positive difference in the quality of life and well-being of patients and families at all stages of the disease. Table 19.3 lists interventions that may take only an estimated 1–10 min, are easily integrated into one's current practice, and can offer significant potential clinical benefits to the patient and or his or her caregiver. These interventions tend to be conducted one-on-one.

Identify those simple but impactful nursing interventions that are easily integrated into one's daily work, and those that are equally essential but are more time consuming, requiring a more flexible staff schedule in order to be sustainable in practice (See below).

Part IV, Chap. 12, discusses how just prior to a medical intervention, verbal suggestions that remind patients of the goals of an impending treatment, can trigger innate healing processes aligned with the goals of medical treatment [58–60]. Strategies include sharing relevant drug-related information and *emphasizing* its clinical benefits while specifically drawing the patient's attention to the current administration of the medication [61, 62]. These simple strategies have been shown to activate the patient's nitric oxide, endogenous morphine, reward and motivation (dopamine) systems which induce a therapeutic response in contrast to patients who were not so informed. Providing information about a drug's therapeutic effect *has been found to enhance the absorption rate* and efficacy of anxiolytics, opioids and muscle relaxants leading to improved clinical outcomes in experimental human studies [60–65]. The findings from these studies suggest that strategies which promote positive cognitive expectations of a treatment benefit also may be effective in minimizing the extent of immune suppression during chemotherapy, although more rigorous human research is needed [59, 66, 67]. What you say, when you say it and as the patient observes it, what you do appear to matter clinically.

Chapter 12 also examines strategies for discussing potential side effects with patients, such as framing, so that the individual remains confidant in the proposed treatment outcomes. A therapeutic outcome is more likely when the nurse's suggestions are consistent with the patient's beliefs and the patient is fully aware of the hoped for clinical benefit of the drug being administered *in the moment* [60, 62, 65].

Table 19.3 Brief impactful nursing interventions

Clinical examples of brief impactful nursing interventions (Part IV)
1. Be fully present-facilitated by ridding negative thoughts, emotions and feelings of stress with two to three deep breaths before entering patient's room (Chaps. 11 and 16).
2. Pull up a chair to patient's bed or clinic chair and sit face-to-face to create healing space (Chap. 11).
3. Respect patient beliefs about his or her desired wellness (Chap. 12).
4. Use verbal suggestions (provide relevant info) that enhance patient's positive cognitive expectations of a treatment benefit or counter negative patient expectations (Chap. 12).
5. Use open treatment approach (i.e., explain what treatment is being given at the time it is administered (Chap. 12).
6. Be aware of clinical environmental stimuli that can foster nocebo effects (Chap. 12).
7. Review recommended changes to the informed consent process to enhance treatment efficacy (Chap. 12).
8. Use of physical touch (Chap. 14).

Further clinical research with respect to cancer-related treatments is needed but converging evidence suggests that a nurse's positive and relevant information about a medication can enhance the clinical efficacy of treatment. Because innate healing processes tend to be triggered by the patient's conscious beliefs and expectations concerning their health outcomes as well as by various clinical environmental factors, modulating these beliefs and environmental factors can take very little time, are very easy to implement, and can make a therapeutic difference (Review Chaps. 8 and 12).

The 30- to 40-min Nursing Interventions

Some clinical approaches are optimally carried out within the therapeutic nurse–patient and caregiver relationship at clinic or in-hospital visits as one-on-one *and* or dyadic interventions. Because these therapeutic interventions take longer than the generally brief nursing interventions discussed in "The 1- to 10-min Nursing Interventions (Table 19.3)", the clinic nurse would likely want to preschedule visits with the patient and or caregiver in the clinic. In hospital units that lack a standard protected time for nurse–patient sessions in their daily staff schedule (see Sect. on Staffing, schedules and assignments, below), the nurse would need to 'carve out' time with the support of a nursing colleague who would monitor his or her other patients on the unit. This has usually been done on an ad hoc basis, a function of clinical urgency rather than reflecting a normative value of professional practice.

Suggested nursing interventions are summarized in Table 19.4. Patients and family caregivers experience moments of vulnerability that require our presence and emotional support. These moments may *happen anytime* but especially occur

Table 19.4 Impactful interventions taking 30–40 min

1. Establish a nurse–patient relationship that fosters the patient being known to the nurse by being fully present, compassionate, and responsive to the individual's concerns, feelings, and emotions (Chap. 8).
2. Discuss treatment goals and manage distorted negative patient beliefs about cancer or treatment, and possible side effects in advance of treatment or during consent process (Chap. 12).
3. Provide needed information and cognitive and behavioral coping strategies to reduce emotional distress, foster self-efficacy (Chap. 9).
4. Strengthen self-efficacy beliefs and self-management skills surrounding for, e.g., clinical aspects of cancer care (Chaps. 9 and 10; Appendices A and B).
5. Promote sense of meaning or purpose; helping patient come to terms with a cancer diagnosis, transition to palliative care (Chap. 10).
6. Promote patient–caregiver supportive communications in one-on-one or within a dyadic context (Chap. 11; Appendix in Chap. 11; Appendix B).
7. Address patient fears, distress, and concerns, and caregiver needs (Chaps. 15–18).
8. Facilitate mind–body therapies, especially relaxation response (mindful meditation), imagery, physical exercise, healthy diet to promote resilience and health (Chaps. 13–18, Appendix C).
9. Use of healing touch in supportive care and the terminal phase (Chap. 14).
10. Encourage a healthy lifestyle (Part V; Appendix C).
11. Being present, active listening and emotional, informational, appraisal and instrumental support in response to the patient and caregiver's special concerns (Chaps. 8 and 11; Appendix B).

around critical transitions along the continuum (the start of chemotherapy, a major operation, a cancer recurrence, transitioning to survivorship or to end of life). With some clinical foresight (albeit with difficulty) setting aside appropriate time with the patient and family caregiver may be scheduled purposefully into your day, something that likely already happens more often than not in many clinical settings; and for all, should become standardized practice.

The length of time of the nurse–patient session will depend on the patient's or caregiver's clinical needs. The patient who is emotionally distressed will obviously take longer than a patient, for instance, who has adapted well to the treatment regimen and is about to receive his or her next chemotherapy. But as will be discussed in the section below, scheduling these sessions especially on a busy in-patient unit requires the collaboration of the whole team.

Regularly Scheduled Nurse-Led Group Workshops (Appendix in Chap. 9; Appendix in Chap. 13; Appendix A)

Some healing- and resilient-promoting strategies may be most amenable to learning within a group. In particular multimodal, multitargeted interventions that consist of more than one strategy may be more optimally delivered to groups of individuals facing the same or similar clinical concerns/threats regarding cancer, upcoming treatments and or vulnerable transitions to palliative care or survivorship. Thoughtfully crafted workshops at key points along the continuum, each one tailored to the needs of the patient and or caregiver with similar clinical status and concerns have been shown to be effective in promoting resilience (Appendix in Chap. 9; Appendix in Chap. 13; Appendix A). The workshops might consist of more than one of the following tailored topics: (1) relevant psychoeducation, (2) cognitive and behavioral coping skills, (3) supportive relationships, (4) communication skills, (5) healthy lifestyle behaviors, (6) useful resources, (7) self-management strategies for practical cancer or treatment-related concerns, and (8) stress-reducing relaxation response technique, relaxation exercises, and/or mindful meditation to reduce emotional distress [5, 25, 31, 32, 68, 69]. The one exception to using workshops might be patients and caregivers approaching the terminal phase who are often too ill and benefit more from one to one care.

The use of regular workshops offers nurses an effective time management strategy that enables patients and caregivers to receive healing- and resilient-promoting information and strategies that otherwise might be difficult to implement across all individuals and their caregivers. Workshops should be led by skilled members of the nursing team on a rotating basis and would need to be integrated into a revised staffing schedule. Nurses more than any other profession with the exception of medicine understand the illness trajectory and its biopsychosocial impact on patients and families, making them the appropriate preceptors of these workshops. The one caveat is that each strategy requires the nurse to develop the clinical expertise to implement these strategies, which tend to be addressed in university nursing classes and clinical rotations, and urgently need to be transferred to the clinical realm of practice.

Staffing, Schedules, and Assignments

The goals, objectives, values, and beliefs about nursing practice will clarify the type of organizational structure that is needed to support whole person care for patients, and family caregivers. It takes team leadership to implement the change that is conducive to a satisfying practice. Creating the desired professional practice will depend on the team working together to design an appropriate organizational structure and schedule that support opportunities for both professional learning and a meaningful clinical practice defined by the goals of the nursing discipline and not just the medical expectations of the unit. Everything should be scrutinized through the prism of the nursing model upon which nursing clinical practice will be based.

Nurse Qualifications

Research findings consistently support the need for university-based staffing ratios with significantly more Master's prepared and specialized nurses *to* baccalaureate nurses (e.g., [41]). A nursing team with advanced degrees is a clinical imperative in providing optimal patient and caregiver quality care within the context of a therapeutic nurse–patient relationship [13, 16]. Part of this determination is an analysis of the nurse's daily work on the unit. Differentiate between activities critical to direct patient care and those that are not. Define complexity of care on the unit and the type of staffing required to meet this challenge effectively. For instance, extraneous activities might consist of administrative related paper work, the distribution of patient trays at mealtime and so on. Delegate those activities to relevant personnel.

Staff Scheduling

The 24-h work schedule might be reviewed as a function of what happens at each 8-h interval on the unit in order to optimize the presence of nurses with advanced practice as a function of patient and caregiver needs, interdisciplinary rounds, journal club and so on. To strengthen inter staff communications about patients and families, it may be possible to ensure that the staffing compositions of day and evening rotations consist of the same group of nurses who pair up across the shifts to care for the same patients and caregivers, enabling a more informed coverage and potentially a more satisfying practice. Nursing notes are obviously an important way of conveying information across shifts. But communicating with the same nurse on the opposite rotation who is also caring for the same patients stimulates more effective problem solving around patient and caregiver concerns and a personal sense of satisfaction. Nurses on the same rotation could determine their daily nursing schedule and expected workload by taking into account their respective patient and family concerns. Each nurse dyad on the *same rotation* could also decide among themselves, the type of quality time with their patient and family each nurse requires, and accordingly cover for one another. These are just suggestions, they may not work for everyone, but they are meant to stimulate problem solving initiatives (See next sect.).

Carve Out Protected Time for Nurses to Engage in Therapeutic Patient/Caregiver

An integral part of restructuring the nurses' daily work schedule must involve establishing daily, protected time for nurses to engage in the therapeutic concerns of patients and caregivers. Different strategies are possible. A nursing intervention study in psychiatric in-patient care showed that carving out protected time for nurses to engage with patients from Monday through Friday was feasible [7]. During this quality time with patients, one or two nurses took charge of the unit's administrative functions, and the unit was closed to all visitors including health professionals who did not "belong" to the unit. The study findings suggested that this structural adaptation might be feasible in other hospital units. It is worth a serious consideration for in-patient cancer care units. It is likely that most palliative care units already have established protected time for nurses to engage therapeutically with patients and families.

The work schedule and organization of the unit should be regularly reviewed and tweaked by the nursing team to address potential inherent stressors that could lead to a sense of demoralization and exhaustion. The process of taking accountability for one's practice is empowering, self-validating, and emotionally restorative.

A University-Affiliated Clinical Learning Environment

A hospital unit or clinical setting that serves as an affiliated university-learning environment for student nurses seeking an advanced nursing degrees provides an invaluable opportunity for nurses on the unit to further their critical analytic and clinical skills. through on-site academic learning opportunities for students and nurses alike. led by relevant experts. Time carved out for bi weekly journal clubs focused on analyzing scientific articles consistent with the key concepts in the model and reviewed by staff *and students* on a rotation basis contributes to the continuous acquisition of relevant knowledge and skills, a hallmark of professional practice [70]. Inviting clinical experts to enhance the psychosocial expertise of staff and students via one-way mirrors, videotaping, and or role playing followed by group discussion should be standard clinical learning in every oncology setting.

Clinical Anecdote 19.2

My first nursing experience was in an adolescent unit with an estimated 30 beds. The unit consisted of patients under medicine, surgery, psychiatry and oncology! Shortly after my arrival, the head nurse resigned. So we were led by a rotating system of team leaders. We were on 12-h shifts, and every day we worked with different nurses. We were exhausted at a time when staff shortages were not the main problem; we were suffering from a lack of professional satisfaction. We did not feel validated in interdisciplinary meetings. We were never asked for our assessment of the patient and his family; only to report on the most basic physical parameters. The question we asked ourselves during a team meeting was: "What aspects of our work make our heart sing?" And unsurprisingly it was the clinical experience of meaningful encounters with our patients, and that our work with family and patients was validated at a minimum by our peers. And we wanted a stronger voice in multidisciplinary meetings.

We were very lucky that for most of the summer, there was NO head nurse. We found our own solutions to our work-related problems. That in itself was energy-producing and empowering, and lifted our spirits immediately! That spiritual lift has informed my work in nursing ever since. Because it told me that individuals who have chosen a career in Nursing wish to be treated as professionals and not constantly told to conform to someone else's expectations of what to do.

Our solution was to create a new staff schedule that ensured we worked with the same colleagues each day, and were buddied up with the same nurse on the opposite shift caring for the same group of adolescents, so that the information we shared during rounds was of greater professional significance. And we did one more thing that humanized and validated our work as professionals—we gave our selves permission to go to the hospital library to read relevant articles that could enhance the quality of our nursing care, and our ability to actively participate in multi disciplinary rounds, supported by relevant articles as evidence of best practices when challenged. It was liberating! Later this way of working together as professionals was developed further in outpatient clinical settings where the nurses were Masters prepared advanced practitioners. These nurses able to practice according to the goals of their discipline became the first in that university hospital to care for their own patients and families. The nurses complemented the work of their medical colleagues, which resulted in mutual respect and colleagueship. To promote our ongoing learning we began our own Journal club. It was 1979.

Today of course many of these staff changes have thankfully become standard practice. I recount this experience mainly to underscore how important it is to enable nurses to feel validated in their work. And if you cannot find a team with the same shared values of professional practice, it is worth seeking another clinical environment of like-minded nurses.

Nurturing the Nurse's Wholeness

Ultimately, the nurse's ability to enhance healing and resilience in patients and family caregivers will depend on the nurse's own state of overall well-being or sense of wholeness (Table 19.5). The quality of the nurse–patient relationship, and by extension the patient's healing capabilities, depends on the nurse's own sense of wholeness [71]. A sense of wholeness has to do with experiencing an overall sense of fulfillment and well-being. This can only be fulfilled through professional self actualization which is the ability to be fully engaged in one's hosen profession to the full extent and depth of the parameters of its discipline. It has to do with how a person feels about him- or herself, his or her self-esteem, sense of purpose and the extent to which he/she feels valued and supported. This is as true for patients as the nurses who care for them. One must be whole within one self in order to foster healing in others (e.g., [71–73]).

Table 19.5 Adopting a conceptual model (CM) of practice: A summary of the key elements suggested in this chapter

1. Committed nursing leadership
2. Review staff values and goals of nursing on unit: Discuss the meaning of professional practice and the key elements
3. Review key elements and benefits of a therapeutic nurse–patient relationship
4. Clarify the main focus of nursing and clinical benefits for patients: the whole person versus mainly tasks and procedures
5. Nurse leader and team discussions: strengths, weaknesses of current practice; the elements of a satisfying practice; benefits and challenges of implementing CM
6. Review goals, objectives, and key concepts of stress, healing and resilience model: discuss obstacles to implementation and problem solve: for example take a stepwise approach based on priorities of learning
7. Nurse leadership facilitates opportunities for nurses to develop critical thinking skills, ability to review relevant research articles during a protected weekly hour such as journal club
8. Review healing-inducing clinical interventions (Part IV): Discuss related clinical research; nurses' current level of clinical skills (such as nurses' communication skills with patients/caregivers); the clinical contexts for each intervention and time required to implement.
9. Prioritize the order of needed clinical interventions—provide opportunities to acquire clinical expertise in identified areas of practice, including clinical interventions
9.1. Facilitate clinical expertise over time via courses, workshops from nurse experts.
10. Prioritize the acquisition and implementation of psychosocial nursing interventions in terms of the length of time required
11. If possible, create new or renegotiate clinical-university learning environments to meet needs of both nurses and students
12. Discuss importance of nurses' nurturing one another's sense of wholeness and professional actualization, and propose tailored strategies to achieve and sustain this goal.

A healing environment cannot stand when the signs of burnout are overlooked, the clinical environment lacks opportunities for nurses to develop their own professional aspirations, and nursing exhaustion is not addressed. An essential component of shared accountability is to look out for one another's health and signs of stress. The team and the head nurse each have the responsibility to identify signs of emotional exhaustion, institute immediate measures to effectively alleviate stress, and to prevent it in the first place. Unaddressed work-related concerns lead to increasingly negative interpersonal team work [74]. Burn out inhibits an otherwise caring nurse from conveying attitudes of compassion and emotional empathy that are the cornerstones of nursing practice. And it results in nurses leaving the profession.

Final Remarks

The way we conceptualize Nursing shapes how patients and family caregivers are cared for. Our thoughts and feelings about the goals of practice, cancer and its treatment modalities, and our knowledge and clinical skills influence the quality of our interactions with the patient and family caregiver. Scientific evidence and clinical skills such as communication skills that we bring to bear in the clinical setting exert a significant impact on the patient's quality of life and well-being, and the ability to sustain a meaningful nurse–patient–caregiver relationship [57].

When we say that we care for the "whole" patient but lack a patient-centered conceptual model, relevant scientific knowledge and clinical expertise, we are unable to care for the whole person resulting in consequential implications for their current and future resilient and healthy capabilities of which we are unlikely to even be cognizant. [75–78]. Concepts of stress, healing, coping, support, and health are fundamental to the substantive practice of nursing and to the care of the whole person with cancer and the family caregiver. The nursing model based on these concepts and further delineated by goals and desired clinical outcomes provide the scientific incentive for nurses to take professional action, all the more so, given their privileged role of knowing the patient and family caregiver better than any other healthcare provider with the possible exception of the oncologist.

By promoting healing and resilient neurobiological and behavioral processes of the whole being we are able to optimize the patient's health. In so doing we complement and support the goals of medical treatment. Through effective psychosocial interventions we facilitate the reduction of damaging stress effects throughout the human organism, optimize the patient's emotion-regulating capabilities and facilitate the ability to tolerate treatment to completion. We may even help to attenuate its toxic effects on critical immune functions. We can do this at the bedside, in the oncology clinic and in an independent practice. Whether nurses act in a comprehensive and timely manner at vulnerable moments along the cancer trajectory will ultimately influence whether the individual will remain at risk for a cancer recurrence or a co morbid disease or even a shortened survival. This is why a biological as well as a psychological healing-enhancing and resilient-promoting nursing approach across the continuum is so important as conceptualized by the healing and resilient model. But of equal note, nurses, who practice according to the goals and values of the nursing discipline are more likely to experience a greater sense of professional fulfillment.

References

1. Ferrell BR, Temel JS, Temin S, Alesi ER, Balboni TA, Basch EM, et al. Integration of palliative care into standard oncology care: American Society of Clinical Oncology clinical practice guideline update. J Clin Oncol. 2017;35(1):96–112. PubMed PMID: 28034065. Epub 2016/12/31. eng.
2. Reeve K, Black PA, Huang J. Examining the impact of a Healing Touch intervention to reduce posttraumatic stress disorder symptoms in combat veterans. Psychol Trauma. 2020;12(8):897–903. PubMed PMID: 33346680. Epub 2020/12/22. eng.
3. Lashbrook MP, Valery PC, Knott V, Kirshbaum MN, Bernardes CM. Coping strategies used by breast, prostate, and colorectal cancer survivors: a literature review. Cancer Nurs. 2018;41(5):E23–39. PubMed PMID: 28723724. Epub 2017/07/21. eng.
4. Ellis KR, Janevic MR, Kershaw T, Caldwell CH, Janz NK, Northouse L. Meaning-based coping, chronic conditions and quality of life in advanced cancer & caregiving. Psycho-Oncology. 2017;26(9):1316–23. PubMed PMID: 27147405. Pubmed Central PMCID: PMC5097695. Epub 2016/05/06. eng.

5. Dionne-Odom JN, Azuero A, Lyons KD, Hull JG, Prescott AT, Tosteson T, et al. Family caregiver depressive symptom and grief outcomes from the ENABLE III randomized controlled trial. J Pain Symptom Manag. 2016;52(3):378–85. PubMed PMID: 27265814. Pubmed Central PMCID: PMC5023481. Epub 2016/06/07. eng.
6. Kwekkeboom K, Zhang Y, Campbell T, Coe CL, Costanzo E, Serlin RC, et al. Randomized controlled trial of a brief cognitive-behavioral strategies intervention for the pain, fatigue, and sleep disturbance symptom cluster in advanced cancer. Psycho-Oncology. 2018;27(12):2761–9. PubMed PMID: 30189462. Pubmed Central PMCID: PMC6279506. Epub 2018/09/07. eng.
7. Molin J, Lindgren B, Graneheim U, Ringner A. Time together: a nursing intervention in psychiatric inpatient care-feasibility and effects. Int J Ment Health Nurs. 2018;27(6):1698–708.
8. Banerjee SC, Manna R, Coyle N, Penn S, Gallegos TE, Zaider T, et al. The implementation and evaluation of a communication skills training program for oncology nurses. Transl Behav Med. 2017;7(3):615–23. PubMed PMID: 28211000. Pubmed Central PMCID: PMC5645276. Epub 2017/02/18. eng.
9. Grossman M, Agulnik J, Batist G. The Peter Brojde lung cancer centre: a model of integrative practice. Curr Oncol. 2012;19(3):e145–59. PubMed PMID: 22670104. Pubmed Central PMCID: PMC3364775. Epub 2012/06/07. eng.
10. Grossman M, Hooton M. The significance of the relationship between a discipline and its practice. J Adv Nurs. 1993;18(6):866–72. PubMed PMID: 8320379. Epub 1993/06/01. eng.
11. Shang J, Friese CR, Wu E, Aiken LH. Nursing practice environment and outcomes for oncology nursing. Cancer Nurs. 2013;36(3):206–12. PubMed PMID: 22751101. Pubmed Central PMCID: PMC3593758. Epub 2012/07/04. eng.
12. Correa VC, Lugo-Agudelo LH, Aguirre-Acevedo DC, Contreras JAP, Borrero AMP, Patiño-Lugo DF, et al. Individual, health system, and contextual barriers and facilitators for the implementation of clinical practice guidelines: a systematic meta review. Health Res Pol Syst. 2020;18(1):74. PubMed PMID: 32600417. Pubmed Central PMCID: PMC7322919. Epub 2020/07/01. eng.
13. Passalacqua R, Annunziata MA, Borreani C, Diodati F, Isa L, Saleri J, et al. Feasibility of a quality improvement strategy integrating psychosocial care into 28 medical cancer centers (HuCare project). Support Care Cancer. 2016;24(1):147–55. PubMed PMID: 25957011. Epub 2015/05/10. eng.
14. Ko W, Kiser-Larson N. Stress levels of nurses in oncology outpatient units. Clin J Oncol Nurs. 2016;20(2):158–64. PubMed PMID: 26991708. Epub 2016/03/19. eng.
15. Melnyk BM, Fineout-Overholt E, Gallagher-Ford L, Kaplan L. The state of evidence-based practice in US nurses: critical implications for nurse leaders and educators. J Nurs Admin. 2012;42(9):410–7. PubMed PMID: 22922750. Epub 2012/08/28. eng.
16. Moreno-Poyato AR, Casanova-Garrigos G, Roldán-Merino JF, Rodríguez-Nogueira Ó. Examining the association between evidence-based practice and the nurse-patient therapeutic relationship in mental health units: a cross-sectional study. J Adv Nurs. 2021;77(4):1762–71. PubMed PMID: 33336475. Epub 2020/12/19. eng.
17. Moreno-Poyato AR, Delgado-Hito P, Leyva-Moral JM, Casanova-Garrigós G, Montesó-Curto P. Implementing evidence-based practices on the therapeutic relationship in inpatient psychiatric care: a participatory action research. J Clin Nurs. 2019;28(9–10):1614–22. PubMed PMID: 30588686. Epub 2018/12/28. eng.
18. Gottlieb L, Rowat K. The McGill model of nursing: a practice derived model. Adv Nurs Sci. 1987;9(4):51–61.
19. Gottlieb L, Gottlieb B. The development/health framework within the McGill Model of Nursing: 'Laws of nature' guiding whole person care. Adv Nurs Sci. 2007;30(1):E43–57.
20. Butts JB, Rich KL. Philosophies and theories for advanced nursing practice. Sudbury, MA; Mississauga, ON; London: Jones & Bartlett Learning; 2011, 665 p.
21. Malakian A, Mohammed S, Fazelzad R, Ajaj R, Artemenko A, Mayo SJ. Nursing, psychotherapy and advanced cancer: a scoping review. Eur J Oncol Nurs. 2022;56:102090. PubMed PMID: 35026499. Epub 2022/01/14. eng.

22. McCorkle R, Dowd M, Ercolano E, Schulman-Green D, Williams AL, Siefert ML, et al. Effects of a nursing intervention on quality of life outcomes in post-surgical women with gynecological cancers. Psycho-Oncology. 2009;18(1):62–70. PubMed PMID: 18570223. Pubmed Central PMCID: PMC4186244. Epub 2008/06/24. eng.
23. Zhang Q, Li F, Zhang H, Yu X, Cong Y. Effects of nurse-led home-based exercise & cognitive behavioral therapy on reducing cancer-related fatigue in patients with ovarian cancer during and after chemotherapy: a randomized controlled trial. Int J Nurs Stud. 2018;78:52–60. PubMed PMID: 28939343. Epub 2017/09/25. eng.
24. Lee V, Cohen SR, Edgar L, Laizner AM, Gagnon AJ. Meaning-making and psychological adjustment to cancer: development of an intervention and pilot results. Oncol Nurs Forum. 2006;33(2):291–302. PubMed PMID: 16518445. Epub 2006/03/07. eng.
25. Dionne-Odom JN, Taylor R, Rocque G, Chambless C, Ramsey T, Azuero A, et al. Adapting an early palliative care intervention to family caregivers of persons with advanced cancer in the rural deep south: a qualitative formative evaluation. J Pain Symptom Manag. 2018;55(6):1519–30. PubMed PMID: 29474939. Pubmed Central PMCID: PMC5951755. Epub 2018/02/24. eng.
26. McCorkle R, Ercolano E, Lazenby M, Schulman-Green D, Schilling LS, Lorig K, et al. Self-management: enabling and empowering patients living with cancer as a chronic illness. CA Cancer J Clin. 2011;61(1):50–62. PubMed PMID: 21205833. Pubmed Central PMCID: PMC3058905. Epub 2011/01/06. eng.
27. McCorkle R, Strumpf NE, Nuamah IF, Adler DC, Cooley ME, Jepson C, et al. A specialized home care intervention improves survival among older post-surgical cancer patients. J Am Geriatr Soc. 2000;48(12):1707–13. PubMed PMID: 11129765. Epub 2000/12/29. eng.
28. Sackett D. Evidence-based medicine. Semin Perinatol. 1997;21(1):3–5.
29. Stannard D. A practical definition of evidence-based practice for nursing. J Perianesth Nurs. 2019;34(5):1080–4. PubMed PMID: 31582131. Epub 2019/10/05. eng.
30. Chan RJ, Teleni L, McDonald S, Kelly J, Mahony J, Ernst K, et al. Breast cancer nursing interventions and clinical effectiveness: a systematic review. BMJ Support Palliat Care. 2020;10(3):276–86. PubMed PMID: 32499405. Epub 2020/06/06. eng.
31. Dionne-Odom JN, Azuero A, Lyons KD, Hull JG, Tosteson T, Li Z, et al. Benefits of early versus delayed palliative care to informal family caregivers of patients with advanced cancer: outcomes from the ENABLE III randomized controlled trial. J Clin Oncol. 2015;33(13):1446–52. PubMed PMID: 25800762. Pubmed Central PMCID: PMC4404423. Epub 2015/03/25. eng.
32. Bakitas MA, Tosteson TD, Li Z, Lyons KD, Hull JG, Li Z, et al. Early versus delayed initiation of concurrent palliative oncology care: patient outcomes in the ENABLE III randomized controlled trial. J Clin Oncol. 2015;33(13):1438–45. PubMed PMID: 25800768. Pubmed Central PMCID: PMC4404422. www.jco.org. Author contributions are found at the end of this article. Epub 2015/03/25. eng.
33. Upton D, Upton P. Development of an evidence-based practice questionnaire for nurses. J Adv Nurs. 2006;53(4):454–8. PubMed PMID: 16448488. Epub 2006/02/02. eng.
34. Beckstrand RL, Collette J, Callister L, Luthy KE. Oncology nurses' obstacles and supportive behaviors in end-of-life care: providing vital family care. Oncol Nurs Forum. 2012;39(5):E398–406. PubMed PMID: 22940519. Epub 2012/09/04. eng.
35. Solans M, Romaguera D, Gracia-Lavedan E, Molinuevo A, Benavente Y, Saez M, et al. Adherence to the 2018 WCRF/AICR cancer prevention guidelines and chronic lymphocytic leukemia in the MCC-Spain study. Cancer Epidemiol. 2020;64:101629. PubMed PMID: 31756676. Epub 2019/11/23. eng.
36. Chan EA, Wong F, Cheung MY, Lam W. Patients' perceptions of their experiences with nurse-patient communication in oncology settings: a focused ethnographic study. PLoS One. 2018;13(6):e0199183. PubMed PMID: 29912967. Pubmed Central PMCID: PMC6005521. Epub 2018/06/19. eng.
37. Harrington KJ, Affronti ML, Schneider SM, Razzak AR, Smith TJ. Improving attitudes and perceptions about end-of-life nursing on a hospital-based palliative care unit. J Hosp Palliat Nurs. 2019;21(4):272–9. PubMed PMID: 30893285. Epub 2019/03/21. eng.

38. Canadas-De la Fuente GA, Gomez-Urquiza JL, Ortega-Campos EM, Canadas GR, Albendin-Garcia L. De la Fuente-Solana EI. Prevalence of burnout syndrome in oncology nursing: a meta-analytic study. Psycho-Oncology. 2018;27(5):1426–33. PubMed PMID: 29314432. Epub 2018/01/10. eng.
39. Gi TS, Devi KM, Neo Kim EA. A systematic review on the relationship between the nursing shortage and nurses' job satisfaction, stress and burnout levels in oncology/haematology settings. JBI Lib Syst Rev. 2011;9(39):1603–49. PubMed PMID: 27819963. Epub 2011/01/01. eng.
40. Thorne S, Hislop TG, Kim-Sing C, Oglov V, Oliffe JL, Stajduhar KI. Changing communication needs and preferences across the cancer care trajectory: insights from the patient perspective. Support Care Cancer. 2014;22(4):1009–15. PubMed PMID: 24287506. Epub 2013/11/30. eng.
41. Thorn H, Uhrenfeldt L. Experiences of non-specialist nurses caring for patients and their significant others undergoing transitions during palliative end-of-life cancer care: a systematic review. JBI Database System Rev Implement Rep. 2017;15(6):1711–46. PubMed PMID: 28628524. Epub 2017/06/20. eng.
42. McAndrew S, Chambers M, Nolan F, Thomas B, Watts P. Measuring the evidence: reviewing the literature of the measurement of therapeutic engagement in acute mental health inpatient wards. Int J Ment Health Nurs. 2014;23(3):212–20. PubMed PMID: 24103061. Epub 2013/10/10. eng.
43. Kelley JM, Kraft-Todd G, Schapira L, Kossowsky J, Riess H. The influence of the patient-clinician relationship on healthcare outcomes: a systematic review and meta-analysis of randomized controlled trials. PLoS One. 2014;9(4):e94207. PubMed PMID: 24718585. Pubmed Central PMCID: PMC3981763 Chairman of Empathetics, LLP. This does not alter the authors' adherence to all the PLOS ONE policies on sharing data and materials. Epub 2014/04/11. eng.
44. Hartley S, Raphael J, Lovell K, Berry K. Effective nurse-patient relationships in mental health care: a systematic review of interventions to improve the therapeutic alliance. Int J Nurs Stud. 2020;102:103490. PubMed PMID: 31862531. Pubmed Central PMCID: PMC7026691. Epub 2019/12/22. eng.
45. Beers E, Lee Nilsen M, Johnson JT. The role of patients: shared decision-making. Otolaryngol Clin N Am. 2017;50(4):689–708. PubMed PMID: 28571664. Epub 2017/06/03. eng.
46. National Breast Cancer Centre and National Centre Control Initiative. Clinical practice guidelines for the psychosocial care of adults; 2003.
47. Pishgooie AH, Atashzadeh-Shoorideh F, Falcó-Pegueroles A, Lotfi Z. Correlation between nursing managers' leadership styles and nurses' job stress and anticipated turnover. J Nurs Manag. 2019;27(3):527–34. PubMed PMID: 30136322. Epub 2018/08/24. eng.
48. Laschinger HK, Wong CA, Cummings GG, Grau AL. Resonant leadership and workplace empowerment: the value of positive organizational cultures in reducing workplace incivility. Nurs Econ. 2014;32(1):5–15, 44; quiz 16. PubMed PMID: 24689153. Epub 2014/04/03. eng.
49. Chadwick A, Zoccola PM, Figueroa WS, Rabideau EM. Communication and stress: effects of hope evocation and rumination messages on heart rate, anxiety, anxiety and emotions after a stressor. Health Commun. 2016;31(12):1447–59.
50. House JS, Landis KR, Umberson D. Social relationships and health. Science (New York, NY). 1988;241(4865):540–5. PubMed PMID: 3399889. Epub 1988/07/29. eng.
51. House J. Work, stress and social support. Reading, MA: Addison-Wesley; 1981.
52. Hostinar CE. Recent developments in the study of social relationships, stress responses, and physical health. Curr Opin Psychol. 2015;5:90–5. PubMed PMID: 26366429. Pubmed Central PMCID: PMC4562328. Epub 2015/09/15. Eng.
53. Hostinar CE, Gunnar MR. Future directions in the study of social relationships as regulators of the HPA axis across development. J Clin Child Adolesc Psychol. 2013;42(4):564–75. PubMed PMID: 23746193. Epub 2013/06/12. eng.
54. Djulbegovic B, Guyatt GH. Progress in evidence-based medicine: a quarter century on. Lancet. 2017;390(10092):415–23. PubMed PMID: 28215660. Epub 2017/02/22. eng.

55. Brown CG. The Iowa Model of evidence-based practice to promote quality care: an illustrated example in oncology nursing. Clin J Oncol Nurs. 2014;18(2):157–9. PubMed PMID: 24675251. Epub 2014/03/29. eng.
56. Ramos-Morcillo AJ, Fernández-Salazar S, Ruzafa-Martínez M, Del-Pino-Casado R. Effectiveness of a brief, basic evidence-based practice course for clinical nurses. Worldviews on evidence-based nursing. Sigma Theta Tau Int Hon Soc Nurs. 2015;12(4):199–207. PubMed PMID: 26220505. Epub 2015/07/30. eng.
57. Wittenberg E, Reb A, Kanter E. Communicating with patients and families around difficult topics in cancer care using the COMFORT communication curriculum. Semin Oncol Nurs. 2018;34(3):264–73. PubMed PMID: 30100368. Pubmed Central PMCID: PMC6156926. Epub 2018/08/14. eng.
58. Finniss DG, Kaptchuk TJ, Miller F, Benedetti F. Biological, clinical, and ethical advances of placebo effects. Lancet. 2010;375(9715):686–95. PubMed PMID: 20171404. Pubmed Central PMCID: PMC2832199. Epub 2010/02/23. eng.
59. Segerstrom SC, Sephton SE. Optimistic expectancies and cell-mediated immunity: the role of positive affect. Psychol Sci. 2010;21(3):448–55. PubMed PMID: 20424083. Pubmed Central PMCID: PMC3933956. Epub 2010/04/29. eng.
60. Colloca L, Barsky AJ. Placebo and nocebo effects. N Engl J Med. 2020;382(6):554–61. PubMed PMID: 32023375. Epub 2020/02/06. eng.
61. Colloca L, Enck P, DeGrazia D. Relieving pain using dose-extending placebos: a scoping review. Pain. 2016;157(8):1590–8. PubMed PMID: 27023425. Pubmed Central PMCID: PMC5364523. Epub 2016/03/30. eng.
62. Colloca L, Lopiano L, Lanotte M, Benedetti F. Overt versus covert treatment for pain, anxiety, and Parkinson's disease. Lancet Neurol. 2004;3(11):679–84. PubMed PMID: 15488461. Epub 2004/10/19. eng.
63. Flaten MA, Simonsen T, Olsen H. Drug-related information generates placebo and nocebo responses that modify the drug response. Psychosom Med. 1999;61(2):250–5. PubMed PMID: 10204979. Epub 1999/04/16. eng.
64. Colloca L, Klinger R, Flor H, Bingel U. Placebo analgesia: psychological and neurobiological mechanisms. Pain. 2013;154(4):511–4. PubMed PMID: 23473783. Pubmed Central PMCID: PMC3626115. Epub 2013/03/12. eng.
65. Ren Y, Xu F. How patients should be counseled on adverse drug reactions: avoiding the nocebo effect. Res Soc Adm Pharm. 2018;14(7):705. PubMed PMID: 29656936. Epub 2018/04/17. eng.
66. Ben-Shaanan TL, Azulay-Debby H, Dubovik T, Starosvetsky E, Korin B, Schiller M, et al. Activation of the reward system boosts innate and adaptive immunity. Nat Med. 2016;22(8):940–4. PubMed PMID: 27376577. Epub 2016/07/05. eng.
67. Ben-Shaanan TL, Schiller M, Azulay-Debby H, Korin B, Boshnak N, Koren T, et al. Modulation of anti-tumor immunity by the brain's reward system. Nat Commun. 2018;9(1):2723. PubMed PMID: 30006573. Pubmed Central PMCID: PMC6045610. Epub 2018/07/15. eng.
68. Antoni MH, Lechner S, Diaz A, Vargas S, Holley H, Phillips K, et al. Cognitive behavioral stress management effects on psychosocial and physiological adaptation in women undergoing treatment for breast cancer. Brain Behav Immun. 2009;23(5):580–91. PubMed PMID: 18835434. Pubmed Central PMCID: PMC2722111. Epub 2008/10/07. eng.
69. Cohen L, Parker PA, Vence L, Savary C, Kentor D, Pettaway C, et al. Presurgical stress management improves postoperative immune function in men with prostate cancer undergoing radical prostatectomy. Psychosom Med. 2011;73(3):218–25. PubMed PMID: 21257977. Epub 2011/01/25. eng.
70. Lehane E, Leahy-Warren P, O'Riordan C, Savage E, Drennan J, O'Tuathaigh C, et al. Evidence-based practice education for healthcare professions: an expert view. BMJ Evid Base Med. 2019;24(3):103–8. PubMed PMID: 30442711. Pubmed Central PMCID: PMC6582731. Epub 2018/11/18. eng.

71. Ross J. Assessing the whole person to improve outcomes. J Perianesth Nurs. 2015;30(2):157–9. PubMed PMID: 25813303. Epub 2015/03/31. eng.
72. Barthow C, Moss C, McKinlay E, McCullough L, Wise D. To be involved or not: factors that influence nurses' involvement in providing treatment decisional support in advanced cancer. Eur J Oncol Nurs. 2009;13(1):22–8. PubMed PMID: 19010732. Epub 2008/11/18. eng.
73. Powazki R, Walsh D, Cothren B, Rybicki L, Thomas S, Morgan G, et al. The care of the actively dying in an academic medical center: a survey of registered nurses' professional capability and comfort. Am J Hospice Palliat Care. 2014;31(6):619–27. PubMed PMID: 24142595. Epub 2013/10/22. eng.
74. Welp A, Meier LL, Manser T. The interplay between teamwork, clinicians' emotional exhaustion, and clinician-rated patient safety: a longitudinal study. Crit Care. 2016;20(1):110. PubMed PMID: 27095501. Pubmed Central PMCID: PMC4837537. Epub 2016/04/21. eng.
75. Fava GA, McEwen BS, Guidi J, Gostoli S, Offidani E, Sonino N. Clinical characterization of allostatic overload. Psychoneuroendocrinology. 2019;108:94–101. PubMed PMID: 31252304. Epub 2019/06/30. eng.
76. Wang M, Zhao J, Zhang L, Wei F, Lian Y, Wu Y, et al. Role of tumor microenvironment in tumorigenesis. J Cancer. 2017;8(5):761–73. PubMed PMID: 28382138. Pubmed Central PMCID: PMC5381164. Epub 2017/04/07. eng.
77. Antoni MH, Lutgendorf SK, Blomberg B, Carver CS, Lechner S, Diaz A, et al. Cognitive-behavioral stress management reverses anxiety-related leukocyte transcriptional dynamics. Biol Psychiatry. 2012;71(4):366–72. PubMed PMID: 22088795. Pubmed Central PMCID: PMC3264698. Epub 2011/11/18. eng.
78. Lutgendorf SK, Andersen BL. Biobehavioral approaches to cancer progression and survival: mechanisms and interventions. Am Psychol. 2015;70(2):186–97. PubMed PMID: 25730724. Pubmed Central PMCID: PMC4347942. Epub 2015/03/03. eng.

Closing Remarks

Rather ten times die in the surf, heralding the way to a new world, than stand idly on the shore—
                                                                                                Florence Nightingale

Epilogue

In essence this book is a call to collective action. Based on an articulated conceptual model of whole person care, it advocates the urgent need for change, a professional imperative in which nurses may find their evidentiary voice in the stated goals, desired outcomes, scientific content, and proposed psychosocial interventions of practice. At its core the model speaks to our collective humanity, and our human need for authentic connections with one another, whether we are a patient, caregiver, or healthcare provider. As an integral part of the human condition, we share the same basic needs for compassion and understanding, the same emotions of hope, joy, suffering, and a shared capacity for healing, throughout our developmental stages that culminate in death.

Much has been written by bards of the past about the ephemeral passage of time, dust-to-dust. Yet our life must *mean* something, however long or short it is—or what's the point. As nurses we do not have far to look for a realizable purpose particularly when the focus of our practice is the whole human being, and techniques and procedures are valued as complementary instruments that support but do not define nursing care. We need more than ever to reexamine our values and beliefs about nursing and to realign our core practice toward caring for the whole person. The conceptual model of whole person care delineates the nature of that practice and provides evidentiary support to justify its goals, desired outcomes, content, and psychosocial nursing interventions.

Knowing the patient and the family caregiver within the context of a connected nurse-patient (caregiver) relationship creates a personalized milieu within which healing and resilient capabilities may flourish or at least improve. We can learn about concepts of stress, healing, resilience, and health, but if we are unable to establish a meaningful connection with our patient and family caregiver, so that they feel *known* by their nurse, critical opportunities to facilitate their innate and self-induced healing processes will never materialize. Martin Buber stated that the "world is not comprehensible, but it is embraceable when we embrace even one human being." We can make the world better one person at a time.

The way we conceptualize Nursing shapes how patients and family caregivers are cared for. Our thoughts and feelings about the work, about cancer, its treatment modalities, the scope and depth of our scientific and clinical competence influence the quality of our interactions with the patient and family caregiver. The scientific knowledge and clinical skills that we bring to bear in caring for patients and their family caregivers are emblematic of our perceived role as clinical nurses with respect to the whole person. For instance, most university-educated nurses have been exposed to different psychosocial interventions from a theoretical perspective. They may have even observed patient-nurse simulations for illustrative purposes, followed by limited role playing. However this pedagogical approach to psychosocial interventions falls far short of normal learning requirements in order to achieve a sense of self-efficacy and behavioral competence. In the main nursing curricula have failed to include student practicums which focus exclusively on the expert acquisition of well-known psychosocial interventions. Yet, psychosocial interventions constitute a significant proportion of whole person care.

When *we say* that we care for the "whole" patient but lack a requisite conceptual model and corresponding scientific knowledge, we do not possess the neurophysiological (and behavioral) basis for meaningfully developing and evaluating the effectiveness of psychological interventions with biobehavioral endpoints that are theoretically or empirically known to be associated with stress, healing, and resilience, and by extension, health. We do not possess adequate knowledge of the widespread effects of current and past, acute and chronic stresses that may continue to influence the disease course, treatment efficacy, surgical recovery time, and even long-term survival. Those days of a one treatment fits all approach are in the past.

It is the author's hope that this book will heighten nurses' cognizant awareness of at least three seminal issues that are relevant for a more effective nursing practice: First is the need to conceptualize practice in terms of the *whole* person. This becomes much clearer when we realize that neurophysiological, molecular, and metabolic processes underlie the manifestation of psychological, emotional, cognitive, physical, behavioral, and spiritual processes. Beliefs, thoughts, feelings, spiritual aspirations, and emotions are communicated throughout the human being as biological substrates. Nurses know this, but I would argue that the clinical implications of that knowledge have yet to be fully integrated or realized in a comprehensive clinical approach to whole patient care.

It is hoped that this book also heightens the nurse's awareness of various social and environmental factors in the clinical setting that can inadvertently exacerbate or facilitate healing processes without the apparent knowledge of either the patient or healthcare team. Research findings have shown that the patient's cognitive expectation for a desired outcome, especially related to symptoms, can either positively or negatively affect healing, resilience, and treatment efficacy. This finding may be leveraged by the nurse to support a positive treatment expectation or counter a negative expectation with empirically known strategies. The nurse's awareness of potential nocebo effects in the clinical environment, such as a clinic wall color, can also be used to mobilize relevant strategies that may help to suppress or counter its deleterious effects on physiological healing and resilience.

Thirdly, it is hoped that the conceptual model can serve as an incentive to develop and evaluate relevant multimodal, multitargeted psychosocial nursing interventions with unique and overlapping endpoints to enhance healing and resilience in patients with cancer and their caregivers across the trajectory.

In closing, the conceptual model served as the organizing scientific predicate for nurses caring for the whole patient with cancer and the family caregiver. Notwithstanding, its core tenets and concepts are equally applicable for nurses with healthy populations, as well as with other chronic illnesses or injuries, supported by scientific evidence tailored to the population of clinical interest.

Clinical Approaches: Appendices

Appendix A

Psychosocial Interventions, Self-Management (SMI) Approaches

Author	Purpose/intervention	Study design	Sample/phase of disease	Outcomes
Kalter et al. [1]	Effects of *psychosocial interventions* (PSI) on quality of life (QOL), emotional (EF) and social function (SF) in patients with cancer: *Interventions assessed:* (a) *information* about cancer, treatment, side effects, consequences; (b) *support* to help patients cope with cancer & treatment: express emotions, decrease sense of isolation, identify unmet needs, take some control over events, deal with family and healthcare givers, enhance acceptance of losses, changed roles; (c) *coping skills training* (CST), i.e., new cognitive behavioral skills, relaxation, mental imaging, thought and affect management, activity planning; (d) *psychotherapy*; (e) *spiritual/existential therapy:* interventions increasing awareness of transcendent power, belonging to a meaningful universe, meditation and/or prayer (as patient preferred), reading, discussion, reflection on spiritual issues	Meta-analysis using 22 RCTs	$N = 4217$ patients with various cancers during different types of treatment	1. **PSI significantly improved QOL, EF, SF** 2. Significant differences in effects of different PSI 3. **CST** significantly increased QOL, EF, SF 4. **Younger patients** had significantly larger effects of CST on EF ($P = 0.01$) and SF ($P = 0.03$) 5. **Patients on chemotherapy** had larger CST effects on QOL and EF 6. **Patients who had surgery** had larger CST effects on SF ($p = 0.04$) 7. Effects on QOL were larger in women who did *not* receive hormone treatment ($p < 0.01$) 8. Effects on QOL were larger in studies that target distress ($p < 0.01$) **Conclusion** (a) Publication bias was not significant according to the funnel plot, Duval and Tweedie's trim and fill procedure, and Egger's test of bias based on the funnel plot

Andersen et al. [2]	To assess psychological intervention in terms of two paths to enhanced health: (1) reducing distress, (2) increasing functional immunity **Intervention** (a) progressive relaxation exercises, (b) positive ways to cope with stress/symptoms, (c) ways to ↑ support, (d) improve diet, exercise, and adherence to treatment	RCT with RA to: (a) clinical intervention (b) assessment only Small group sessions, (a) weekly for 4 months, (b) then monthly for 8 months	227 newly diagnosed postsurgical patients with regional breast cancer	**Intervention group** 1. Path analyses showed significant improvement in health at 12 months 2. Intervention significantly decreased stress at 4 months which contributed to improved health at 12 months ($p < 0.05$) 3. Increased levels of T cell blastogenesis 4–12 months after entry into study **Controls** 1. Functional status decreased 2. Symptoms increased by 29% compared to 14% in the intervention group **Conclusion:** Intervention-related behavioral change accounted for improvements in symptoms
Andersen et al. [3]	Same intervention as Andersen 2007 Designed to assess the effect of intervention on emotional distress, health behaviors, and immune responses (WBC, T lymphocytes, T cell subsets, NK cells with relevant cell surface markers **Intervention**—small groups, 1 weekly session for 4 months (a) progressive relaxation exercises, (b) positive ways to cope with symptoms, (c) ways to ↑ support, (d) improve diet, exercise, and adherence to treatment, (e) ways to improve mood, health behaviors, adhere to cancer treatment, (f) strategies to reduce stress	RCT with RA to: (a) clinical intervention (b) assessment only Small group sessions, (a) weekly for 4 months	227 newly diagnosed postsurgical patients with regional breast cancer	1. Intervention group demonstrated significant reductions in anxiety levels ($p < 0.05$) 2. Improved perceived support ($p < 0.05$) 3. Improved dietary habits ($p < 0.05$) 4. Reduced smoking ($p < 0.05$) 5. Better adherence to treatment 6. T lymphocyte blastogenesis increased over course of treatment in intervention group and declined in assessment group at 4 months

(continued)

Author	Purpose/intervention	Study design	Sample/phase of disease	Outcomes
Andersen et al. [4]	**Follow-up study to Andersen's 2004 RCT** Assessed effects of a psychological intervention conducted in newly diagnosed postsurgical patients who now had a cancer recurrence a median of 11 years later **Hypothesis** Intervention group would demonstrate a longer survival than the assessment group **Intervention** *See Andersen 2004 above*	Patients with cancer recurrence (with RA to): (a) clinical intervention (b) assessment only Small group sessions, (a) weekly for 4 months, (b) then monthly for 8 months	Originally, 227 newly diagnosed postsurgical patients with regional breast cancer Followed over the years, and at a median of 11 years, 41/62 people with a cancer recurrence evaluated (Intervention=n = 23; Assessment group n = 18)	1. After median of 11 years, intervention group had a decreased risk of recurrence (hazard ration, 0.55; p = 0.034) 2. All patients were psychologically distressed after diagnosis of recurrence 3. Intervention group showed reduced risk of death after recurrence based on intent-to-treat analysis (HR: 0.41; P = 0.014) 4. Intervention group showed 56% decrease in risk of dying of breast cancer 5. Intervention group were more successful obtaining and maintaining support which may have buffered effects of stress of cancer recurrence 6. Patients in intervention group with the highest baseline levels of support survived the longest

Author	Purpose/intervention	Study design	Sample/phase of disease	Outcomes
Cohen (2011)	To assess whether a pre-/postsurgical stress management (SM) intervention improves immune functions in *men undergoing surgery for prostate cancer* **Intervention** 1. *CBT consisted of:* (a) *2-session presurgical intervention* info about prostate cancer and surgery, discussed concerns about surgery; taught diaphragmatic breathing, guided imagery, relaxation skills (b) *session 2*—imagined what the surgery would be like; learned problem-solving coping skills, support seeking behaviors, realistic expectations (c) booster sessions on the morning of surgery, and 48 hrs postsurgery to boost problem-solving approaches, and use of relaxation exercises 2. *Supportive attention* (SA) (a) 2 sessions provided empathy, detained psychosocial interview, reflective listening skills, discussed patient concerns (b) Brief boosters on the morning of surgery, 48 h postsurgery	159 RA to: (a) stress management (SM) (b) supportive attention (SA) (c) standard care (SC)	Men with early-stage prostate cancer	***The SM intervention*** 1. SM group showed significantly higher levels of NK cell cytotoxicity ($p = 0.04$) 2. Increased levels of circulating pro-inflammatory cytokines (IL-12p70) ($p = 0.02$); IL-1b ($p = 0.02$); TNF-α ($p = 0.05$) compared to ***SA group*** 48 h postsurgery 3. SM group had higher levels of NK cell cytotoxicity ($p = 0.02$) and IL-1B ($p = 0.05$) compared to SC 4. Immune parameters increased for SM group; but decreased or stayed the same for SA and SC groups 5. SM group had significantly better mood scores than SC group ($p = 0.006$) 6. Changes in mood were not related to immune outcomes ***Conclusion*** Results show potential psychological and immune benefits of presurgical SM intervention (a) Only research assistant blind to group alignment (b) Patients not blinded, does not state whether MDs, statistician blinded to groups or goals of treatment (c) Clinical significance of findings not reported

Author	Purpose/intervention	Study design	Sample/phase of disease	Outcomes
Dionne-Odom et al. [5]	To assess **after-death caregiver depressive symptoms and grief scores** for *early* compared to *delayed* receipt of a palliative care intervention for caregivers (ENABLE III) **Self-management Intervention** Involved **one on one telephone sessions** for caregivers in rural community *Session 1*—described caregiver role, defined palliative/supportive care, introduced problem-solving approach based on COPE (McMillan 2006) *Session 2*—caregiver self-care (healthy eating, exercise, relaxation) and partnering in patient symptom assessment/management *Session 3*—how to build a support team, decision making, decision support, advance care planning *Also:* patients and caregivers given their own nurse to discuss feelings and thoughts -3 weekly CG educational sessions, then monthly to address concerns until end of study or patient had died; in which case nurse made a bereavement call to offer condolences and address grief issues	122 Caregivers RA to (a) early PC (i.e., immediately after randomization) ($n = 61$) (b) 3 months after randomization of caregivers of patients newly diagnosed with advanced cancer, cancer recurrence, or progression of advanced cancer ($n = 61$) 8–12 weeks post death of loved one, 44 caregivers of 70 patients who died completed after-death questionnaires (early group: $n = 19$; delayed group: $n = 25$)	Caregivers after the death of patients	NS differences between groups on measures of depression, grief scores (a) Mean depressive symptom scores for early and late caregiver groups were: 14.6 (SD = 10.7) and 17.6 (SD 11.8) respectively (b) Mean grief scores for the early and late caregiver groups were: 22.7 (SD = 4.9) and 24.9 (SD 6.9) respectively (c) Adjusted between group differences were NS for either depressed scores ($d = 0.07$, $p = 0.88$) or grief ($d = -0.21$, $p = 0.51$) Summary After decedents' death there was no difference on measures of either grief or depression 8 to 12 weeks afterward (a) No control group was possible given patient's stage of illness, and known reciprocal interdependent effects between patient and caregiver

| Dionne-Odom et al. [6] | To investigate effects of early versus later start of a palliative care intervention for family members of patients with advanced cancer (ENABLE 111 RCT Self-management Intervention (SMI) topics

Involved one on one telephone sessions for caregivers in rural community led by own nurse

Session 1—described caregiver role, defined palliative/supportive care, introduced problem-solving approach based on COPE (McMillan 2006)

Session 2—caregiver self-care (healthy eating, exercise, relaxation) and partnering in patient symptom assessment/management

Session 3—how to build a support team (strengthen communication skills), decision making, decision support, advance care planning

Also: patients and caregivers also could discuss feelings and thoughts

-3 weekly CG educational sessions, then monthly to address concerns until end of study or patient had died: in which case nurse made a bereavement call to offer condolences and address grief issues | 122 Caregivers RA to
(a) early PC (i.e., immediately after randomization) ($n = 61$)
(b) later PC (i.e., 3 months after randomization)
(c) patients were newly diagnosed with advanced cancer, cancer recurrence, or progression of advanced cancer ($n = 61$) | Mostly female (78.7%) caregivers of patients with advanced and terminal phase cancer | 1. *Between-group differences between the two groups from enrollment to 3 months:*
(a) early group had significantly lower depression scores compared to the late group: (mean difference −3.4; SE, 1.5; $d = -0.32$, $P = 0.02$)
(b) NS differences were shown for quality of life (Mean diff: Mean diff −2; SE 2.3, $d = -0.13$, $p = 0.39$); burden (Mean diff 0.3, SE 0.7; $d = 0.09$, $p = 0.64$); stress (Mean diff −0.5; SE 0.5; $d = -0.2$; $p = 0.29$); and demand (Mean diff: =0; SE 0.7; $d = -0.01$; $p = 0.97$) at 3 months
2. *In terminal decline phase*
(a) the early group showed significantly *less depression* than late phase (mean difference −3.8; SE, 1.5; $d = -0.39$; $P = 0.02$)
(b) early group also showed significantly *less stress burden* than late group (mean difference −1.1; SE, 0.4; $d = -0.44$; $P = 0.01$)
(c) NS difference for quality of life ($P = 0.07$), objective burden ($P = 0.27$), or demand burden ($P = 0.22$)
Conclusion Clear benefits to caregivers when palliative care initiated as early as possible at 3 months
The early group also showed better scores on depression and stress burden during the terminal phase |

Author	Purpose/intervention	Study design	Sample/phase of disease	Outcomes
Dionne-Odom et al. [7]	To adapt content, format, and delivery of a 6-session palliative care *telehealth SMI intervention for family caregivers* with monthly follow-ups in order to increase self-care and care giving skills	Qualitative study of semistructured interviews with 18 people with metastatic cancer and the patient's 20 family caregivers and 26 lay patient navigators shown an outline of the family caregiver intervention	Rural living caregivers of patients with advanced/terminal cancer	1. Recommendations: from participants (a) intervention should be flexible, adaptable format based on regular needs assessment (b) sessions should be a minimum of 20 minutes with preference for one on one rather than via telehealth (c) faith important to address but should not be a main objective

Author	Purpose/intervention	Study design	Sample/phase of disease	Outcomes
Bakitas et al. [8]	To investigate effects of **early versus later** start of palliative care intervention **for patients with advanced cancer on quality of life, symptom impact, mood, 1-year survival, and resource use** (ENABLE III RCT) **Self-management (SMI) Intervention** **Sessions 1–3**: focus was on problem-solving, symptom management, self-care, coordination of local resources, communication, decision making, advance care planning **Sessions 4–6**: included life review aimed at framing illness challenges as personal growth opportunities, outlook, based on their booklet *Charting Your Course* **Sessions afterward**: monthly follow-ups to reinforce content and address new challenges. Sessions lasted 30–45 min delivered by telehealth	RCT to (a) early group (b) late entry group 3 months after enrollment (see [6]) Both groups received usual care Patients assessed at baseline, 6, 12, 18, and 24 weeks after enrollment; then every 12 weeks afterward till patient death or end of study	Rural living caregivers of patients with advanced/terminal cancer	1. Patient reported outcomes after enrollment were NS for quality of life ($p = 0.34$), symptom impact ($p = 0.09$), mood ($p = 0.33$) or **before death, NS for QOL** ($p = 0.73$), and mood ($p = 0.82$) 2. 1-year survival rates in the early group were 63% and 48% in the later start group, significant at $p = 0.03$. 3. All other analyses were NS, including resource use, hospitalizations, ER visits, and home deaths **Conclusion** There was no usual care group (a) No clinical benefit in starting the palliative care intervention either immediately after diagnosis or three months later (b) When the same intervention was assessed compared to a usual care group, significant differences were found in patient outcomes [9]

(continued)

Author	Purpose/intervention	Study design	Sample/phase of disease	Outcomes
Bakitas et al. [9]	To determine effect of a palliative care SMI intervention on quality of life, symptom intensity, mood and resource utilization (*ENABLE II*) based on a chronic care model and principles of self-management **Intervention: *Psychoeducational palliative care based on a Self-Management model of care, led by an advanced practice nurse*** (a) phone based, educational approach to encourage patient activation, empowerment, and self-management (b) *on-going assessment and coaching in problem solving*, advance care planning, family and healthcare team communication strategies, symptom management, crisis prevention, timely referral to palliative care Specifically (a) *Assessments Distress thermometer*—11 point 90-100 (recommended by Allen 2014, NCCN guidelines): if > 3, then assessed in 5 areas: practical problems, family problems, emotional problems, spiritual/religious, physical problems (b) *4 structured modules given weekly:* (1) problem solving, (2) communication and social support, (3) symptom management, (4) advance care planning, unfinished business and list of useful resources (Education manual-guided interventions: *Charting your course*: An intervention for people and families living with cancer developed during ENABLE 1 (obtained from author). (c) then monthly telephone follow-ups until end of study or patient's death	RCT of 322 patients to (a) palliative care (b) usual care	Patients with advanced disease of gastrointestinal (41%), lung (36%), genitourinary (12%), breast cancer (10%)	1. *Estimated treatment effects:* (intervention minus usual care) was 4.6 ($P = 0.02$) for quality of life (a) symptom intensity was -27.8 ($p = 0.06$) (b) depressed mood was -1.8 ($p = 0.02$) 2. *Estimated treatment effects in persons who died:* (a) for quality of life was 8.6 ($p = 0.02$) (b) for symptom intensity -24.2 ($p = 0.24$), (c) for depressed mood -2.7 ($p = 0.03$) 3. Days in hospital, ICU, ED visits were all NS **Conclusion** Compared to usual care, persons who received intervention to improve physical, psychosocial, and care coordination with oncology care showed higher quality of life and mood

Author	Purpose/intervention	Study design	Sample/phase of disease	Outcomes
Temel et al. [10]	Evaluated impact of early integrated palliative care in patients with newly diagnosed incurable lung and GI cancer **Psychosocial Interventions** (a) Communications about prognosis, treatment goals, care preferences over time (b) Facilitated illness understanding, treatment decisions, advance care planning (c) Symptom management (d) Establishing a "rapport" with patient and caregiver (e) Facilitating coping addressing mood, redirecting hope, counseling, behavioral coping, spiritual coping, life review, coping with family, patient and or caregiver referrals	RCT RA 350 patients with lung or GI cancer 1. early integrated palliative care group 2. usual care	175 patients with lung and GI cancer	Compared to usual care, intervention patients reported: 1. Significant improvement in QOL at 24 weeks (1.59 v-3.40; $p = 0.010$) but not at 12 weeks When patients with lung and GI analyzed separately: 2. Patients with lung cancer reported significant improvements in QOL and mood at 12 and 24 weeks whereas usual care patients did more poorly (deteriorated) 3. GI patients in both intervention and usual care groups improved at 12 weeks in QOL but still NS 4. Only patients in the intervention group with lung cancer also had significantly higher QOL and lower depression levels at 2, 4, and 6 months before death 5. The main symptoms patients experienced included: pain (58.4%), fatigue (52.1%0), nausea (21.7%), and anxiety (18.1%) 6. The topics included managing symptoms (74.7%), coping (70.2%), establishing a rapport (44.4%), treatment decisions (16.35%), advance care planning (14.2%), and disposition (2.1%). When facilitating coping was the focus of the healthcare intervention, the most frequent strategies were redirecting hope (71.1%), coping counseling (67.0%), behavioral coping (65.4%), spiritual coping (18.3%), and conducting a life review (9.8%) (Temel 2016 **Conclusion** (a) Differential results depending on cancer site, with GI patients doing more poorly overall (b) No discussion of how data to be assessed for risk of bias which appears to exist (c) Patients and clinicians were not blinded to group assignment, underpowered to do analyses of patients with lung or GI cancer separately. Possible confounding due to the fact that usual group met regularly with palliative care team for first 24 days of study

(continued)

Author	Purpose/intervention	Study design	Sample/phase of disease	Outcomes
Kim et al. [11]	To evaluate the effects of *self-management interventions* (SMI) for cancer *survivors after treatment* **Intervention** Self-management interventions aimed at empowering patients and caregivers to improve their health and well-being while living with cancer by developing a set of practical skills that can be applied in daily life and enhance self-efficacy and competence [12]: (a) provide education (b) supportive interventions (c) develop SMI skills and plan of action to assess and manage health-related problems, deal with changes in life roles, as well as manage emotions related to their cancer [12]	12 systematic reviews of self-management content and meta-analysis using 9 RCT SMI compared to usual care, attention control, or waitlist group (a) Cochrane collaboration tool to assess risk of bias (b) Studies selected based on PRISMA guidelines	N-2804 cancer survivors after treatment Most common cancer was breast cancer ($n = 6$); others were hematologic, gynecologic, and prostate cancers	1. ***Qualitative synthesis*** showed that the major study population were breast cancer survivors (a) SMIs centered on medical, emotional, and behavioral management (b) Most common mode of delivery was web-based 2. Meta-analysis of 9 trials showed a significant medium increase on HRQOL ($d = 0.55$, $p = 0.046$, chi square = 92%), and a large effect size reduction on fatigue that almost attain statistical significance ($d = -1.17$, $p = 0.058$, chi square = 98%) (a) NS on anxiety, depression, self-efficacy posttreatment, but a small effect size increase in self-efficacy long term ($d = 0.27$, $p = 0.021$ chi square = 44.9%) 3. Systematic review of 12 studies showed majority of survivors had breast cancer; most common delivery was web-based; SMI content consisted of medical/behavioral and emotional management **Conclusion** Substantial heterogeneity limits interpretation of the findings. Need further studies to determine the most effective content and mode of delivery 2. ***Quantitative results*** (a) showed a significant medium effect on HRQOL ($d = 0.55$, $p = 0.046$, $X^2 = 92\%$) (b) a NS effect on fatigue ($d = -1.17$, $p = 0.058$, $X^2 = 98\%$) (c) significant small effect of SMI on self-efficacy ($k = 5$) ($d = 0.27$, $p = 0.021$, $X^2 = 44.9\%$) (d) effects on anxiety, depression, were NS 3. ***Content and delivery of interventions*** Varied across studies and points of emphasis shaped by different or no theoretical underpinnings 4. ***Focus of interventions*** (a) 7 studies focused on management of distress and emotions, uncertainty, empowerment (b) 4 trials focused on medical/behavioral management such as symptoms (e.g., fatigue), exercise, and diet (c) 1 trial consisted of medical issues, role, and emotional management 5. ***Self-management skill-related interventional components*** (a) Problem solving most frequently included (n-10) (b) Taking action ($n = 9$), use of resources ($n = 8$), forming partnerships ($n = 8$), decision making ($n = 7$) **Conclusion** SMI had a significant medium effect on HRQOL but studies were associated with high risk of bias (heterogeneity), lacked standard interventional components, methodological limitations of design, measurement. Finally conceptual overlap between stress coping and self-management components

Author	Purpose/intervention	Study design	Sample/phase of disease	Outcomes
Cuthbert et al. [13]	To evaluate evidence for self-management interventions for cancer SURVIVORS and describe its components	Systematic review Included experimental and quasiexperimental designs Systematic review followed Cochrane Handbook and PRISMA guidelines Unable to do meta-analysis due to high heterogeneity of studies Study quality based on Cochrane risk of bias tool for RCTS, another tool for nonrandomized studies Data synthesis included narrative and tabular summary of results	Based on 41 studies ($n = 6038$) adults who completed treatment for primary cancer	1. *Interventional aspects and sample* (a) 41 Studies included and majority were based on breast cancer patients (b) More than 50% of studies lacked a theoretical framework, which varied greatly across studies when present (c) Main outcomes were: self-efficacy, clinical outcomes, quality of life, healthcare utilization (d) Duration ranged from one session to many over 12 months (e) 72% of studies included standardized training for the HCP 2. *Content* (a) Psychoeducational interventional components varied across studies (b) Most included combinations of: • education about cancer in general or a specific type and treatment • education on health behaviors such as stress management, diet, physical activity • coping skills training to manage cancer and life-related issues • information about managing physical aspects of cancer, e.g., dressings, medications, symptom management • coping skills to manage psychological impact of cancer, communication skills, problem-solving skills 3. Clinical outcomes difficult to assess: (a) QOL—15/26 reported statistical improvement, one reported worsened QOL, 10 reported NS differences (b) others reported significant improvements in depression (k=2), anxiety (k=1), distress (k=2), fatigue (k=3), self-efficacy (k=1), illness adjustment (k=2), support (k=1), but these initial improvements were generally not sustained (c) only 3 outcomes showed consistent improvements: self-reported physical activity levels, knowledge, and disease progression (?) *Conclusion* The lack of a standardized theory guiding key components of the intervention, plus variable frequency and duration of the intervention, weak designs and lack of standard and validated measurements all contribute to high risk of bias, and difficulty interpreting findings (a) Need to develop a tailored SMI intervention evaluated by rigorously designed RCT focusing on patients/caregivers based on one cancer type, and at similar stage of disease

Author	Purpose/intervention	Study design	Sample/phase of disease	Outcomes
Kavalieratos et al. [14]	Assess the relationship of palliative care (PC) with quality of life, survival, mood, for people with life-limiting disease and their caregivers based on *a self-management intervention* (SMI) model	Meta-analysis of 43 RCTs	(a) 12,731 adults with self-limiting disease: 69.7% were patients with cancer 32.5% had heart failure (b) 24479 caregivers	1. PC was associated with statistical and significant clinical improvements in patient QOL at the 1–3 months follow-up (SMD 0.46; 95% CL, 0.08 to 0.83) and symptom burden (SMD −0.66; 95% CL, −1.25 to −0.07) 2. In trials of low risk of bias (*n* = 5) the relationship between palliative care and QOL was decreased but significant (SMD 0.20; 95% CL, 0.06 to 0.34) but association with symptom burden was NS (−0.21; 95% CL, −0.42 to 0.00) 3. NS between palliative care and survival (Hazard ratio: 0.90; 95% CL, 0.69 to 1.17) 4. PC was associated with improvement in advance care planning, patient and caregiver satisfaction, lower health care utilization consistent with goals of SMI 5. Caregiver outcomes were inconsistent (15 trials) **Summary** Quality evidence was generally low to moderate No distinction between early and later palliative care contrary to findings by Dionne-Dom (2015, 2016 and Bakistas 2010)

Northouse et al. [15]	To determine the types of interventions provided to family caregivers and their effectiveness on health-related outcomes	Meta-analysis of 29 RCTs (caregivers/study ranged between 14 and 329) Sample included caregiver-patient dyads and just caregivers as target of interventions	Caregivers of cancer patients Not specified; appears to include dyads across stages of disease	1. Identified 3 interventions for caregivers: (a) ***psychoeducation*** (e.g., info about managing patient symptoms, physical aspects; attention to emotional, psychosocial needs of patients, caregivers, marital/family relationship) (b) **Skills training** (k=9, 25.7%) (development of coping, communication, problem-solving skills) (c) ***Therapeutic counseling*** (k=6, 17.1%) (development of therapeutic relationship to address concerns about cancer and care giving)Results 2. Interventions had small to medium effects that significantly decreased caregiver burden, increased their ability to cope, increased self-efficacy and aspects of quality of life 3. 2/3rd of the interventions given to caregiver/patient dyads (k=22; 62.9%) and 1/3rd given to caregivers alone (k=13; 37.5%) 4. Majority of interventions given face to face (k=24; 68.6%; by telephone (k=7; 20%), and by group meeting (k=4; 11.3%) 5. Nurses delivered interventions in 52% of the studies

(continued)

Author	Purpose/intervention	Study design	Sample/phase of disease	Outcomes
Northouse et al. [16]	Assessed whether a brief or extensive dyadic intervention for caregivers and patients with advanced cancer at home is effective in improving QOL and other health-related outcomes **Intervention for the dyads: Original FOCUS intervention:** (a) To provide information, support, reduce stress and maintain hope (b) home-based (c) addressed 5 areas: family involvement, optimistic attitude, coping effectiveness, uncertainty reduction, symptom management (d) delivered by nurses (received 40 h training)	RCT RA dyads to: (a) Brief dyadic intervention (2–90 min home visits plus one 30 min phone call) (b) Extensive dyadic intervention (4–90 min home visits, plus 2 30 min telephone sessions) c) Usual care for dyads Assts at baseline, 3 and 6 months later	Final sample: 302/484 patient/caregiver dyads of patients with **advanced** cancer Stage III-IV breast, prostate, lung, or colorectal cancer 66% patients were currently on treatment 66% of caregivers had comorbid conditions	1. Significant **group by time interactions** with improvement in dyadic coping ($p < 0.05$), self-efficacy ($p < 0.05$), and social quality of life ($p < 0.01$) 2. Univariate analysis demonstrated significant effects on avoidant coping and healthy behaviors 3. Simple effects showed control dyads' avoidant coping did not change across baseline, 3 and 6 months follow-ups. 4. Dyads in both extensive and brief interventions showed significant reduction in use of avoidant coping from baseline to 3 months follow-up; and at 6 months only for those in the brief intervention 5. Only dyads in the brief intervention showed significant improvement in their use of healthy behaviors (**nutrition and exercise**) at 3 months ($p < 0.001$) only even as some patients were deteriorating **RE Self-efficacy** 1. Simple effects showed that controls and brief dyads' self-efficacy did not change significantly from baseline to 3 or 6 months **Re Social QOL** 1. Simple effects showed that control dyads had a significant decrease in social QOL at 3 months 2. In contrast, simple effects showed that brief and extensive dyads maintained their social QOL at 3 and 6 months from baseline **Re Emotional QOL** 1. Significant improvement in brief and extensive group caregivers' emotional QOL but not control caregivers ($p < 0.05$) 2. Significant improvement in controls, brief and extensive group patients emotional QOL at 3 months **Summary** 1. Most effects were found at 3 months after baseline 2. Both brief and extended interventions had positive but not sustainable effects on patient-caregiver dyads 3. May be difficult to sustain improvements as patients' disease advances and caregiver burden increases

Author	Purpose/intervention	Study design	Sample/phase of disease	Outcomes
Badger et al. [17]	To test effectiveness of two telephone-based interventions (a) an interpersonal counseling (TIP-C) (b) *health education* attention condition (HEAC)	A three-wave repeated measures experimental design	71 prostate cancer survivors and 70 family partners	**Re Cancer survivors:** (a) ***Survivors in the HEAC group*** showed significant improvements in quality of life outcomes for: depression ($F(1,69) = 12.31, P < 0.001$) negative affect ($F(1, 69) = 15.72, P < 0.001$) perceived stress ($F(1, 69) = 15.72, P < 0.001$) fatigue ($F(1,69)\ 9.61, P = <0.01$) spiritual well-being ($F(1,69) = 10.34, P < 0.01$) compared to the TIP-C counseling group (b) ***Partners in HEAC group showed*** significant improvements in quality of life outcomes for : depression ($F(1,69) = 4.54, P < 0.05$) fatigue ($F(1,69) = 10.28, P < 0.01$) social support from family ($F(1,69) = 6.47, P < 0.05$) social well-being ($F(1,69) = 7.67, P < 0.01$) spiritual well-being ($F(1,69) = 11.31, P < 0.01$) compared to those in the TIP-C condition **Conclusion** Results underscore importance of providing relevant information about the cancer, treatment, and ways to strengthen health to survivors and their partners

(continued)

Author	Purpose/intervention	Study design	Sample/phase of disease	Outcomes
Galway et al. [18]	To assess effects of psychosocial interventions to increase quality of life and reduce emotional distress in the *first 12 months after diagnosis*. Interventions within a supportive nurse–patient relationship could consist of: (a) CBT (14 studies) (b) counseling (8 studies) (c) brief preparatory interventions offered immediately prior to treatment and a combination of counseling, psychotherapy, and relaxation techniques (d) psychoeducation (e) meaning making (1 study)	Cochrane review 30 trials	First 12 months of newly diagnosed patients with diverse cancers	1. Psychosocial interventions had a small significant improvement in quality of life based on cancer-specific measures (SMD, 0.16, 95% CI 0.02 to 0.30, 6 studies) 2. General distress was significantly reduced, when "mood measures" were used (SMD, −0.81, 95% CI, −1.44 to −0.18, 8 studies) 3. Psychosocial interventions for newly diagnosed distressed cancer patients showed no effect based on measures of either anxiety (SMD 0.05, 95% CI, −0.13 to 0.22, 4 studies) or depression (SMD, 0.12, 95% CI, 0-0.07 to 0.31, 6 studies) 4. Nurse-administered face-to-face and telephone interventions consisting of psychoeducational information provided within a supportive nurse–patient relationship showed a significant small increased effect on quality of life in patients with breast cancer (SMD 0.23, 95% CI, 0.04 to 0.43, 2 studies)

Fulton [19]	Investigated effects of *integrated palliative-oncology care*	Systematic review of 11 companion papers and 10 RCTs and quasiexperimental studies in meta-analysis Median time of start of interventions between 8–12 weeks since diagnosis	2385 Patients of diverse cancers diagnosed as advanced, cancer recurrence, or cancer progression	1. ***Results of integrated palliative care (IPC) on quality of life***
				   (a) IPC increased quality of life in the short term compared to standard oncology care ($n = 9$; SMD 0.24; 95% CI 0.13 to 0.35; I2 = 0.0%) with small to moderate effects in 8/9 studies
				 2. ***RE Symptom burden***
				   (a) 1–3 months after randomizations IPC patients showed small but NS improvements in symptom burden compared to controls ($n = 6$; SMD −0.17; 95% CI −0.45 to 0.11; I2 =62%) though moderate heterogeneity observed across studies (5/6 showed improvements but one study was an outlier)
				 3. ***Psychological symptom outcomes***
				   (a) 6 studies that reported effects on depression were NS with depression severity a continuous clinical outcome ($n = 4$; SMD −0.09: 95% CI −0.32 to 0.13; I2 =0%)
				   (b) 1/2 studies reporting proportion of patients attaining clinical cut off (≥) for depression showed an intervention effect ($n = 104$; 4% vs 17%; $p = 0.04$)
				   (c) Similar proportional analysis was NS for anxiety
				 4. ***Survival outcomes***
				   (a) When sensitivity analysis limited studies to those with greater homogeneity, all-cause mortality was significantly reduced ($n = 4$; HR, 0.77; 95% CI, 0.61 to 0.98, I2 =0.0% showing a small effect.
				 5. ***End of life outcomes***
				   (a) In studies following patients from 6 to 35 months, patients receiving PC more likely to die at home ($n = 3$; RR 1.19; 95% CI, 1.05 to 1.36; I2 =0.0% compared to standard care
				   (b) Patients in IPC were less likely to receive aggressive end of life care compared to usual care (33% vs 54%, $p = 0.05$)
				 6. ***Caregiver and patient experience outcomes***
				   (a) 3 trials patients in IPC reported better caregiver experience at 3 months; at 4 months trend was still better though NS
				   (b) Caregiver quality did not change between groups

(continued)

Author	Purpose/intervention	Study design	Sample/phase of disease	Outcomes
Temel [20]	To investigate effect of an early palliative care *(EPC)* intervention on patient outcomes and end of life care in newly diagnosed ambulatory patients with metastatic non-small cell lung cancer	RCT RA to: (a) standard care (b) EPC	151 newly diagnosed ambulatory patients with metastatic lung cancer 27 patients died by 12 weeks	1. *Quality of life* (a) Patients in the EPC had better quality of life (FACT-L) than standard care patients with higher scores denoting higher quality of life (EPC: 98.0 vs SC 91.5, $p = 0.03$) 2. *Depressed symptoms* (a) EPC had fewer patients with depressed symptoms compared to SC (16% vs 38%, $p = 0.01$) 3. *Survival outcomes* (a) Fewer EPC patients experienced aggressive treatment than those in SC (33% vs 54%, $p = 0.05$) (b) But EPC patients lived significantly longer than SC patients ($p = 0.02$) as evidenced by median survival (11.6 months: 95% CI, 6.4 to 16.9, $n = 77$) compared to (8.9 months, 95% CI, 6.3 to 11.4, $n = 74$) *Conclusion* Patients with non-small cell lung cancer had less symptoms of depression (PHQ-9), better quality of life, and lived longer than those receiving standard care, despite receiving less aggressive end of life treatment

References

1. Kalter J, Verdonck-de Leeuw IM, Sweegers MG, Aaronson NK, Jacobsen PB, Newton RU, et al. Effects and moderators of psychosocial interventions on quality of life, and emotional and social function in patients with cancer: an individual patient data meta-analysis of 22 RCTs. Psychooncology. 2018;27(4):1150–61; PubMed PMID: 29361206. Pubmed Central PMCID: PMC5947559. Epub 2018/01/24. eng.
2. Andersen BL, Farrar WB, Golden-Kreutz D, Emery CF, Glaser R, Crespin T, et al. Distress reduction from a psychological intervention contributes to improved health for cancer patients. Brain Behav Immun 2007;21(7):953–61; PubMed PMID: 17467230. Pubmed Central PMCID: PMC2039896. Epub 2007/05/01. eng.
3. Andersen BL, Farrar WB, Golden-Kreutz DM, Glaser R, Emery CF, Crespin TR, et al. Psychological, behavioral, and immune changes after a psychological intervention: a clinical trial. J Clin Oncol 2004;22(17):3570–80; PubMed PMID: 15337807. Pubmed Central PMCID: PMC2168591. Epub 2004/09/01. eng.
4. Andersen BL, Thornton LM, Shapiro CL, Farrar WB, Mundy BL, Yang HC, et al. Biobehavioral, immune, and health benefits following recurrence for psychological intervention participants. Clin Cancer Res 2010;16(12):3270–8; PubMed PMID: 20530702. Pubmed Central PMCID: PMC2910547. Epub 2010/06/10. eng.
5. Dionne-Odom JN, Azuero A, Lyons KD, Hull JG, Prescott AT, Tosteson T, et al. Family caregiver depressive symptom and grief outcomes from the ENABLE III randomized controlled trial. J Pain Symptom Manage 2016;52(3):378–85; PubMed PMID: 27265814. Pubmed Central PMCID: PMC5023481. Epub 2016/06/07. eng.
6. Dionne-Odom JN, Azuero A, Lyons KD, Hull JG, Tosteson T, Li Z, et al. Benefits of early versus delayed palliative care to informal family caregivers of patients with advanced cancer: outcomes from the ENABLE III randomized controlled trial. J Clin Oncol 2015;33(13):1446–52; PubMed PMID: 25800762. Pubmed Central PMCID: PMC4404423. Epub 2015/03/25. eng.
7. Dionne-Odom JN, Taylor R, Rocque G, Chambless C, Ramsey T, Azuero A, et al. Adapting an early palliative care intervention to family caregivers of persons with advanced cancer in the rural deep south: a qualitative formative evaluation. J Pain Symptom Manage 2018;55(6):1519–30; PubMed PMID: 29474939. Pubmed Central PMCID: PMC5951755. Epub 2018/02/24. eng.
8. Bakitas MA, Tosteson TD, Li Z, Lyons KD, Hull JG, Li Z, et al. Early versus delayed initiation of concurrent palliative oncology care: patient outcomes in the ENABLE III randomized controlled trial. J Clin Oncol 2015;33(13):1438–45; PubMed PMID: 25800768. Pubmed Central PMCID: PMC4404422. Epub 2015/03/25. eng.
9. Bakitas M, Lyons KD, Hegel MT, Balan S, Brokaw FC, Seville J, et al. Effects of a palliative care intervention on clinical outcomes in patients with advanced cancer: the Project ENABLE II randomized controlled trial. JAMA 2009;302(7):741–9; PubMed PMID: 19690306. Pubmed Central PMCID: PMC3657724. Epub 2009/08/20. eng.

10. Temel JS, Greer JA, El-Jawahri A, Pirl WF, Park ER, Jackson VA, et al. Effects of early integrated palliative care in patients with lung and GI cancer: a randomized clinical trial. J Clin Oncol. 2017;35(8):834–41; Pubmed Central PMCID: PMC5455686. Epub 2016/12/29. eng.
11. Kim SH, Kim K, Mayer DK. Self-management intervention for adult cancer survivors after treatment: a systematic review and meta-analysis. Oncol Nurs Forum. 2017;44(6):719–28; PubMed PMID: 29052663. Epub 2017/10/21. eng.
12. McCorkle R, Ercolano E, Lazenby M, Schulman-Green D, Schilling LS, Lorig K, et al. Self-management: enabling and empowering patients living with cancer as a chronic illness. CA Cancer J Clin 2011;61(1):50–62; PubMed PMID: 21205833. Pubmed Central PMCID: PMC3058905. Epub 2011/01/06. eng.
13. Cuthbert CA, Farragher JF, Hemmelgarn BR, Ding Q, McKinnon GP, Cheung WY. Self-management interventions for cancer survivors: A systematic review and evaluation of intervention content and theories. Psychooncology 2019;28(11):2119–40; PubMed PMID: 31475766. Epub 2019/09/03. eng.
14. Kavalieratos D, Corbelli J, Zhang D, Dionne-Odom JN, Ernecoff NC, Hanmer J, et al. Association between palliative care and patient and caregiver outcomes: a systematic review and meta-analysis. JAMA 2016;316(20):2104–14; PubMed PMID: 27893131. Pubmed Central PMCID: PMC5226373. Epub 2016/11/29. eng.
15. Northouse LL, Katapodi MC, Song L, Zhang L, Mood DW. Interventions with family caregivers of cancer patients: meta-analysis of randomized trials. CA Cancer J Clin 2010;60(5):317–39; PubMed PMID: 20709946. Pubmed Central PMCID: PMC2946584. Epub 2010/08/17. eng.
16. Northouse LL, Mood DW, Schafenacker A, Kalemkerian G, Zalupski M, LoRusso P, et al. Randomized clinical trial of a brief and extensive dyadic intervention for advanced cancer patients and their family caregivers. Psychooncology. 2013;22(3):555–63; PubMed PMID: 22290823. Pubmed Central PMCID: PMC3387514. Epub 2012/02/01. eng.
17. Badger TA, Segrin C, Figueredo AJ, Harrington J, Sheppard K, Passalacqua S, et al. Psychosocial interventions to improve quality of life in prostate cancer survivors and their intimate or family partners. Qual Life Res 2011;20(6):833–44; PubMed PMID: 21170682. Pubmed Central PMCID: PMC3117079. Epub 2010/12/21. eng.
18. Galway K, Black A, Cantwell M, Cardwell CR, Mills M, Donnelly M. Psychosocial interventions to improve quality of life and emotional well-being for recently diagnosed cancer patients. Cochrane Database Syst Rev. 2012;11(11):CD007064; PubMed PMID: 23152241. Pubmed Central PMCID: PMC6457819. Epub 2012/11/16. eng.
19. Fulton JJ, LeBlanc TW, Cutson TM, Porter Starr KN, Kamal A, Ramos K, et al. Integrated outpatient palliative care for patients with advanced cancer: a systematic review and meta-analysis. Palliat Med 2019;33(2):123–34; PubMed PMID: 30488781. Pubmed Central PMCID: PMC7069657. Epub 2018/11/30. eng.
20. Temel JS, Greer JA, Muzikansky A, Gallagher ER, Admane S, Jackson VA, et al. Early palliative care for patients with metastatic non-small-cell lung cancer. N Engl J Med 2010;363(8):733–42; PubMed PMID: 20818875. Epub 2010/09/08. eng.

Appendix B

Nursing Strategies (Review chaps. 12, 13 and 14)

Psychosocial Interventions that facilitate Psychological Adjustment to the Cancer or Treatment-Related Threat

Nursing objectives	Content/various strategies	Clinical outcomes	References
1. Cognitive–approach (includes problem-solving, emotion-focused and meaning making coping strategies)	Suggested overall approach (a) Set meaningful patient-centered (or caregiver) goals, identify problem/challenge/source of stress (b) Provide relevant information regarding illness, prognosis, and treatment goals (c) Promote a combination of problem-focused, emotion-focused, and meaning-making coping efforts to manage/resolve beliefs and thoughts about the cancer-related or treatment-related threats, and the accompanying negative emotional reactions (d) Encourage storytelling and or deliberate rumination to facilitate the individual's reintegration of the threat (cognitive processing) (e) Find out what is important to the individual and if possible turn it into a goal and work together to make it happen	↑ed QOL[2,6]; ↓depression[2,3,6] ↓pain, fatigue, anxiety[2,3,5,6] ↓ers mood disturbance[2], ↑emotional well-being[1] ↓ed intrusive thoughts[4] ↓ed expression of pro-inflammatory & metastases-related genes[5] ↓ed NFKB/rel factors	[1–6]
(a) *Cognitive-oriented* coping approaches to manage the threat	(a) Provide relevant information (b) Use of reframing such as, reframing a nonmetastatic diagnosis "as a challenge or a wake up call to live a healthy life" (c) Use cognitive restructuring to dispel distorted beliefs and encourage positive reappraisals (d) Manage cognitive threats via one or more strategies: brainstorming, problem-solving, perspective taking to consider the consequences of a coping response such as a problem-solving approach (e) Deconstruct (breaking down) global, hyperbolic words (f) Facilitate deliberate rumination, purposeful narratives	Psychological and biological adjustment/adaptation	[7–11]

(continued)

Nursing objectives	Content/various strategies	Clinical outcomes	References
(b) Emotion-oriented coping approaches to manage emotional reactions to threats	(a) Normalize feelings of worry and anxiety (b) Reframe, focus on the positive, *encourage positive emotions*[7,8,9] (c) Encourage use of distraction (pleasant activity, hobby, TV, and/or being with friends)[5] (d) Use *positive affirmations*, encourage *positive self-talk* (e) Encourage a present-oriented focus (f) Relaxation exercises, mindful meditation, or engaging in physical exercise to reduce the intensity of emotional distress (g) Celebrate family occasions and being with friends (h) Support patient hope, and help patients find hope in changing clinical status (i) use of cognitive restrucuring to link effects of thoughts and behaviors on emotions		[7, 9, 10, 12–18]
(c) Meaning-focused coping strategies	***Manualized interventions*** (a) meaning-making intervention (b) life review intervention ***Individual strategies*** (a) reframing (b) find clinical benefits in light of reality (c) facilitate positive reappraisals (d) propose alternative explanations, interpretations (e) ***use of storytelling, narratives to integrate cancer into the person's life story to facilitate acceptance and or new purpose and meanings*** (f) infuse ordinary daily events with positive meaning (g) discuss changes in individual's basic goals, values since diagnosis with a goal of reprioritizing patient goals, and reaffirming values intrinsic to the person ***Indicators of meaning found given clinical reality*** (a) acceptance (b) found benefits, new meaning, purpose (c) reprioritized goals and values	↑QOL, ↑ meaning in life ↑hope ↑ self-esteem[1], optimism[1], self-efficacy ↓ depression, ↓ anxiety	[19–27]

(d) *Behavioral coping strategies*	(a) Relaxation exercises[7,8] (b) Mindful meditation[4,10] (c) Relaxation response technique[6] (d) Combined strategy: Relaxation, imagery, and distraction[5] *Other strategies:* (e) Massage[1] (f) Reiki/therapeutic touch[2] (g) Acupuncture[3] (h) Reflexology[9]	↑es QOL[10], spirituality[10] Improves negative emotional reactions to cancer-related experiences of uncertainty[4], fear of recurrence[4], loss of control[4] ↓ depression[4,10], anxiety[4], fatigue[4,5], insomnia[4,5] ↓ pain[3,5] Minimizes treatment-related suppression of natural killer cell cytotoxicity[4]	[5, 28–34]
2. Self-management interventions	Managing the *practical problems arising from the cancer or treatment* (a) Education, providing relevant resources, and supportive interventions that enhance the individual's self-efficacy beliefs (confidence) (b) Involves patient/caregiver with nurse assessing, problem, developing, goal, desired outcomes and action plan (steps to achieve outcome), implementing, and evaluating problem-solving interventions around health-related issues (e.g., symptom management, adhering to treatment schedule) associated with the treatment or cancer (c) Collaborative nurse–patient or caregiver approach: Practical problems may include: (d) Dealing with changes in life roles (e) Managing emotions related to cancer (f) Developing effective communication skills with the patient, family, healthcare providers symptom management	↑ed self-efficacy ↑ed well-being ↓ed stress response ↓depression	[10, 35–37]

Nursing objectives	Content/various strategies	Clinical outcomes	References
3. Strengthen supportive relationships	Strengthen supportive relationships via (a) Active listening, use of paraphrasing, reflective feedback, and acknowledging the pain and emotion behind hurtful verbalizations (b) Encourage patient, family caregiver basic *communication skills*: Nonjudgmental sharing of thoughts, feelings, and experiences, the ability to discuss issues without hurting one another; refrain from accusation, blame. Start sentence with I feel rather than you always… (c) Encourage active listening, emotional, informational, appraisal, instrumental forms of support that validate each person and enhance feelings of safety, security, and being cared for (d) Tangible/instrumental support may include doing errands for loved one, but also physical caring activities within the context of protecting and ensuring caregiver health (e) Promote displays of affectionate behavior, use of touch of loved one, lean toward one another, maintain eye contact (f) Convey your desire to help one another or support each other better (g) Use clinical anecdotes that underscore the support-related topic as a focus of discussion	Improved quality of life, overall well-being, and being understood and cared for	[7, 10, 34, 38, 39]

References

1. Antoni MH, Lechner S, Diaz A, Vargas S, Holley H, Phillips K, et al. Cognitive behavioral stress management effects on psychosocial and physiological adaptation in women undergoing treatment for breast cancer. Brain Behav Immun. 2009;23(5):580–91. https://doi.org/10.1016/j.bbi.2008.09.005.
2. Badr H, Smith CB, Goldstein NE, Gomez JE, Redd WH. Dyadic psychosocial intervention for advanced lung cancer patients and their family caregivers: results of a randomized pilot trial. Cancer. 2015;121(1):150–8. https://doi.org/10.1002/cncr.29009
3. Eileen M, Benson H, Stuart RN. The wellness book. 1993.
4. Jassim GA, Whitford DL, Hickey A, Carter B. Psychological interventions for women with non-metastatic breast cancer. Cochrane Database Syst Rev. 2015;5:CD008729. https://doi.org/10.1002/14651858.CD008729.pub2.
5. Lau BHP, Chow AYM, Ng TK, Fung YL, Lam TC, So TH, et al. Comparing the efficacy of integrative body-mind-spirit intervention with cognitive behavioral therapy in patient-caregiver parallel groups for lung cancer patients using a randomized controlled trial. J Psychosoc Oncol.2020;38(4):389–405. https://doi.org/10.1080/07347332.2020.1722981.
6. Matthews H, Grunfeld EA, Turner A. The efficacy of interventions to improve psychosocial outcomes following surgical treatment for breast cancer: a systematic review and meta-analysis. Psychooncology. 2017;26(5):593–607. https://doi.org/10.1002/pon.4199.
7. Benson H, Stuart E. The wellness book: the comprehensive guide to maintaining health and treating stress-related illness. New York: Simon and Schuster;1992.
8. Folkman S, Greer S. Promoting psychological well-being in the face of serious illness: when theory, research and practice inform each other. Psychooncology. 2000;9(1):11–9. https://doi.org/10.1002/(sici)1099-1611(200001/02)9:1<11::aid-pon424>3.0.co;2-z.
9. Jacobsen J, Brenner K, Greer JA, Jacobo M, Rosenberg L, Nipp RD, Jackson VA. When a patient is reluctant to talk about it: a dual framework to focus on living well and tolerate the possibility of dying. J Palliat Med. 2018;21(3):322–7. https://doi.org/10.1089/jpm.2017.0109.
10. Meichenbaum D. A clinical handbook for assessing and treating adults with post -traumatic stress disorder (PTSD). Waterloo, ON: Institute Press;1994.
11. Park CL, Edmondson D, Fenster JR, Blank TO. Meaning making and psychological adjustment following cancer: the mediating roles of growth, life meaning, and restored just-world beliefs. J Consult Clin Psychol. 2008;76(5):863–75. https://doi.org/10.1037/a0013348.
12. Antoni MH, Lutgendorf SK, Blomberg B, Carver CS, Lechner S, Diaz A, et al. Cognitive-behavioral stress management reverses anxiety-related leukocyte transcriptional dynamics. Biol Psychiatry. 2012;71(4):366–72. https://doi.org/10.1016/j.biopsych.2011.10.007.
13. Carlson LE, Zelinski E, Toivonen K, Flynn M, Qureshi M, Piedalue KA, Grant R. Mind-body therapies in cancer: what is the latest evidence? Curr Oncol Rep. 2017;19(10):67. https://doi.org/10.1007/s11912-017-0626-1.

14. Dunkel-Schetter C, Feinstein LG, Taylor SE, Falke RL. Patterns of coping with cancer. Health Psychol. 1992;11(2):79–87. https://doi.org/10.1037//0278-6133.11.2.79.
15. Greer JA, Applebaum AJ, Jacobsen JC, Temel JS, Jackson VA. Understanding and addressing the role of coping in palliative care for patients with advanced cancer. J Clin Oncol.2020;38(9):915–25. https://doi.org/10.1200/jco.19.00013.
16. Greer JA, Park ER, Prigerson HG, Safren SA. Tailoring cognitive-behavioral therapy to treat anxiety comorbid with advanced cancer. J Cogn Psychother. 2010;24(4), 294–313. https://doi.org/10.1891/0889-8391.24.4.294.
17. Greer JA, Traeger L, Bemis H, Solis J, Hendriksen ES, Park ER, et al. A pilot randomized controlled trial of brief cognitive-behavioral therapy for anxiety in patients with terminal cancer. Oncologist. 2012;17(10), 1337–45. https://doi.org/10.1634/theoncologist.2012-0041.
18. Segerstrom SC, Sephton SE. Optimistic expectancies and cell-mediated immunity: the role of positive affect. Psychol Sci. 2010;21(3):448–55. https://doi.org/10.1177/0956797610362061.
19. Beesley VL, Smith DD, Nagle CM, Friedlander M, Grant P, DeFazio A, Webb PM. Coping strategies, trajectories, and their associations with patient-reported outcomes among women with ovarian cancer. Support Care Cancer. 2018;26(12):4133–42. https://doi.org/10.1007/s00520-018-4284-0.
20. Haber D. Life review: implementation, theory, research, and therapy. Int J Aging Hum Dev. 2006;63(2):153–71. doi: https://doi.org/10.2190/da9g-rhk5-n9jp-t6cc
21. Lee V, Cohen SR, Edgar L, Laizner AM, Gagnon AJ. Meaning-making and psychological adjustment to cancer: development of an intervention and pilot results. Oncol Nurs Forum. 2006;33(2):291–302. https://doi.org/10.1188/06.onf.291-302.
22. Park CL. Making sense of the meaning literature: an integrative review of meaning making and its effects on adjustment to stressful life events. Psychol Bull. 2010;136(2):257–301. https://doi.org/10.1037/a0018301.
23. Park C, Folkman S. Meaning in the context of stress and coping. Rev General Psychol. 1997;1:115–44. https://doi.org/10.1037/1089-2680.1.2.115.
24. Teo I, Baid D, Ozdemir S, Malhotra C, Singh R, Harding R, et al. Family caregivers of advanced cancer patients: self-perceived competency and meaning-making. BMJ Support Palliat Care. 2020;10(4):435–42. https://doi.org/10.1136/bmjspcare-2019-001979.
25. Vos J, Vitali D. The effects of psychological meaning-centered therapies on quality of life and psychological stress: a metaanalysis. Palliat Support Care. 2018;16(5):608–32. https://doi.org/10.1017/s1478951517000931.
26. Zhang H, Zhao Q, Cao P, Ren G. Resilience and quality of life: exploring the mediator role of social support in patients with breast cancer. Med Sci Monit. 2017;23:5969–79. https://doi.org/10.12659/msm.907730.
27. Zhang J, Yin Y, Wang A, Li H, Li J, Yang S, et al. Resilience in patients with lung cancer: structural equation modeling. Cancer Nurs. 2021;44(6):465–72. https://doi.org/10.1097/ncc.0000000000000838

28. Alimi D, Rubino C, Pichard-Leandri E, Fermand-Brule S, Dubreuil-Lemaire ML, Hill C. Analgesic effect of auricular acupuncture for cancer pain: a randomized, blinded, controlled trial. J Clin Oncol. 2003;21(22):4120–6. https://doi.org/10.1200/jco.2003.09.011.
29. Kwekkeboom KL, Cherwin CH, Lee JW, Wanta B. Mind-body treatments for the pain-fatigue-sleep disturbance symptom cluster in persons with cancer. J Pain Symptom Manage. 2010;39(1):126–38. https://doi.org/10.1016/j.jpainsymman.2009.05.022.
30. Kwekkeboom K, Zhang Y, Campbell T, Coe CL, Costanzo E, Serlin RC, Ward S. Randomized controlled trial of a brief cognitive-behavioral strategies intervention for the pain, fatigue, and sleep disturbance symptom cluster in advanced cancer. Psychooncology. 2018;27(12):2761–9. https://doi.org/10.1002/pon.4883.
31. Lee PL, Tam KW, Yeh ML, Wu WW. Acupoint stimulation, massage therapy and expressive writing for breast cancer: a systematic review and meta-analysis of randomized controlled trials. Complement Ther Med.2016;27:87–101. https://doi.org/10.1016/j.ctim.2016.06.003.
32. Lutgendorf SK, Sood AK, Antoni MH. Host factors and cancer progression: biobehavioral signaling pathways and interventions. J Clin Oncol. 2010;28(26):4094–9. https://doi.org/10.1200/jco.2009.26.9357.
33. Mantoudi A, Parpa E, Tsilika E, Batistaki C, Nikoloudi M, Kouloulias V, et al. Complementary therapies for patients with cancer: reflexology and relaxation in integrative palliative care. A randomized controlled comparative study. J Altern Complement Med. 2020;26(9):792–8. https://doi.org/10.1089/acm.2019.0402.
34. Schellekens MPJ, Tamagawa R, Labelle LE, Speca M, Stephen J, Drysdale E, et al. Mindfulness-based cancer recovery (MBCR) versus supportive expressive group therapy (SET) for distressed breast cancer survivors: evaluating mindfulness and social support as mediators. J Behav Med. 2017;40(3):414–22. https://doi.org/10.1007/s10865-016-9799-6.
35. Kim SH, Kim K, Mayer DK. Self-management intervention for adult cancer survivors after treatment: a systematic review and meta-analysis. Oncol Nurs Forum. 2017;44(6):719–28. doi: https://doi.org/10.1188/17.onf.719-728.
36. Leventhal H, Phillips LA, Burns E. The common-sense model of self-regulation (CSM): a dynamic framework for understanding illness self-management. J Behav Med. 2016;39(6):935–46. https://doi.org/10.1007/s10865-016-9782-2.
37. McCorkle R, Ercolano E, Lazenby M, Schulman-Green D, Schilling LS, Lorig K, Wagner EH. Self-management: enabling and empowering patients living with cancer as a chronic illness. CA Cancer J Clin. 2011;61(1):50–62. https://doi.org/10.3322/caac.20093.
38. House JS. Work, stress and social support. Reading, MA: Addison-Wesley; 1981.
39. Jacobsen J, Kvale E, Rabow M, Rinaldi S, Cohen S, Weissman D, Jackson V. Helping patients with serious illness live well through the promotion of adaptive coping: a report from the improving outpatient palliative care (IPAL-OP) initiative. J Palliat Med. 2014;17(4):463–8. https://doi.org/10.1089/jpm.2013.0254.

Appendix C

Clinical Interventions to Promote Healthy Lifestyle Behaviors

Cancer Survivors

Authors	Purpose/intervention	Study design	Sample/phase of disease	Outcomes
Schwingshackl et al. [1]	To assess effects of a *Mediterranean diet (MedD)* on the risk of overall cancer mortality, risk of individual cancers and mortality, and risk of cancer recurrence *in cancer survivors*	Systematic review and meta-analysis of RCTs and cohort observational and case/control studies: total number of studies = 83	$N = 2,139,753$	1. MedD had a significantly lower risk of overall cancer mortality (RR_{cohort} 0.86, 95% CI, 0.81 to 0.91, $I^2 = 82\%$; $n = 14$ studies) than the lowest MedD group 2. MedD produced a significant lower risk for: (a) Colorectal cancer ($RR_{observational}$ = 0.82, 95% CI 0.75 to 0.88, $I^2 = 73\%$; $n = 11$ studies) (b) Breast cancer (RR_{RCT}: 0.43, 95% CI, 0.21 to 0.88, $n = 1$ study) ($RR_{observational}$: 0.92, 95% CI 0.87 to 0.96, $I^2 = 22\%$, $n = 16$ studies) (c) Gastric cancer ($RR_{observational}$: 0.72, CI 95% 0.60 to 0.86, $I^2 =55\%$, $n = 4$ studies) (d) Liver cancer ($RR_{observational}$: 0.58, 95% CI 0.46 to 0.73, $I^2 =$)%, $n = 2$ studies) (e) Head/neck cancer ($RR_{observational}$: 0.49, 95% CI 0.37 to 0.66, $I^2 = 87\%$; $n = 7$ studies) (f) Prostate cancer ($RR_{observational}$: 0.96, 95% CI 0.92 to 1.00, $I^2 = 0\%$; $n = 6$ studies) 3. ***In cancer survivors:*** (a) highest adherence to MedD on cancer mortality and cancer recurrence was nonsignificant in cancer survivors (RR: 0.95, 95% CI, 0.82 to 1.12; $I^2 = 5\%$, $n = 4$ studies) 4. ***Pooled analyses:*** (a) fruit intake significantly reduced cancer risk (RR: 0.93, 95% CI, 0.89 to 0.97, $I^2 = 60\%$, $n = 13$) (b) as did vegetable consumption (RR: 0.96, 95% CI, 0.93 to 0.98, $I^2 = 0\%$, $n = 14$ studies) (c) whole grain intake (RR: 0.91, 95% CI, 0.87 to 0.95, $I^2 =31\%$, $n = 9$ studies)

	Purpose	Study type / Sample	Results
	Investigated the effects of diet quality based on the Healthy Eating Index (HEI), Alternate Healthy Eating Index (AHEI), and Dietary Approaches to Stop Hypertension Score (DASH) on all-cause mortality and cancer mortality among *cancer survivors*	$N = 1{,}670{,}179$ people with various cancers and cancer survivors as well as cardiovascular disease incidence followed between 3 and 24 years	5. Individuals who adhered to the Healthy Eating Index (HEI), Alternate Healthy Eating Index (AHEI), and/or Dietary Approaches to Stop Hypertension (DASH) Score were shown to significantly reduce the risk for: (a) all-cause mortality (RR 0.78; 95% CI, 0.82 to 0.87; $I^2 = 59\%$; $n = 13$) (b) cancer (incidence or mortality) (RR 0.84, 95% CI, 0.82 to 0.87; $I^2 = 66\%$; $n = 31$), as well as other chronic illnesses specifically type 2 diabetes, cardiovascular and neurodegenerative diseases (Schwingshackl et al. [11]) (c) cancer survivors who adhered to these quality diets showed a significant reduction in all-cause mortality (RR 0.88, 95% CI, 0.81 to 0.95; $I^2 = 38\%$; $n = 7$) and cancer mortality (RR 0.90, 95% CI, 0.83 to 0.98; $I^2 = 0\%$, $n = 7$)
Smits et al. [2]	To assess effectiveness of *lifestyle interventions* in increasing quality of life of endometrial and ovarian cancer *survivors* *The interventions* consisted of home-based exercise and/or nutrition; 1/3 studies also included hospital/group counseling. Exercise was mainly aerobics with or without resistance training	Systematic review and meta-analysis of 3 RCTs and 5 nonrandomized studies	Survivors of mainly endometrial and ovarian cancer	1. Meta-analysis of 3 RCT studies suggested that the lifestyle interventions failed to increase global QOL (1.16 (95% CI, −5.91 to −8.23), $p = 0.75$) at 3 months and at 6 months (2.48 (95% CI, −4.63 to 9.58), $p = 0.49$) 2. The data was subject to high risk of bias, partially due to the heterogeneous make up of lifestyle in each study

(continued)

Authors	Purpose/intervention	Study design	Sample/phase of disease	Outcomes
Gao et al. [3]	To investigate effects of exercise on survivors of colorectal cancer after treatment **Exercise intervention** 60–150 min of moderate and high intensity aerobic exercise	Systematic review and meta-analysis of 20 studies ($N = 1223$)	Colorectal cancer survivors	1. **Types of exercise** (a) 14 studies: aerobic; 5 studies—walking; 1 study—hatha yoga; 2 cycle ergometrics; 6 studies combined aerobic/resistance 2. **Frequency of exercise** (a) ranged from 3 to 7 times/week; 60–300 min/week 3. **Intensity** 6 studies-moderate intensity; 1 study low intensity; 2 studies alternated hi/mod intensity; controls—moderate 4. **Supervision** (a) *5 studies: aerobic under supervision; 9 studies: home-based aerobic* 5. **Findings** (a) exercise was significantly more effective than either usual care or usual lifestyle in increasing VO_{2peak} ($n = 107$, SMD = 0.72, 95% CL, 0.32 to 1.11; $I^2 = 41\%$, $P = 0.0004$) (b) exercise significantly decreased fasting insulin levels ($n = 150$, SMD = -0.55, 95% CL = -0.88 to -0.23, $I^2 = 0\%$, $P = 0.0009$) and insulin resistance ($n = 150$, SMD = -0.62, 95% CL = 0.95 to -0.29, $I2 = 0\%$, $P = 0.0002$) in survivors of colorectal cancer (insulin and insulin resistance are mediators of colorectal carcinogenesis) (c) also shown to decrease levels of sICAM-1 (intercellular adhesion molecule that is overexpressed in pathological states) (SISAM-1 and SVCAM-1 are endothelial cell adhesion molecules that facilitate cancer progression) (d) moderate-intensity exercise was related to a more pro-inflammatory immune state, resulting in increased oxidative DNA damage **Conclusion** Findings suggest that exercise may be effective for improving tumor-related biomarkers, metabolism as well as overall cardiopulmonary fitness in survivors of colorectal cancer (a) A range of heterogeneity across studies ranged from none to moderate levels

| Schwedhelm et al. [4] | Investigate relationship between food intake and dietary patterns and risk of mortality and or cancer recurrence among cancer survivors | Systematic view and 9 studies in meta-analysis **Participants/study** (R = 57 to 22,890) *Follow-up* Range: *1.2 to 16 years* *Different guidelines* in 9 studies used in meta-analysis, e.g., Healthy Eating Index (n = 7) 9 studies in meta-analysis had assessed effects of dietary patterns on overall mortality or cancer recurrence and *used principal components analysis to identify* dietary patterns: (a) called whole foods/ prudent or healthy when there was high intake in fruits, vegetables, low fat dairy, and whole grains, and low in processed meat, refined grains, processed fat foods, sugars, desserts, and high fat dairy (b) unhealthy patterns labeled: unhealthy or western diet: high fat, sugar, snacks, processed meat and foods, refined grains and sugar, fat dairy, etc. | 117 studies that enrolled 209 597 survivors of cancer Types of cancer (number of studies) (a) 41 breast cancer; 18 colorectal; 16 head and neck, 13 gastro-esophageal | *Results* 1. Inverse relationship between **higher intake of vegetables and risk of mortality** (RR 0.86, 95% CI, 0.79 to 0.94; $I^2 = 43\%$) and higher intake of **fish and risk of mortality** (RR 0.85, 95% CI, 0.78 to 0.93; $I^2 = 0\%$) 2. **Alcohol intake** was related to increased risk of mortality (RR 1.08, 95% CI, 1.02 to 1.16, $I^2 = 70\%$) (a) NS risk of mortality for dairy, meat, cereal, bread, eggs, tea, red meat, processed meat) 3. Adherence to **high quality diet** was inversely related to overall mortality (RR, 0.78; 95% CI 0.72 to 0.85, $I^2 = 0$) (a) Effects related to overall mortality remained when only diet postdiagnosis analyzed: (RR, 0.79; 95% CI 0.71 to 0.89, $I^2 = 0\%$) 4. **Regarding highest category of healthy diet pattern** was inversely related to overall mortality (RR 0.89, 95% CI 0.67 to 0.98, $I^2 = 44\%$) (a) Remained same finding when only postdiagnosis dietary pattern analyzed (RR 0.77, 95% CI, 0.60 to 0.99; $I^2 = 56\%$) 5. Highest pattern of adherence to *western diet* was related to **increased** risk of mortality (RR 1.46, 95% CI, 1.27 to 1.68 (n = 8); $I^2 = 0$–68%) (a) Same finding for post-diagnosis dietary pattern (RR 1.51; 95% CI, 1.24 to 1.85; $I^2 = 17\%$) (n = 6) 6. Highest category of adherence to healthy dietary pattern was not associated with any significant effects on cancer recurrence compared to lowest category of adherence (RR; 0.94, 95% CI, 0.74 to 1.24, $I^2 = 19\%$) (a) western diet also was not associated with any significant effects on cancer recurrence Conclusion (a) Risk of bias ranged from minimal to moderate depending on the analysis— contributing factors may include differences in types of cancer, timing of measurement after diagnosis, sex and age, and the dietary indicators used across studies (b) Further studies needed to assess contribution of postdiet and dietary patterns on cancer survival and cancer recurrence |

During Treatment

Authors	Purpose/intervention	Study design	Sample/phase of disease	Outcomes
de van der Schueren et al. [5]	To assess the effects of (a) dietary counseling (DC) (b) high energy oral nutritional supplements (ONS) to improve intakes, or (c) ONS replete with protein and n-3 polyunsaturated fatty acids (PUFA) aiming to regulate cancer-related metabolic changes **During treatment** malnutrition caused by poor nutritional intake and metabolic treatment and/or cancer-induced changes during treatment **Interventions** (a) dietary counseling (DC) (b) high energy oral nutritional supplements (ONS) or (c) ONS with added protein and n-3 polyunsaturated fatty acids to regulate cancer-related metabolic changes	Systematic review and meta-analyses of 11 RCTs	Patients on chemoradiotherapy	1. 11 studies showed significant improvement in body weight during chemoradiotherapy (+1.31 kg, 95% CI 0.24–2.38, $p = 0.02$, heterogeneity $Q = 21.1$, $p = 0.007$) 2. High protein, n-3 PUFA-enriched intervention in contrast to isocaloric controls was shown to have a significant effect on lean body mass loss and quality of life (+1.89 kg, 95% CI 0.51–3.27, $p = 0.02$, $Q = 3.1$, $p = 0.37$) (a) The high protein n-3 PUFA intervention shown to reduce lean body mass loss ($N = 2$) and improve aspects of QOL ($N = 3$) 3. Subanalysis showed that the overall positive clinical outcomes were mainly the result of the high protein, n-3 PUFA interventions, suggesting their potential value of targeting metabolic alterations 4. DC and or high energy ONS showed nonsignificant effects on (+ 0.80 kg, 95% CI −1.14 to −2.74, $p = 0.32$, $Q = 10.5$, $p = 0.03$) Limitations (a) Small number of studies, poor quality evidence, and underpowered to show effects on treatment toxicity and survival

| Custódio et al. [6] | To evaluate relationship between consumption of food groups, patients dietary inflammatory index (DII) and their nutritional status during chemotherapy (CT) | Prospective study Patients assessed at 3 points using anthropometric and dietary measures T0 that is the baseline measure after 1st CT cycle T1: is the time 'point' after the intermediate CT cycle T2: is the point of measurement after the last CT cycle | 55 women with breast cancer receiving chemotherapy | 1. Significant increase in weight, body mass index, and waist circumference
2. T1 >T2: consumption of eggs, poultry
3. T0 > T1 and T2: total fruit and vegetables consumed
4. Diet increasingly pro-inflammatory over study ($X^2_{(2)} = 61.127$) and was attributed to abdominal adiposity
5. Total fruit: T0 = R^2 = 0.208, T1: R^2 = 0.095; T2: R^2 =0.120 predicted **DII** changes at three assessment points
6. Total vegetable consumption (T0 R^2=0.284; T1: R^2= 0.365; T^2= 0.580) predicted DII changes at three assessment points
7. Grain consumption significantly related to T1 (R^2=0.084) and T^2 (R^2=0.118)
8. Consumptions of simple sugars also significantly related at T0 (R^2=0.137) and T1 (R^2=0.126)
Summary
(a) Changes in food consumption resulted in a higher inflammatory index for diet Suggests importance of using guidelines to optimize patients diet during and after chemotherapy |

(continued)

Authors	Purpose/intervention	Study design	Sample/phase of disease	Outcomes
Custódio et al. [7]	Impact of chemotherapy (CT) on diet and nutritional status in women with breast cancer **during treatment**	Prospective study 1-year study Data collected at three points T0: baseline measure after 1st CT cycle T1: after intermediate CT cycle T2: after last CT cycle	55 women with breast cancer receiving chemotherapy	1. Majority of women had a diet requiring modification at the start (T0: 58.2%, $n = 32$) and during treatment (T1: 54.5%, $n = 30$) 2. At end of treatment T2: 49.1%, $n = 27$ still deemed to have an inadequate diet: total fruit, dark green and orange vegetables ($p = 0.043$) and legumes decreased significantly over treatment ($p = 0.026$) 3. Significant reduction in macronutrients and micronutrients 4. 56% ($n = 31$) were overweight 5. Weight, BMI, and waist circumference increased significantly over treatment, indicating a worsening nutritional status **Conclusion** (a) Chemotherapy interferes with patient's diet which negatively impacts quality and quantity of macronutrients and micronutrients taken, and BMI and waist measurements worsen

Exercise Before, During, and/or After Treatment

Authors	Purpose/intervention	Study design	Sample/phase of disease	Outcomes
Mishra et al. [8]	To assess the effect of exercise on overall health-related quality of life (HRQOL) *in adults with cancer before, during, and after treatment* Types of exercise intervention (a) Walking and/or cycling, resistance training, strength training (b) resistance training (c) strength training (d) cycling (e) yoga (f) qigong	Meta-analysis (Cochrane review) of patients with breast, prostate, gynecological, hematologic, and others RA to: (a) exercise ($n = 2286$) comparison ($n = 1985$)	56 trials ($N = 4826$) 36/56 based on patients during active treatment 10/56 based on patients during and after treatment 10/56 based on those awaiting treatment (prehabilitation phase)	1. Positive impact on overall HRQOL *from baseline to 12 weeks* (SMD 0.33; 95% CI, 0.12 to 0.55) 2. Exercise significantly improved *over usual care* at 12 weeks (SMD 0.47; 95% CI, 0.16 to 0.79) 3. ***Physical functioning from baseline to 12 weeks*** significantly improved: (SMD 0.69; 95% CI 0.16 to 1.22); also at 6 months *over baseline* (SMD 0.28; 95% CI 0.00 to 0.55) (a) Significant improvement *over usual care* at 12 weeks (SMD 0.28; 95% CI, 0.11 to 0.45) or at 6 months (SMD 0.29; 95% CI, 0.07 to 0.50) 4. **Role function from baseline to 12 weeks**: (SMD: 0.48; 95% CI, 0.07 to 0.90) (a) Significant improvement *over usual care* at 12 weeks (SMD 0.17; 95% CI, 0.00 to 0.34) or at 6 months (SMD 0.32; 95% CI, 0.03 to 0.61) 5. **Social functioning**: At 12-week follow-up *over baseline*: (SMD 0.54; 95% CI, 0.03 to 1.05) (a) Significant improvement when *compared to usual care* at 12 weeks (SMD 0.16; 95% CI, 0.04 to 0.27) and at 6 months (SMD 0.24; 95% CI 0.03 to 0.44) 6. ***Significant decrease in fatigue over baseline at 12 weeks***: (SMD −0.73; 95% CI, −1.14 to −0.31) 7. *RE subgroup analysis* (a) Greater reduction in anxiety for survivors of breast cancer (b) Greater reduction for depression, fatigue, sleep disturbances and increase in HRQOL, emotional well-being, physical functioning and role functioning for survivors of other cancers *except breast cancer* (c) Greater improvements in HRQOL, physical functioning and reduction in anxiety, fatigue and sleep disturbances when prescribed a *moderate to vigorous exercise* versus a mild exercise program **Conclusion** Exercise may improve QOL of patients right after exercise program ends; reduced fatigue during and after end of exercise; positive effects when exercise was more intense; problem is that forms of exercise varied across studies – need to identify optimal time to start exercise, duration and frequency, type of exercise

Prehabilitation

Authors	Purpose/intervention	Study design	Sample/phase of disease	Outcomes
Moran et al. [9]	To assess whether **prehabilitation** influences postoperative outcomes after intra-abdominal operations ***Interventions*** (a) inspiratory muscle training (b) aerobic exercise, and/or (c) resistance training	Systematic review and meta-analysis of 9 RCTs	435 presurgical individuals with colorectal, abdominal, upper gastrointestinal, and liver cancers, and open bariatric operations	1. Prehabilitation appears to decrease postoperative complications after surgery (OR; 0.59, 95% CI, 0.38 to 0.91, $p = 0.03$) 2. Based on only 4 studies, unable to determine whether the intervention could shorten postoperative length of stay 3. No postoperative mortality was reported, but conclusion relating the intervention to mortality was not possible 4. High risk of bias across the studies ***Conclusion*** Higher quality studies required to validate its use in the preoperative diagnostic phase

Treanor et al. [10]	To assess *prehabilitation programs* for new patients with cancer during diagnostic phase **Interventions:** One or more of the following: (a) psychological support (b) education (c) exercise	Systematic review and meta-analysis of 18 RCTs evaluating prehabilitation programs	$N = 1381$ patients with diverse cancers	*RE Exercise/physical resistance training* 1. ***Prostate cancer:*** meta-analysis of 3/18 RCTs showed that *pelvic floor muscle training* (PFMT) exercises were effective significantly increasing the odds of *continence* at 3 months postsurgery (OR = 3.29, 95% CI =1.57 to 6.91, $I^2 = 14\%$) compared to usual care (a) A meta-analysis of two/18 studies showed a trend toward increased continence compared to usual care, based on the amount of daily pad use at 6 months for prostate cancer (MD = −0.96, 95% CI, = −2.04 to 0.12, $I^2 = 90\%$) (b) Stress management intervention significantly improved mood, physical well-being, and immune function 2. ***Lung cancer*** Presurgical exercise significantly decreased hospital length of stay (MD = −4.18, 95% CI = −5.43 to −2.93) and (a) Presurgical exercise also significantly reduced the odds of postsurgical complications (OR = 0.25, 95% CI = 0.10 to 0.66) 3. ***Breast cancer*** Psychology-based intervention improved fatigue and psychological outcomes with a trend toward an increase in quality of life (a) Psychosocial interventions consisted mainly of stress-based psychoeducation, problem solving, relaxation skills, and supportive discussions ***Conclusion*** More studies based on rigorous methodology and design with low risk of bias in order to conduct meta-analyses with high quality evidence for interventions in the prehabilitation phase

(continued)

Authors	Purpose/intervention	Study design	Sample/phase of disease	Outcomes
Trépanier et al. [11]	To assess the effect of a *prehabilitation intervention* (based on combined exercise and nutritional programs)	Pooled data (2 RCTs and 1 cohort) Primary outcomes: (a) 5-year disease-free survival **(DFS)** (b) Overall survival (OS)	202 patients grouped into intervention versus usual care to have elective, biopsy-proven, primary nonmetastatic colorectal cancer surgery	1. Postoperative complications and time to start chemotherapy postsurgery were similar 2. Prehabilitation duration was a median of 29 days (range 20–40) 3. Mean duration of study follow-up was 60.3 months (SD 26.2) 4. Whereas DFS was similar for stages 1–3 ($p = 0.244$), prehabilitation had a significant and increased effect of DFS in stage 3 patients compared to usual care (73.4% vs 50.9%, $p = 0.044$) 5. NS difference in OS ($p = 0.226$) 6. Prehabilitation predicted a significantly improved DFS (hazard ratio 0.45, 95% CI, 0.21 to 0.93) after adjusting for stage and other confounding variables **Conclusion** Prehabilitation had a positive and improved effect on DFS in patients with stage III colorectal cancer

Prehabilitation with Neoadjuvant Treatment

Authors	Purpose/intervention	Study design	Sample/phase of disease	Outcomes
Ngo-Huang et al. [12]	To investigate effects of a **home-based prehabilitation exercise** program on (a) physical activity (b) changes in physical function and (c) health-related quality of life (HRQOL). Program is for preoperative patients with pancreatic cancer. **The intervention** Each week complete: (a) ≥60 min of moderate-intensity aerobic exercise and (b) ≥60 min of strengthening exercises	Prospective single-arm study 1. *Activity level* measured by self-reports, accelerometers of (a) moderate to vigorous physical activity (MVPA) (b) light physical activity (LPA) (c) sedentary activity (SA) 2. *Physical function measures at baseline and follow-up* included: (a) 6-minute walk test (6MWT) (b) 5 sit-to-stand positions asap (eg 95 x STS) (c) handgrip strength (HGS) (d) 3-min walk for speed (GS) (e) Physical Function Short Form (PROMIS) (f) HRQOL	50 patients during preoperative treatment for pancreatic cancer during preoperative chemotherapy or chemoradiation	1. The 6MWT ($p < 0.001$), 5xSTS ($p = 0.049$), and the GS ($P = 0.009$) significantly improved at follow-up over baseline measures 2. *Significant improvements in the 6-minute walk* were related to self-reported increases in aerobic exercise ($\beta = 0.19$, $p = 0.048$), moderate-to-vigorous physical activity (MVPA) ($\beta = 0.18$, $p = 0.03$) and light physical activity (LPA) ($\beta = 0.08$, $p = 0.03$) 3. *An increase in weekly LPA* was related to a significant increase in health-related quality of life (HRQOL) ($\beta = 0.03$, $p = 0.02$) 4. An increase in weekly sedentary activity was significantly associated with decreased HRQOL **Conclusion** This intervention was associated with significant improvements in physical function and HRQOL; and patients awaiting resectable pancreatic surgery also demonstrated improvement in some measures for physical functioning

During Chemotherapy

Authors	Purpose/intervention	Study design	Sample/phase of disease	Outcomes
van Waart et al. [13]	To evaluate the effectiveness of two types of physical exercise programs in increasing or maintaining physical fitness, decreasing fatigue, increasing health-related quality of life, and improving chemotherapy completion rates in patients during adjuvant chemotherapy for breast cancer	RCT with RA to 3 arms: (a) a low intensity, home-based physical activity program (OncoMove), (b) moderate to high intensity with supervised resistance and aerobic exercise program (OnTrack), or (c) usual care Assts: baseline, at the end of chemotherapy, and at the 6-month follow-up	230 patients with breast cancer	(a) Compared to usual care the OncoMove and OnTrack programs led to less decrease in cardiorespiratory fitness ($p < 0.001$), improved physical functioning ($p \leq 0.001$), less nausea ($p = 0.029$), and vomiting (p 0.031) (b) OnTrack also showed better muscle strength ($p = 0.002$), and less physical fatigue ($p < 0.001$) (c) At 6 months: most outcomes had returned to their baseline values in all three groups (d) Both programs resulted in a faster return to work and with more work hours a week ($p = 0.014$) **Conclusion** (a) Both programs were effective in improving health-related outcomes, including the home low intensity physical activity program (b) Discussions around blinding or other ways to assess for risk of bias, not located (c) More than half of eligible subjects declined to participate suggesting the need to identify potential causes that might be addressed

Adjuvant Chemotherapy

Authors	Purpose/intervention	Study design	Sample/phase of disease	Outcomes
van Vulpen et al. [14]	To assess the effects of physical exercise on different types of fatigue during adjuvant therapy for breast cancer	Meta-analysis	Pooled effects of 6 exercise programs for 784 patients	(a) Compared to controls, exercise showed significant benefits on general fatigue (ES: −0.22, 95% CI, −0.38 to −0.05), physical fatigue (ES: −0.35, 95% CI, −0.49 to −0.21) (b) Physical exercise also was shown to significantly improve the fatigue subscales "reduced" activity (ES: −0.22, 95% CI, −0.38 to −0.05) and improve "reduced motivation" (ES: −0.18, 95% CI −0.35 to −0.01) (c) NS effects on cognitive fatigue and affective fatigue (d) Based on 4 studies examining "supervised" exercises only: "slightly bigger" pooled effect estimates were shown for general fatigue (ES: −0.25, 95% CI −0.47 to −0.04) and physical fatigue (ES: −0.39, 95% CI −0.56 to −0.23) ***Conclusion*** (a) Physical exercise during adjuvant chemotherapy has beneficial effects on general and physical fatigue, reduced activity and reduced motivation, but is NS for cognitive and affective fatigue (b) Seems that physical exercise is a viable intervention to improve general and physical fatigue

(continued)

Authors	Purpose/intervention	Study design	Sample/phase of disease	Outcomes
Juvet et al. [15]	To assess the efficacy of physical exercise on fatigue and self-reported physical functioning in patients with breast cancer during and after adjuvant chemotherapy and at 6-month follow-up	Meta-analysis Assessed for quality of RCTs using an 8-point criteria (randomization procedure, allocation concealment, performance bias, blinding, intent to treat, loss of participants to follow-up): ≥8: high quality; 507 moderate quality; ≤4, poor quality (a) Used Cochrane's I^2 statistic to assess for heterogeneity among studies	25 RCTs ($n = 3418$ patients with breast cancer) during and after treatment	(a) Compared to controls, physical exercise (PE) showed a significant improvement in physical functioning (SMD: 0.27, 95% CI, 0.12 to 0.41) (b) PE also showed a significant improvement in fatigue (SMD: −0.32, 95% CI, −0.49 to −0.14) (c) Patient who received PE after the end of adjuvant chemotherapy showed a small improvement in both fatigue and physical functioning levels over patients who received the PE during adjuvant treatment (d) The 6-month assessment showed that the PE group maintained a small but significant improvement in both measures compared to controls Conclusion (a) Physical exercise has clinical benefits in enhancing physical functioning and decreasing fatigue (b) The studies were shown to have moderate to high quality evidence (c) A number of studies of breast cancer were small, underpowered

McTiernan et al. [16]	To update evidence in the relationships between physical activity and risk for cancer, and for mortality in persons with cancer	45 reports of systematic reviews of meta-analyses, systematic reviews, and polled analyses of data up to December 2016. An updated analyses of 5 meta-analyses and 25 papers also done between January 2017 and February 2018	(a) 45 reports consisting of hundreds of studies and millions of study participants (b) 5 meta-analyses	(a) Showed strong evidence that compared to the lowest physical activity levels, the highest physical activity levels were significantly related to reduced risks for breast, bladder, endometrial, colon, renal, esophageal, and gastric cancers, with an estimated 10–20% reduction in risk (b) Based on 18 meta-analyses and systematic reviews, the report also showed moderate to limited relationships between higher levels of physical activity and lower reductions in all-cause and cancer-specific mortality in people with breast, prostate, and colorectal cancers, with a 40–50% reductions in relative risk (c) A further analysis of the 2017-2018 5 meta-analyses and 25 studies showed consistent findings with those reported above ***Conclusion*** (a) Levels of physical activity as reported in the WCRF 2018 guidelines are related to a reduced risk of colorectal, prostate, and breast cancer and longer survival (b) Need to investigate associations between physical activity and other cancer populations

References

1. Schwingshackl L, Bogensberger B, Hoffmann G. Diet quality as assessed by the healthy eating index, alternate healthy eating index, dietary approaches to stop hypertension score, and health outcomes: an updated systematic review and meta-analysis of cohort studies. J Acad Nutr Diet. 2018;118(1):74–100.e11. https://doi.org/10.1016/j.jand.2017.08.024.
2. Smits A, Lopes A, Das N, Bekkers R, Massuger L, Galaal K. The effect of lifestyle interventions on the quality of life of gynaecological cancer survivors: a systematic review and meta-analysis. Gynecol Oncol. 2015;139(3):546–52. https://doi.org/10.1016/j.ygyno.2015.10.002.
3. Gao R, Yu T, Liu L, Bi J, Zhao H, Tao Y, et al. Exercise intervention for post-treatment colorectal cancer survivors: a systematic review and meta-analysis. J Cancer Surviv. 2020;14(6):878–93. https://doi.org/10.1007/s11764-020-00900-z.
4. Schwedhelm C, Boeing H, Hoffmann G, Aleksandrova K, Schwingshackl L. Effect of diet on mortality and cancer recurrence among cancer survivors: a systematic review and meta-analysis of cohort studies. Nutr Rev. 2016;74(12):737–48. https://doi.org/10.1093/nutrit/nuw045.
5. de van der Schueren MAE, Laviano A, Blanchard H, Jourdan M, Arends J, Baracos VE. Systematic review and meta-analysis of the evidence for oral nutritional intervention on nutritional and clinical outcomes during chemo(radio)therapy: current evidence and guidance for design of future trials. Ann Oncol. 2018;29(5):1141–53. https://doi.org/10.1093/annonc/mdy114.
6. Custódio IDD, Franco FP, Marinho EDC, Pereira TSS, Lima MTM, Molina Mdcb, et al. Prospective analysis of food consumption and nutritional status and the impact on the dietary inflammatory index in women with breast cancer during chemotherapy. Nutrients. 2019;11(11):2610. https://doi.org/10.3390/nu11112610.
7. Custódio ID, Marinho Eda C, Gontijo CA, Pereira TS, Paiva CE, Maia YC. Impact of chemotherapy on diet and nutritional status of women with breast cancer: a prospective study. PLoS One. 2016;11(6):e0157113. https://doi.org/10.1371/journal.pone.0157113.
8. Mishra SI, Scherer RW, Snyder C, Geigle PM, Berlanstein DR, Topaloglu O. Exercise interventions on health-related quality of life for people with cancer during active treatment. Cochrane Database Syst Rev. 2012;2012(8):CD008465. https://doi.org/10.1002/14651858.CD008465.pub2.
9. Moran J, Guinan E, McCormick P, Larkin J, Mockler D, Hussey J, et al. The ability of prehabilitation to influence postoperative outcome after intra-abdominal operation: a systematic review and meta-analysis. Surgery. 2016;160(5):1189–201. https://doi.org/10.1016/j.surg.2016.05.014.
10. Treanor C, Kyaw T, Donnelly M. An international review and meta-analysis of prehabilitation compared to usual care for cancer patients. J Cancer Surviv. 2018;12(1):64–73. https://doi.org/10.1007/s11764-017-0645-9.
11. Trépanier M, Minnella EM, Paradis T, Awasthi R, Kaneva P, Schwartzman K, et al. Improved disease-free survival after prehabilitation for colorectal

cancer surgery. Ann Surg. 2019;270(3):493–501. https://doi.org/10.1097/sla.0000000000003465.
12. Ngo-Huang A, Parker NH, Bruera E, Lee RE, Simpson R, O'Connor DP, et al. Home-based exercise prehabilitation during preoperative treatment for pancreatic cancer is associated with improvement in physical function and quality of life. Integr Cancer Ther. 2019;18:1534735419894061. https://doi.org/10.1177/1534735419894061.
13. van Waart H, Stuiver MM, van Harten WH, Geleijn E, Kieffer JM, Buffart LM, et al. Effect of low-intensity physical activity and moderate- to high-intensity physical exercise during adjuvant chemotherapy on physical fitness, fatigue, and chemotherapy completion rates: results of the PACES randomized clinical trial. J Clin Oncol. 2015;33(17):1918–27. https://doi.org/10.1200/jco.2014.59.1081.
14. van Vulpen JK, Peeters PH, Velthuis MJ, van der Wall E, May AM. Effects of physical exercise during adjuvant breast cancer treatment on physical and psychosocial dimensions of cancer-related fatigue: a meta-analysis. Maturitas. 2016;85:104–11. https://doi.org/10.1016/j.maturitas.2015.12.007.
15. Juvet LK, Thune I, Elvsaas IkØ, Fors EA, Lundgren S, Bertheussen G, et al. The effect of exercise on fatigue and physical functioning in breast cancer patients during and after treatment and at 6 months follow-up: a meta-analysis. Breast. 2017;33:166–77. https://doi.org/10.1016/j.breast.2017.04.003.
16. McTiernan A, Friedenreich CM, Katzmarzyk PT, Powell KE, Macko R, Buchner D, et al. Physical activity in cancer prevention and survival: a systematic review. Med Sci Sports Exerc. 2019;51(6):1252–61. https://doi.org/10.1249/mss.0000000000001937.

GPSR Compliance

The European Union's (EU) General Product Safety Regulation (GPSR) is a set of rules that requires consumer products to be safe and our obligations to ensure this.

If you have any concerns about our products, you can contact us on ProductSafety@springernature.com

In case Publisher is established outside the EU, the EU authorized representative is:

Springer Nature Customer Service Center GmbH
Europaplatz 3
69115 Heidelberg, Germany

Batch number: 07961527

Printed by Printforce, the Netherlands